This book is to be returned on or before
the last date stamped below.

0 5 JAN 2009

THE YEARBOOK

OF

OBSTETRICS AND GYNAECOLOGY

VOLUME 11

The Yearbook of
OBSTETRICS
and
GYNAECOLOGY

Volume 11

Edited by
Tim Hillard and David Purdie

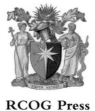

RCOG Press

Published by the **RCOG Press** at the Royal College of Obstetricians and Gynaecologists, 27 Sussex Place, Regent's Park, London NW1 4RG

www.rcog.org.uk

Registered charity no. 213280

First published 2004

ISBN 1 900364 82 4

RCOG Press Editor: Margaret Carver
Index: Catherine Topliff
Design by FiSH Books, London
Printed by Latimer Trend & Co Ltd. Estover Road, Plymouth PL6 7PL

Contents

Contributors

Vasanth Andrews
Clinical Research Fellow
Mayday University Hospital
London Road
Croydon
Surrey CR7 7YE
UK

Hailegiorgis Atenfesu
Staff Specialist
Fistula Hospital
PO Box 3609
Addis Ababa
Ethiopia

Adam H Balen FRCOG
Consultant in Reproductive Medicine and
Surgery
Department of Reproductive Medicine
Clarendon Wing
Leeds General Infirmary
Leeds LS2 9NS
UK

Adrian Bianchi
Specialist Paediatric and Neonatal Surgeon
Neonatal Surgical Unit
St Mary's Hospital
Hathersage Road
Manchester M13 0JH
UK

Lesley L Breech
Assistant Professor
Department of Gynecology and Obstetrics
Emory University School of Medicine
69 Jesse Hill Jr., Dr., SE
Atlanta
GA 30303
USA

Andrew Browning MRCOG
Staff Specialist
Addis Ababa Fistula Hospital
PO Box 3609
Addis Ababa
Ethiopia

Shiao Chan MRCOG
Clinical Research Fellow
Department of Fetal Medicine, Level 3
Birmingham Women's Hospital
Metchely Park Road
Edgbaston
Birmingham B15 2TG
UK

Lucy Chappell PhD MRCOG
Subspecialty Trainee in Maternal and Fetal
Medicine
Centre for Fetal Care
Queen Charlotte's Hospital
Du Cane Road
London W12 0HS
UK

Charles Coutelle MD DSc
Professor and Head of Gene Therapy
Research Group
2nd Floor, Sir Alexander Fleming Building
Imperial College
South Kensington
London SW7 2AZ
UK

Hilary Critchley FRCOG
Professor of Reproductive Medicine
Centre for Reproductive Biology
The Chancellor's Building
University of Edinburgh
49 Little France Crescent
Edinburgh EH16 4SB
UK

Anna L David MRCOG
Clinical Academic Research Fellow
Department of Obstetrics and Gynaecology
86–96 Chenies Mews
London WC1E 6HX
UK

Colin J Davis MD MRCOG
Consultant Obstetrician and Gynaecologist
Directorate of Women and Children
2nd Floor, East Wing
The Royal London Hospital
Whitechapel
London E1 1BB
UK

Kara Dent MRCOG
Specialist Registrar in Obstetrics and
Gynaecology
University Hospital of North Staffordshire
Stoke-on-Trent ST4 6QG
UK

Andrew J Drakeley MRCOG
Subspeciality Fellow, Reproductive Medicine
Reproductive Medicine Unit
Liverpool Women's Hospital
Crown Street
Liverpool L8 7SS
UK

James Drife FRCOG
Professor of Obstetrics and Gynaecology
Department of Obstetrics and Gynaecology
The General Infirmary at Leeds
Clarendon Wing
Belmont Grove
Leeds LS2 9NS
UK

Sean Duffy FRCOG
Senior Lecturer
Department of Obstetrics and Gynaecology
Level 9, Gledhow Wing
St James's University Hospital
Beckett Street
Leeds LS9 7TF
UK

Diana M Eccles
Consultant and Honorary Senior Lecturer in
Clinical Genetics
Wessex Clinical Genetics Service
Level G
Princess Anne Hospital
Coxford Road
Southampton SO16 5YA
UK

Maeve Eogan MRCOG
Special Lecturer
UCD Department of Obstetrics and
Gynaecology
National Maternity Hospital
Holles Street
Dublin 2
Ireland

Elisabet Epstein
Specialist in Obstetrics and Gynaecology
Department of Obstetrics and Gynaecology
Malmö University Hospital
SE-205 02 Malmö
Sweden

Ayman AA Ewies MRCOG
Specialist Registrar
The James Cook Hospital
Marton Road
Middlesbrough T53 4BW
UK

Glenn Gardener
Consultant in Obstetrics and Fetal Medicine
Fetal Medicine Unit
Elizabeth Garrett Anderson and Obstetric
Hospital
Huntley Street
London WC1E 6DH
UK

Chris Griffin FRANZCOG MMED CMFM DDU
Consultant Obstetrician
Princess of Wales Women's Unit
Heartlands Hospital
Birmingham B9 5SS
UK

E Catherine Hamlin
Chief Executive Officer
Addis Ababa Fistula Hospital
PO Box 3609
Addis Ababa
Ethiopia

Catherine J Hayden
Research Fellow
Department of Reproductive Medicine
Clarendon Wing
Leeds General Infirmary
Leeds LS2 9NS
UK

Barbara Hewson
Barrister
Hardwicke Civil
Hardwicke Building
New Square
Lincoln's Inn
London WC2A 3SB
UK

Jonathan T Hindley MRCOG
Research Fellow in Gynaecology
Interventional MRI
St Mary's Hospital
Praed Street
London W2 1NY
UK

Gordon Hosker
Consultant Clinical Scientist (Physiological
Measurement)
The Warrell Unit
St Mary's Hospital
Hathersage Road
Manchester M13 0JH
UK

Jon A Hyett MRCOG
Consultant in Obstetrics and Fetal Medicine
King's College Hospital London
Denmark Hill
London SE5 9RS
UK

Tal Z Jacobson MA MRCOG
Fellow in Endoscopic Gynaecological Surgery
Department of Obstetrics and Gynaecology
The Royal London Hospital
Whitechapel
London E1 1BB
UK

Ruhi Jawad MRCOG
Forensic Gynaecologist
The Haven – Camberwell
King's College Hospital
15–22 Caldecot Road
London SE5 9RS
UK

Davor Jurkovic MRCOG
Consultant Obstetrician and Gynaecologist
Early Pregnancy and Gynaecology Assessment
Unit
Suite 8, Golden Jubilee Wing
King's College Hospital
Denmark Hill
London SE5 8RX
UK

Christine Kettle
Specialist Midwife
North Staffordshire Hospital NHS Trust
The Academic Unit of Obstetrics and
Gynaecology
City General Hospital
Newcastle Road
Stoke-on-Trent ST4 6QG
UK

Charles R Kingsland FRCOG
Consultant Gynaecologist
Reproductive Medicine Unit
Liverpool Women's Hospital
Crown Street
Liverpool L8 7SS
UK

**Sailesh Kumar DPhil (Oxon) FRCS
FRANZCOG MMed (ORG) MRCOG**
Consultant in Fetal Medicine and Honorary
Senior Lecturer
Centre for Fetal Care
Queen Charlotte's and Chelsea Hospital
Du Cane Road
London W12 0HS
UK

Ronald F Lamont FRCOG
Consultant and Honorary Reader
Department of Obstetrics and Gynaecology
Northwick Park Hospital
Watford Road
Middlesex HA1 3UJ
UK

Frank Lawton FRCOG
Consultant Gynaecological Cancer Surgeon
Department of Obstetrics and Gynaecology
King's College Hospital
Denmark Hill
London SE5 8RX
UK

Christopher Lee
Department of Obstetrics and Gynaecology
King's College Hospital
Denmark Hill
London SE5 8RX
UK

Adam Magos MD FRCOG
Consultant Gynaecologist
The Royal Free Hospital
Pond Street
London NW3 2QG
UK

Isaac Manyonda MRCOG
Consultant Obstetrician and Gynaecologist
Department of Obstetrics and Gynaecology
St George's Healthcare NHS Trust
Blackshaw Road
Tooting
London SW17 0QT
UK

Michael Maresh FRCOG
Consultant Obstetrician
St Mary's Hopsital
Whitworth Park
Manchester M13 0JH
UK

Jo Marsden FRCS
Surgical Fellow
Academic Department of Surgery
The Royal Marsden Hospital Trust
Fulham Road
London SW3 6JJ
UK

M Ruth Mason
Specialist Registrar Obstetrics and
Gynaecology
Department of Obstetrics and Gynaecology
Poole Hospital NHS Trust
Longfleet Road
Poole
Dorset BH15 2JB
UK

Joanna Mesquita-Guimarães
Research Fellow
Department of Reproductive Medicine
Clarendon Wing
Leeds General Infirmary
Leeds LS2 9NS
UK

Mulu Muleta
Medical Director
Addis Ababa Fistula Hospital
PO Box 3609
Addis Ababa
Ethiopia

Marie-Louise Newell
Professor
Centre for Paediatric Epidemiology and
Biostatistics
Institute of Child Health
University College London
30 Guilford Street
London WC1N 1EH
UK

Shaughn O'Brien FRCOG
Professor and Head of Academic Department
of Obstetrics and Gynaecology
Academic Unit
University Hospital of North Staffordshire
Stoke-on-Trent ST4 6QG
UK

**Colm O'Herlihy MD FRCPI FRCOG
FRANZCOG**
Professor and Head of Department
UCD Department of Obstetrics and
Gynaecology
National Maternity Hospital
Holles Street
Dublin 2
Ireland

Karl S Oláh FRCS MRCP(I) FRCOG
Consultant and Honorary Senior Lecturer
Department of Obstetrics and Gynaecology
Warwick Hospital
Lain Road
Warwick CV34 5BW
UK

Nicholas Panay MRCOG
Consultant Obstetrician and Gynaecologist
Queen Charlotte's and Chelsea Hospital
Du Cane Road
London W12 0HS
UK

Michael Pawson FRCOG
Consultant Gynaecologist (retired)
Department of Gynaecology
Chelsea and Westminster Hospital
369 Fulham Road
London SW
UK

Catherine Peckham FRCOG
Professor
Centre for Paediatric Epidemiology and
Biostatistics
Institute of Child Health
University College London
30 Guilford Street
London WC1N 1EH
UK

Prakashbhan S Persad MRCOG
Consultant Gynaecologist
San Fernando General Hospital
Independence Avenue
San Fernando
Trinidad and Tobago

Samantha J Pretlove MRCOG
Research Fellow in Obstetrics and
Gynaecology
Birmingham Women's Hospital
Metchley Park Road
Edgbaston
Birmingham B15 2TG
UK

Margaret CP Rees FRCOG
Reader in Reproductive Medicine
Nuffield Department of Obstetrics and
Gynaecology
John Radcliffe Hospital
Headley way
Headington
Oxford OX3 9DU
UK

Lesley Regan FRCOG
Professor of Obstetrics and Gynaecology
Department of Obstetrics and Gynaecology
St Mary's Hospital
Mint Wing
South Wharf Road
London W2 1NY
UK

Sylvia Rimmer
Consultant Radiologist
St Mary's Hospital
Whitworth Park
Manchester M13 0JH
UK

John A Rock
Chancellor, Professor of Obstetrics and
Gynecology
Louisiana State University Health Sciences
Center
433 Bolivar Street
New Orleans
Louisiana 70112
USA

Charles H Rodeck FRCOG
Professor of Obstetrics and Gynaecology
Department of Obstetrics and Gynaecology
University College London
86–96 Chenies Mews
London WC1E 6HX
UK

Lynne Rogerson MRCOG
Department of Obstetrics and Gynaecology
Level 9, Gledhow Wing
St James's University Hospital
Beckett Street
Leeds LS9 7TF
UK

Nigel Sacks MS FRCS FRACS
Consultant Breast and Endocrine Surgeon
The Royal Marsden Hospital NHS Trust
Fulham Road
London SW3 6JJ
UK

Robert Sawers FRCOG
Consultant Obstetrician and Gynaecologist
Department of Obstetrics and Gynaecology
Birmingham Women's Hospital
Edgbaston
Birmingham B15 2TG
UK

Neil K Shah MRCOG
Specialist Registrar in Obstetrics and
Gynaecology
Princess of Wales Women's Unit
Heartlands Hospital
Birmingham B9 5SS
UK

Malini Sharma MRCOG
Clinical Research Fellow
Minimally Invasive Therapy Unit and
Endoscopy Training Centre
University Department of Obstetrics and
Gynaecology
The Royal Free Hospital
Pond Street
London NW3 2QG
UK

Laurence Shaw FRCOG
Consultant Obstetrician and Gynaecologist
East Kent Hospitals NHS Trust
Queen Elizabeth the Queen Mother Hospital
St Peters Road
Margate
Kent CT9 4AN
UK

Abdul H Sultan MRCOG
Consultant Obstetrician and Gynaecologist
Mayday University Hospital
London Road
Croydon
Surrey CR0 5PR
UK

Biruk Tafesse
Staff Specialist
Addis Ababa Fistula Hospital
PO Box 3609
Addis Ababa
Ethiopia

Tommy Tang
Research Fellow
Department of Reproductive Medicine
Clarendon Wing
Leeds General Infirmary
Leeds LS2 9NS
UK

Alexander Taylor
Clinical Research Fellow
University Department of Obstetrics and
Gynaecology
Royal Free Hospital
Pond Street
Hampstead
London NW3 2QG
UK

Ranee Thakar MRCOG
Consultant Obstetrician and Gynaecologist,
Urogynaecology Subspecalist
Mayday University Hospital
London Road
Croydon
Surrey CR7 7YE
UK

Michael Themis
Research Lecturer
2nd Floor, Sir Alexander Fleming Building
Imperial College
South Kensington
London SW7 2AZ
UK

Pat Tookey
Senior Lecturer
Centre for Paediatric Epidemiology and
Biostatistics
Institute of Child Health
University College London
30 Guilford Street
London WC1N 1EH
UK

Philip M Toozs-Hobson MD MRCOG
Consultant in Obstetrics and Gynaecology
Birmingham Women's Hospital
Metchley Park Road
Edgbaston
Birmingham B15 2TG
UK

Lil Valentin
Professor of Obstetrics and Gynaecology
Department of Obstetrics and Gynecology
Malmö University Hospital
SE-205 02 Malmö
Sweden

Vineeta Verma MRCOG
Specialist Registrar Obsterics and
Gynaecology
Queen Charlotte's and Chelsea Hospital
Du Cane Road
London W12 0HS
UK

Jan Welch
Clinical Director
The Haven
King's College Hospital
15–22 Caldecot Road
London SE5 9RS
UK

Alec Welsh PhD MRCOG FRANZCOG
Staff Specialist in Obstetrics and Fetal
Medicine
Royal Prince Alfred Hospital
Missenden Road
Camperdown
New South Wales 2050
Australia

Zita West SRN SCM LIC AC
Midwife Acupuncturist
Zita West Clinic
144 Harley Street
London W1
UK

Catherine Williamson
Senior Lecturer in Obstetric Medicine
IRDB
Imperial College
Hammersmith Campus
Du Cane Road
London W12 0NN
UK

Ambaye Woldemicheal
Medical Director
Fistula Hospital
PO Box 3609
Addis Ababa
Ethiopia

Foreword

This 11th edition of the *Yearbook in Obstetrics and Gynaecology* has once again drawn together authoritative contributions from across the spectrum of our specialty. It has been nearly 2 years since the last *Yearbook*, and this bumper edition, which contains over 40 chapters, has been released to coincide with the 75th anniversary celebrations of the College.

In these days of increasing specialisation, more and more of us spend our time reading specialist journals, attending specialist society meetings and following guidelines and recommendations from regulatory bodies. It is thus refreshing to sit back and reflect on the varied subjects of the 42 chapters in this volume and admire the breadth and depth of our specialty. Whatever your special interest, you will find topics of direct and overlapping relevance to your work, as well as many chapters of general interest such as the feedback from the workforce survey and the implications of the Human Rights Act. Some of the chapters are based on eponymous College lectures, others are comprehensive reviews complementing those that are published in *The Obstetrician & Gynaecologist* journal, and others are unique opportunities to get acquainted with subjects that might otherwise pass us by.

There are several chapters on the ever-increasing capacity of ultrasound for prenatal diagnosis at seemingly ever earlier gestations, chapters on the role of thyroid hormone in the development of the fetal cortex, on fetal gene therapy and on fetal reduction. There are excellent reviews of the management of cholestasis and HIV in pregnancy, the impact of pregnancy on the urinary system, the role of anti-oxidants in pre-eclampsia, the choice of instrumental delivery and the diagnosis and management of obstetric perineal trauma. Other chapters look at the possible implication of bacterial vaginosis in late miscarriage and premature labour, new systems for CTG monitoring and the thorny problem of how to manage ovarian cysts in pregnancy. There are fascinating 'must-read' chapters on topics many of us rarely see such as conjoined twins, abdominal pregnancy and obstetric fistula.

From the surgical perspective there are authoritative reviews of the McIndoe vaginoplasty and endometrial carcinoma with further chapters on subtotal abdominal hysterectomy, vaginal hysterectomy and vaginal myomectomy. The trend towards increasing outpatient procedures and 'one-stop' clinics is reflected with chapters on the ultrasonic assessment of postmenopausal bleeding, outpatient hysteroscopy and thermal ablation of uterine fibroids. There is an excellent review of urodynamics, a look at the psychological impact of subfertility and a practical insight into the world of forensic gynaecology.

Our close relationship with other species is highlighted in a fascinating look at the anthropology of the menopause, another 'must-read' chapter. Continuing the endocrinological theme, there are chapters on polycystic ovary syndrome, the endometrium and intrauterine progestogens. Unlike some of our European gynaecological colleagues, we are not usually directly involved in the management of breast problems, but breast cancer is never far from our thoughts and it often overlaps into our clinical practice, as highlighted by the excellent overview of the genetic testing for breast cancer and other gynaecological cancers. There is a critical review of the data behind the recent hormone replacement therapy and breast cancer controversies and a look at the options for the management of the menopause in those with previous breast cancer. In our everyday clinical practice we are constantly reminded of the limitations of our traditional therapeutic options. In recent years there has been a welcome increase in the scientific evaluation of complementary medicines and acupuncture, both of which are reviewed in this volume.

In keeping with previous *Yearbooks*, the majority of the contributors in this edition are Fellows and Members of our College. Many of the contributors are established or up-and-coming experts in their field and will be well-known to you. We are grateful to them for giving up their time in their busy schedules to produce such high quality work. I would also like to thank Professor David Purdie for his contribution from the outset in commissioning these chapters and Professor Mary Anne Lumsden and Peter O'Donovan for their help in reviewing some of the earlier chapters. Whether you are preparing for the MRCOG, in training, or however far along the path of 'lifetime learning' you are, I am sure that you will find this book a valuable addition to your personal library. I hope you enjoy it.

Tim Hillard
July 2004

1

Instrumental vaginal delivery: forceps or ventouse?

James Drife

Based on a lecture given on 15 February 2002 at the Modern Management of Labour course in the Royal College of Obstetricians and Gynaecologists.

INTRODUCTION

In 1993 the Royal College of Obstetricians and Gynaecologists (RCOG) stated that the vacuum extractor, or ventouse, 'is the instrument of first choice for assisted delivery'.[1] Afterwards, the use of the ventouse increased in the UK. In some hospitals, staff were instructed to use it for every assisted delivery.[2] Ten years on, have women or babies benefited? This chapter takes a critical look at the College's recommendation.

RATES OF INSTRUMENTAL DELIVERY

Assisted vaginal delivery is a subject of major importance to pregnant women, although, strangely, it is rarely discussed in the antenatal clinic.[3] Data from Aberdeen published in 2001[4] show that a primigravid woman in her mid-thirties has a one in three chance of having her baby delivered by either forceps or ventouse, and, even for a multigravid woman aged over 40, the chance is still as high as one in ten.

Variations

Instrumental delivery rates, however, vary widely between hospitals, as much as, if not more than, caesarean section rates. In the 1980s instrumental delivery rates varied between 4% and 26% in different areas of Scotland, and in England they varied from 10% in Yorkshire to 24% in East Anglia.[3] At the same time the rates were 1.5% in the Czech Republic and 15% in Australia and Canada.[5]

The reasons for these variations are unknown. Nor do we know why the rate rises with increasing maternal age.[6] The main indications for assisted delivery are delay in the second stage of labour and fetal distress, both of which can be defined in different ways and are to some extent subjective.

The variations have implications for research. Entry criteria for randomised controlled trials (RCTs) should be clearly defined[7] and we ought to understand the reasons for using instruments before conducting RCTs on which instruments to use.[3] Ill-defined indications for intervention, however, mean that entry criteria for RCTs comparing vacuum and forceps deliveries have been at best pragmatic. The trials on which the RCOG recommendation was based may have included easy (perhaps even unnecessary) instrumental deliveries and an under-representation of difficult cases in which assisted delivery really was indicated.

BACKGROUND TO THE RCOG RECOMMENDATION

Debate about the relative merits of forceps and vacuum delivery has continued for decades. In the mid-19th century James Young Simpson designed forceps that are still in use but he abandoned his 'air tractor' soon after demonstrating it in 1849.[8]

The introduction of vacuum extraction

The first widely used vacuum extractor was developed by Malmstrom of Sweden in the 1950s.[9] There were some enthusiastic advocates in the UK, one of whom was JA ('Hamish') Chalmers, an obstetrician in Worcester, who died in 1998. Chalmers was concerned that the ventouse gained acceptance in Europe but not in the UK. His *BMJ* obituary, written by Richard Johanson[10] (now himself deceased at a tragically early age) tells how Chalmers had been deeply affected by witnessing misuse of the forceps early in his career. 'His student memories of traumatic labours remained real: he once saw a woman die after 17 different applications of forceps.' During the 1960s Chalmers wrote several articles about the ventouse[11–13] and he developed a lasting friendship with Malmstrom.

The first RCTs

Hamish Chalmers' son Iain (later Sir Iain) became director of the National Perinatal Epidemiology Unit, which was established in Oxford in 1978. In 1981 the Unit collaborated with St Mary's Hospital, Portsmouth, in organising an RCT comparing forceps with vacuum extraction. There had been only one previous similar RCT, conducted by Lasbrey *et al.*[14] in South Africa and published in 1964. It had concluded that:

1.   The vacuum extractor, if used with the head engaged and the cervix fully dilated, provides a mode of delivery as safe for the baby as forceps, more comfortable and less traumatic to the mother, and simpler for the obstetrician.
2.   Because of the incidence of cap haematoma, forceps delivery is probably preferable in cases where the occiput is anterior, the head is at the pelvic outlet, and local anaesthesia is adequate for forceps delivery.'

Lasbrey *et al.* also concluded that forceps delivery was preferable when a severely ill mother had to avoid bearing down, and that Kielland's forceps were more effective in rotating the fetal head, but should be reserved for fetuses that do not easily descend and rotate with two or three pulls of the vacuum extractor.

When the Portsmouth operative delivery trial was published in 1983[15] it claimed that the South African study had failed to examine the babies born by forceps, making impossible a comparison of the effects on fetal trauma. It also suggested that the vacuum had improved since the 1960s, the Malmstrom cup having been replaced by the Bird cup. The Portsmouth trial randomised 304 women requiring operative delivery. (The instrumental delivery rate in the hospital at that time was 10.7%.) Of the 304 deliveries, 106 were conducted by obstetric senior house officers (SHOs), 101 by GP trainees, 64 by registrars and 15 by senior registrars or consultants. Eighteen women randomised in the trial had spontaneous vertex deliveries. The results showed that vacuum extraction caused significantly less maternal trauma but there was an increase in mild neonatal jaundice compared with forceps. The authors concluded that the study was too small to rule out a clinically important effect on serious neonatal morbidity and that another trial was needed.

In 1987 the North Staffordshire/Wigan trial was organised by Richard Johanson.[16] A total of 264 women were randomised to delivery either by Kobayashi silicone cup ventouse or forceps. This group represented 68% of the 390 instrumental deliveries carried out during the study period in the two hospitals involved. Of the other 126 deliveries, 103 were by forceps and 23 by the ventouse. Of the 264 deliveries in the study, 125 were performed by SHOs, 132 by registrars, two by senior registrars and one by a consultant. (The other four women delivered normally.) The failure rates were 27% with the vacuum and 10% with forceps. There was significantly more maternal morbidity with forceps compared with the vacuum, and no differences in neonatal morbidity were detected.

Interpreting the RCTs

When this trial was published in May 1989 it was accompanied by a commentary by Hamish and Iain Chalmers entitled: 'The obstetric vacuum extractor is the instrument of first choice for operative vaginal delivery'.[17] The authors concluded that there was evidence that the vacuum extractor resulted in a substantial reduction in maternal morbidity and there was no evidence that forceps had any compensating advantages. (They appeared to ignore the failure rates in the North Staffordshire trial.) On the basis of the two UK trials, they calculated that continued preference for the forceps would result in 10 000 women unnecessarily experiencing moderate or severe pain during childbirth each year in the UK and 3500 women suffering unnecessarily from severe pain for several days after delivery.

The rise of evidence based medicine

The year in which these articles appeared, 1989, was an important one for obstetrics. It saw the publication of *A Guide to Effective Care in Pregnancy and Childbirth,* (known as ECPC), edited by Murray Enkin, Marc Keirse and Iain Chalmers.[18] The section on assisted delivery, written by Aldo Vacca and Marc Keirse, concluded that 'for most instrumental rotational deliveries vacuum extraction is to be preferred over forceps. The same may hold, albeit to a lesser extent, for most other operative vaginal deliveries as well.' However, they counselled that skills with both instruments should be maintained. 'Reserving one instrument for routine applications and the other for especially difficult situations would be ill-advised.'[18]

In 1990 ECPC was the subject of a commentary in the *British Journal of Obstetrics and Gynaecology* (*BJOG*), of which Iain Chalmers was then an assistant editor. The commentary hailed it as 'probably the most important book in obstetrics to appear this century'.[19] Again, the timing was significant. Obstetricians, at the end of an historic transformation in the safety of childbirth in the UK,[20] were receiving an unexpected backlash of criticism for being unsympathetic to women. This came not only from consumer groups but also from other doctors.[21] Both ECPC and the *BJOG* criticised obstetricians for failing to base their practice on RCT evidence.

When some correspondents to the *BJOG* criticised the Chalmers' commentary,[22–24] the authors responded that the only way to rebut their conclusion was for others to conduct their own RCTs and come up with their own evidence.[25] It is interesting to note that no one at that time criticised the quality of the RCTs that had already been carried out. Obstetricians, on the defensive and perhaps still unfamiliar with RCT methods, used other arguments to try to counter the Chalmers' conclusions, but accepted that the RCTs had been well designed. It would be several years before their quality was examined critically.

The West Midlands trial

After the North Staffordshire trial, Johanson et al.[26] formulated a policy of using Silc cup extraction for straightforward lift-out deliveries and Bird cups for those that were more difficult. In June 1993 they published an RCT comparing this new policy with 'the standard forceps policy'.[26] The West Midlands trial randomised 607 women to either vacuum or forceps delivery. The failure rate was 15% with the vacuum and 10% with forceps. Anal sphincter damage or upper vaginal extensions were found in 11% of the vacuum group and 17% of the forceps group, and less analgesia was used in the vacuum group. Cephalhaematoma was found in 9% of babies delivered by the vacuum and in 3% delivered by forceps. The study concluded that the vacuum was again associated with less maternal trauma than the forceps, but that further studies were needed to assess neonatal morbidity accurately. Within months, however, the RCOG recommendation had appeared.

THE CHANGE IN UK PRACTICE

UK practice had begun to change in 1990, soon after the Chalmers' commentary. Meniru, studying routine reports from hospitals to the RCOG, found that between 1989 and 1993 the rate of vacuum extraction rose from 1.37% to 3.5%, while the forceps rate fell from 8.62% to 6.62%.[27] The slight overall rise in the instrumental delivery rate, from 9.99% to 10.12%, was not significant. Meniru also sent a questionnaire to 252 maternity units in 1992. This produced only a 40% response, but 67% of respondents replied that they would allow the use of vacuum extraction before full dilatation,[27] a prospect that many would view with alarm.[28]

After 1993 the change accelerated. In one hospital in which a new policy in line with the RCOG recommendation was introduced, the vacuum extraction rate increased from 0 in 1994 to 4.2% in 1996, with a corresponding fall in the forceps rate from 5.7% to 3.8%. Thus, by 1996 in that hospital, vacuum deliveries outnumbered forceps deliveries, the overall instrumental delivery rate had increased from 5.7% to 8.0%, and the failure rate of the vacuum was 26% (the same as in the North Staffordshire trial). When the indication was 'failure to progress', however, the failure rate of the vacuum was as high as 33%. The overall failure rate of forceps at the same time was 4%.[2]

COMPLICATIONS OF VACUUM EXTRACTION

In 1996 the *BJOG* had a new editor, John Grant, who took a particular interest in the use of RCT evidence.[7] He commissioned two commentaries on the vacuum versus forceps debate, expecting them to discuss it from opposing viewpoints, but received only one manuscript.[3] This came from the present writer, who was at that time one of the Journal's scientific editors. This was the first time I had looked carefully at the RCTs. Like many other busy readers, I had accepted their findings, assuming that their design was beyond reproach.

Neonatal damage

The first surprise was that vacuum extraction carried risks of serious neonatal damage. At that time the risks of forceps damage to the baby were well known but the vacuum was generally felt to be safe. Enthusiasts of the ventouse had suggested that reports of neonatal injury were few and anecdotal.[21] In fact, neonatal complications of vacuum extraction were being reported mainly in paediatric journals. It was only in the late 1990s that they began to appear in obstetric journals.[29-31] The list of complications includes cranial fracture, retinal haemorrhage, jaundice, extracranial trauma and intracranial trauma.[32] There are wide variations in their reported incidence.[3] Jaundice ranged from 2.4% to 28% in different trials and scalp trauma from 6% to 37%. Cephalhaematoma affects about 8% of babies.[3] Bleeding around the tentorium has been detected by CT scanning, but the occurrence rate is unclear.[33] In a report on 27 infants with subgaleal bleeding, Govaert et al.[34] commented: 'There is little doubt that difficult, often elective vacuum extraction is the main cause of this neonatal emergency.'

Failure

The other important complication of vacuum extraction is failure. One difficulty in assessing failure rates is that the design of the vacuum cup changed in successive studies, Malmstrom's cup being followed by the Bird cup and then by the Silc cup. Detachment rates as low as 4% have been reported with the metal cup[35] and failure rates as high as 27% with the silicone cup.[16] It has been argued that failure of suction is a useful mechanism to prevent excessive traction,[21] but serious questions need to be asked about an instrument that fails on more than 25% of the occasions on which it is used. Vacca[36] concluded in 2002 that: 'The soft cups are inefficient devices that have unacceptably high failure rates and they do not reduce the incidence of cephalhaematomas or subgaleal haemorrhages.' He advises restricting their use to outlet and low occipito-anterior positions when the fetal caput is visible.

COMPARATIVE TRIALS AND THEIR LIMITATIONS

As the disadvantages of the vacuum extractor became apparent, the RCTs comparing vacuum and forceps were scrutinised more critically. These included RCTs carried out in the USA[37,38] as well as the UK trials referred to above.

Maternal soft tissue damage and pain

A consistent finding has been that maternal soft tissue damage is more common and more severe with forceps than with the vacuum. Such damage, however, is assessed subjectively by the operator and rates vary between different trials. Rates in one US trial were 36% in the vacuum group and 49% in the forceps group.[37] In the UK trials, anal sphincter damage or a high vaginal tear occurred in 9–11% of the vacuum group and 17–22% of the forceps group.[3]

Maternal pain is also difficult to quantify objectively. The use of anaesthesia was assessed in the West Midlands trial,[26] but this was decided in advance by the operator. In the North Staffordshire trial, 'unbearable' pain at delivery was reported by 18% of the vacuum group and 27% of the forceps group.[39] The West Midlands trial reported severe pain at delivery in 52% of both groups, and at 24–48 hours in 10% of the vacuum group and 13% of the forceps group.[40] 'Unbearable' pain during instrumental delivery raises issues that are discussed later in this chapter.

Fetal damage

The incidence of fetal damage varies between different studies. Superficial scalp changes have been reported in 44% of vacuum deliveries and 71% of forceps deliveries,[37] cephalhaematomas in 9–14% of vacuum deliveries and 2–3% of forceps deliveries,[26,37] and fetal lacerations or abrasions in 7% of both groups.[41] Retinal haemorrhages have been reported in 34–64% of babies delivered by vacuum and 16–38% of those delivered by forceps. Neonatal jaundice is more likely after vacuum extraction.[3] The importance of these complications is uncertain and it is generally believed that they have no long-term significance. Nevertheless, a study of boys aged 18 found higher intelligence among those delivered by forceps than those delivered spontaneously or by vacuum.[42]

Delay in delivery

When ECPC was published in 1989 it concluded that: 'The widely held belief that vacuum extraction is too slow to be useful when rapid delivery is required for fetal distress can now firmly be laid to rest. With proper technique, the interval between deciding on the need for instrumental delivery and delivery itself is no longer with vacuum extraction than with forceps.'[18]

This conclusion was questioned by an observational study in Oxford in 2000.[43] In cases without fetal distress the decision to delivery time was about 40 minutes, whether forceps or ventouse was used. In cases with fetal distress, the decision to delivery time was 29.2 minutes with the vacuum and 23.3 minutes with forceps. Both these figures are probably higher than most obstetricians would have imagined, but they suggest that, when necessary, rapid delivery can be achieved more quickly with forceps than with the vacuum.

Flaws and limitations of the trials

One problem with the RCTs of forceps versus vacuum delivery is the grouping of different types of forceps and different types of vacuum cup. There is a great deal of difference between rotation with Kielland's forceps and a 'lift out' with Wrigley's forceps, and it is now clear that there are major differences between metal and Silc cups. This raises again the question of entry criteria into the RCTs.

Entry criteria

As mentioned above, the North Staffordshire trial included only two-thirds of the instrumental deliveries in the hospital during the study period. Of the other one-third, over 80% were delivered by forceps.[16] In the West Midlands trial, cases were entered only when the obstetrician was unsure which instrument to use, and the 607 cases randomised represented about half the instrumental deliveries in the hospitals over the study period. The mode of delivery in the other half is not recorded.[26] The proper conclusion from these RCTs, therefore, is that the vacuum is the instrument of choice in equivocal cases.[44] Results from this subset cannot be applied to all assisted deliveries.

Lack of blinding

Both the obstetrician and the woman knew which instrument was used. Maternal outcome, the most significant outcome measure in all the RCTs, should have been assessed by independent observers. Apart from the long-term studies mentioned below, however, maternal soft tissue damage was assessed by the operator who carried out the delivery. Prior expectations could have influenced the operator and might even have affected the woman's assessment of her experience. The same applies to the finding that women required less analgesia before vacuum extraction than before forceps delivery.

Observer bias

The comparative trials have been organised by enthusiasts for the vacuum. There is nothing wrong with that, and indeed few if any research projects are initiated by people who are indifferent to their outcome. This is why meticulous protocols regarding entry criteria, randomisation and blinding are necessary. When entry criteria are debatable and blinding is omitted, consistency of results across different trials becomes much less convincing.

Generalisability

An assumption underlying the UK RCTs is that instrumental deliveries are carried out by doctors in training. The lack of consultant presence in the delivery suite in the 1980s and 1990s in the UK was well known but it was still surprising when studies showed just how inexperienced the doctors were who carried out many of the instrumental deliveries. In one study, when SHOs at the end of their jobs were questioned about training in the use of forceps, 23% said they had had no training and 35% of the remainder thought their training had been less than adequate.[45] In another, less than 40% of GP trainees believed at the end of six months that they were competent to perform a simple forceps delivery.[46]

This pattern is now undergoing a major change, driven not by RCTs but by clinical governance, complaints, litigation and observational studies.[47] Consultant presence on the labour ward is now belatedly becoming the norm.[48] The results of RCTs involving so many doctors at an early stage in their training cannot necessarily be applied to the practice of trained obstetricians, either in the UK or abroad.

LONG-TERM EFFECTS ON THE PELVIC FLOOR

The studies discussed so far have been of the short-term effects of assisted delivery. Later in the 1990s further studies were published of the medium and long-term effects. Only one was an RCT, but others give relevant background information.

Physiological studies

Sultan et al.[49] used anal endosonography and anorectal neurophysiological tests to study 202 women six weeks before delivery, 150 of them six weeks after delivery, and 32 with abnormal findings six months after delivery. Six weeks after delivery, 13% of primiparous women (and 23% of multiparous women) who delivered vaginally had anal incontinence or faecal urgency. At six months, sphincter defects were found in 35% of primiparous women and 44% of multiparous women. Defects were found in eight of the ten women who had forceps delivery but in none of the five who had vacuum extraction and none of the 23 who underwent caesarean section.

Interview studies

MacLennan et al.,[50] as part of the 1998 South Australian Health Omnibus Survey, interviewed 3010 men and women aged 15–97 years. The prevalence of urinary incontinence was 35.3% in women and 4.4% in men. Pregnancy, regardless of mode of delivery, increased the risk of pelvic floor dysfunction, defined as any form of prolapse or incontinence, including that of flatus. Pelvic floor dysfunction affected 12.4% of nulliparous women, 43% of those who had undergone a caesarean section, 58% after spontaneous delivery and 64% after instrumental delivery.

MacArthur et al.[51] interviewed 906 women ten months after delivery in a maternity hospital in Birmingham. Among other questions about postpartum morbidity, they were asked about faecal incontinence, soiling and urgency. Thirty-six (4%) had developed new faecal incontinence after the birth, of whom 22 had unresolved symptoms. The risk of faecal incontinence was 10% after instrumental delivery, 5% after emergency caesarean section, 3% after spontaneous vaginal delivery and 0% after elective caesarean section. Of the 18 women delivered by vacuum extraction, 22% had symptoms, compared with 7% of the 110 women delivered by forceps. This difference was not statistically significant.

Meyer *et al.*[52] prospectively studied 151 pregnant women in Lausanne, using history, clinical and ultrasound examination, and urodynamic testing. Twenty-five had forceps and 82 a spontaneous delivery. Ten months later, the incidence of faecal incontinence was 4% after forceps and 5% after spontaneous delivery. Stress incontinence affected 20% of the forceps group and was 15% after spontaneous delivery. Sexual responsiveness was diminished in 12% after forceps and 18% after spontaneous delivery.

Long-term follow-up of a randomised trial

A five-year follow-up of the women in the North Staffordshire trial was published in 1999.[53] Of 306 questionnaires, 228 were returned, giving a 74.8% response rate. Five years after delivery, 47% of the women had urinary incontinence, 44% had bowel urgency and 20% had faecal incontinence 'often' or 'sometimes'. There were no significant differences between the groups but there was a surprising trend. The proportion of women reporting faecal incontinence sometimes or frequently was 26% in the vacuum group and 15% in the forceps group. The *P*-value for this difference was 0.06, just outside the accepted level of significance.

Vacuum extraction and forceps delivery therefore have similar long-term effects on the pelvic floor. What is of concern is the apparently high incidence of pelvic floor problems, including occasional faecal incontinence, and the consistent finding that the risk is highest with instrumental delivery and lowest with elective caesarean section.

LESSONS FROM THE DEBATE

This has been a story of research, controversy and strong personalities. It teaches several lessons. One is that, when the time is right, changes in clinical practice can be brought about by a small number of people, provided they feel strongly enough.

The vacuum versus forceps debate has indeed raised strong feelings. At its outset, an older generation of authority figures disparaged the vacuum[36] and a new generation became determined to prove them wrong.[54] The new generation, in its turn, responded emotionally to articles and presentations that questioned the robustness of their research findings.[3,55] Our patients may be surprised that such a basic issue cannot be resolved by more dispassionate discussion.

Guidelines

Guidelines are now in general being scrutinised with increasing scepticism.[56] John Grant believes that they are a transient phenomenon and that 'the culture of guidelines is the antithesis to the ethos of medicine'.[57] Nevertheless, at present they are surprisingly popular with clinicians. The people who write them, however, are not immune from the pressures of scientific fashion. The task of reviewing the literature is increasingly being carried out by nonclinicians or by doctors who have temporarily or permanently ceased clinical practice. It is essential that working clinicians are fully involved in guideline writing and refereeing, and that the clinicians who use guidelines should scrutinise them carefully, whenever possible reviewing the original articles on which they are based. A particular danger signal, perhaps, is when a guideline can be summed up in a single sentence.

The real issues

Perhaps the most important question raised by this debate is whether or not we should be carrying out instrumental delivery at all. As mentioned above, we rarely discuss assisted delivery with women antenatally, despite its high incidence. This may be because we instinctively fear that after such a discussion a woman will ask for an elective caesarean section. How else to react to discussion of a 36–49% risk of soft tissue damage, an 18–27% risk of 'unbearable' pain and a 10% risk of faecal incontinence? Today, however, the most emotional issue in obstetrics is the question of caesarean section on demand.[58] The RCT we really need is one comparing abdominal and vaginal operative delivery,[59] but the time is not yet right, and perhaps we are afraid of what the result may be.

CONCLUSION

When trying to answer the question 'vacuum or forceps?' our knowledge has not advanced much since Lasbrey summed up his conclusions after the first RCT in 1964. We know a little more about the results of changing vacuum cup designs, and a lot more about the long-term effects of instrumental, and indeed normal, delivery.

We are re-learning the need for good training and clinical expertise. It is now agreed that the obstetrician needs to be equally skilled with vacuum and forceps. There are excellent teaching articles[5] and computer assisted learning programmes[60] about the vacuum, but skills with forceps are atrophying and alarm bells are ringing about the disappearance of Kielland's forceps.[61] It is to be hoped that, with consultants now present in the labour ward, trainees will be carefully taught how and when to use both instruments and, more importantly, when not to use them.

References

1. Royal College of Obstetricians and Gynecologists Audit Committee. *Procedures Suitable for Audit*. London: RCOG Press; 1993.
2. Tuffnell DJ, Wright A. Choice and instrumental delivery. *Br J Obstet Gynaecol* 1997;104:507–8.
3. Drife JO. Choice and instrumental delivery. *Br J Obstet Gynaecol* 1996;103:606–11.
4. Bell JS, Campbell DM, Graham WJ, Penney GC, Ryan M, Hall MH. Can obstetric complications explain the high levels of obstetric interventions and maternity service use among older women? A retrospective analysis of routinely collected data. *BJOG* 2001;108:910–18.
5. Johanson R. Ventouse delivery. *The Diplomate* 1994;1:186–91.
6. Rosenthal AN, Paterson-Brown S. Is there an incremental rise in the risk of obstetric intervention with increasing maternal age? *Br J Obstet Gynaecol* 1998;105:1064–9.
7. Grant JM. Multicentre trials in obstetrics and gynaecology. Smaller explanatory trials are required. *Br J Obstet Gynaecol* 1996;103:599–602.
8. Eustace DL. James Young Simpson: the controversy surrounding the presentation of his Air Tractor (1848–1849). *J R Soc Med* 1993;86:660–3.
9. Malmstrom T. The vacuum extractor. An obstetrical instrument. *Acta Obstet Gynecol Scand Suppl* 1957;36 Suppl 3:7–50.
10. Johanson R. James Alexander ('Hamish') Chalmers. *BMJ* 1998;317:1019.
11. Chalmers JA. The vacuum extractor (Ventouse) – an alternative to the obstetric forceps. *Proc R Soc Med* 1960;53:753–6.
12. Chalmers JA. The vacuum extractor in difficult delivery. *J Obstet Gynaecol Br Cwlth* 1965;72:889–91.
13. Chalmers JA. *The Ventouse*. Chicago, IL: Year Book; 1971.

14.   Lasbrey AH, Orchard CD, Crichton D. A study of the relative merits and scope for vacuum extraction as opposed to forceps delivery. *S Afr J Obstet Gynaecol* 1964;2:1–3.

15.   Vacca A, Grant A, Wyatt G, Chalmers I. Portsmouth operative delivery trial: a comparison of vacuum extraction and forceps delivery. *Br J Obstet Gynaecol* 1983;90:1107–12.

16.   Johanson R, Pusey J, Livera N, Jones P. North Staffordshire/Wigan assisted delivery trial. *Br J Obstet Gynaecol* 1989;96:537–44.

17.   Chalmers JA, Chalmers I. The obstetric vacuum extractor is the instrument of first choice for operative vaginal delivery. *Br J Obstet Gynaecol* 1989;96:505–9.

18.   Vacca A, Keirse M. Instrumental vaginal delivery. In: Enkin M, Keirse MJNC, Chalmers I, editors. *A Guide to Effective Care in Pregnancy and Childbirth*. Oxford: Oxford University Press; 1989. p. 243–6.

19.   Paintin DB. Effective care in pregnancy and childbirth. *Br J Obstet Gynaecol* 1990;97:967–73.

20.   Turnbull A. Overview. In: Department of Health. *Report on Confidential Enquiries in Maternal Deaths in England and Wales 1982–84*. London: HMSO; 1989. p. 140–51.

21.   Savage A. Personal view. *BMJ* 1985;290:1584.

22.   Greenwood PA. Correspondence. *Br J Obstet Gynaecol* 1989;96:1454–5.

23.   Goodlin RC. Correspondence. *Br J Obstet Gynaecol* 1989;46:1455–6.

24.   Purdey JM, Stirrat GM, James DK. Correspondence. *Br J Obstet Gynaecol* 1989;96:1456.

25.   Chalmers JA, Chalmers I. Authors' reply. *Br J Obstet Gynaecol* 1989;96:1457–8.

26.   Johanson RB, Rice C, Doyle M, Arthur J, Anyanwu L, Ibrahim J, *et al.* A randomised prospective study comparing the new vacuum extractor policy with forceps delivery. *Br J Obstet Gynaecol* 1993;100:524–30.

27.   Meniru GI. An analysis of recent trends in vacuum extraction and forceps delivery in the United Kingdom. *Br J Obstet Gynaecol* 1996;103:168–70.

28.   Ugwumadu AHN, Thakar BR, Manyonda IT. An analysis of recent trends in vacuum extraction and forceps delivery in the United Kingdom. *Br J Obstet Gynaecol* 1996;103:937–8.

29.   Stewart KJ, Acolet D, Peterson D. Leptomeningocoele: a rare complication of ventouse delivery. *BJOG* 2000;107:1173–5.

30.   Kent A, Lemyre B, Loosley-Millman M, Paes B. Posterior fossa haemorrhage in a preterm infant following vacuum assisted delivery. *BJOG* 2001;108:1008–10.

31.   Choy CMY, Tam WH, Ng PC. Skull fracture and contralateral cerebral infarction after ventouse extraction. *BJOG* 2001;108:1298–9.

32.   Drife J. Intracranial haemorrhage in the newborn: obstetric aspects. *Clinical Risk* 1998;4:71–4.

33.   Avrami E, Frishman E, Minz M. CT demonstration of intracranial haemorrhage in term newborn following vacuum extractor delivery. *Neuroradiology* 1993;35:107–8.

34.   Govaert P, Vanhaesebrouck P, De Praeter C, Moens K, Leroy J. Vacuum extraction, bone injury and neonatal subgaleal bleeding. *Eur J Paediatr* 1992;151:432–5.

35.   Lim FTH, Holm JP, Schuitemaker NWE, Jansen FHM, Hermans J. Stepwise compared with rapid application of vacuum in ventouse extraction procedures. *Br J Obstet Gynaecol* 1997;104:33–6.

36.   Vacca A. In praise of Kielland's forceps. *BJOG* 2002;109:1417.

37.   Dell DC, Sightle SE, Plauche WC. Soft cup vacuum extraction: a comparison of outlet delivery. *Obstet Gynecol* 1985;66:624–8.

38.   Williams MC, Knappell RA, O'Brien WF, Weiss A, Kanarek KS. A randomised comparison of assisted vaginal delivery by obstetric forceps and polyethylene vacuum cup. *Obstet Gynecol* 1991;78:789–94.

39. Pusey J, Hodge C, Wilkinson P, Johanson RB. Maternal impressions of forceps or the Silc-cup. *Br J Obstet Gynaecol* 1991;98:4887–8.

40. Johanson RB, Wilkinson P, Bastible A, Ryan S, Murphy H, Redman CWE, *et al.* Health after assisted vaginal delivery: follow-up of a random controlled study. *J Obstet Gynaecol* 1993;13:242–6.

41. Achanna S, Monga D. Outcome of forceps delivery versus vacuum extraction – a review of 200 cases. *Singapore Med J* 1994;35:605–8.

42. Nilson ST. Boys born by forceps and vacuum extraction examined at 18 years of age. *Acta Obstet Gynecol Scand* 1984;63:549–54.

43. Okunwobi-Smith Y, Cooke I, MacKenzie IZ. Decision to delivery intervals for assisted vaginal vertex delivery. *BJOG* 2000;107:467–71.

44. Cox J, Paterson-Brown S. Choice and instrumental delivery. *Br J Obstet Gynaecol* 1996;103:1269–73.

45. Ennis M. Training and supervision of obstetric senior house officers. *BMJ* 1991;303:1442–3.

46. Smith LFP. GP trainees' views on hospital obstetric vocational training. *BMJ* 1991;303:1447–50.

47. Drife J. Reducing risk in obstetrics. In: Vincent C, editor. *Clinical Risk Management.* 2nd ed. London: BMJ Books; 2001. p. 77–94.

48. Royal College of Obstetricians and Gynaecologists and Royal College of Midwives. *Towards Safer Childbirth: Minimum Standards for the Organisation of Labour Wards.* London: RCOG Press; 1999.

49. Sultan AH, Kamm MA, Hudson CN, Thomas JM, Bartram CI. Anal-sphincter disruption during vaginal delivery. *N Engl J Med* 1993;329:1905–11.

50. MacLennan AH, Taylor AW, Wilson DH, Wilson D. The prevalence of pelvic floor disorders and their relationship to gender, age, parity and mode of delivery. *BJOG* 2000;107:1460–70.

51. MacArthur C, Bick DE, Keighley MRB. Faecal incontinence after childbirth. *Br J Obstet Gynaecol* 1997;104:46–50.

52. Meyer S, Hohfeld P, Achtari C, Russolo A, De Grandi P. Birth trauma: short and long term effects of forceps delivery compared with spontaneous delivery on various pelvic floor parameters. *BJOG* 2000;107:1360–5.

53. Johanson RB. Maternal and child health after assisted vaginal delivery: five-year follow up of a randomised controlled study comparing forceps and ventouse. *Br J Obstet Gynaecol* 1999;106:544–9.

54. Drife JO. Loving the vacuum. *BMJ* 1985;290:1823.

55. Grant JM. Too little evidence. *Br J Obstet Gynaecol* 1998;105 Suppl 17:1.

56. Johnson N. Guidelines on using guidelines. *BJOG* 2002;109:495–7.

57. Grant JM. Editor's choice: medicine as ritual. *BJOG* 2002;109:[un-numbered].

58. Groom KM, Paterson-Brown S. Caesarean section on demand. In: Sturdee D, Oláh K, Purdie D, Keane D, editors. *The Yearbook of Obstetrics and Gynaecology,* Vol. 10. London: RCOG Press; 2002. p. 175–85.

59. Grant JM. Editor's choice: mistakes with meta-analysis. *Br J Obstet Gynaecol* 1996;103:ix.

60. Vacca A. Choice and instrumental delivery. *Br J Obstet Gynaecol* 1996;103:1269.

61. Oláh K. In praise of Kielland's forceps. *BJOG* 2002;109:492–4.

2

Diagnosis of obstetric anal sphincter trauma

Vasanth Andrews, Ranee Thakar and Abdul H Sultan

INTRODUCTION

Obstetric anal sphincter trauma is a major cause of anal incontinence in women.[1] Trauma may be mechanical and/or neurological. Until ten years ago many women were thought to have purely neurogenic faecal incontinence. With the advent of anal sphincter imaging, especially anal endosonography, it has been shown that many of these women who were thought to have only neurological damage have evidence of anal sphincter defects.[2-5] Sonographic anal sphincter defects that were not identified clinically have been detected in about one-third of women having their first vaginal delivery.[1] There is a strong association between anal sphincter damage and defaecatory symptoms.[1] In the UK, anal incontinence is believed to affect 40 000 mothers (5%) annually.[6] This chapter includes an overview of anal sphincter anatomy, classification of perineal tears, pathogenesis and risk factors for sphincter damage and, finally, techniques used in the diagnosis of anal sphincter injury.

ANATOMY AND PHYSIOLOGY OF THE ANAL SPHINCTER

The anal canal is the distal continuation of the rectum and measures about 3.5 cm in length. Compared with the male, the female anal sphincter is shorter anteriorly.[7] The external anal sphincter is made up of striated muscle and is subdivided into subcutaneous, superficial and deep layers (Figure 1). However, there is considerable controversy about whether these subdivisions exist.[7] The external anal sphincter is innervated by the pudendal nerve, which is a mixed sensory and motor nerve; it contracts voluntarily or reflexly during a sudden rise in intra–abdominal pressure such as coughing. The internal anal sphincter is a thickened continuation of the circular smooth muscle of the bowel. It contributes about 70% of the resting pressure and is under autonomic control. It is separated from the external sphincter by the conjoint longitudinal muscle that is a continuation of the longitudinal smooth muscle of the bowel.

PATHOGENESIS

The mechanisms that maintain anal continence are complex and are affected by many factors including lack of compliant rectal reservoir, changes in stool consistency and volume, diminished anorectal sensation, enhanced colonic transit, and disordered mental function. However, the ultimate barrier to rectal contents is provided by the puborectalis sling and the anal sphincter. Obstetric trauma is by far the most frequent cause of anal incontinence.

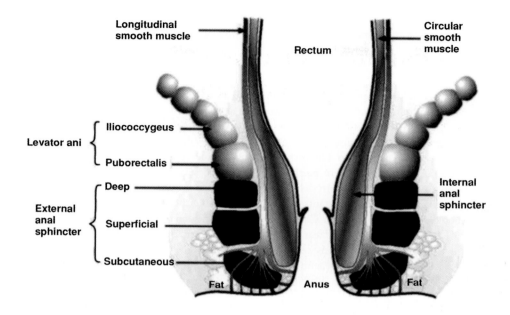

Figure 1 *Diagrammatic representation of the anal sphincter (reproduced from Sultan AH, Thakar R. Lower genital tract anal sphincter trauma.* Best Pract Res Clin Obstet Gynaecol *2002;16:99–116, with permission from Baillière Tindall)*

Neurogenic trauma

Prospective studies have shown an increase in fibre density of anal sphincter striated muscle after vaginal delivery, indicating evidence of re-innervation following denervation.[8,9] The fibre density was not increased after caesarean section. The maximum resting pressure (indicative of internal sphincter function) does not change following vaginal delivery. However, the maximal squeeze pressure has been shown to be reduced two months after delivery, indicating persistent weakness of the external sphincter. Snooks *et al.*[8] have shown prolonged pudendal nerve terminal motor latency at 48 hours, although another study found no significant change.[9] The nerve conduction delay is attributed to direct compression of or traction injury to the pudendal nerve as it changes direction around the ischial spine. Multiparity, forceps delivery, increased duration of the second stage, third degree perineal tears and high birthweight are important factors associated with pudendal nerve damage.

Occult anal sphincter trauma

Until the advent of anal endosonography, anal incontinence was largely attributed to neurogenic trauma. However, Sultan *et al.*,[1] in 1993, found that 33% of women sustain damage to the anal sphincter that is not recognised at delivery. These findings have been confirmed by a further five prospective studies that report occult sphincter rates of between 19% and 40%.[10–14] One-third of these women are symptomatic in the short term, but longer term follow-up is awaited to see if this group is at higher risk of incontinence later in life. It also remains to be established whether 'occult sphincter' tears are truly 'occult' or also include damage to the anal sphincter that is 'missed' owing to confusion over classification and lack of training of doctors and midwives.

Instrumental delivery

Women who have an instrumental delivery are at greater risk of perineal trauma than after a normal delivery. Donnelly et al.[10] found that instrumental delivery was more likely to lead to faecal incontinence: 23% versus 1.4% ($P < 0.001$) for normal vaginal deliveries.

There have been two large randomised controlled trials evaluating perineal trauma associated with forceps and vacuum extraction. The first study was conducted in the UK by Johanson et al.[15] in 1993. Mediolateral episiotomies were performed and led to severe vaginal laceration in 17% of forceps compared with 11% of vacuum deliveries. No long-term sequelae in terms of neurological development or visual acuity of the infants was associated with either instrument in the trial.[16] Bofill et al.[17] conducted the second study in Canada, where midline episiotomies are carried out. They reported a 29% third or fourth degree tear rate with forceps compared with 12% with vacuum.

The Royal College of Obstetricians and Gynaecologists (RCOG) and the Cochrane Review of controlled trials recommend that vacuum extraction should be the instrument of choice.[18]

CLASSIFICATION OF PERINEAL TEARS

There is lack of consistency in the classification of obstetric anal sphincter injuries. Sultan and Thakar[19] reviewed every obstetric text in the library of the RCOG and found that 17% did not mention any classification and 22% classified anal sphincter injury as 'second degree'.

Fernando et al.[6] surveyed 672 consultants in active obstetric practice and found that 33% classified a complete or partial external sphincter tear as 'second degree'. There was regional variation in the 'misclassification', with up to a ten-fold difference between regions. A far higher proportion of consultant obstetricians in the northern parts of the UK considered a complete external anal sphincter tear to be a 'second degree tear'. This may reflect the teachings of Professor Ian Donald.[20]

In order to standardise the classification of perineal trauma, Sultan proposed the following classification now adopted by the RCOG (Guideline 29) and internationally.[21,22]

- first degree: laceration of the vaginal epithelium or perineal skin only

- second degree: involvement of the perineal muscles but not the anal sphincter

- third degree: disruption of the anal sphincter muscles, which should be further subdivided into:
  3a: <50% thickness of external sphincter torn
  3b: >50% thickness of external sphincter torn
  3c: internal sphincter also torn

- fourth degree: a third degree tear also with disruption of the anal epithelium.

Isolated tears of the anal epithelium without involvement of the anal sphincters (buttonhole) are rare. To avoid confusion, they are not included in the above classification.

CLINICAL ASSESSMENT OF ANAL SPHINCTER DAMAGE

Clinical examination at the time of delivery remains the cornerstone of diagnosis of anal sphincter damage. Careful examination of the perineum and vagina should be performed on all women after delivery. Every woman who has had an episiotomy or sustains a perineal tear should have a rectal examination to exclude rectal or anal sphincter injury. Any first or second degree perineal tear that extends to the anal verge must be assumed to be a third degree tear until verified by an experienced doctor or midwife.

It is essential that there is adequate exposure and lighting for inspection of the perineum. If exposure is inadequate, examination should be performed in the lithotomy position. First the apex of the vaginal laceration must be identified. A rectal examination should then be performed to exclude injury to the anorectal mucosa and anal sphincter. Diagnosis of anal sphincter disruption requires clear visualisation and confirmation is by palpation. By inserting the index finger in the anal canal with the thumb in the vagina, the anal sphincter can be palpated by performing a pill rolling motion. If in doubt, the woman can be asked to contract the anal sphincter and, if it is disrupted, there will be absence of puckering on the perianal skin anteriorly. As the external anal sphincter is in a state of tonic contraction, disruption results in retraction of the sphincter ends, which therefore need to be grasped and retrieved. The internal anal sphincter should also be identified and repaired separately. This is a circular muscle and appears paler than the external sphincter. Under normal circumstances, the distal end of the internal sphincter lies a few millimetres proximal to the distal end of the external sphincter. However, if the external sphincter is relaxed after regional or general anaesthesia, the distal end of the internal sphincter will appear to be at a lower level. If the internal anal sphincter is visible the external sphincter is invariably torn.

The necessity for adequate training cannot be overemphasised. This is highlighted by a study involving 75 doctors working in obstetrics and gynaecology and 75 qualified midwives in London.[23] No doctor could name the muscles routinely cut during an uncomplicated episiotomy (the superficial transverse perineal and bulbospongiosus muscles). More than half the doctors and midwives who named the muscles wrongly believed that the levator ani muscle was cut routinely during an uncomplicated episiotomy. One doctor believed that the gluteus maximus was routinely divided in a mediolateral episiotomy, and a further two named the external anal sphincter. There was considerable variation in what they thought constituted a third degree tear.

Groom et al.[24] showed that, when women delivering vaginally had the perineum inspected for anal sphincter damage by a clinical research fellow, the overall rate of third degree tears diagnosed by birth attendants rose from 2.5% to 9.3%. This was due to increased vigilance by birth attendants once they became aware that their practice was being independently reviewed. Furthermore, the rate of third degree tears picked up by the clinical research fellow and subsequently verified by an experienced obstetrician was 14.9%. This study clearly demonstrates that, with increased vigilance and knowledge, it is possible to improve the clinical diagnosis.

PHYSIOLOGICAL ASSESSMENT OF ANAL SPHINCTER DAMAGE

There are many tests of anorectal physiology, including perineometry, anal manometry, pudendal nerve terminal latency studies, electromyographic studies and mucosal electrosensitivity. Continence is dependent on multiple factors, so no single test can be definitive, and therefore a number of tests are performed. However, anal manometry and anal ultrasound are complementary and essential in the initial assessment of anal incontinence.

There are many devices to measure anal pressure, each of which has merits and limitations. This also reflects that no method is ideal and difficulties arise when trying to compare studies from different centres. The standard method of performing anorectal manometry is with the person lying in the left lateral position. The catheter is introduced through the anal canal into the rectum (up to the 7 cm mark). The station pull through technique involves gentle withdrawal of the catheter at intervals of 0.5 cm until the cranial end of the canal is identified.

The catheter is then withdrawn at 1 cm stations and the resting pressure measured. Movement of the catheter can stimulate the sphincter, so a stabilisation period of 30 seconds is allowed at each station. The highest recorded pressure is termed the maximum resting pressure and is a reflection predominantly of internal sphincter function. The same procedure is then repeated with the person squeezing the sphincter tightly at each station. The highest reading is termed the maximum voluntary contraction pressure and is a reflection of external anal sphincter function. The maximum squeeze and resting pressures are lower in women than in men and decrease with age in both sexes.

RADIOLOGICAL ASSESSMENT OF ANAL SPHINCTER DAMAGE

Anal endosonography

Following the original description of anal sphincter anatomy by endosonography by Law and Bartram[2] in 1989, Sultan et al.[3,7] validated and clarified the endosonographic anatomy by in vivo and in vitro studies.

At present, B & K Medical (Naerum, Denmark) is the only company manufacturing the specialised rotating probe that provides a 360-degree image. The probe has a hard sonolucent cone. This is filled with degassed water for acoustic coupling. Care must be taken to ensure that no air bubbles are present in the probe because this can lead to sonographic artefacts. Ideally, anal endosonography is performed with the woman lying prone. However, it was originally described in the left lateral position, which is essential in pregnant women. Anal endosonographic images have been orientated such that anterior is to the right; however, by convention, most scans are now performed with anterior orientated superiorly.

The probe is withdrawn down the anal canal and images of the puborectalis, external sphincter, internal sphincter and longitudinal muscle are visualised. It is not possible to see the planes of cleavage between the components of the external anal sphincter with anal endosonography. However the trilaminar (deep, subcutaneous, superficial) pattern of the external sphincter can be deduced by the changing pattern seen at different levels.[7] The internal anal sphincter and subepithelial tissues can also be easily identified in both sexes. In men, the longitudinal muscle layer can also be identified because it is relatively hyperechoic compared with the external anal sphincter, but it is discernible in only 40% of women.[7]

Defects are recorded in a circumferential pattern and best described as hour readings from a clock face (Figure 2). In the longitudinal axis they are described according to the level of the various components of the external sphincter (deep, superficial and subcutaneous). Thirdly, defects are described as either partial or full thickness.

Three-dimensional endosonography

Three-dimensional endosonography has been introduced in the past five years,[25] allowing for computer aided multiplanar reconstruction of the anal canal. Three-dimensional endosonography uses an identical probe to that for two-dimensional scanning. The probe is mounted on a hand held mechanical rig, which moves the probe in a caudal direction at a constant velocity when in use and constructs a three-dimensional image of the canal from the images collected. After the image is produced it can be manipulated so that sections can be taken in any plane and accurate measurements of any injury can be documented (Figure 3).

With three-dimensional imaging, longitudinal measurements pre- and post-parturition can be obtained. Work by Williams et al.[26] has shown that the sphincter shortens after parturition and the angle it makes with the anal canal axis increases. The significance of these findings is not known.

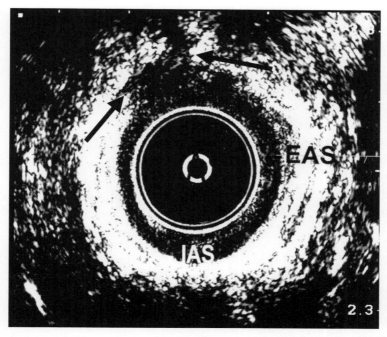

Figure 2 *Endoanal scan demonstrating an external sphincter defect (between arrows): EAS = external anal sphincter; IAS = internal anal sphincter (reproduced from Thakar R, Sultan AH. Management of obstetric anal sphincter injury.* The Obstetrician & Gynaecologist *2003;5:72–8)*

Compared with axial ultrasound (two-dimensional ultrasonography), three-dimensional ultrasonography has not been shown to increase the rate of detection of anal sphincter damage.[27] Its diagnostic potential, therefore, has yet to be realised, although it may aid the elucidation of obstetric tears and fistulas that are difficult to interpret with axial imaging.

Transperineal ultrasound

The transducer used for transperineal ultrasonography is one that is frequently used and is commonly available with most obstetric ultrasound scanners. By contrast, endoanal scanners are more specialised and exclusive to one company (B & K Medical).

A prospective study published in 2002 has shown that, if anal endosonography is taken as a reference method for diagnosing anal sphincter defects, the sensitivity of transperineal ultrasound is 50% and the specificity is 84%.[28]

This method has not been found to be useful in visualising the internal anal sphincter in the immediate postpartum period if any damage has occurred; this is thought to be due to the presence of oedema.[29] Compared with anal endosonography, studies have shown that the internal anal sphincter is thicker with transperineal ultrasound, which is thought to be because of the absence of endoluminal distension when using this method.[29] Further evaluation of this more accessible form of ultrasound is needed by comparing scan findings with histological findings to verify and validate imaging with this modality.

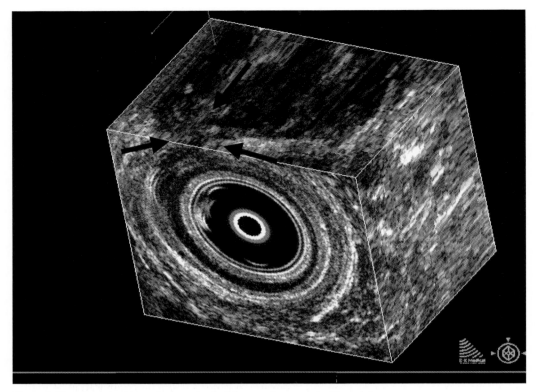

Figure 3 *Three-dimensional image demonstrating the full extent of an external sphincter defect*

Magnetic resonance imaging

Magnetic resonance imaging (MRI) has long been established as a diagnostic radiological tool. Its use in endoanal imaging however has only emerged since the mid-1990s. MRI has been shown to be accurate in demonstrating the anatomy of the anal sphincter complex.[30–34]

MRI can be used to identify external anal sphincter atrophy. This has been validated histologically after anterior sphincteroplasty on women suffering from faecal incontinence after childbirth.[35] Diagnosis of sphincter atrophy is less accurate with endoanal ultrasound because the outer border of the external sphincter muscle in atrophy is replaced with fat and the outer reflection is lost. This makes it difficult to determine the outer border from the ischio-anal fat. MRI is a valuable pre-operative tool to exclude significant atrophy prior to sphincter repair.

To date there have been two studies comparing MRI with endoanal ultrasonography. Rociu *et al.*,[36] in 1999, compared ultrasonography and MRI imaging in 22 women with faecal incontinence who underwent sphincter repair, and then reviewed the results retrospectively. They performed MRI and ultrasonography prior to surgery. The findings were evaluated separately and validated with surgical results. These authors found that there was better correlation with injuries to both the external and internal sphincters found at surgery and MRI compared with ultrasound. This study included only a few women and none of the results were statistically significant.

A larger prospective study of 52 consecutive women with faecal incontinence by Malouf et al.[37] did not confirm these findings. Each woman underwent endoanal MRI and interobserver variation was assessed. These authors found moderate correlation between the two observers for both imaging modalities; there was more interobserver agreement using anal endosonography than MRI.

These studies are conflicting and it has been suggested that this in part may be explained by differences in the study populations, study design and experience with the technique.[38] Larger prospective studies are needed to evaluate both diagnostic modalities and these are continuing.

MANAGEMENT

The management of obstetric anal sphincter trauma is not discussed in this chapter. The reader is referred to an article, by Thakar and Sultan[39] for comprehensive coverage of this aspect.

CONCLUSIONS AND RECOMMENDATIONS

Anal incontinence is an embarrassing and socially debilitating condition affecting women, but it is grossly under reported. Childbirth is a major aetiological factor in causing disruption of the anal sphincter. It would appear that most injuries are clinically apparent but are not recognised or documented because of misclassification or lack of training. It is possible that if all clinical tears are identified the prevalence of true occult injuries may diminish.

Anal endosonography is the gold standard technique for the diagnosis of anal sphincter defects. However, its value as a diagnostic tool in the immediate postpartum period needs to be established.

Many cases of litigation relate to missed third degree tears giving rise to faecal incontinence. There is a need for more intense and focused training of doctors and midwives in recognising the full extent of perineal injury. Anal sphincter disruption is not a common complication of vaginal delivery, so training may be suboptimal and therefore hands-on workshops using specially designed models and fresh animal tissue is the way forward.[40]

References

1.   Sultan AH, Kamm MA, Hudson CN, Thomas JM, Bartram CI. Anal sphincter disruption during vaginal delivery. *N Engl J Med* 1993;329:1905–11.
2.   Law BJ, Bartram CI. Anal endosonography: technique and normal anatomy. *Gastrointest Radiol* 1989;14:349–53.
3.   Sultan AH, Nicholls RJ, Kamm MA, Hudson CN, Benyon J, Bartram CI. Anal endosonography and correlation with *in vitro* and *in vivo* anatomy. *Br J Surg* 1993;80:508–11.
4.   Law PJ, Kamm MA, Bartram CI. Anal endosonography in the investigation of faecal incontinence. *Br J Surg* 1991;78:312–14.
5.   Burnett SJ, Spence-Jones C, Speakman CT, Kamm MA, Hudson CN, Bartram CI. Unsuspected sphincter damage following childbirth revealed by anal endosonography. *Br J Radiol* 1991;64:225–7.
6.   Fernando RJ, Sultan AH, Radley S, Jones PW, Johanson RB. Management of obstetric anal sphincter injury: a systematic review & national practice survey. *BMC Health Serv Res* 2002;2:9.
7.   Sultan AH, Kamm MA, Hudson CN, Nicholls JR, Bartram CI. Endosonography of the anal sphincters: normal anatomy and comparison with manometry. *Clin Radiol* 1994;49:368–74.

8.   Snooks SJ, Setchell M, Swash M, Henry MM. Injury to innervation of pelvic floor sphincter musculature in childbirth. *Lancet* 1984;ii:546–50.

9.   Allen RE, Hosker GL, Smith AR, Warrell DW. Pelvic floor damage and childbirth: a neurophysiological study. *Br J Obstet Gynaecol* 1990;97:770–9.

10. Donnelly V, Fynes M, Campbell D, Johnson H, O'Connell PR, O'Herlihy C. Obstetric events leading to anal sphincter damage. *Obstet Gynecol* 1998;92:955–61.

11. Rieger N, Schloithe A, Saccone G, Wattchow D. A prospective study of anal sphincter injury due to childbirth. *Scand J Gastroenterol* 1998;33:950–5.

12. Zetterstrom J, Mellgren A, Jensen LJ, Wong WD, Kim DG, Lowry AC, *et al.* Effect of delivery on anal sphincter morphology and function. *Dis Colon Rectum* 1999;42:1253–60.

13. Fynes M, Donnelly V, Behan M, O'Connell PR, O'Herlihy C. Effect of second vaginal delivery on anorectal physiology and faecal incontinence: a prospective study. *Lancet* 1999;354:983–6.

14. Abramowitz L, Sobhani I, Ganansia R, Vuagnat A, Benifla JL, Darai E, *et al.* Are sphincter defects the cause of anal incontinence after vaginal delivery? Results of a prospective study. *Dis Colon Rectum* 2000;43:590–8.

15. Johanson RB, Rice C, Doyle M, Arthur J, Anyanwu L, Ibrahim J, *et al.* A randomised prospective study comparing the new vacuum extractor policy with forceps delivery. *Br J Obstet Gynecol* 1993;100:524–30.

16. Johanson RB, Heycock E, Carter J, Sultan AH, Walklate K, Jones PW. Maternal and child health after assisted vaginal delivery: five-year follow up of a randomised controlled study comparing forceps and ventouse. *Br J Obstet Gynaecol* 1999;106:544–9.

17. Bofill JA, Rust OA, Schorr SJ, Brown RC, Martin RW, Martin JN Jr, *et al.* A randomised prospective trial of the obstetric forceps versus the M-cup vacuum extractor. *Am J Obstet Gynecol* 1996;175:1325–30.

18. Johanson RB, Menon BK. Vacuum extraction versus forceps for assisted vaginal delivery. *Cochrane Database Syst Rev* 2000;(2):CD00006.

19. Sultan AH, Thakar R. Lower genital tract and anal sphincter trauma. *Best Practice Res Clin Obstet Gynaecol* 2002;16:99–115.

20. Donald I. *Practical Obstetric Problems.* 5th ed. London: Lloyd-Luke; 1979. p. 811.

21. Sultan AH. Obstetric perineal injury and anal incontinence. *Clin Risk* 1999;5:193–6.

22. Royal College of Obstetricians and Gynaecologists. *Management of Third and Fourth Degree Perineal Tears Following Vaginal Delivery.* Guideline No. 29. London: RCOG Press; 2002.

23. Sultan AH, Kamm MA, Hudson CN. Obstetric perineal trauma: an audit of training. *J Obstet Gynaecol* 1995;15:19–23.

24. Groom KM, Paterson-Brown S. Can we improve on the diagnosis of third degree tears? *Eur J Obstet Gynecol Reprod Biol* 2002;101:19–21.

25. Gold DM, Bartram CI, Halligan S, Humphries KN, Kamm MA, Kmiot WA. Three-dimensional endoanal sonography in assessing anal canal injury. *Br J Surg* 1999;86:365–70.

26. Williams AB, Bartram CI, Halligan S, Marshall MM, Spencer JA, Nicholls RJ, *et al.* Alteration of anal sphincter morphology following vaginal delivery revealed by multiplanar anal endosonography. *BJOG* 2002;109:942–6.

27. Williams AB, Bartram CI, Halligan S, Spencer JA, Nicholls RJ, Kmiot WA. Anal sphincter damage after vaginal delivery using three-dimensional endosonography. *Obstet Gynecol* 2001;97:770–5.

28. Lohse C, Bretones S, Boulvain M, Weil A, Krauer F. Trans-perineal versus endo-anal ultrasound in the detection of anal sphincter defects. *Eur J Obstet Gynecol* 2002;103:79–82.

29. Shobeiri SA, Nolan TE, Yordan-Jovet R, Echols KT, Chesson RR. Digital examination

compared to trans-perineal ultrasound for the evaluation of anal sphincter repair. *Int J Gynaecol Obstet* 2002;78:31–6.

30. Hussain SM, Stoker J, Lameris JS. Anal sphincter complex: endoanal MR imaging of normal anatomy. *Radiology* 1995;197:671–7.

31. Hussain SM, Stoker J, Zwamborn AW, Den Hollander JC, Kuiper JW, Entius CA, *et al.* Endoanal MRI of the anal sphincter complex: correlation with cross-sectional anatomy and histology. *J Anat* 1996;189:677–82.

32. deSouza NM, Puni R, Gilderdale DJ, Bydder GM. Magnetic resonance imaging of the anal sphincter using an internal coil. *Magn Reson Q* 1995;11:45–56.

33. deSouza NM, Puni R, Zbar A, Gilderdale DJ, Coutts GA, Krausz T. MR imaging of the anal sphincter in multiparous women using an endoanal coil: correlation with *in vitro* anatomy and appearances in faecal incontinence. *AJR Am J Roentgenol* 1996;167:1465–71.

34. Stoker J, Lameris JS. Endoanal magnetic resonance imaging. *Acta Gastroenterol Belg* 1997;60:274–7.

35. Briel JW, Zimmerman D, Stoker J, Rociu E, Lameris JS, Mooi WJ, *et al.* Relationship between sphincter morphology on endoanal MRI and histopathological aspects of the external anal sphincter. *Int J Colorectal Dis* 2000;15:87–90.

36. Rociu E, Stoker J, Eijkemans MJ, Schouten WR, Lameris JS. Fecal incontinence: endoanal US versus endoanal MR imaging. *Radiology* 1999;212:453–8.

37. Malouf AJ, Halligan S, Williams AB, Bartram CI, Dhillon S, Kamm MA. Prospective assessment of interobserver agreement for endoanal MRI in fecal incontinence. *Abdom Imaging* 2001;26:76–8.

38. Stoker J, Bartram CI, Halligan S. Imaging of the posterior pelvic floor. *Eur Radiol* 2002;12:779–88.

39. Thakar R, Sultan AH. Management of obstetric anal sphincter injury. *Obstet Gynaecol* 2003;5:72–8.

40. Thakar R, Sultan AH, Fernando R, Monga A, Stanton SL. Can workshops on obstetric anal sphincter rupture change practice? *Int Urogynecol J Pelvic Floor Dysfunct* 2001;12:55.

3

Oral hypoglycaemics and polycystic ovary syndrome

Adam H Balen, Joana Mesquita-Guimarães, Tommy Tang and Catherine J Hayden

INTRODUCTION

Polycystic ovary syndrome (PCOS), as first described by Stein and Leventhal,[1] was defined as the clinical association of amenorrhoea, hirsutism, obesity and infertility, together with demonstrably enlarged polycystic ovaries. PCOS is now known as a heterogeneous condition with a spectrum of symptoms, pathology and laboratory findings.[2] PCOS is one of the most common endocrine disorders, affecting approximately 1–15% of women of reproductive age.[2,3]

PCOS AND INSULIN RESISTANCE

The association between insulin resistance, compensatory hyperinsulinaemia and hyperandrogenism has provided insight into the pathogenesis of PCOS.[2] The cellular and molecular mechanisms of insulin resistance in PCOS have been extensively investigated and it is evident that the major defect is a decrease in insulin sensitivity secondary to a post-binding abnormality in insulin receptor mediated signal transduction, with a less substantial, but significant, decrease in insulin responsiveness.[4,5] It appears that decreased insulin sensitivity in PCOS is potentially an intrinsic defect in genetically susceptible women, since it is independent of obesity, metabolic abnormalities, body fat topography and sex hormone levels. There may be genetic abnormalities in the regulation of insulin receptor phosphorylation, resulting in increased insulin independent serine phosphorylation and decreased insulin dependent tyrosine phosphorylation.[4,5]

Although the insulin resistance may occur irrespective of body mass index (BMI), the common association of PCOS and obesity has a synergistic deleterious impact on glucose homeostasis and can worsen both hyperandrogenism and anovulation. An assessment of BMI alone is not thought to provide a reliable prediction of cardiovascular risk. It has been reported that the association between BMI and coronary heart disease almost disappeared after correction for dyslipidaemia, hyperglycaemia and hypertension.[6] Some women have profound metabolic abnormalities in the presence of a normal BMI and others have few risk factors with an elevated BMI.[7,8] It has been suggested that, rather than BMI itself, it is the distribution of fat that is important, with android obesity being more of a risk factor than gynecoid obesity.[7] Hence the value of measuring the waist:hip ratio, or waist circumference, which detects abdominal visceral fat rather than subcutaneous fat. It is the visceral fat that is metabolically active and, when increased, results in higher rates of insulin resistance, type II diabetes, dyslipidaemia, hypertension and left ventricular enlargement.[7] Exercise has a significant effect on reducing both visceral fat and cardiovascular risk.

Lord and Wilkin[7] have found a closer link between waist circumference and visceral fat mass, as assessed by CT scan, than between visceral fat mass and waist:hip ratio or BMI. Waist circumference should ideally be less than 79 cm, while a measurement that is greater than 87 cm carries a significant risk.

Insulin acts through multiple sites to increase endogenous androgen levels (Figure 1). Increased peripheral insulin resistance results in a higher serum insulin concentration. Excess insulin binds to the insulin–like growth factor-I (IGF-I) receptors, which enhances androgen production in the theca cells in response to luteinising hormone (LH) stimulation.[9] Hyperinsulinaemia also decreases the synthesis of sex hormone binding globulin (SHBG) by the liver. There is therefore an increase in serum concentrations of free testosterone and consequent peripheral androgen action.[5,10–15] In

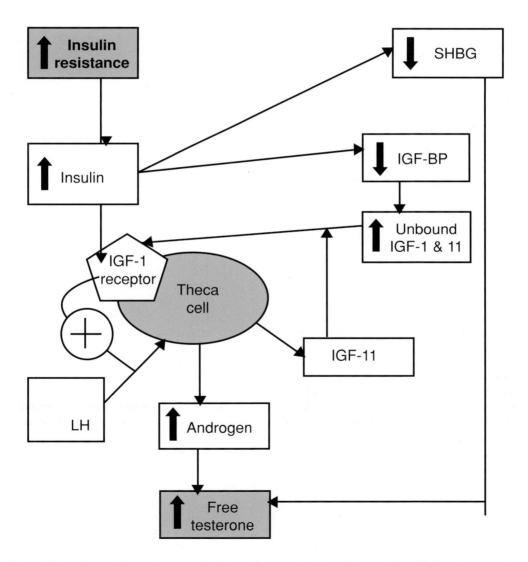

Figure 1 *The mechanism of hyperinsulinaemia induced hyperandrogenism; SHBG = sex hormone binding globulin; IGF-BP = insulin-like growth factor binding protein; IGF = insulin-like growth factor; LH = luteinising hormone*

addition, hyperinsulinaemia inhibits the hepatic secretion of insulin-like growth factor binding protein-I (IGFBP-I), leading to increased bioavailability of IGF-I and II,[15–17] the important regulators of ovarian follicular maturation and steroidogenesis.[18] Together with more IGF-II secretion from the theca cells, IGF-I and II further augment ovarian androgen production by acting on IGF-I receptors.[19,20]

Insulin may increase endogenous androgen concentrations by increased cytochrome P450c17α enzyme activity, which is important for ovarian and adrenal steroid hormone biosynthesis. Insulin induced overactivity of P450c17α and exaggerated serum 17-hydroxyprogesterone (17-OHP) response to stimulation by gonadotrophin-releasing hormone (GnRH) agonist have also been demonstrated.[15,21,22]

Chronic hyperandrogenaemia is thought by some to affect the secretion of gonadotrophins in favour of an increase in LH, which is typical in PCOS and contributes to the mechanism of anovulation.[10–13,23–26] There are many other potential mechanisms for hypersecretion of LH, which are beyond the scope of this chapter (for a contemporary review see Balen and Rose, 1994[27]). Intraovarian androgen excess is responsible for anovulation by acting directly on the ovary, promoting the process of follicular atresia,[28,29] and is characterised by apoptosis of granulosa cells. As a consequence there is an increasingly larger stromal compartment, which retains LH responsiveness and continues to secrete androgens.

PCOS, INSULIN RESISTANCE AND HEALTH RISKS

The sequelae of PCOS are far beyond reproductive health; women with this syndrome have increased relative risks for cardiovascular disease and type II diabetes mellitus. Hyperinsulinaemia was established in 2000 as a pivotal factor for myocardial infarction, hypertension, and ischaemic heart and thromboembolic disease to occur at an unusually young age.[30] As a consequence of insulin resistance, women with PCOS exhibit an atherogenic lipid profile (elevated levels of total and low-density lipoprotein cholesterol and triglycerides with decreases in high-density lipoprotein cholesterol) and a raised concentration of plasminogen activator inhibitor-1 (PAI-1), the major inhibitor of fibrinolysis.[31–33] Increased serum concentrations of homocysteine and uric acid have also been observed in women with PCOS compared with a control group of similar body mass and older age.[34] Although the metabolic changes reported in women with PCOS undoubtedly lead to an increased risk for type II diabetes, the evidence for higher mortality from cardiovascular disease is conflicting.[30]

The majority of studies that have identified the risk factors of obesity and insulin resistance in women with PCOS have investigated adult populations, commonly including women who have presented to specialist endocrine or reproductive clinics. However, PCOS has been identified in much younger populations,[35] in which women with increasing symptoms of PCOS have been found to be insulin resistant. These data emphasise the need for long-term prospective studies of young women with PCOS in order to clarify the natural history of the condition and to determine which women will be at risk of diabetes and cardiovascular disease later in life, and also at what stage abnormalities in cardiovascular risk factors develop. A study of women with PCOS and a mean age of 39 years, who were followed over a period of six years, revealed that 9% of those with normal glucose tolerance developed impaired glucose tolerance and 8% developed type II diabetes,[36] and 54% of women with impaired glucose tolerance at the start of the study had type II diabetes at follow-up. The risks of disease progression, not surprisingly, were greatest in those who were overweight. These data are supported by a study on 53 women with PCOS and a mean age of 41 years, in whom it was reported that obesity, rather than menstrual cycle pattern, correlated most closely with hyperinsulinaemia, dyslipidaemia and hypertension.[37]

Although the serious long-term health implications associated with PCOS are substantial, most women are not aware of these risks. Indeed, in the vast majority of gynaecological practice, medical care of these women has been limited mainly to symptomatic control of cosmetic concerns, menstrual dysfunction and infertility. Over the past ten years there has been an increasing awareness among clinicians of the association between PCOS and hyperinsulinaemia. Furthermore, many women are themselves well informed through support groups and websites and come requesting treatment with insulin sensitising agents.

APPROACHES TO THE MANAGEMENT OF PCOS

Although obesity worsens the symptoms,[38] the metabolic scenario conspires against weight loss, which should be considered first-line therapy. Management is then symptom orientated with anti-androgen therapy, either alone or, more often, in combination with oral contraceptives, which is effective in correcting the hallmark of the syndrome, hyperandrogenism. Menstrual cycle disturbances are usually managed by cyclical oestrogen/progestogen preparations and, when fertility is required, ovulation may be induced by clomiphene citrate (CC), gonadotrophin therapy or laparoscopic ovarian diathermy. The recognition of the critical role of hyperinsulinaemia has provided the rationale for the use of insulin sensitising agents in the management of each of the above mentioned symptoms.

PCOS is the most common cause of anovulatory infertility. Obese women with this syndrome often require multiple courses and high doses of CC or gonadotrophins to induce ovulation.[12,39] Increasing obesity is associated with elevated hyperinsulinaemia, so the high degree of hyperinsulin-aemia in obese women with the PCOS may account for their poor responsiveness to ovulation induction and, consequently, for their increased requirement of follicle-stimulating hormone (FSH) for follicular maturation. In theory, hyperinsulinaemia could adversely affect folliculogenesis and ovulation by increasing intraovarian androgen production, altering gonadotrophin secretion, or directly affecting follicular development. Insulin resistance may also be implicated in the ovarian hyper-responsiveness observed in women with polycystic ovaries.

Weight loss

With respect to reproductive function, the woman's BMI correlates with both an increased rate of cycle disturbance and infertility,[40,41] secondary to disturbances in insulin metabolism.[42] Even moderate obesity (BMI $> 27 \, \text{kg/m}^2$) is associated with a reduced chance of ovulation[43] and a body fat distribution leading to an increased waist:hip ratio appears to have a more important effect than body weight alone.[44] Obese women (BMI $> 30 \, \text{kg/m}^2$) should be encouraged to lose weight. A study by Clark et al.[45] looked at the effect of a weight loss and exercise programme on women with anovulatory infertility, clomiphene resistance and a BMI $> 30 \, \text{kg/m}^2$. The emphasis of the study was a realistic exercise schedule combined with positive reinforcement of a suitable eating programme over a six-month period. Thirteen of the 18 women enrolled completed the study. Weight loss had a significant effect on endocrine function, ovulation and subsequent pregnancy. Fasting insulin and serum testosterone concentrations fell, and 12 of the 13 women resumed ovulation; 11 became pregnant (five spontaneously). An extension of this study, in women with a variety of diagnoses, demonstrated that in 60 of 67 participants weight loss resulted in spontaneous ovulation with lower than anticipated rates of miscarriage and a significant saving in the cost of treatment.[46]

A reduction in body weight of 5–10% will cause a 30% reduction in visceral fat, which is often sufficient to restore ovulation and reduce markers for metabolic disease.[8] Weight loss should also be encouraged prior to ovulation induction treatments because they appear to be less effective when the BMI is greater than 28–30 kg/m². [47] Much has been written about diets that are said to be particularly helpful for women with PCOS. In reality, however, there is no evidence that women with PCOS require anything different in their diet than overweight women with normal ovaries. [7] The aim is to eat foods that produce a 'low glycaemic response', such as vegetables, fruit, fibre, protein and fat. Refined foods high in carbohydrate cause an increased glycaemic response and also reduce satiety, which results in overeating.

Exercise is important in helping to achieve weight loss, and improve insulin sensitivity and reproductive function. Visceral fat is affected more than subcutaneous fat and as little as two hours of exercise a week may be sufficient. A study of 970 female twins reported that physical activity was the strongest independent predictor of central abdominal fat and total fat mass. [48] A difference of one hour's exercise between twins was found to account for a 1 kg difference in body fat. Regular aerobic exercise is most beneficial and a strategy should be developed to maintain exercise activity.

Insulin sensitising agents

The use of troglitazone, the first oral thiazolidinedione approved for the treatment of type II diabetes, has a beneficial effect upon insulin resistance in PCOS. [49] In some studies [50,51] it was found that administration at a dose of 400 mg daily improved total body insulin sensitivity, lowered circulating insulin levels, and ameliorated the metabolic and hormonal derangements in obese PCOS women. Unfortunately troglitazone has been removed from clinical practice because of its hepatotoxicity. Later generations of thiazolidinediones, such as rosiglitazone [52] and pioglitazone, may have a role in the future, although there is natural reluctance to introduce them for the treatment of women of reproductive years because of the uncertainty regarding long-term adverse effects and teratogenicity.

Metformin has been extensively used in the management of insulin resistant states and has been most thoroughly investigated for the management of PCOS. This biguanide is a nonsteroidal compound that appears both indirectly and directly to influence ovarian function. Metformin is claimed to have a multifactorial action with primary effects on insulin sensitivity. It lowers blood glucose mainly by enhancing peripheral glucose uptake and inhibiting hepatic glucose production. Metformin also enhances insulin sensitivity at post-receptor levels and stimulates insulin mediated glucose disposal without affecting pancreatic insulin secretion. [53–55]

There is evidence that metformin also has a direct effect on androstenedione and testosterone production by theca cells *in vitro* by inhibiting the expression of steroidogenic acute regulatory protein and 17-alpha-hydroxylase. [56]

The major concern with biguanides has been the risk of lactic acidosis. This is a rare and serious metabolic complication of metformin therapy, occurring mainly in women with renal impairment, with an incidence of approximately 8 per 100 000 patient years. [57] Lactic acidosis does not appear to be a problem for otherwise fit women with PCOS who are not frankly diabetic and who have normal renal and liver function.

The most commonly reported minor adverse effects of metformin include bloating, nausea, vomiting, flatulence and diarrhoea. These symptoms appear to be dose dependent and may be substantially minimised by taking the tablet with meals. It is likely that an incremental dosage protocol (500 mg up to 850 mg, initially once and then twice daily) will be helpful for acclimatisation and to minimise undesirable gastrointestinal complaints.

These women are also encouraged to implement a structured exercise and supervised hypo-caloric diet programme when metformin treatment begins. Although weight reduction in women with PCOS is difficult to achieve and maintain – in part due to the anabolic effects of insulin, androstenedione, testosterone and dehydroepiandrosterone sulphate (DHEAS) – it is known to be associated with substantial improvements in spontaneous ovulation, menstrual regularity, ovulation induction efficiency and conception.[58,59]

THE EFFECTS OF METFORMIN IN PCOS

In the past few years a number of mostly uncontrolled short-term studies have assessed the effects of metformin on insulin sensitivity and endocrine profile in women with PCOS. Velazquez *et al*.[31] demonstrated that an improvement in insulin sensitivity induced by 1500 mg of metformin a day for eight weeks leads to a favourable change in serum concentrations of androgens, SHBG and gonadotrophins. Metformin resulted in a rapid fall in insulin and the insulin:glucose ratio with a concurrent significant decrease in serum concentrations of testosterone, free testosterone, DHEAS and androstenedione. A significant increase in the concentration of SHBG was also noted. As far as gonadotrophin concentrations were concerned there was a significant decrease in LH concentration, an increase in FSH, and normalisation of the LH:FSH ratio.

These results are in agreement with Diamanti-Kandarakis *et al*.,[14] who found improvement in insulin sensitivity matched by significant reductions in ovarian hyperandrogenism, in particular in the key biological markers of free testosterone and androstenedione. The reduction in free testosterone levels was clearly due to an increase in SHBG concentration after metformin treatment, although these effects appeared to be independent of weight loss.

In a controlled study in 25 obese women with PCOS, four to eight weeks of metformin (500 mg three times a day) led to significant reductions in serum insulin, free testosterone and LH, and to an increase in SHBG.[60] These women also showed an attenuation in the serum 17-OHP response to GnRH agonist stimulation, a proposed hallmark feature of ovarian hyperandrogenism. These effects were independent of changes in body weight, confirming that metformin activity is not dependent on weight loss. These data are consistent with the results of a study by Moghetti *et al*.,[10] in which metformin treatment for six months led to significant reductions in serum concentrations of free testosterone as well as in the serum 17-OHP response to GnRH agonist stimulation.

More recently, in 2000, it was demonstrated that metformin-induced insulin reduction is associated with increases in SHBG and IGFBP-I, and a reduced IGF-I:IGFBP-I ratio, which may be partly responsible for the reduction in plasma androgen levels in women with PCOS. Metformin, by reducing the IGF-I availability to the ovaries, may modify the hyperandrogenic intrafollicular milieu so characteristic of PCOS.[17]

Not all the data, however, have been so encouraging. Two trials[61,62] with essentially identical recruitment criteria and using slightly higher doses of metformin (850 mg twice and three times a day) over similar lengths of time, showed little or no benefit with respect to insulin metabolism, hormone concentrations or lipid variables. In a study that was designed to balance dietary intake and sustain body weight, Ehrmann *et al*.[62] found that hyperinsulinaemia and androgen excesses in obese nondiabetic women with PCOS were not improved by the administration of high-dose metformin, and both basal and stimulated LH and FSH levels were unaffected. A further trial showed that metformin therapy had no additional benefit over the effect of a low-calorie diet that induced weight loss.[63] The reasons for these disagreements are unclear but they could be due to different methods used to assess insulin action and large BMI differences (29 versus 39 kg/m^2) between the study groups. It has been claimed that the ability of metformin to alter insulin sensitivity in individuals with major obesity (BMI of 40 kg/m^2 and above) is limited.[64]

It has been proposed that increased ovarian cytochrome P450c17α activity is a feature of the PCOS. Cytochrome P450c17α is a key enzyme in ovarian androgen steroidogenesis. Decreasing serum insulin concentrations with metformin reduces ovarian P450c17α enzyme activity, as demonstrated by a significant reduction in the responses of 17-OHP to the administration of human chorionic gonadotrophin, and ameliorates hyperandrogenism.[22,60] In contrast, in two other studies,[65,66] there was no effect in terms of 17-OHP response to buserelin, suggesting that insulin may have differential effects on the hyperandrogenaemia of PCOS other than on P450c17α enzyme activity.

Metformin, by reducing fasting insulin and the insulin response to glucose in hyperinsulinaemic women with PCOS, reduces the hyperinsulinaemia-driven hyperandrogenism and can reverse the endocrinopathy, which is often enough to allow regular menstrual cycles, reversal of infertility, and spontaneous pregnancy. The achievement of normal menstrual cycles may also reduce the risk of endometrial hyperplasia and adenocarcinoma associated with PCOS.[67]

As previously stated, PCOS may be associated with a substantially increased risk of heart attack and stroke, although there is debate over whether the major risk is PCOS itself or obesity in these women. The risk of cardiovascular disease is mostly related to alterations in plasma lipids, lipoproteins, apoproteins, PAI-1 and blood pressure.[30] Several authors[13,24,31,32,59] have shown that metformin therapy is associated with improvements in lipid profile, fibrinolytic activity, and systolic and diastolic blood pressure, providing considerable potential cardioprotection.

METFORMIN AND REPRODUCTIVE FUNCTION

Evidence supporting ovarian responsiveness to metformin has accumulated from several institutions through small studies published during the past decade. For example, among 22 women with PCOS who received metformin for six months, Velazquez et al.[13] demonstrated a restoration of menstrual cyclicity in 96% of those who were oligo/amenorrhoeic. This menstrual regularisation was accompanied by an ovulatory response in 87% of those with regular menses, and by a pregnancy rate of 19%. All women who had normalisation of menstrual irregularities showed a metformin induced reduction in insulin levels at baseline and after a glucose load that was associated with a substantial decrease in serum concentrations of free testosterone and the LH:FSH ratio.

Similarly, an extensive two-year investigation of 43 amenorrhoeic, hyperinsulinaemic women with PCOS who were treated with metformin demonstrated the return of normal menses in more than 90%.[24] Many other studies[10,12,13,26,60,68] have, to varying degrees (between 44% and 96%), shown improvements in both spontaneous and drug-induced ovulatory function, development of normal menses, and restoration of fertility, which were independent of changes in body weight. Indeed, a significant decline in serum concentrations of testosterone and LH occurred within one week in a small group of women,[68] indicating a rapid effect of metformin on ovarian function. The reasons for the striking differences in clinical response to metformin may reflect the heterogeneity in the pathogenesis of the syndrome and different populations.

Metformin is not an ovulation induction agent. Unlike gonadotrophins or CC, metformin does not accelerate ovarian follicular recruitment or growth. The physiological aim of metformin therapy in PCOS is the resumption of normal, monofollicular gonadal function. Metformin has no known direct stimulant effect on the ovarian stromal or germ cell compartment. There is therefore no associated increased risk for multiple gestation when metformin is used to enhance fertility in PCOS. Although many women with PCOS may benefit from treatment with insulin-lowering agents, the ideal candidates for such therapy are probably those who are overweight with elevated serum androgen concentrations and/or fasting insulin levels greater than or equal to 10 mU/l.

Metformin can increase the frequency of induced ovulation in previously CC resistant women. The administration of metformin to 11 CC resistant women with a mean BMI of 38 kg/m^2 was shown to increase the number of ovulatory cycles induced with CC by almost three-fold and increase the pregnancy rate by almost eight-fold compared with a control group given a placebo.[69] In addition, a conception rate of 21% after ovulation, similar to normal cycle fecundity, was observed, suggesting that combined metformin and CC use have no adverse effects on postovulatory reproductive events.

An often quoted study by Nestler et al.[12] involved the prescription of metformin (500 mg three times daily) or placebo to 61 women with a mean BMI of 32 kg/m^2 for 35 days, by which time 12 of the 35 who received metformin had ovulated (34%) compared with only 1 of the 26 given placebo (4%, $P < 0.001$). On day 35 of the study all those who had yet to ovulate were given CC (50 mg for five days) and progesterone levels were measured after 11 and 19 days, when the study was stopped. Of the 21 who received metformin and CC, 19 had ovulated (90%) compared with only 2 of the 25 given placebo and CC (8%, $P < 0.001$). This study provided striking results in the absence of a change in BMI, yet criticisms have been made about the study design (with assessment finishing 19 days after CC administration) and the surprisingly low rate of ovulation in the CC/placebo group.

There are now a number of small, double blind placebo controlled trials of metformin at different doses in women with anovulatory PCOS. One such study from Hong Kong found no benefit, although the women had a normal BMI and there were only ten in each group.[70] A larger study from Turkey with 28 obese women per group reported a rate of ovulation of 78% in those treated with 850 mg metformin twice daily versus 14% in the control group.[71]

A further study from Turkey using metformin 850 mg twice daily versus placebo in 32 obese CC resistant women reported that 6/16 of those treated ovulated compared with 1/16 in the placebo group.[72] Additional treatment with recombinant FSH in those who were still anovulatory (10 metformin treated versus 15 placebo) led to similar rates of ovulation (94% versus 75%), but again the small numbers may account for the lack of significance.

A group of 20 CC resistant women with PCOS and moderate obesity were prescribed metformin (1500 mg daily) prior to treatment with FSH and were found to have a more orderly follicular growth, with less likelihood of overstimulation than when treated with FSH alone.[23]

The largest prospective randomised controlled trial to date is that of Fleming et al.,[73] who randomised 94 women to receive either metformin 850 mg twice daily or placebo. It is interesting that significantly more women withdrew in the metformin arm owing to adverse effects (15 versus 5, $P < 0.05$). Those treated with metformin were found to have an increased rate of ovulation (23% versus 13%, $P < 0.01$) and a quicker first time to ovulation (24 versus 42 days, $P < 0.05$). Significant weight loss was reported in the treated group, while the placebo group gained weight ($P < 0.05$) over the 14 weeks of therapy. Glucose tolerance was not improved in either group. This study also reported an inverse relationship between body mass and efficacy of metformin.

Improvements in ovulatory function in women given metformin plus CC or FSH may be due to a decrease in the direct effects of insulin on the ovaries, to the normalisation of clomiphene induced gonadotrophin secretion, or to a direct tissue sensitising effect of the drug at the ovarian level. Differences in the reported studies may be due to variation in populations, definitions of PCOS, degrees of obesity and insulin resistance, and the definition of CC resistance (i.e. failure of response or failure of conception).

We are currently coordinating a large multicentre study of metformin (850 mg twice daily) versus placebo for six months in anovulatory women with a BMI of more than 30 kg/m^2, the results of which are expected in 2003.

METFORMIN AND SUPEROVULATION FOR ASSISTED CONCEPTION

In vitro fertilisation (IVF) is an effective treatment for women with PCOS who are refractory to standard ovulation induction treatments or who have coexisting infertility problems, as shown in a study where significantly more oocytes were recovered per cycle in a group of women with PCOS than in a control group of normo-ovulatory women with tubal factor infertility (19.4% versus 5.4%, $P < 0.004$).[74] The fertilisation rates (40.4% versus 67.6%) and cleavage rates (34.4% versus 65.6%) were also lower in women with PCOS than in the control group. These data suggest that the quality of oocytes retrieved from women with PCOS are poorer than those from normal women.[75] Another study[76] noted a significantly higher incidence of embryo transfer cancellations in the PCOS group owing to failure of either oocyte recovery or fertilisation. However, the mean number of embryos transferred and the pregnancy rates per embryo transferred did not differ between the two groups.

The follicular endocrine microenvironment may affect oocyte quality in women undergoing IVF.[77] Testosterone concentration in the follicular fluid was significantly elevated in PCOS follicles compared with those from women without PCOS, and significantly higher levels of follicular testosterone were found in those follicles with meiotically incompetent oocytes than in follicles with meiotically competent oocytes in PCOS. It was concluded that the excess follicular androgen concentration could affect oocyte quality. Metformin may reduce the follicular androgen level and improve the outcome of IVF treatments. A retrospective study reported the use of metformin at differing doses in 30 cycles of IVF with intracytoplasmic sperm transfer in CC resistant women with PCOS compared with a historical 'control' group with CC resistant PCOS.[78] The impression was of a lower total follicle count, yet there was a similar number of more mature oocytes and developing embryos, with higher fertilisation and pregnancy rates. Caution is required, however, when interpreting retrospective data.

We are currently assessing the effect of metformin versus placebo in a prospective study of women with PCOS undergoing IVF. The endpoints are follicular response and rates of ovarian hyperstimulation syndrome.

MISCARRIAGE/TERATOGENICITY

Because of the introduction over the past eight years of insulin lowering agents in gynaecological practice, many successful conceptions are occurring while women are receiving metformin. The clinician must therefore consider the appropriateness of continuing therapy in pregnancy. Some researchers have reported evidence that continuation of metformin during early pregnancy may confer some protection against miscarriage. As high insulin and high LH levels have been associated with significant pregnancy loss,[24] the putative beneficial effect of metformin in decreasing miscarriage in PCOS may derive from a generalised improvement of endocrine function centred on correction of abnormal insulin metabolism. In addition, the ability of metformin to lower PAI-1 activity should reduce the rate of first trimester spontaneous abortion.[49,79] Abnormally high activity of PAI-1 promotes miscarriage, probably through thrombotic induction of placental microvascular disease.

In an uncontrolled study comparing pregnancies that occurred with and without metformin, the rate of first trimester spontaneous abortion was reduced from 73% to 10%.[33] These data are difficult to interpret because the participants were used as their own historical controls. It is important that there was no evidence of teratogenicity or maternal complications. An extension of this study by the same group[80] reported a reduced rate of gestational diabetes when metformin was continued through pregnancy: 33% compared with 67% in previous pregnancies. In contrast to the miscarriage data of the earlier work,[33] a study of 48 anovulatory women treated with increasing doses of metformin revealed that 40% resumed spontaneous menses, 31% required clomiphene (of whom 67% then ovulated), and a total of 42% conceived, among whom there was a miscarriage rate of 35%.[81]

Metformin does not appear to have a deleterious effect on mouse embryo development at high doses[82] and the data on human teratogenicity also seem reassuring. Furthermore, metformin has been used for many years in South Africa in the management of both diabetes during pregnancy and gestational diabetes, without deleterious effect.[83]

CONCLUSION

In conclusion, treatment with the insulin sensitising agent metformin provides a safe, effective and physiologically rational approach in women with PCOS. The numerous reports of the short- and long-term beneficial endocrine and metabolic effects of metformin appear to outweigh the negative trials.[84,85] In the context of infertility there is evidence that metformin may enhance reproductive function and may also augment the effects of drugs that induce ovulation, such as CC and gonadotrophins.[85,86] A Cochrane review of the current evidence is continuing.[87] Large randomised controlled studies are still required to determine the ability of metformin to influence the occurrence of hirsutism and acne. Metformin has been shown to reduce progression to type II diabetes by 31% in high-risk individuals (defined by a history of gestational diabetes, impaired glucose tolerance, or a first degree relative with diabetes).[88] In women with PCOS, prolonged studies are still required to determine the putative benefits for long-term health.

FOOTNOTE

This chapter was written in early 2002. Much relevant material has been published subsequently, to which we have not been able to make reference. Currently, a Cochrane review has confirmed a beneficial effect of metformin in improving rates of ovulation when compared with placebo, and also in improving rates of both ovulation and pregnancy when used with CC compared with CC alone.[89] The total number of women included in the Cochrane series was 310 and the largest study was on 92 women,[73] although the majority were much smaller. The data indicate that serum concentrations of insulin and androgens improve, although, contrary to popular belief, body weight does not fall.

References

1. Stein IF, Leventhal ML. Amenorrhea associated with bilateral polycystic ovaries. *Am J Gynecol* 1935;29:181–91.
2. Balen AH. The pathogenesis of polycystic ovary syndrome – the enigma unravels? *Lancet* 1999;354:966–7.
3. Franks S. Polycystic ovary syndrome. *N Engl J Med* 1995;333:853–61.
4. Dunaif A. Insulin resistance in polycystic ovary syndrome. *Ann NY Acad Sci* 1993;28:60–4.
5. Dunaif A. Insulin resistance and the polycystic ovary syndrome: mechanism and implications for pathogenesis. *Endocr Rev* 1997;18:774–800.
6. Ashton WD, Nanchahal K, Wood DA. Body mass index and metabolic risk factors for coronary heart disease in women. *Eur Heart J* 2001;22:46–55.
7. Lord J, Wilkin T. Polycystic ovary syndrome and fat distribution: the central issue? *Hum Fertil (Camb)* 2002;5:67–71.
8. Despres JP, Lemieux I, Prud'homme D. Treatment of obesity: need to focus on high risk abdominally obese patients. *BMJ* 2001;322:716–20.

9.   Bergh C, Carlsson B, Olsson JH, Selleskog U, Hillensjo T. Regulation of androgen production in cultured human thecal cells by insulin-like growth factor I and insulin. *Fertil Steril* 1993;59:323–31.

10.   Moghetti P, Castello R, Negri C, Tosi F, Perrone F, Caputo M, *et al*. Metformin effects on clinical features, endocrine and metabolic profiles, and insulin sensitivity in polycystic ovary syndrome: a randomized, double-blind, placebo-controlled 6-month trial, followed by open, long-term clinical evaluation. *J Clin Endocrinol Metab* 2000;85:139–46.

11.   Hasegawa I, Murakawa H, Suzuki M, Yamamoto Y, Kurabayashi T, Tanaka K. Effect of troglitazone on endocrine and ovulatory performance in women with insulin resistance-related polycystic ovary syndrome. *Fertil Steril* 1999;71:323–7.

12.   Nestler JE, Jakubowicz DJ, Evans WS, Pasquali R. Effects of metformin on spontaneous and clomiphene-induced ovulation in the polycystic ovary syndrome. *N Engl J Med* 1998;338:1876–80.

13.   Velazquez E, Acosta A, Mendoza SG. Menstrual cyclicity after metformin therapy in polycystic ovary syndrome. *Obstet Gynecol* 1997;90:392–5.

14.   Diamanti-Kandarakis E, Kouli C, Tsianateli T, Bergiele A. Therapeutic effects of metformin on insulin resistance and hyperandrogenism in polycystic ovary syndrome. *Eur J Endocrinol* 1998;138:269–74.

15.   Nestler JE, Jakubowicz DJ. Lean women with polycystic ovary syndrome respond to insulin reduction with decreases in ovarian P450c17 alpha activity and serum androgens. *J Clin Endocrinol Metab* 1997;82:4075–9.

16.   LeRoith D, Werner H, Beitner-Johnson D, Roberts CT Jr. Molecular and cellular aspects of the insulin-like growth factor I receptor. *Endocr Rev* 1995;16:143–63.

17.   De Leo V, La Marca A, Orvieto R, Morgante G. Effect of metformin on insulin-like growth factor (IGF) I and IGF-binding protein I in polycystic ovary syndrome. *J Clin Endocrinol Metab* 2000;85:1598–600.

18.   Adashi E. Intraovarian regulation: the proposed role of insulin-like growth factors. *Ann NY Acad Sci* 1993;687:10–12.

19.   Voutilainen R, Franks S, Mason HD, Martikainen H. Expression of insulin-like growth factor (IGF), IGF-binding protein, and IGF receptor messenger ribonucleic acids in normal and polycystic ovaries. *J Clin Endocrinol Metab* 1996;81:1003–8.

20.   Erickson GF, Magoffin DA, Cragun JR, Chang RJ. The effects of insulin and insulin-like growth factors-I and II on estradiol production by granulosa cells of polycystic ovaries. *J Clin Endocrinol Metab* 1990;70:894–901.

21.   Rosenfield RL, Barnes RB, Cara JF, Lucky AW. Dysregulation of cytochrome P450c 17 alpha as the cause of polycystic ovarian syndrome. *Fertil Steril* 1990;53:785–91.

22.   La Marca A, Egbe TO, Morgante G, Paglia T, Ciani A, De Leo V, *et al*. Metformin treatment reduces ovarian cytochrome P450c 17 alpha response to human chorionic gonadotrophin in women with insulin resistance-related polycystic ovary syndrome. *Hum Reprod* 2000;15:21–3.

23.   De Leo V, la Marca A, Ditto A, Morgante G, Cianci A. Effects of metformin on gonadotropin-induced ovulation in women with polycystic ovary syndrome. *Fertil Steril* 1999;72:282–5.

24.   Glueck CJ, Wang P, Fontaine R, Tracy T, Sieve-Smith L. Metformin-induced resumption of normal menses in 39 of 43 (91%) previously amenorrheic women with the polycystic ovary syndrome. *Metabolism* 1999;48:511–19.

25.   Nestler JE, Jakubowicz DJ, Reamer P, Gunn RD, Allan G. Ovulatory and metabolic effects of D-chiro-inositol in polycystic ovary syndrome. *N Engl J Med* 1999;340:1314–20.

26.   Morin-Papunen LC, Koivunen RM, Ruokonen A, Martikainen HK. Metformin therapy improves the menstrual pattern with minimal endocrine and metabolic effects in women

with polycystic ovary syndrome. *Fertil Steril* 1998;69:691–6.

27. Balen AH, Rose M. The control of leuteinising hormone secretion in the polycystic ovary syndrome. *Contemp Rev Obstet Gynaecol* 1994;6:201–7.

28. Hsueh AJ, Billig H, Tsafiri A. Ovarian follicle atresia: a hormonally controlled apoptotic process. *Endocr Rev* 1994;15:707–24.

29. Uilenbroek JTJ, Woutersen PJ, van der Schoot P. Atresia in preovulatory follicles: gonadotropin binding in steroidogenic activity. *Biol Reprod* 1980;23:219–29.

30. Rajkowha M, Glass MR, Rutherford AJ, Michelmore K, Balen AH. Polycystic ovary syndrome: a risk factor for cardiovascular disease? *BJOG* 2000;107:11–18.

31. Velazquez EM, Mendoza SG, Hamer T, Sosa F, Glueck CJ. Metformin therapy in polycystic ovary syndrome reduces hyperinsulinemia, insulin resistance, hyperandrogenemia and systolic blood pressure, while facilitating normal menses and pregnancy. *Metabolism* 1994;43:647–54.

32. Velazquez EM, Mendoza SG, Wang P, Glueck CJ. Metformin therapy is associated with a decrease in plasma plasminogen activator inhibitor-1, lipoprotein(a), and immunoreactive insulin levels in patients with the polycystic ovary syndrome. *Metabolism* 1997;44:454–7.

33. Glueck CJ, Phillips H, Cameron D, Sieve-Smith L, Wang P. Continuing metformin throughout pregnancy in women with polycystic ovary syndrome appears to safely reduce first-trimester spontaneous abortion: a pilot study. *Fertil Steril* 2001;75:46–52.

34. Yarali H, Yildirir A, Aybar F, Kabakci G, Bukulmez O, Akgul E, et al. Diastolic dysfunction and increased serum homocysteine concentrations may contribute to increased cardiovascular risk in patients with polycystic ovary syndrome. *Fertil Steril* 2001;76:511–16.

35. Michelmore KF, Balen AH, Dunger DB, Vessey MP. Polycystic ovaries and associated clinical and biochemical features in young women. *Clin Endocrinol (Oxf)* 1999;51:779–86.

36. Norman RJ, Masters L, Milner CR, Wang JX, Davies MJ. Relative risk of conversion from normoglycaemia to impaired glucose tolerance or non-insulin dependent diabetes mellitus in polycystic ovary syndrome. *Hum Reprod* 2001;16:1995–8.

37. Elting MW, Korsen TJ, Shoemaker J. Obesity, rather than menstrual cycle pattern or follicle cohort size, determines hyperinsulinaemia, dyslipidaemia and hypertension in ageing women with polycystic ovary syndrome. *Clin Endocrinol (Oxf)* 2001;55:767–76.

38. Balen AH, Conway GS, Kaltsas G, Techatrasak K, Manning PJ, West C, et al. Polycystic ovary syndrome: the spectrum of the disorder in 1741 patients. *Hum Reprod* 1995;10:2107–11.

39. Dale PO, Tanbo T, Haug E, Abyholm T. The impact of insulin resistance on the outcome of ovulation induction with low-dose follicle stimulating hormone in women with polycystic ovary syndrome. *Hum Reprod* 1998;13:567–70.

40. Kiddy DS, Hamilton-Fairley D, Bush A, Short F, Anyaoku V, Reed MJ, et al. Improvement in endocrine and ovarian function during dietary treatment of obese women with polycystic ovary syndrome. *Clin Endocrinol (Oxf)* 1992;36:105–11.

41. Balen AH, Conway GS, Kaltsas G, Techatraisak K, Manning PJ, West C, et al. Polycystic ovary syndrome: the spectrum of the disorder in 1741 patients. *Human Reprod (Oxf)* 1995;10:2705–12

42. Conway GS. Insulin resistance and the polycystic ovary syndrome. *Contemp Rev Obstet Gynaecol* 1990;2:34–9.

43. Grodstein F, Goldman MB, Cramer DW. Body mass index and ovulatory infertility. *Epidemiology* 1994;5:247–50.

44. Zaazdstra BM, Seidell JC, Van Noord PA, te Velde ER, Habbema JD, Vrieswijk B, et al. Fat and female fecundity: prospective study of effect of body fat distribution on conception rates. *BMJ* 1993;306:484–7.

45. Clark AM, Ledger W, Galletly C, Tomlinson L, Blaney F, Wang X, et al. Weight loss results in

significant improvement in pregnancy and ovulation rates in anovulatory obese women. *Hum Reprod* 1995;10:2705–12.

46. Clark AM, Thornley B, Tomlinson L, Galletley C, Norman RJ. Weight loss in obese infertile women results in improvement in reproductive outcome for all forms of fertility treatment. *Hum Reprod* 1998;13:1502–5.

47. Hamilton-Fairley D, Kiddy D, Watson H, Paterson C, Franks S. Association of moderate obesity with poor pregnancy outcome in women with polycystic ovary syndrome treated with low dose gonadotrophins. *Br J Obstet Gynaecol* 1992;99:128–31.

48. Samaras K, Kelly PJ, Chiano MN, Spector TD, Campbell LV. Genetic and environmental influences on total-body and central abdominal fat: the effect of physical activity in female twins. *Ann Intern Med* 1999;130:873–82.

49. Diamanti-Kandarakis E, Zapanti E. Insulin sensitizers and antiandrogens in the treatment of polycystic ovary syndrome. *Ann NY Acad Sci* 2000;900:203–12.

50. Dunaif A, Scott D, Finegood D, Quintana B, Whitcomb R. The insulin-sensitizing agent troglitazone improves metabolic and reproductive abnormalities in the polycystic ovary syndrome. *J Clin Endocrinol Metab* 1996;81:3299–306.

51. Ehrmann DA, Schneider DJ, Sobel BE, Cavaghan MK, Imperial J, Rosenfield RL, et al. Troglitazone improves defect in insulin action, insulin secretion, ovarian steroidogenesis, and fibrinolysis in women with polycystic ovary syndrome. *J Clin Endocrinol Metab* 1997;82:2108–16.

52. Cataldo NA, Abbasi F, McLaughlin TL, Lamendola C, Reaven GM. Improvement in insulin sensitivity followed by ovulation and pregnancy in a woman with polycystic ovary syndrome who was treated with rosiglitazone. *Fertil Steril* 2001;76:1057–9.

53. Bayley CJ. Metformin and its role in the management of type II diabetes. *Curr Opin Endocrinol Diabetes* 1997;4:40–7.

54. Dunn CJ, Peters DH. Metformin. A review of its pharmacological properties and therapeutic use in non-insulin-dependent diabetes mellitus. *Drugs* 1995;49:721–49.

55. Perriello G. Mechanisms of metformin action in non-insulin dependent diabetes mellitus. *Diabetes Metab Rev* 1996;11 Suppl 1:S51–6.

56. Attia GR, Rainey WE, Carr BR. Metformin directly inhibits androgen production in human thecal cells. *Fertil Steril* 2001;76:517–24.

57. Bailey CJ. Metformin – an update. *Gen Pharmacol* 1993;24:1299–309.

58. Clark AM, Ledger W, Galletly C, Tomlinson L, Blaney F, Wang X, et al. Weight loss results in significant improvement in pregnancy and ovulation rates in anovulatory obese women. *Hum Reprod* 1995;10:2705–12.

59. Pasquali R, Casimirri R, Vicennati V. Weight control and its beneficial effect on fertility in women with obesity and polycystic ovary syndrome. *Hum Reprod* 1997;12 Suppl 1:82–7.

60. Nestler JE, Jakubowicz DJ. Decreases in ovarian cytochrome P450c 17 alpha activity and serum free testosterone after reduction of insulin secretion in polycystic ovary syndrome. *N Engl J Med* 1996;335:617–23.

61. Açbay Ö, Gündogdu S. Can metformin reduce insulin resistance in polycystic ovary syndrome? *Fertil Steril* 1996;65:946–9.

62. Ehrmann DA, Cavaghan MS, Imperial J, Sturis J, Rosenfield R, Polonsky KS. Effects of metformin on insulin secretion, insulin action and ovarian steroidogenesis in women with polycystic ovary syndrome. *J Clin Endocrinol Metab* 1997;82:524–30.

63. Crave JC, Fimbel S, Lejeune H, Cugnardey N, Dechaud H, Pugeat M. Effects of diet and metformin administration on sex hormone-binding globulin, androgens and insulin in hirsute and obese women. *J Clin Endocrinol Metab* 1995;80:2057–62.

64. Kahn SE, Prigeon RL, McCulloch DK, Boyco EJ, Bergman RN, Schwartz MW, et al. Quantification of the relationship between insulin sensitivity and beta-cell function in human subjects. Evidence for a hyperbolic function. *Diabetes* 1993;42:1663–72.

65. Unlühizarci K, Kelestimur F, Bayram F, Sahin Y, Tutus A. The effects of metformin on insulin resistance and ovarian steroidogenesis in women with polycystic ovary syndrome. *Clin Endocrinol (Oxf)* 1999;51:231–6.

66. Sahin Y, Ayata D, Kelestimur F. Lack of relationship between 17-hydroxyprogesterone response to buserelin testing and hyperinsulinemia in polycystic ovary syndrome. *Eur J Endocrinol* 1997;136:410–15.

67. Balen AH. Polycystic ovary syndrome and cancer. *Hum Reprod Update* 2001;7:522–5.

68. Pirwany IR, Yates RW, Cameron IT, Fleming R. Effects of the insulin sensitizing drug metformin on ovarian function, follicular growth and ovulation rate in obese women with oligomenorrhoea. *Hum Reprod* 1999;14:2963–8.

69. Vandermolen DT, Ratts VS, Evans WS, Stovall DW, Kauma SW, Nestler JE, et al. Metformin increases the ovulatory rate and pregnancy rate from clomiphene citrate in patients with polycystic ovary syndrome who are resistant to clomiphene citrate alone. *Fertil Steril* 2001;75:310–15.

70. Ng EH, Wat NM, Ho PC. Effects of metformin on ovulation rate, hormonal and metabolic profiles in women with clomiphene-resistant polycystic ovaries: a randomized, double-blinded placebo-controlled trial. *Hum Reprod* 2001;16:1625–31.

71. Kocak M, Caliskan E, Simsir C, Haberal A. Metformin therapy improves ovulatory rates, cervical scores, and pregnancy rates in clomiphene citrate-resistant women with polycystic ovary syndrome. *Fertil Steril* 2002;77:101–6.

72. Yarali H, Yildiz BO, Demirol A, Zeyneloglu HB, Yigit N, Bukulmez O, et al. Co-administration of metformin during rFSH treatment in patients with clomiphene citrate-resistant polycystic ovary syndrome: a prospective randomized trial. *Hum Reprod* 2002;17:289–94.

73. Fleming R, Hopkinson ZE, Wallace AM, Greer IA, Sattar N. Ovarian function and metabolic factors in women with oligomenorrhoea treated with metformin in a randomized double blind placebo-controlled trial. *J Clin Endocrinol Metab* 2002;87:569–74.

74. Dor J, Shulman A, Levran D, Ben-Rafael Z, Rudak E, Mashiach S. The treatment of patients with polycystic ovarian syndrome by *in-vitro* fertilization and embryo transfer: a comparison of results with those of patients with tubal infertility. *Hum Reprod* 1990;5:816–18.

75. Buylalos RP, Lee C. Polycystic ovary syndrome: pathophysiology and outcome with *in vitro* fertilization. *Fertil Steril* 1996;65:1–10.

76. Kodama H, Fukuda J, Kanube H, Matsui T, Shimizu Y, Tanaka T. High incidence of embryo transfer cancellations in patients with polycystic ovary syndrome. *Hum Reprod* 1995;10:1962–7.

77. Teissier M, Chable H, Paulhac S, Aubard Y. Comparison of follicle steroidogenesis from normal and polycystic ovaries in women undergoing IVF: relationship between steroid concentrations, follicle size, oocyte quality and fecundability. *Hum Reprod* 2000;15:2471–7.

78. Stadtmauer LA, Toma SK, Riehl RM, Talbert LM. Metformin treatment of patients with polycystic ovary syndrome undergoing *in vitro* fertilization improves outcomes and is associated with modulation of the insulin-like growth factors. *Fertil Steril* 2001;75:505–9.

79. Glueck CJ, Phillips H, Cameron D, Tracy T, Sieve-Smith L, Wang P. Continuing metformin through pregnancy in women with polycystic ovary syndrome appears to safely reduce first-trimester spontaneous abortion: a pilot study. *Fertil Steril* 2001;75:46–52.

80. Glueck CJ, Wang P, Kobayashi S, Phillips H, Sieve-Smith L. Metformin therapy throughout

pregnancy reduces the development of gestational diabetes in women with polycystic ovary syndrome. *Fertil Steril* 2002;77:520–5.

81. Heard MJ, Pierce A, Carson SA, Buster JE. Pregnancies following use of metformin for ovulation induction in patients with polycystic ovary syndrome. *Fertil Steril* 2002;77:669–73.

82. Bedaiwy MA, Miller KF, Goldberg JM, Nelson D, Falcone T. Effect of metformin on mouse embryo development. *Fertil Steril* 2001;76:1078–9.

83. Coetzee EJ, Jackson WP. The management of non-insulin-dependent diabetes during pregnancy. *Diabetes Res Clin Pract* 1986;1:281–7.

84. Homburg R. Should patients with polycystic ovary syndrome be treated with metformin? A note of cautious optimism. *Hum Reprod* 2002;17:853–6.

85. Nestler JE, Stovall D, Akhter N, Iuorno MJ, Jakubowicz DJ. Strategies for the use of insulin-sensitizing drugs to treat infertility in women with polycystic ovary syndrome. *Fertil Steril* 2002;77:209–15.

86. Nestler J. Should patients with polycystic ovarian syndrome be treated with metformin? An enthusiastic endorsement. *Hum Reprod* 2002;17:1950–3.

87. Lord JM, Norman R, Flight I. Insulin-sensitising drugs (metformin, troglitazone, rosiglitazone, pioglitazone, D-chiro-inositol) for polycystic ovary syndrome. *Cochrane Database Syst Rev* 2003;(3):CD003053.

88. Knowler WC, Barrett-Connor E, Fowler SE, Hamman RF, Lachin JM, Walker EA, *et al.* Reduction in the incidence of type 2 diabetes with lifestyle intervention or metformin. *N Engl J Med* 2002;346:393–403.

89. Lord JM, Flight IHK, Norman RJ. Metformin in polycystic ovary syndrome: systematic review and meta-analysis. *BMJ* 2003;327:951–5.

4

Conjoined twins

Adrian Bianchi, Michael Maresh and Sylvia Rimmer

INTRODUCTION

The management of a pregnancy with conjoined twins causes enormous difficulties for the parents and the team involved with their care. In addition, the enormous media interest causes stresses on the hospital itself and can affect anyone working within the hospital, from the domestic staff to the chief executive. Ethical and legal issues may arise as in the case of Jodie and Mary in 2000. This article reviews the management of conjoined twins with particular reference to the experience of the Manchester team over the last 14 years.

INCIDENCE AND TYPES OF CONJOINED TWINS

Conjoined twins are said to arise because of an incomplete division of the inner cell mass at 13–16 days of gestation. They are therefore not only monozygotic, and of identical sex and karyotype, they also share the same amniotic space and yolk sac. However it has also been suggested that they arise through fusion of two originally separate monovular embryonic discs.[1]

The number of conjoined twins born in England and Wales reported to the National Congenital Anomaly System is currently about two per annum, giving a reported incidence of about 1 in 300 000 births.[2] Between 1964 and 1978, when ultrasound was not widely used in the antenatal period, the incidence was reported to be 1 in 87 000 births.[3] This is likely to be a more accurate estimate because, with nearly all women having at least one ultrasound scan in pregnancy, almost all cases should be diagnosed antenatally and many women are likely to opt for a termination of pregnancy. This certainly has been our experience in Manchester, with 10/15 of the cases presenting to us resulting in termination.

The present working classification is that of Potter and Craig,[4] which classifies the varieties according to the anatomical site of union (Table 1). It can be seen that by far the most common type is the combined thoraco-omphalopagus twinning at 75%, which also carries the worst

Table 1 *Classification of conjoined twins (Potter and Craig, 1975)*[4]

Type	%	Organs shared
Thoracopagus	74	Bowel, heart, liver
Pyopagus	17	Genitourinary tract, rectum, spine
Ischiopagus	6	Bowel, genitourinary tract, liver (bipus, tripus, tetrapus), pelvis
Craniopagus	2	Brain
Omphalopagus	1	Bile ducts, bowel, liver
Heteropagus	<1	Epigastrium, lower chest

prognosis for survival because of the fused abnormal hearts and the high incidence of associated abnormalities, particularly tracheal and pulmonary, hepatic and intestinal, and possibly chromosomal.

ANTENATAL DIAGNOSIS

Although in the past conjoined twins often were not diagnosed before birth, with the routine use of antenatal diagnostic ultrasound all cases should now be identified. The diagnosis should be considered in any set of monochorionic, monoamniotic twins, particularly when the fetuses bear a constant relationship to each other. Persistent continuity of the skin surfaces at the site of fusion should be visualised to avoid false positive diagnoses. Variable presentation of the twins relative to each other does not exclude the diagnosis and may occur where the junction is a narrow pedicle, which may allow rotation. This can occur in omphalopagus twins with a cephalic–breech presentation and result in a false negative diagnosis. Other diagnostic features include both heads persistently at the same level, constant bi-breech or bi-cephalic presentation, and a single umbilical cord containing more than three vessels.[5,6]

With increasing use of late first trimester ultrasound scanning it should be feasible to diagnose conjoined twins or certainly be highly suspicious at this stage of pregnancy. In our own series the majority of women did not have first trimester scanning, but in the five women who did the diagnosis was made at this stage. In one of our cases from 1989, a single large shared heart with five chambers was clearly visible at 12 weeks. With advances in imaging techniques there have been reports of more detailed assessment of cardiovascular anatomy by using Doppler ultrasound at this stage[7] and of the evaluation of brain sharing (craniopagus) using three-dimensional ultrasound.[8] More detailed assessment using imaging is discussed below.

INITIAL POSTDIAGNOSIS MANAGEMENT AND THE MULTIDISCIPLINARY TEAM

Once the diagnosis has been made the critical next step is to give these women the best possible information about the particular type of condition and the prognosis. This is best given by specialists in a regional or supraregional perinatal centre with experience of managing conjoined twins. The subject of termination of pregnancy needs to be raised, and in some cases with major cardiac involvement, the woman may opt rapidly for a termination after counselling at her first detailed consultation, when it is clear that prognosis and quality of life are so poor. However, the best information can be given only by those with experience in the field once as many details as possible have been obtained through antenatal imaging. Accordingly, if the woman is uncertain about whether to continue with the pregnancy or is sure that she wishes to continue, then members of the multidisciplinary team need to be involved. The question of karyotyping should also be raised. Although there is no increased risk of chromosomal abnormality with conjoined twins, the additional presence of an abnormal karyotype may alter the decision of whether or not the pregnancy should continue.

The initial members of the team who will need to be involved include the obstetrician/fetal specialist, the ultrasonologist, the neonatologist and the specialist neonatal surgeon. Of equal immediate relevance are clinical (often midwives) and lay (including religious) counsellors who, together with the family and trusted close friends, will support the prospective parents. The team will need to expand when it is clear that the pregnancy is continuing and as the nature of the anomalies becomes clearer. Medically, obstetric and neonatal anaesthetists need to be involved. Other specialists such as a cardiologist, a neurosurgeon, an orthopaedic surgeon and a plastic surgeon may well be required. Midwife counsellors have even more of a role as the pregnancy continues, often becoming the trusted confidants of the prospective parents and providing valuable insights to the team. Hospital managers require early notification to assist in ensuring that confidentiality is maintained and to enable them to handle the intense media interest that always occurs if it becomes known that conjoined twins are expected to be or have been born. They also need to agree to accept the woman and that her care is to be provided by the hospital because this will be costly and potentially disruptive to the general running of the hospital. Ethical, moral and legal issues arise, particularly if it is necessary to consider the possible loss of one twin, as occurred in one of our cases in 2000 (Jodie and Mary). The hospital legal team will therefore need to be consulted at an early stage.

PUBLICITY, THE PRESS AND THE MEDIA

The enormous media interest that is generated by the birth of conjoined twins puts even greater pressures on the parents, the hospital and the team. For that reason the hospital must take measures to ensure that information leaks do not occur. Consideration of the use of an alias and reminders to all staff of the problems if the information becomes public knowledge are required. Most parents do not initially favour publicity, and it is particularly important to the development of a trusting relationship that team members respect their decision. They may eventually change their minds, and it is equally relevant that the team, through its leaders, supports and assists the parents with measured but accurate and reliable information. The hospital's public relations officer will act as a 'protective shield' as well as a liaising with the press and other media, maintaining close cooperation with the clinicians while releasing sensitive information only with the express approval of the parents and the hospital's legal advisers. The hospital's public relations officer should also guide the team and the parents in their associations with the press and other media. The team leaders may be asked to speak directly to the press and the public, and should embrace such opportunity for public education.

LEGAL ISSUES

In English law a woman has absolute right over her own body, and her fetuses are not recognised separately. Thus the issue of termination of the pregnancy is determined by the wishes of the woman once she has been fully informed and understands the implications. Once born, the twins immediately acquire legal rights, separate from the mother and from each other. Conflicts of interest may arise (e.g. the loss of one twin in favour of the other, or limb and organ allocation). This may necessitate recourse to the law. In this situation, as occurred in the case of Jodie and Mary in 2000, each twin will require separate representation, which will also be separate from the parents and the carers (i.e. potentially four separate legal teams). Time should be allowed antenatally for in-depth discussion and clarification so that there are few 'surprises' at sensitive times after the birth. Such difficult situations, faced openly together, enhance the relationship between the team and the parents.

POSTDIAGNOSIS ANTENATAL CARE AND COUNSELLING

Termination of pregnancy

Termination of pregnancy does need to be raised sensitively with all women known to be carrying conjoined twins and, as mentioned above, some may come quickly to the decision that this is their preferred option. For those who have difficulty in making a decision, referral is advisable at this stage to a centre where expertise in this field is available. This will allow for further evaluation of the fetal condition and counselling by those with previous experience. If a clear diagnosis has been made by about 12 weeks of pregnancy and the woman has decided on a termination, a standard suction termination of pregnancy by an experienced operator is likely to be the best option. With a singleton pregnancy, once past about 12–13 weeks, few gynaecologists perform suction terminations, preferring medical methods. Medical termination should be with antiprogesterone priming and then prostaglandins. There should be no need to consider hysterotomy. At 22 weeks of pregnancy the total weight of the conjoined twins should not exceed 1 kg and the combined dimensions should be less than a term fetus. We have not experienced difficulties with terminating pregnancies with conjoined twins at this stage. After 22 weeks, feticide would be advised, and the later the pregnancy is terminated the more chance that a caesarean delivery will be required. These two procedures, feticide and caesarean section, may well make a woman decide to continue with the pregnancy.

Detailed antenatal imaging

Conventional detailed ultrasound assessment at about 20 weeks of gestation should demonstrate the extent of cranial, skeletal and soft tissue fusion. Anomalies will not necessarily be restricted to the region of the join (e.g. ischiopagus twins) and, as always, a thorough visualisation of all areas is required. With thoracopagus twins, detailed fetal cardiac assessment is necessary. Separate hearts will beat asynchronously. Their anatomy is best demonstrated by using two-dimensional colour and spectral Doppler ultrasound (Figure 1). Pericardial sharing occurs in about 20% of cases, but this cannot be demonstrated on ultrasound either ante- or postnatally, nor may it be seen on postnatal magnetic resonance imaging (MRI).

With the advent of ultrafast imaging sequences, fetal MRI has become a useful additional technique for demonstrating the anatomy in conjoined twins. We have used it in 2000 with a case of ischiopagus twins particularly with regard to confirming abnormal intracranial anatomy and others reported its use with thoracopagus twins in 2001.[9]

For cases of thoracopagus and omphalopagus twinning, a full assessment of the gastrointestinal tracts, the hepatobiliary systems and the hepatic venous drainage is not achievable antenatally (Figure 2). Similarly, with cases of pyopagus and ischiopagus twins, precise details of the lowest parts of the genitourinary and gastrointestinal tracts (e.g. urethra, vagina, rectum) may need to await postdelivery examination (see below).

Sequential ultrasound scans should be made at appropriate intervals (usually at least every 3–4 weeks) to assess fetal growth and ensure no significant change in fetal organ function, such as the heart. Polyhydramnios may well develop, particularly with thoracopagus twins, so that assessment of fetal growth is totally dependent on ultrasound measurements.

General antenatal care

Once it is clear that the woman is continuing with the pregnancy, care should be totally transferred to a team at a specialist perinatal centre. Being such a rare condition it is best that only a few teams in a country take such referrals. Routine antenatal care should not be forgotten and, as with any twin pregnancy, almost every antenatal complication is more common when compared with a singleton pregnancy. The risk of preterm labour is clearly high, particularly in the presence of polyhydramnios. Elective early admission to hospital is often used, particularly as it is likely that the woman will not live near to the perinatal centre. It also protects the woman from well meaning questions about her pregnancy. Hospitalisation makes it easier to detect any signs of preterm

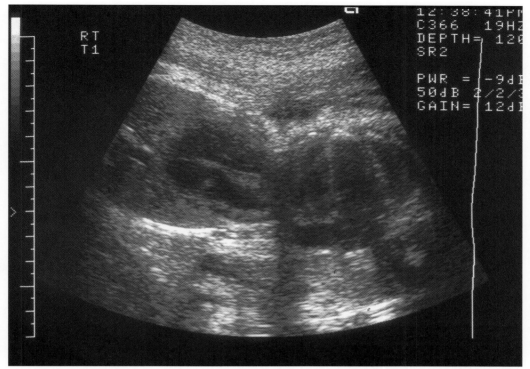

Figure 1 *Antenatal ultrasound scan of the thorax of thoracopagus conjoined twins who had separate hearts but were subsequently found to have a shared pericardium*

labour. It also facilitates the development of a trusting relationship with the prospective parents and in particular with the ward midwifery team who will also care for their emotional and psychological needs.

Looking after such pregnancies may also be stressful for members of the team. Regular briefings allow participants to express views and to work through emotional issues towards one common team approach. All carers should be allowed freely to volunteer to serve or to opt out without prejudice. The development of a trusting relationship between team members and between the team and the parents is fundamental to a successful outcome. Team leaders are required and their roles will evolve, as determined by the stage of the pregnancy and the nature of the anomalies. Such leaders have a major and onerous coordinating role, taking cognisance of the opinions of diverse colleagues and carers, and progressing them, with the approval of all, into an overall action plan. This will involve the organisation of frequent team briefings and discussion sessions, liaison with the parents, dissemination of information, and the coordination of compromise among specialists. Even after delivery and after separation, a team spokesperson and the hospital public relations officer will continue to be required for comment for months or even years.

PLACE, TIMING AND MODE OF DELIVERY

There can be little argument that delivery should take place adjacent to an area where two teams

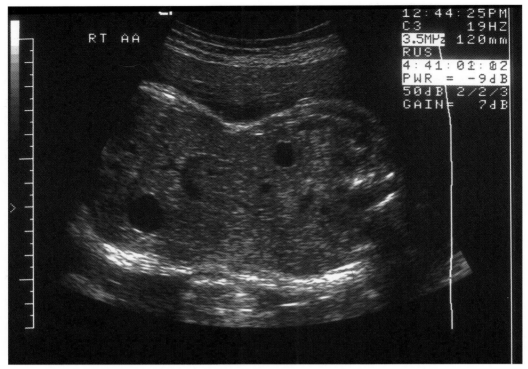

Figure 2 *Transverse antenatal ultrasound scan of thoracopagus conjoined twins showing a shared liver, with portal veins and both stomachs demonstrated*

(one for each child) of neonatal anaesthetists, surgeons and physicians can work together to attempt to resuscitate and stabilise the babies. Such resources should be available in a specialist perinatal centre, to which the woman should be transferred, ideally well in advance of delivery.

Timing of delivery has to be individualised. In thoracopagus cases associated with poly-hydramnios, the decision is often taken out of our hands by the onset of preterm labour. With ultrasound monitoring of fetal growth we have not found it necessary to intervene early and have not electively delivered any thoraco-omphalopagus or ischiopagus twins before 36 weeks.

With regard to the mode of delivery, the vaginal route is probably best avoided apart from in preterm ischiopagus twins, where it certainly could be contemplated. Caesarean section is normally required and with term thoracopagus and omphalopagus twins the classical incision is usually required. With ischiopagus twins successful delivery can be accomplished through a transverse incision in a well developed lower uterine segment. The decision about the method of anaesthesia used should, as always, result from discussions between the woman and the anaesthetist, taking into account maternal safety and wishes.

Prior to delivery the prospective parents need to be reminded that some types of respiratory tract and cardiac anomalies are associated with rapid death after birth, and they should determine before-hand the nature of any religious provision that they wish to be immediately available to the children.

NEONATAL ASSESSMENT

After stabilisation, both children need to be transferred to the appropriate neonatal facility (medical or surgical) for continuing monitoring and assessment. The parents should be closely involved and given access to their children as soon as possible and at any time. This is often a shocking and bewildering time for the parents, who will require space, encouragement and support to come to terms with the state of their children. No amount of antenatal preparation and counselling can ever adequately prepare them for the eventual postnatal reality.

Early ultrasound scanning will provide confirmation and updated information, particularly relating to vital structures such as brain, heart, liver and kidneys. Basic radiology can initially confirm antenatal imaging (Figure 3). Contrast radiology such as micturating cystograms, intravenous urograms and gastrointestinal contrast studies may all be necessary to evaluate abdominal and pelvic anatomy and the extent of organ sharing (Figure 4). This is followed by detailed computed tomographic, three-dimensional computed tomographic and MRI scanning as dictated by the nature of the anomalies. Angiography may be relevant to assessment of the blood supply, particularly the venous drainage, of the conjoined livers. Expert cardiac specialist services will be required for a full assessment, particularly for fused abnormal hearts. Genetic and chromosomal review may be relevant, together with further orthopaedic and neurological investigations.

The team leaders are responsible for coordinating all investigations and collating information for discussion at team briefings and with the parents. At this time the neonatal nursing staff have an increasing role, taking over from the midwives in supporting the parents and assisting the team in planning.

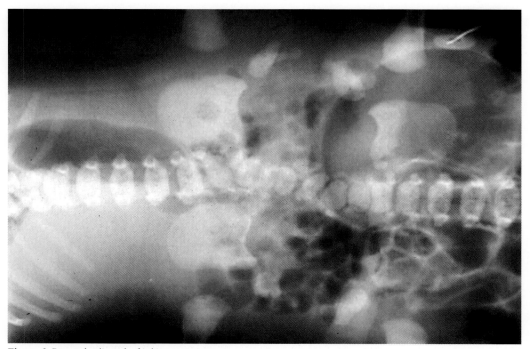

Figure 3 *Postnatal radiograph of ischiopagus twins*

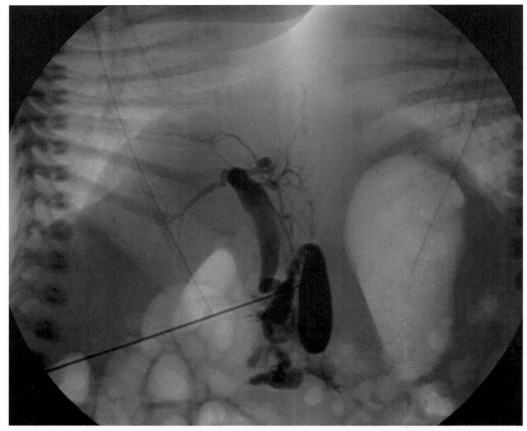

Figure 4 *Postnatal fine needle percutaneous transhepatic cholangiogram of thoracopagus twins demonstrating puncture of one of the four gall bladders and showing partially obstructed bile ducts; also showing gas in the stomach and small bowel of the twins*

PLANNING AND SEPARATION

The issue of separation of the twins will already have been discussed in depth antenatally, but will now need careful re-evaluation in the light of the postnatal knowledge and the condition of the twins. The risk to both or either of the twins may be considerable, and neither may survive. Equally, it may again become necessary to reconsider the issue of the loss of one twin in favour of the other. Ethical and legal considerations may need to be rehearsed and recourse to the courts may become necessary for direction and for consent for separation. It is always preferable to proceed at all times with the full approval and consent of the parents, for whom such circumstances are particularly stressful.

Emergency crash separation because of the death or impending loss of one twin or some major life threatening condition (e.g. necrotising enterocolitis, heart failure) carries a high mortality rate,[10] which even for ischiopagus twinning is quoted at 64%.[11] In contrast, planned elective separation has a much lower mortality rate; for ischiopagus twins this is 5%.[11] It is therefore far better, and indeed more logical, to allow a period of stabilisation and growth, during which time a better understanding of the children and their anomalies is obtained. In the meantime operative interventions other than separation may be relevant (e.g. relief of bowel or urinary obstruction). The timing and nature of elective separation will be determined largely by the stability of the vital organs and the eventual potential psychological impact of excessive delay on the children. Consideration may need to be given to a serialised approach rather than a single operative intervention. Given a stable situation and growing twins, then separation should be considered at some time during the first year of life, preferably after the early risks of life threatening conditions such as brain haemorrhage and necrotising enterocolitis have receded. An accurate understanding of existent anatomy should have been obtained such that there are few surprises at surgery. Issues such as limb (ischiopagus tripus or bipus) and perineal structure (genitalia, anal sphincter) allocation, organ donation (heart, bladder, gonads) and the need for tissue expansion to allow wound closure should already have been resolved (Figure 5).

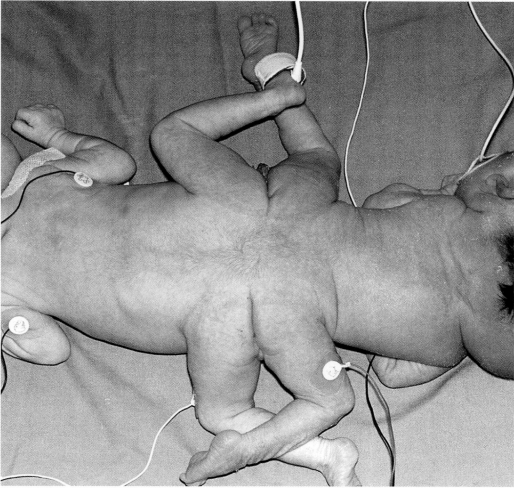

Figure 5 *Ischiopagus conjoined twins postdelivery*

Surgical and anaesthetic planning involves the provision of a full surgical, nursing and anaesthetic team for each twin. A second fully equipped operating room must be available once the separation has occurred. Each surgical and anaesthetic team must have a clear understanding of their area of responsibility and must accept the considered decisions of the team leaders, whose judgements at the time of surgery have to be final. Of particular relevance and requiring coordination is the nature of the anaesthesia for each twin. This cannot be discussed in detail in a brief review. The operative intervention, if single, will be long and arduous and as such is best phased with rest periods for the children and the surgical teams. Each twin is separately monitored and prepared as for any major surgical intervention. The neonatal surgical unit should be prepared to receive both twins postoperatively. Even in the event of the sacrifice and the expected death of one twin, it is essential to endeavour to offer the maximum opportunity for survival to both twins at all times and until death has occurred. In the event of agreed sacrifice, then the wishes of the parents with regard to the deceased child must be followed in full. For the survivors, postoperative care is routine as for any major operative intervention. Clearly, issues of hospital security will continue to occupy the hospital security officers throughout the period and well into the postoperative time, when public interest is often maximal.

THE LONG-TERM PROGNOSIS

The long-term prognosis for survival will depend on the severity of the associated anomalies and the impact on organ function, particularly after birth. The twins' quality of life will be affected also by the nature of the union. Similar considerations will apply if separation of the twins is to be considered. It is well accepted that the survival of conjoined twins rarely depends on the actual operation for separation, but rather on the 'nature of the anatomy'. Most of the anomalies are potentially correctable and the surgical reconstructive procedures are the standard ones for the various anomalies encountered, but modified to fit the particular individual circumstances. Most authorities would therefore recommend separation, particularly if the expected quality of life is good. This recommendation remains valid even if only one twin is expected to survive, rather than allowing the inevitable death of both babies.

Clearly, the outcome for each variety of conjoined twinning will depend on the nature of the conjoin and the impact on vital organs after separation. Thoracopagus twins with an abnormal fused heart do particularly badly (Figure 1), whereas lesser unions (e.g. omphalopagus, pyopagus) and those not involving vital organs (e.g. ischiopagus; 5% mortality at elective separation[11]) will fare rather better. Such figures do not take account of the quality of life, both physical and psychological, in the longer term.

The long-term outlook will again be determined by the nature of the congenital anomalies and the operative intervention. Further surgical adjustments may be necessary to ensure the best achievable quality of life. Thus it is possible for conjoined twins to have relatively normal, good quality lives after separation. However, consideration of 'quality of life' must be placed also against the expected quality and expectancy of a conjoined life, particularly should early death not occur. Equally, the issue of quality must be considered against a separate life of reduced potential, as for example with a reduced number of limbs, the absence of a bladder, no anal sphincters or absent genital structures or gonads.

CONCLUSION

The management of conjoined twins is a major undertaking involving a large number of highly specialised departments and taking up expensive and precious hospital resources. It demands a healthy understanding and interaction among medical, nursing and management colleagues, with expert 'public relations' and full legal and social backup. The level of expertise among obstetric, fetal, surgical, anaesthetic and nursing colleagues must be considerable, and borne out of constant interaction and involvement with the management of similar anomalies in singleton pregnancies. Such expertise will be concentrated in major tertiary centres combining highly specialised services. It is therefore appropriate and preferable for conjoined twins to be managed only at selected designated centres with the appropriate skill base. However, in any one country it is preferable for there to be an alternative centre offering a choice of management team and venue to the parents. Furthermore, this provides opportunity for professional discussion, sharing and healthy competition towards the better care of the mother with a complex pregnancy and the best possible outcome for her conjoined twins.

References

1. Spencer R. Theoretical and analytical embryology of conjoined twins: part I: embryogenesis. *Clin Anat* 2000;13:36–53.
2. Physick N, The National Congenital Anomaly System, Office of National Statistics, London: personal communication, 2001.
3. Lawson GW. Conjoined twins. *J Obstet Gynaecol* 1982;2:165–8.
4. Potter EL, Craig JM. *Pathology of the Fetus and Infant.* 3rd ed. Chicago, IL: Year Book; 1975.
5. Gore RM, Filly RA, Parer JT. Sonographic antepartum diagnosis of conjoined twins. Its impact on obstetric management. *JAMA* 1982;247:3351–3.
6. Maggio M, Callan NA, Hamod KA, Sanders RC. The first-trimester ultrasonographic diagnosis of conjoined twins. *Am J Obstet Gynecol* 1985;152:833–5.
7. Ohkuchi A, Minakami H, Sato I, Nakano T, Tateno M. First-trimester ultrasonographic investigation of cardiovascular anatomy in thoracoabdominally conjoined twins. *J Perinat Med* 2001;29:77–80.
8. Bega G, Wapner R, Lev-Toaff A, Kuhlman K. Diagnosis of conjoined twins at 10 weeks using three-dimensional ultrasound: a case report. *Ultrasound Obstet Gynecol* 2000;16:388–90.
9. Spielmann AL, Freed KS, Spritzer CE. MRI of conjoined twins illustrating advances in fetal imaging. *J Comput Assist Tomogr* 2001;25:88–90.
10. O'Neill JA. Conjoined twins. In: O'Neill JA, editor. *Pediatric Surgery,* Vol. 2. St Louis, MO: Mosby-Year Book; 1998. p. 1925–38.
11. Hoyle RM, Thomas CG Jr. Twenty-three-year follow-up of separated ischiopagus tetrapus conjoined twins. *Ann Surg* 1989;210:673–9.

5

McIndoe vaginoplasty: timeless and effective

Lesley L Breech and John A Rock

INTRODUCTION

Congenital vaginal agenesis is a relatively uncommon condition. The reported incidence is 1 in 4000 to 10 000 female births.[1] The Mayer–Rokitansky–Kuster–Hauser (Rokitansky) syndrome involves vaginal agenesis with a normal vulva, normal secondary sexual development, müllerian dysplasia (with uterine aplasia or hypoplasia and hypoplastic fallopian tubes), normal ovaries, and a normal karyotype.[2-5] The general gynaecologist is likely to encounter this condition sometime in his or her professional career; familiarity with its current management is therefore important. The descriptions of attempts to correct vaginal agenesis date to Hippocrates.[6] Ideally, the optimal procedure to create a neovagina would be at low risk to the woman and would form a vaginal canal of adequate size and function to allow intercourse to occur. The McIndoe vaginoplasty is the most commonly used vaginoplasty procedure throughout the world. No associated deaths have been reported, functional success rates are excellent, and complication rates are minimal. Currently, there is no consensus regarding the best surgical option. All would agree, however, the best initial management should be an attempt at passive dilatation.

NONSURGICAL APPROACH

In 1938, Frank[7] described a method of creating an artificial vagina without surgery. In 1940, he reported excellent results in eight women treated by this method.[8] His follow-up study demonstrated that a vagina formed in this manner remained permanent in depth and calibre, even in women who neglected dilatation for more than a year. Rock and associates at the Johns Hopkins Hospital[9] reported that an initial trial of vaginal dilatation was successful in 9 of 21 women. Ingram[10] also described a passive dilatation technique for creating a neovagina. This avoided some of the challenges of Frank's method, including the necessary awkward position for proper dilatation. Ingram was able to produce satisfactory vaginal depth and coital function in 10 of 12 women with vaginal agenesis and 32 of 40 with various types of stenosis. The major advantage of this technique is that the woman is not required physically to press the dilator against the vaginal pouch. Careful instruction on the proper use of the dilators is essential. A dilator is put in place and tight underclothes worn while the woman sits on a racing-type bicycle seat that is placed on a stool 24 inches above the floor, which allows the flexibility to do other things during dilatation. The woman is instructed to sit leaning forward with the dilator in place for at least two hours per day at intervals of 15–30 minutes. Roberts *et al.*[11] reported the largest series of women with vaginal agenesis who used the Ingram method of dilatation to create a neovagina. The records of 51 women with müllerian agenesis were reviewed; 37 attempted vaginal dilatation and 14 young women underwent a surgical intervention. Functional success was defined as satisfactorily achieving intercourse or accepting the largest dilator without discomfort during the clinic visit. All women were followed up for at least two years and for an average of 9.25 years. Functional success was achieved in 91.9% of those that attempted dilatation (Table 1), supporting the benefit of an attempt at dilatation before surgery.

Women with a flat perineum with no dimple or pouch may have no alternative other than the surgical creation of a neovagina for comfortable sexual relations. For women who are unable or unwilling to obtain a neovagina using dilatation methods, the McIndoe vaginoplasty is our recommended procedure of choice. It is a safe, simple surgical technique that avoids the disadvantages of laparotomy. When performed by a competent specialist, the morbidity is minimal and the functional success rate outstanding.

SURGICAL APPROACH

Surgical reconstruction should be deferred until the woman is psychologically ready. Social and sexual maturity are important components to the success of any vaginoplasty procedure. Often women undergo surgery in the early teenage years, when they are not motivated for the crucial postoperative care of the neovagina. The postoperative therapy may be quite intensive and they must be willing and able to comply or risk failure of the vaginoplasty. In our practice, we recommend deferring the procedure until late adolescence or early adulthood. Patients should be assisted by a professional team; psychological support should be available both pre-operatively and postoperatively to deal with the emotional and physical reality of a neovagina. In their review of long-term results after operative correction of vaginal aplasia, Mobus et al.[12] also recognised the importance of delaying surgical intervention and providing comprehensive support for these women throughout the process.

Historical background

The currently most popular operation for creating a neovagina, the McIndoe vaginoplasty, began with simple attempts to create a space between the rectum and the bladder.[13] With the early attempts, the space would constrict because the surgeon would fail to recognise the importance of continued dilatation until the constrictive phase of healing was complete. At the Johns Hopkins Hospital in 1938, Wharton[14-16] combined adequate dissection of the vaginal space with continuous dilatation with a balsa-wood form that was covered with a thin rubber sheath. The balsa form was left in place; however, a skin graft was not used. He based his procedure on the principle that the vaginal epithelium would proliferate into the space, and would, therefore, within a relatively short time, cover the raw surfaces. This may be satisfactory as long as the space is kept dilated long enough to allow the epithelium to grow in. Even after several years, however, the vault of the

Table 1 *Dilatation success and failure rates (adapted from Roberts CP, Haber MJ, Rock JA. Vaginal creation for müllerian agenesis. Am J Obstet Gynecol 2001;185:1349–52,[11] with permission from Elsevier Science)*

Group	No. ($n = 37$)	%
Successful dilatation	34	91.9
Failed dilatation	3	8.1

vagina occasionally remains without epithelial covering. Coital bleeding and leucorrhoea result from persistent granulation tissue, and the neovagina may be constricted by scarring in the upper portion. In Counsellor's 1948 report from the Mayo Clinic,[17] 100 operations to construct a neovagina were reported; 14 were performed by Wharton's method, all with excellent results. The authors stated that the disadvantages of persistent granulation tissue with bleeding and leucorrhoea were of no consequence. This has not been the experience of the authors of this chapter.

The Abbe–Wharton–McIndoe operation

When inlay skin grafts were first used to construct a neovagina, the results were poor because the necessity for continuing dilatation of the new vagina was again not recognised. Severe contraction, uncontrolled by continuous or intermittent dilatation, almost invariably spoiled the results. Although Abbe[13] and others preceded him by many years in using a skin-covered prosthesis in neovaginal construction, it was Sir Archibald McIndoe,[18,19] at the Queen Victoria Hospital (England), who popularised the method and gave it a substantial clinical trial. He emphasised the three important principles used today in successful operations for vaginal agenesis:

- dissection of an adequate space between the rectum and the bladder
- inlay split-thickness skin grafting
- the cardinal principle of continuous and prolonged dilatation during the contractile phase of healing.

Other tissues such as amnion and peritoneum have been used to line the new vaginal space, but they have not had substantial success. However, Tancer et al.[20] reported good results with human amnion. Karjalainen et al.[21] noted that a more physiological result was achieved with an amnion graft than with a skin graft. Nevertheless, concerns about the transmission of HIV with human amnion now limit this option.

Several series have reported satisfactory short-term results using regenerated oxidised cellulose (Interceed, Absorbable Adhesion Barrier, Ethicon, Inc., Somerville, NJ) as the vaginal lining.[22] More experience with this technique will be important to assess success.

TECHNIQUE OF ABBE–WHARTON–MCINDOE

Operation

Taking the graft

After a careful pelvic examination under anaesthesia to verify previous findings, the woman is positioned for the taking of a skin graft from the buttocks. For cosmetic reasons, the graft should not be taken from the thigh or hip unless for some reason it cannot be obtained from the buttocks. The woman may be asked to sunbathe in a brief bathing suit before coming to the hospital so that its outline can be seen. An attempt should be made to take the graft from both buttocks within these borders. The quality of the graft determines to a great extent the success of the operation. We have found the Padgett electrodermatome to be the most satisfactory instrument for taking the graft. With relatively little experience and practice, a gynaecological surgeon can successfully cut a graft of controlled width and thickness. The instrument is set and checked for taking a graft approximately 0.45 mm thick and 9 cm wide. The total graft length should be 16–20 cm. If the entire graft cannot be taken from one buttock, then a graft 8–10 cm long will be needed from each side.

The skin of the donor site is prepared with an antiseptic solution, chlorhexidine (in lieu of povidone-iodine solution, to minimise irritation), which is then thoroughly washed away. The skin is then lubricated with mineral oil as assistants steady and stretch the skin tight. Considerable pressure should be applied uniformly across the dermatome blade. The thickness of the graft must have minimal variation. A graft that is a little too thick is better than one that is a little too thin. There should be no breaks in the continuity of the graft. The graft is placed between two layers of moist gauze and the donor sites are dressed. The donor site is soaked with a dilute solution of adrenaline for haemostasis and a sterile dressing is applied. A pressure dressing is then placed over the site and can be removed on the seventh postoperative day. The sterile dressing will dry in place over the donor site and ultimately will fall off by itself. Moistened areas on the dressing can be dried with cool air. If there is separation and evidence of some superficial infection, then mebromin can be applied to these areas.

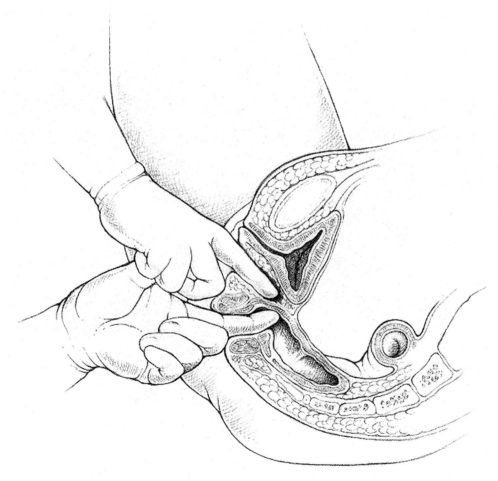

Figure 1 *The neovaginal space is developed between the bladder and the rectum, using both sharp and blunt dissection; the dissection is extended laterally first, then towards the midline; a finger in the rectum during dissection is helpful to protect the rectum from injury (reproduced from: Rock JA, Morley GW. Construction of a neovagina with a split thickness graft. In:* Obstetrics and Gynecology Illustrated. *New York: LTI Medica; 1987, with permission from Learning Technology Inc.)*

Creating the neovaginal space

The woman is placed in the lithotomy position and a transverse incision is made through the mucosa of the vaginal vestibule. The space between the urethra and bladder anteriorly and the rectum posteriorly is dissected until the under surface of the peritoneum is reached (Figure 1). This step may be safer with a catheter in the urethra and sometimes a finger in the rectum to guide the dissection in the proper plane. After incising the mucosa of the vaginal vestibule transversely, the surgeon is often able to create a channel on each side of a median raphe, starting with blunt dissection and then dilating each channel with Hegar dilators or with finger dissection. In some instances it may be necessary to develop the neovaginal space by dissecting laterally and bringing the fingers towards the midline. The median raphe is then divided, thus joining the two channels. This manoeuvre is helpful in dissecting an adequate space without causing injury to surrounding structures.

To avoid subsequent narrowing of the vagina at the level of the urogenital diaphragm, it may be helpful to incise the puborectalis muscles bilaterally along the mid-portion of the medial margins. Although useful in all circumstances, incision of the puborectalis muscles is more important in women with androgen insensitivity syndrome with an android pelvis, in which the levator muscles are more taut against the pelvic diaphragm, than in those with a gynaecoid pelvis. Incision of the puborectalis muscles causes no difficulty with faecal continence, significantly improves the ease with which the vaginal form can be inserted into the canal in the postoperative period, and has eliminated the problem of contracture of the upper vagina caused by a poorly applied form. The dissection should be carried as high as possible without entering the peritoneal cavity and without cleaning away all tissue beneath the peritoneum. A split-thickness skin graft will not take well when applied against a base of thin peritoneum. All bleeding points should be ligated by clamping and tying them with fine sutures. It is essential that the vaginal cavity be dry to prevent bleeding beneath the graft. Bleeding will cause the graft to separate from its bed, resulting in its inevitable failure to implant in that area and in local graft necrosis.

Preparing the vaginal form

Early skin grafts were formed over balsa, which has the advantages of being an inexpensive, easily available, lightweight wood that can be sterilised without difficulty. It also can be whittled easily in the operating room to a proper shape to fit the new vaginal space. However, uneven pressure from the form can cause a skin graft to slough in places, and pressure spots are also associated with an increased risk of fistula formation. The Counseller–Flor modification of the McIndoe technique uses, instead of the rigid balsa form, a foam rubber mould shaped to the vaginal cavity from a foam rubber block and covered with a condom.[23] The foam rubber is gas sterilised in blocks measuring approximately $10 \times 10 \times 20$ cm. The block is shaped with scissors to approximately twice the desired size, compressed into a condom, and placed into the neovaginal space. The form is left in place for 20–30 seconds with the condom open to allow the foam rubber to expand and conform to the neovaginal space. The condom is then closed and the form is withdrawn. The external end is tied with no. 2-0 silk, and an additional condom is placed over the form and tied securely.

Sewing the graft over the vaginal form

The skin graft is then placed over the form and its under surface exteriorised and sewn over the form with interrupted vertical mattress no. 5-0 nonreactive sutures (Figure 2). Where the graft is approximated, the under surfaces of the sutured edges are also exteriorised. The graft should not be 'meshed' to make it stretch further, and the edges of the graft should be approximated meticulously around the form, without gaps. Granulation tissue develops at any site where the form is not covered with skin. Contraction usually occurs where granulation tissue forms. After the form has been placed in the neovaginal space, the edges of the graft are sutured to the skin edge with no. 5-0 nonreactive absorbable sutures, with sufficient space left between sutures for drainage to occur. The surgeon must be careful not to have the form so large that it causes undue pressure on the urethra or rectum. A balsa form should have a groove to accommodate the urethra. With a foam rubber form, this is unnecessary. A suprapubic silicone catheter is placed in the bladder for drainage. The form can be held in place by suturing the labia together with two or three nonreactive sutures.

Replacing with a new form

After 7–10 days, the form is removed and the vaginal cavity is irrigated with warm saline solution and inspected. This is usually performed with mild sedation and without an anaesthetic. The cavity

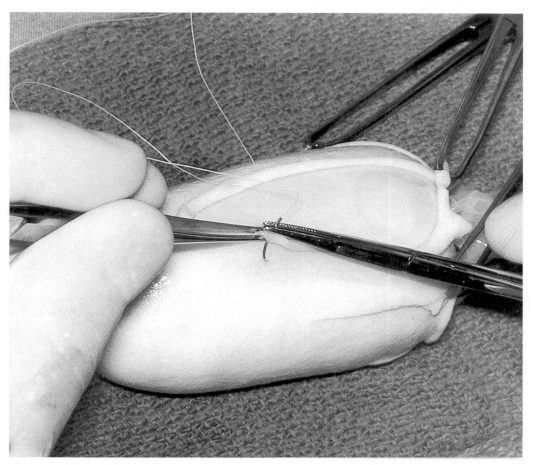

Figure 2 *The skin graft is sewn over the condom-covered form with the dermis side exteriorised (reproduced from: Rock JA, Morley GW. Construction of a neovagina with a split thickness graft. In:* Obstetrics and Gynecology Illustrated. *New York: LTI Medica; 1987, with permission from Learning Technology Inc.)*

should be inspected carefully to determine if the graft has taken satisfactorily in all areas of the new vagina. Any undue pressure by the form should be noted and corrected. It is especially important that there is not too much pressure superiorly against the peritoneum of the cul-de-sac. Such a constant upward pressure could result in weakness with subsequent enterocoele formation. The new vaginal cavity must be inspected frequently to detect and to prevent pressure necrosis of the skin graft.

The woman is given instructions on daily removal and reinsertion of the form and is taught how to administer a low-pressure douche of clear warm water. She is advised to remove the form at the time of urination and defaecation, but otherwise to wear it continuously for 6 weeks. A neoprene form, which is much easier to remove and keep clean than foam rubber, is substituted for the original after 6 weeks. The woman is instructed to use the form during the night for the next 12 months. If there has been no change in the calibre of the vagina by that time, then it is unlikely to occur later, and insertion of the form at night can be carried out intermittently until coitus is a frequent occurrence. However, if there is the slightest difficulty in inserting the form, then the woman should be advised to use it continuously again. Most women are able to maintain the form in place simply by wearing tight fitting underclothes and a perineal pad. Douches are advisable while there is residual vaginal healing and discharge.

RESULTS AND COMPLICATIONS

Several authors of large studies using split-thickness skin grafts to cover the mould have published good functional results. Rates of perioperative and postoperative morbidity have also been excellent. The most common complication is failure of the graft to take, ranging from small areas of granulation tissue to complete failure. Re-operation is reported to vary from less than 1%[24] to 65%.[25] The fistula rate ranges from 1% to 4%.

Results with the McIndoe operation have improved over time and reported levels of satisfactory results have ranged from 80% to 100%. The serious complications formerly associated with the McIndoe operation have been significantly reduced by improvements in technique and greater experience. Serious complications do still occur, however, including postoperative fistulas (urethrovaginal, vesicovaginal and rectovaginal), postoperative infection, and intraoperative and postoperative haemorrhage. Failure of graft take is also still reported as an occasional complication. This failure will often lead to the development of granulation tissue, which may require re-operation, curettage of the granulation tissue down to a healthy base, or even regrafting. Minor degrees of granulation can be treated by the application of silver nitrate. The functional result is more important than the anatomical result in evaluating the success of this operation.

The postoperative results have improved significantly since the foam rubber form replaced the balsa vaginal form. Between 1950 and 2000 the McIndoe operation was performed on 94 women at the Johns Hopkins Hospital and on an additional 50 at Emory University Hospital. During these 50 years, 96% of the 144 women had at least an 80% take of the graft; in only six was there a significant area over which the graft failed.[26]

Urethrovaginal fistula has become even more infrequent since the introduction of the suprapubic catheter and the foam rubber form. The catheter is removed when the woman is voiding well and has no residual urine. In general, she will be able to void without difficulty within the first few days of the procedure. Prophylactic broad spectrum antibiotics started within 12 hours of surgery and continued for seven days are valuable in reducing the incidence of graft failure from infection at the operative site.

It is important that a McIndoe operation be performed correctly the first time. If the vagina becomes constricted because of granulation tissue formation, injury to adjacent structures, or failure to use the form properly, then subsequent attempts to create a satisfactory vagina will be more difficult. Appropriate dissection of the rectovaginal space and the ability to achieve adequate haemostasis may be impaired. The first operation has the best chance of success.

Ozek et al.,[27] like many other surgeons, modified the McIndoe procedure by describing an X-type perineal incision and the use of a perforated vaginal mould during the postoperative period. They postulated that this incision minimised stricture at the vaginal introitus and provided greater ease of dissection of the vaginal cavity. They emphasised that the overall procedure is simple with a generally uneventful postoperative course. Complications included infection, failure of skin graft take, stress urinary incontinence, partial graft loss and vaginal stricture. All women were treated satisfactorily except one with stress urinary incontinence.

Despite minor modifications of the McIndoe vaginoplasty, the essential components of dissection of an adequate space, split-thickness skin grafting, and continuous dilatation during the contractile phase of healing, remain unchanged. Templeman et al.'s review[28] continues to support the safety and efficacy of the procedure. Hojsgaard and Villadsen[25] reported 26 women who underwent vaginoplasty, 18 of whom had Rokitansky syndrome. All were recorded as having a satisfactory result with complete graft take, adequate vaginal dimensions, and no strictures or fistulas giving symptoms. Complete take was achieved in 33% within a week postoperatively; after one further grafting procedure, an additional 38% had complete take. The intraoperative and early postoperative complications were one perforation of the rectum (3.8%) and three occurrences of postoperative bleeding (11.5%). The late complications were vaginal stricture in three women (11.5%), urethrovaginal fistula in two (7.7%), and rectovaginal fistula in one (3.8%). Allessandrescu et al.[24] described the surgical management of 201 women with Rokitansky syndrome. The surgeon substituted a modified transverse perineal incision and a perforated, rigid plastic mould. Intraoperative and postoperative complications consisted of two rectal perforations (1%), eight graft infections (4%), and 11 infections of graft site origin (5.5%). Sexual satisfaction was investigated with both objective and subjective criteria. Among the 201 women, 83.6% had anatomical results evaluated as 'good', 10% as 'satisfactory', and 6.5% as 'unsatisfactory'. More than 71% of these women rated their sexual life as 'good' or 'satisfactory' and reported that they had been able to experience orgasms related to vaginal intercourse. Twenty-three percent reported the ability to have sexual intercourse but could not achieve orgasm and only 5% expressed dissatisfaction with their sexual performance.

Buss and Lee[29] added a review to the previously reported Mayo experience with the McIndoe vaginoplasty.[23,30,31] They reviewed the outcomes of 50 additional women with vaginal agenesis. Forty-seven were located and responded to a questionnaire. The mean duration of follow-up was 6.5 years. Reported complications included two rectovaginal fistulas and one graft failure. Five women required additional reconstructive procedures. Operative vaginoplasty was considered to be functionally successful by 40 of the 47 (85%). Ninety percent of the women who were able to have sexual intercourse rated vaginal function and sexual response as 'satisfactory' or 'good'.

Strickland et al.[32] reported on the coital satisfaction, perception of vaginal competence, and impact on lifestyle of adult females undergoing vaginoplasty as adolescents. Ten of 22 women underwent McIndoe vaginoplasty. All of the women had sexual experience and 80% were sexually active at the time of evaluation. The most frequent difficulty reported was vaginal dryness and lack of lubrication with sexual intercourse. Ninety percent of the women expressed satisfaction that sexual ability was acceptable. This experience also supports the role of the McIndoe vaginoplasty in providing young women with vaginal agenesis with long-term coital ability and minimal disability.

Development of malignancy

Malignant transformation of the neovaginal epithelium has been reported with all types of vaginoplasty, including split-thickness skin grafting. At least ten case reports exist of malignant disease developing in a neovagina. In these women, the type of carcinoma may be related to the type of tissue used for the reconstruction. Hiroi et al.[33] reported seven women with a skin graft neovagina who developed squamous cell carcinoma, while three who had undergone an intestinal transplant developed adenocarcinoma. These findings suggest that epithelium transplanted to the vagina can assume the oncogenic potential of the lower reproductive tract. It is therefore important that women undergo long-term follow-up examinations after split-thickness skin graft vaginoplasty.

ALTERNATIVE PROCEDURES

Alternative surgical procedures include: the use of materials other than split-thickness skin grafts to cover the mould placed into the rectovaginal space, colonic interposition, vulvovaginoplasty using the labia minora, and laparoscopic modifications of previously reported techniques.

In 1907, Baldwin[34] used a double loop of ileum to line a space dissected between the rectum and the bladder, leaving the mesentery connected to the bowel. An end to end re-anastomosis was used to maintain the continuity of the intestinal tract. Baldwin reported this as a normal vagina. In 1910, Popaw[35] constructed a vagina by moving a portion of the rectum anteriorly. Schubert[36] modified the procedure in 1911. The rectum was severed above the anal sphincter and moved anteriorly to serve as the vagina. The sigmoid colon was sutured to the anus to re-establish the integrity of the intestinal tract. Both operations had exceedingly high morbidity and mortality and the use of the procedure declined. Sigmoid colon segments are currently more often used for bowel vaginoplasty owing to the adverse effects associated with small bowel segments. Today, intestinal segments may be used for paediatric patients undergoing complex reconstructive procedures that include a vaginoplasty. Colonic segments have historically been used in young patients because of the proposed advantage that the vagina will 'grow' with them. Additionally, bowel vaginoplasty may have a role in the treatment of women with failure of other attempts, or after treatment for malignancy.

The Vecchietti operation, introduced in Italy by Giusseppe Vecchietti,[37] involves placing surgically an olive-shaped acrylic dilator on the perineum. The olive is connected by a suture, which is passed retroperitoneally, to a traction device placed on the lower abdomen. Postoperatively, progressive continuous traction is applied to the olive, which creates a neovagina by invagination within 6–9 days. The original procedure was performed through an abdominal incision; however laparoscopic modifications have been described with comparable functional success.[38,39]

Davydov[40] developed a three-stage operation involving dissection of the rectovesical space, abdominal mobilisation of the peritoneum with creation of vaginal fornices, and attachment of the peritoneum to the introitus. The laparoscopic modification involves placement of the purse-string suture at the abdominal end of the neovagina using laparoscopic instrumentation. In the largest published series of this procedure including 324 women with vaginal agenesis who underwent vaginal reconstruction using peritoneum, 27 had laparoscopically assisted surgery and the remainder had the procedure completed transvaginally.[31,41,42] The laparoscopic assisted procedure resulted in a shorter operating time, a lower intraoperative complication rate, and shorter hospital stay. The follow-up period was shorter in the laparoscopic group (range 6–24 months compared with 2–11 years in the group undergoing an abdominal operation). The procedure was similarly successful in both groups when assessed by vaginal structure (depth, width, scarring) and function (satisfactory intercourse). In order to achieve success with performance of the laparoscopic modification, it is essential that the surgeon be competent with intracorporal suturing.

Less successful procedures involve dissection of the space between the rectum and the bladder, then lining the space with flaps of skin from the labia or inner thighs. The major drawback is the resultant scarring. The best surgical option is likely to be the one with which the attending surgeon has the most experience.

Even though it is an older technique, McIndoe vaginoplasty is a safe surgical procedure that offers young women the opportunity for a neovagina without the morbidity associated with other alternative methods. The overall complication rate is low and functional success rates are excellent. In most women the graft site is not objectionable. According to a review of 19 studies and 1229 patients, Tolhurst *et al.*[43] note that the majority of young women (83%) are able to achieve normal, good or satisfactory sexual relationships. These statistics compare favourably with the population at large, validating the success of this timeless procedure.

References

1. Evans JN, Poland ML, Boving RL. Vaginal malformations. *Am J Obstet Gynecol* 1981;141:910–20.
2. Mayer CAJ. Uber Verdopplungen des Uterus und ihre Arten, nebst Bemerkungen uber Hasenscharte und Wolfsrachen. *J Chir Augenheilkd* 1829;13:525–64.
3. Rokitansky C. Uber die sogenannten Verdopplungen des Uterus. *Med JB Ost Staat* 1838;26:39–77.
4. Kuster H. Uterus bipartitus solidus rudimentarius cum vagina solida. *Z Geburtshilfe Gynakol* 1910;67:692–718.
5. Hauser GA, Schreiner WE. Das Mayer–Rokitansky–Kuster Syndrom: Uterus bipartitus solidus rudimentarius cum vagina solida. *Schweiz Med Wochenschr* 1961;12:381–4.
6. Goldwynn RM. History of attempts to form a vagina. *Plast Reconstr Surg* 1977;59:319–29.
7. Frank RT. The formation of an artificial vagina without operation. *Am J Obstet Gynecol* 1938;35:1053–5.
8. Frank RT. The formation of an artificial vagina without operation. *N Y State J Med* 1940;40:1669–70.
9. Rock JA, Reeves LA, Retto H, Baramki TA, Zacur HA, Jones HW. Success following vaginal creation for müllerian agenesis. *Fertil Steril* 1983;39:809–13.
10. Ingram JM. The bicycle seat stool in the treatment of vaginal agenesis and stenosis: a preliminary report. *Am J Obstet Gynecol* 1984;140:867–71.
11. Roberts CP, Haber MJ, Rock JA. Vaginal creation for müllerian agenesis. *Am J Obstet Gynecol* 2001;185:1349–52.
12. Mobus VJ, Kortenhorn K, Kreienberg R, Friedberg V. Long-term results after operative correction of vaginal aplasia. *Am J Obstet Gynecol* 1996;175:617–24.
13. Abbe R. New method of creating a vagina in a case of congenital absence. *Med Rec* 1898;54:836.
14. Wharton LR. A simple method of constructing a vagina. *Ann Surg* 1938;107;842–54.
15. Wharton LR. Further experiences in construction of the vagina. *Ann Surg* 1940;111:1010–20.
16. Wharton LR. Congenital malformations associated with developmental defects of the female reproductive organs. *Am J Obstet Gynecol* 1947;53:37.

17.   Counseller VS. Congenital absence of the vagina. *JAMA* 1948;136:861–6.

18.   McIndoe AH, Banister JB. An operation for the cure of congenital absence of the vagina. *J Obstet Gynaecol Br Emp* 1938;45:490–4.

19.   McIndoe AH. The treatment of congenital absence and obliterative conditions of the vagina. *Br J Plast Surg* 1950;2:254–67.

20.   Tancer ML, Katz M, Veridiano NP. Vaginal epithelialization with human amnion. *Obstet Gynecol* 1979;54:345–9.

21.   Karjalainen O, Myllynen L, Kajanoja P, Tennhunen A, Perola E, Timonen S. Management of vaginal agenesis. *Ann Chir Gynaecol* 1980;69:37–41.

22.   Jackson ND, Rosenplatt PL. Use of Interceed Absorbable Adhesion Barrier for vaginoplasty. *Obstet Gynecol* 1994;84:1048–50.

23.   Counseller VS, Flor FS. Congenital absence of the vagina: further results of treatment and a new technique. *Surg Clin North Am* 1957;37:1107–18.

24.   Alessandrescu D, Peltecu GC, Buhimschi CS, Buhimschi IA. Neocolpopoiesis with split-thickness skin graft as a surgical treatment of vaginal agenesis: retrospective review of 201 cases. *Am J Obstet Gynecol* 1996;175:131–8.

25.   Hojsgaard A, Villadsen I. McIndoe procedure for congenital vaginal agenesis: complications and results. *Br J Plast Surg* 1995;48:97–102.

26.   Rock JA, unpublished data.

27.   Ozek C, Gurler T, Alper M, Gundogan H, Bilkay U, Songur E, *et al*. Modified McIndoe procedure for vaginal agenesis. *Ann Plast Surg* 1999;43:393–6.

28.   Templeman CL, Lam AM, Hertweck SP. Surgical management of vaginal agenesis. *Obstet Gynecol Surv* 1999;54:583–91.

29.   Buss JG, Lee RA. McIndoe procedure for vaginal agenesis: results and complications. *Mayo Clin Proc* 1989;64:758–61.

30.   Cali RW, Pratt JH. Congenital absence of the vagina. *Am J Obstet Gynecol* 1968;100:752–63.

31.   Pratt JH, Field CS, Symmonds RE. Congenital absence of the vagina. *Excerpta Medica Int Congress Ser* 1977;412:343–8.

32.   Strickland JL, Cameron WJ, Krantz KE. Long-term satisfaction of adults undergoing McIndoe vaginoplasty as adolescents. *Adolesc Pediatr Gynecol* 1993;6:135–7.

33.   Hiroi H, Yasugi T, Matsumoto K, Fujii T, Watanbe T, Yoshikawa H, *et al*. Mucinous adenocarcinoma arising in a neovagina using the sigmoid colon thirty years after operation: a case report. *J Surg Oncol* 2001;77:61–4.

34.   Baldwin JF. Formation of an artificial vagina by intestinal transplantation. *Am J Obstet Gynecol* 1907;56:636–40.

35.   Popaw DD. Utilization of the rectum in construction of a functional vagina. *Russk Virach St Peter* 1910;43:1512.

36.   Schubert G. *Uber Scheidenbildung bei angeborenom Vaginaldefekt. Zentralbl Gynäk* 1911;35:1017–25.

37.   Vecchietti G. Neovagina nella sindrome di Rokitansky Kuster Hauser [Creation of an artificial vagina in Rokitansky Kuster Hauser syndrome]. *Attual Obstet Ginecol* 1965;11:131–47.

38.   Veronikis DS, McClure GB, Nichols DH. The Vecchietti operation for constructing a neovagina: indications, instrumentation, and techniques. *Obstet Gynecol* 1997;90:301–4.

39.   Borruto F, Chasen ST, Chervenak FA, Fedele L. The Vecchietti procedure for surgical treatment of vaginal agenesis: comparison of laparoscopy and laparotomy. *Int J Gynaecol Obstet* 1999;64:153–8.

40.   Davydov SN. Colpopoiesis from the peritoneum of the utero-rectal space. *Akush Ginecol (Mosk)* 1969;12:55–7.

41. Adamyan LV. Laparoscopic management of vaginal aplasia with or without functional noncommunicating rudimentary uterus. In: Arregui ME, Fitzgibbons RJ, Kathouda N, McKernan JB, Reich H, editors. *Principles of Laparoscopic Surgery: Basic and Advanced Techniques.* New York: Springer-Verlag; 1995. p. 646–51.
42. Adamyan LV. Therapeutic and endoscopic perspectives. In: Nichols DH, Clarke-Pearson DL, editors. *Gynecologic, Obstetric, and Related Surgery.* 2nd ed. St Louis, MO: Mosby; 2000. p. 1209-17.
43. Tolhurst DE, van der Helm TW. The treatment of vaginal atresia. *Surg Gynecol Obstet* 1991;172:407–14.

6

Early expression of thyroid hormone deiodinases and receptors in human fetal cerebral cortex

Shiao Chan

The critical role of thyroid hormones in the normal growth and development of the human central nervous system (CNS) is well recognised, with notable neurological deficits seen in children with untreated congenital hypothyroidism and iodine deficiency.[1] Even with prompt thyroxine (T_4) supplementation from the early postnatal period resulting in the aversion of overt cretinism,[2] these children still demonstrate subtle neurodevelopmental deficits.[3,4] This implies that brain development may be thyroid hormone sensitive not only in the neonatal period but also prior to birth.[5]

EPIDEMIOLOGICAL EVIDENCE

Traditionally, maternal thyroid hormones have not been thought to play a major role in fetal CNS development. However, epidemiological evidence emerging since 1991 suggests that even mild maternal hypothyroxinaemia may adversely affect the long-term neurodevelopment of the offspring despite a euthyroid status in the early neonatal period.[6–8] In two surveys conducted in nonendemic areas, subclinical hypothyroidism, defined as having an elevated thyrotrophin (TSH) level but normal free T_4 concentrations, was found in over 2% of pregnancies,[9,10] which represents a sizeable proportion of the pregnant population.

A group in Maine (USA) studied 62 children of women with elevated TSH concentrations (at or above the 98th centile) at 16 weeks of gestation. These children, who were assessed between seven and nine years of age, performed less well on all 15 of the neuropsychological tests used and had on average a four-point lower IQ score on the Wechsler Intelligence Scale for Children compared with the 124 matched controls.[7] The children of a subgroup of 48 biochemically hypothyroid women who were not treated during the pregnancy because they were clinically euthyroid, performed less well. They had significantly lower IQ scores, with an average reduction of seven points compared with controls and 19% of them scored 85 or less. It is interesting that the serum total T_4 and free T_4 concentrations in the treated and the nontreated clinically euthyroid women were similar during pregnancy. This study has identified both the long-term consequences of subclinical maternal hypothyroidism on offspring as well as the benefits of T_4 treatment during pregnancy, even when supplementation is inadequate. These results confirm findings of an earlier study in the USA, which showed that mothers who had a low serum butanol-extractable iodine level (a measure of circulating thyroid hormones employed in the 1960s) before 24 weeks of gestation, and who were not adequately treated, had infants with lower developmental scores on the Bayley Scale. These children, when tested again at four and seven years of age, demonstrated an increased incidence of subnormal intelligence, specific visuospatial and oculomotor disabilities, more inactivity and slowness on timed tasks.[8]

Not only the severity of maternal hypothyroidism but the timing of it is also important. In the Netherlands, a series of studies found that the strongest predictor of infant mental development was a low maternal free T_4 concentration (at or below the 10th centile) at 12 weeks of gestation rather than at 32 weeks.[6] Furthermore, the infants of women with low free T_4 levels throughout pregnancy were most likely to show delayed development on the Bayley Developmental Scale, while offspring of women whose free T_4 levels were normal at 12 weeks but declined subsequently in pregnancy were moderately at risk. These studies show the importance of normal maternal thyroxinaemia throughout pregnancy, particularly in the first trimester, in attaining normal neurodevelopment. Even though a group in Japan found that two-thirds of subclinical hypothyroidism cases in pregnancy may resolve spontaneously within ten weeks of diagnosis,[11] damage to fetal CNS development during this period may be irreversible despite subsequent restoration of normal thyroxinaemia.

In Toronto, Rovet's group tested the offspring of women who demonstrated a period of thyroid hormone insufficiency during the pregnancy. They have reported that brief periods of hypothyroxinaemia at different gestations gave rise to selective deficits in aspects of visuospatial[12] and auditory discrimination,[7,13] and in attention performance,[14] which are parameters predictive of later cognitive function.[15] Hence different areas of ability were associated with the timing and duration of maternal thyroid hormone deficiency,[16,17] leading to the start of mapping out when particular neuroanatomical structures may be thyroid hormone dependent during the course of gestation.[18]

As studies to date have not examined the full range of offspring competencies in detail, a complete picture of the effects of an altered maternal thyroid hormone economy may be more extensive than initially thought. In addition, many chemicals, both natural and manufactured, that are commonly found in the environment, such as polychlorinated biphenyls, have been shown to alter the expression of thyroid hormone responsive genes in the developing brain in animal studies. The presence of such chemicals may further disrupt thyroid hormone dependent CNS development and exacerbate the consequences of maternal hypothyroxinaemia.[19]

THYROID HORMONES IN THE FETUS

There is evidence that maternal thyroid hormones do cross the placenta in early gestation before the human fetus initiates endogenous thyroid hormone synthesis at the start of the second trimester.[20,21] The fetal thyroid gland begins to release appreciable amounts of hormone only from about 16 weeks of gestation onwards.[22,23] However, thyroid hormones have been found in fetal embryonic fluids[24] and fetal tissues[23,25] in the first trimester. It is interesting to note that the T_4 concentrations in exocoelomic fluids in the first trimester[26] and fetal cerebral cortices at 15–18 weeks of gestation[23] have been strongly correlated with maternal thyroxinaemia, thus supporting the idea that they are maternally derived. The first conclusive evidence of the maternal-fetal transfer of thyroid hormones in humans was reported in the late 1980s. Circulatory thyroid hormone concentrations of around 25–50% of those of normal infants were reported in athyroid fetuses at term, and these were shown to be of maternal origin.[27]

It therefore appears that the fetus is normally completely dependent for optimal development on the maternal supply of thyroid hormones in the first trimester. In the next two trimesters, circulatory fetal thyroid hormones are of both maternal and fetal origin, with approximately 30% of thyroid hormones in cord blood at term still derived from the mother.[27,28] Both fetal circulatory T_4 and triiodothyronine (T_3) levels increase with gestation.[29] While serum free T_4 concentrations approach adult levels by 36 weeks of gestation,[30] fetal serum free T_3 concentrations are still two- to three-fold less than those in the mother at full-term birth and rise towards adult levels only several weeks later.[28] Circulating thyroid hormones comprise protein-bound and free unbound forms, with only the latter being available for tissue uptake. Most circulating thyroid hormone is in the form of T_4 rather than T_3. In the fetus an increasing proportion of thyroid hormones become protein bound as thyroid binding protein concentrations increase with advancing gestation.[26,30]

The placenta plays a role in maintaining the requisite levels of fetal circulating thyroid hormones by its differential expression of iodothyronine deiodinase enzymes throughout gestation.[31,32] Although these enzymes metabolise most of the thyroid hormones presented to the placenta,[33] it is postulated that physiologically critical amounts of maternal thyroid hormones still cross transplacentally.[28] The free T_4 concentrations reached in the human fetal fluids in the first trimester are similar to those capable of exerting biological effects in adults.[26] Thus the early human fetus is exposed to physiologically relevant amounts of free T_4, which could potentially exert thyroid hormone effects within fetal tissues, despite a low total T_4 level. A similar situation has been observed in rodent studies, with T_4 and T_3 levels in fetal rat brain found to be higher than expected from their low circulating levels.[34] Furthermore, thyroid hormones can be found in the human fetal brain in the first trimester but not in other fetal organs at this stage.[35] This suggests a specific role for maternal thyroid hormones in early CNS development.

Unlike in the adult, there are also high levels of reverse T_3 (rT_3) and conjugated thyroid hormones (e.g. glucuronide-added or sulphated T_4) in the fetal circulation.[32,36] These metabolites are physiologically inactive but they may serve as a reservoir of potentially active thyroid hormones for tissues that possess appropriate enzymes for their activation,[37] for example sulphatases in the fetal brain.[37,38]

Although circulating concentrations of the various thyroid hormones are major determinants of the cellular uptake of thyroid hormones into tissues, other factors may modulate local thyroid hormone action, for example, the differential expression and function of thyroid hormone receptors (TR) and thyroid hormone metabolism by enzymes such as the iodothyronine deiodinases and sulfotransferases.

IODOTHYRONINE DEIODINASES

These deiodinases are selenocysteine-containing enzymes that are pre-receptor regulators of local thyroid hormone concentrations.[39] As most of the circulating thyroid hormones are in the form of the prohormone, T_4, local tissue deiodinase action is required to convert it to the active ligand, T_3. Type I (D1) and type II (D2) deiodinases are capable of this conversion − which involves phenolic (outer) ring monodeiodination[40,41] − and are thus regarded as the activating enzymes. Conversely, type III (D3) deiodinase, which has the preferred action of tyrosyl (inner) ring monodeiodination, inactivates T_4 and T_3 to rT_3 and 3,3`-diiodothyronine (T_2) respectively,[42] so the balance of these enzymes can modulate the local T_3 concentrations (Figure 1).

D1, which is found predominantly in kidney, liver and thyroid tissues, is mainly responsible for the supply of circulatory T_3.[43] D1 activity has been documented in the adult rat brain,[44] but it has not been detectable in human cerebral cortex samples from both fetuses and adults.[45,46] Even though our group has detected a limited amount of D1 mRNA in about 50% of fetal and adult cerebral cortex samples by using sensitive techniques,[45] the lack of D1 activity suggests that this subtype is unlikely to play a significant role in the human CNS.

However, D2 and D3 enzymes, with K_m values in the low nanomolar ranges,[40,41,47] are thought to be critically important in the fine homeostatic regulation of intracellular T_3 concentrations in tissues[48] like the CNS,[46,49,50] placenta,[31–33] pituitary gland[51,52] and brown adipose tissue.[53,54] Most of this evidence has been derived from rodent models and a similar homeostatic mechanism is postulated to occur in humans.[55] Furthermore, the deiodinases may have a critical role to play in directing

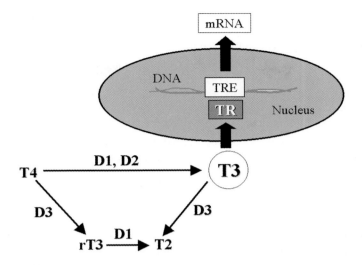

Figure 1 *The predominant reactions of the iodothyronine deiodinase enzymes (D1, D2, D3) and their role as pre-receptor regulators of thyroid hormone action; T_4 = thyroxine; T_3 = triiodothyronine; rT_3 = reverse T_3; T_2 = diiodothyronine; TR = thyroid hormone receptor; TRE = thyroid response element*

normal development. This has been best studied in amphibian metamorphosis, where timely coordinated tissue-specific expressions of D2 and D3 ensure that requisite levels of intracellular T_3 are attained at different developmental stages, regardless of circulating levels of thyroid hormone,[56] in order to regulate normal thyroid hormone-dependent development.

In the brain, approximately 80% of T_3 is derived locally through D2 activity,[57] so local homeostatic mechanisms are particularly important in regulating thyroid hormone action. In the adult human CNS, for example, an inverse relationship between D3 activity and T_3 content has been found,[49] suggesting that D3 contributes to the local regulation of T_3. In rodent studies, fetal hypothyroxinaemia in rats, caused by maternal subtotal thyroid ablation, resulted in enhanced D2 activity and decreased D3 activity in the fetal brain, reflecting an attempt to maintain adequate local T_3 concentrations in the face of limited T_4.[34] Meanwhile, peripheral D1 activity is reduced to help to maintain circulatory T_4 levels for uptake by the more important thyroid dependent tissues.[58,59] Furthermore, the increase in D2 expression was found to be regionally selective in hypothyroidism. For example, during postnatal rat development, which corresponds to the third trimester of human pregnancy in terms of neurodevelopment,[22] there were marked increases in D2 expression documented in the relay nuclei and cortical targets of primary somatosensory and auditory pathways. This suggests that these regions are T_3 responsive and require particular protection against low T_3 levels at this stage of development.[60] It may also suggest that the visual cortical pathways may be more vulnerable to insufficient thyroid hormones than the auditory pathways during development. This idea is reflected by the results of neuropsychological studies of infant visual processing in humans reported in 2002.[12]

Our group in Birmingham has studied the ontogeny of all the deiodinase subtypes in a relatively large group of 67 human fetal cerebral cortices between 7 and 20 weeks of gestation. We found both D2 and D3 mRNA and activity in the fetal cerebral cortex from 7–8 weeks of gestation. Despite significantly increased D2 mRNA levels at 15–16 weeks of gestation compared with adult cortices, there was no significant difference in fetal D2 activity throughout gestation and when compared with the adult.[45] In contrast, another research group has reported a doubling of D2 activity between 11 and 14 weeks and 15 and 18 weeks of gestation, with further increases at 19–22 weeks.[23] This contrast may be ascribed to the smaller sample numbers used by the latter group or different cortical areas being sampled, as well as possible methodological differences because the D2 activity levels reported by the latter group were many times higher than those our group has found. However, they reported D3 activity levels that were more akin to our values. Although we found significantly decreased D3 mRNA expression in fetal cortices compared with adults, there were significantly increased D3 activities in fetal cortices from 11 to 16 weeks of gestation compared with adult samples[45] (Figure 2). This suggests post-transcriptional regulation in the synthesis of the active D3 enzyme. The other group reported peak D3 activities from 15 to 22 weeks of gestation.[23] Nonetheless, despite all these differences in our findings, it can be concluded that the early developing human CNS possesses mechanisms capable of generating and regulating T_3 concentrations locally.

It has also been reported that, under iodine deficient conditions, there are significant increases in D2 activity in the first and early second trimester human fetal cerebral cortices.[23] This suggests that a compensatory mechanism similar to the one seen in rodents under similar conditions[61] is operational in human fetuses too. However, deiodinase activities alone are insufficient to ensure requisite tissue concentrations of T_3 in the human CNS and it is most likely that other thyroid hormone metabolic pathways are involved in T_3 regulation.[37,38,62]

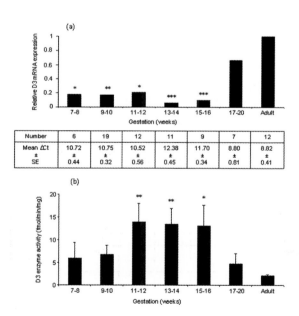

Figure 2 *(a) Relative expression of mRNA encoding iodothyronine deiodinase type III (D3) in human fetal cerebral cortex from 7 to 20 weeks of gestation compared with the adult cerebral cortex, given an arbitrary value of 1: *P < 0.01; **P < 0.001; ***P < 0.0001 compared with adults; the number of samples expressing the mRNA and the mean ΔCt values and standard errors obtained using quantitative RT-PCR for each group are given in the corresponding columns in the table below the graph; (b) Mean iodothyronine deiodinase type III (D3) enzyme activity in human fetal cerebral cortex from 7 to 20 weeks of gestation and in the adult cerebral cortex: *P < 0.01; **P < 0.001 compared with adult (Ct values are the cycle numbers at which logarithmic PCR plots cross a calculated threshold line during real-time quantitative RT-PCR; ΔCt values = Ct of target gene minus Ct of control gene, 19S) (Reprinted from: Chan S, Kachilele S, McCabe CJ, Tannahill LA, Boelaert K, Gittoes NJL, et al. Early expression of thyroid hormone deiodinases and receptors in human fetal cerebral cortex. Brain Res Dev Brain Res 2002;138:109–16,[45] with permission from Elsevier Science)*

THYROID HORMONE RECEPTORS

In both adult humans and rodents, specific regions of the CNS, including the cerebral cortex, hippocampus and cerebellum, are known to express deiodinase enzymes. These areas also co-express TRs, thus suggesting anatomically coordinated expressions of deiodinases and TRs in the CNS.[63,64]

TRs are nuclear transcription factors encoded by the Erb-A α and β genes, each producing two major isoforms by alternative splicing.[65] TRα1, TRβ1 and TRβ2 all bind T_3 to form complexes, which can regulate the transcription of thyroid hormone responsive genes.[66] These genes contain thyroid response elements in their promoter regions to which the T_3-TR complexes may bind (Figure 1). Many such genes have been identified, such as myelin basic protein[67] and neurogranin[68] in the CNS. The nonligand binding α2 isoform, however, may modulate the actions of the other TRs through competitive inhibition.[66,69]

Our group has found mRNA encoding TR isoforms α1, α2 and β1 in a large group of human fetal cortical samples from as early as 7–8 weeks of gestation using the quantitative reverse transcriptase polymerase chain reaction (RT-PCR).[45] TRα1 mRNA expression in fetal cortices was significantly increased about eight-fold at 9–10 and 15–16 weeks compared with adult samples. Conversely, α2 and TRβ1 mRNA expressions in fetal cortices were generally lower compared with adult cortices, reaching significance at 17–20 weeks for α2, and at 9–12 and 17–20 weeks for TRβ1 (Figure 3). However, only 26% of fetal samples between 7 and 20 weeks of gestation had detectable TRβ2 mRNA compared with 62% of adult samples. It is interesting that,

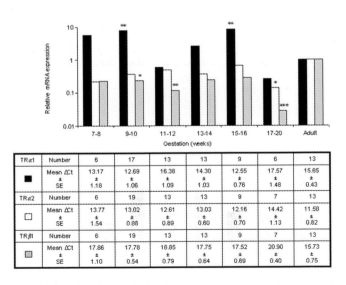

Figure 3 *The relative expressions of mRNA encoding thyroid receptor isoforms α1, α2 and β1 in human fetal cerebral cortex from 7 to 20 weeks of gestation compared with adult cerebral cortex, given an arbitrary value of 1: *P < 0.05; **P < 0.01; ***P < 0.0001 compared with adults; the number of samples expressing the mRNA and the mean ΔCt values and standard errors obtained using quantitative RT-PCR for each group are given in the corresponding columns in the table below the graph (Ct values are the cycle numbers at which logarithmic PCR plots cross a calculated threshold line during real-time quantitative RT-PCR; ΔCt values = Ct of target gene minus Ct of control gene, 19S) (Reprinted from: Chan S, Kachilele S, McCabe CJ, Tannahill LA, Boelaert K, Gittoes NJL, et al. Early expression of thyroid hormone deiodinases and receptors in human fetal cerebral cortex. Brain Res Dev Brain Res 2002;138:109–16,[45] with permission from Elsevier Science)*

even though TRβ2 mRNA levels were at the limits of detection in most samples, of those that did express TRβ2, levels of expression were generally higher in fetal than in adult samples.

These results generally agree with those reported by others who have used conventional RT-PCR to study TR mRNA expression in human fetal cerebral cortices, in particular that the α1, α2 and β1 isoforms were expressed from early gestation and that the β2 isoform was detectable in only some samples, albeit after high numbers of PCR cycles.[70]

We have also used immunocytochemistry to study protein expression of all the TR isoforms from 7 weeks of gestation onwards.[71] Thyroid hormone receptor immunostaining was most marked in the pyramidal neurons. Within these cells immunostaining was predominantly nuclear, exhibiting a reticular pattern, with some granular staining in the cytoplasm[71] (Figure 4). The staining was semiquantitatively scored as percentage immunopositive cells per high-powered field. In the first trimester, TRα1 and α2 were the predominant isoforms expressed with about 20% cellular immunopositivity, while TRβ1 and TRβ2 expressions were low (less than 5% immunopositivity). By the early second trimester, the expressions of all the TR isoforms had increased dramatically with an approximately three-fold and 15-fold increase in the α and β isoforms respectively (Figure 5). Further increases could be observed in the third trimester. As TRs are preferentially expressed by neurons rather than by astrocytes and glia,[72] it is thought that the increase in TR expression over the first half of pregnancy could be due in part to the rising ratio of neurons to glia with gestation.[73,74] In addition, a pattern of a relatively delayed protein expression of the TRβ isoforms compared with the TRα isoforms has also been reported in the developing rat.[75]

In summary, while TRα1 mRNA was variably expressed at higher levels in fetal life than in adult cortex, α2 and TRβ1 mRNA were generally lower. Such a varied ontogeny of mRNA expression among the TR isoforms appears to differ from the pattern of an increasing TR protein expression with gestation for all isoforms. This may be due partly to the discrepancy in the sensitivity of methods used to assess mRNA and protein, with the former being more sensitive. Furthermore, we were unable accurately to quantify protein levels using semiquantitative

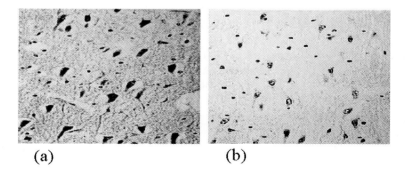

(a)   **(b)**

Figure 4 *Immunostaining of the pyramidal neurons of the fetal cerebral cortex using rabbit polyclonal antibodies against (a) human specific thyroid hormone receptor α1, showing predominantly nuclear localization, compared with (b) control, performed using nonimmune serum (Reprinted from: Kilby MD, Gittoes N, McCabe C, Verhaeg J, Franklyn JA. Expression of thyroid receptor isoforms in the human fetal central nervous system and the effects of intrauterine growth restriction. Clin Endocrinol (Oxf) 2000;53:469–77,[71] with permission from Blackwell Publishing)*

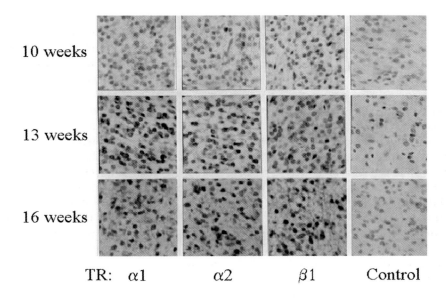

10 weeks

13 weeks

16 weeks

TR: α1   α2   β1   Control

Figure 5 *Immunostaining of the pyramidal neurons of the fetal cerebral cortex using rabbit polyclonal antibodies against human specific thyroid hormone receptors; the expression of TR isoforms α1, α2 and β1 at 10, 13 and 16 weeks of gestation are compared with controls, performed using nonimmune serum (Reprinted from: Kilby MD, Gittoes N, McCabe C, Verhaeg J, Franklyn JA. Expression of thyroid receptor isoforms in the human fetal central nervous system and the effects of intrauterine growth restriction. Clin Endocrinol (Oxf) 2000;53:469–77,[71] with permission from Blackwell Publishing)*

immunocytochemistry analysis. However, a significant increase, in the region of ten-fold, in T_3 binding to fetal cerebral nuclei between the first and early second trimesters of human pregnancy have been described previously,[23,76] lending indirect support to the magnitude of increase in TR protein expression with gestation reported here. Like deiodinases, post-transcriptional regulation of TR expression is likely to be operational because apparent discrepancies between TR protein and mRNA expressions have previously been noted in various tissues.[77–80]

Nevertheless, we can conclude that from an early gestational age the human fetal cerebral cortex is a potentially thyroid hormone responsive tissue because it expresses TRs. It is possible that TRα isoforms have an earlier role to play in cerebral cortex development than the TRβ isoforms. Furthermore, TRα1 may be the predominant isoform mediating T_3-dependent fetal CNS development, while TRβ2 may play a much smaller or a redundant role.

From animal studies, we know that TR expression is tissue specific and temporally regulated, with differential expression patterns observed in specific areas of the developing fetal CNS.[81] These differences are likely to reflect the variable end-organ responses required of thyroid hormone action through the modulation of gene transcription.[66] For example, during the development of the outer nuclear layer of the fetal chick retina, TRβ2 expression during early gestation coincides with rod and cone proliferation and differentiation, while TRα expression in the same layer later in gestation coincides with photoreceptor synaptogenesis and myelination.[82] In addition, the ability of cultured oligodendrocytes to increase myelin basic protein expression in response to T_3 coincides with the appearance of TRβ1.[83]

In rodent models of altered thyroid hormone economy, changes in the timing and level of expression of thyroid hormone responsive genes have also been observed. For example, the expression of Purkinje cell protein-2, a known T_3 responsive gene,[84] is delayed in hypothyroid neonatal rats, resulting in an irreversible deficit in cerebellar Purkinje cell maturation.[75] Hypothyroid neonatal rats also show a marked reduction in myelin basic protein transcripts in the striatum and cerebral cortex but only a modest reduction in the caudal brain regions.[85] This is an example of the differential effects of thyroid hormones on specific CNS areas at particular time points of development.

Of particular current interest is the finding that maternal hypothyroidism can result in altered expressions of thyroid hormone responsive genes in specific regions of the fetal rat CNS at a time before the onset of endogenous fetal thyroid hormone production, which is on gestational day 17 (G17).[86,87] For example, neurogranin (which has a role in synaptic functioning)[88,89] expression was downregulated in the fetal rat brains on G16 when there was maternal hypothyroidism.[86] In a similar experiment, hypothyroid pregnant dams were given an injection of T_4 at G16 and the transcripts of another thyroid hormone responsive gene, neuroendocrine-specific protein-A, were found to be significantly reduced 36 hours later.[90] Such studies demonstrate the potential for maternal thyroid hormones to directly regulate genes in the fetal CNS and provide a possible molecular basis for the epidemiological link between maternal hypothyroxinaemia and neurodevelopmental deficits observed in the offspring.

In rodents, altered gene expressions in fetal hypothyroxinaemia are also accompanied by abnormal histological features within the CNS, including reduced neuronal proliferation, altered dendritic branching, defective synaptogenesis, abnormal neurocytoarchitecture, deficient myelination and impaired cell migration.[91–93]

It is likely that the human fetal CNS also shows similarly variable expression patterns of TR isoforms and thyroid hormone responsive gene expressions, and cytoarchitectural changes in response to hypothyroxinaemia.

CONCLUSION

All this work has led to the hypothesis that there may be a specific and crucial role for thyroid hormones in early human fetal brain development, even before the onset of fetal thyroid function, and that the transplacental passage of maternal thyroid hormones occurs to influence fetal CNS development. The local expression of thyroid hormone deiodinases and receptors, together with normal maternal thyroxinaemia, are therefore required for physiologically optimal thyroid hormone action in the developing fetal brain, particularly during early gestation.[45] Possible pre-receptor regulation of thyroid hormone supply by deiodinases and the expression of the TRs that are available to interact with T_3 to affect the expression of T_3 responsive genes, make the human fetal cerebral cortex a potentially thyroid hormone responsive organ from the first trimester,[45] and hence susceptible to hypothyroxinaemia. Differential patterns of deiodinase subtype and TR isoform expressions throughout gestation are likely to reflect changing T_3 requirements of the cerebral cortex during development. Particularly in early gestation, the thyroid hormones available to affect neurodevelopment would be derived from the maternal circulation. Hence maternal thyroid dysfunction in early pregnancy may be an important factor in the maldevelopment of the fetal brain in humans.

Despite good evidence that maternal thyroid hormones may affect fetal brain development directly, there are likely to be other confounding factors and indirect mechanisms through which maternal hypothyroxinaemia may also impact on the neurodevelopment of the child. These include the secondary effects of maternal hypothyroidism (such as metabolic impairments and maternal anaemia),[94] impaired placental function, maternofetal transfer of antithyroid antibodies,[95] obstetric complications[96,97] and postnatal depression,[98] all of which are known to have an increased incidence in maternal hypothyroidism.

There is much left to be discovered in exploring our hypothesis. Further experiments are being conducted to localise better the expression of deiodinases and TRs within the CNS at different gestational ages, identify the particular T_3 responsive genes that are operational in these thyroid hormone responsive neurostructures, define the precise timing of their thyroid hormone dependency, explore the role played by the T_3 responsive gene products during development, and examine the subsequent neurobehavioural sequelae generated. The mechanisms underlying the regulation of the transplacental passage of maternal thyroid hormones is also being studied in our laboratory.

CLINICAL IMPLICATIONS

Even though there is clinical evidence pointing towards a critical role for maternal thyroid hormones in fetal brain development, with supporting evidence emerging at histological and molecular levels, there is still insufficient evidence to warrant wide scale screening of women before pregnancy or antenatally. A case, however, could be made for screening women with risk factors such as a personal history of thyroid disease, related autoimmune disorders or iodine deficiency, or a positive family history. Issues like the timing and frequency of screening,[99] which hormones ($TSH/T_4/T_3$) to screen,[100,101] what concentrations are acceptable,[101-103] and how and when to treat abnormalities[104-109] are still being debated. It is clear that more comprehensive and larger scale prospective studies of maternal thyroid hormone screening, the effects on offspring, the epidemiological impact this will have on the prevalence of neurodevelopmental delay in the population, and its overall cost effectiveness, are required at this stage. Good cooperation between clinicians, psychologists and scientists from different disciplines will be required for such a major and long-term undertaking. In the meantime there is still much room for progress at a molecular level in our laboratories to help us to understand further the role of thyroid hormones in fetal CNS development.

Acknowledgements

This work has been funded by the MRC, the Mason Medical Research Foundation and the Endowment fund for the former United Birmingham Hospitals. I would like to thank Professor Mark Kilby, Professor Jayne Franklyn, Dr Kachilele, Dr McCabe, Dr Visser and Miss Verhaeg for their contribution to this study.

References

1. Legrand J. [Thyroid hormones and maturation of the nervous system.] *J Physiol (Paris)* 1982;78:603–52.
2. Fisher DA, Dussault JH, Foley TP Jr, Klein AH, LaFranchi S, Larsen PR, *et al*. Screening for congenital hypothyroidism: results of screening one million North American infants. *J Pediatr* 1979;94:700–5.
3. Heyerdahl S, Kase BF, Lie SO. Intellectual development in children with congenital hypothyroidism in relation to recommended thyroxine treatment. *J Pediatr* 1991;118:850–7.

4. Rovet JF. Long-term neuropsychological sequelae of early-treated congenital hypothyroidism: effects in adolescence. *Acta Paediatr Suppl* 1999;88:88–95.

5. Chan S, Kilby MD. Thyroid hormone and central nervous system development. *J Endocrinol* 2000;165:1–8.

6. Pop VJ, Kuijpens JL, van Baar AL, Verkerk G, van Son MM, de Vijlder JJ, *et al.* Low maternal free thyroxine concentrations during early pregnancy are associated with impaired psychomotor development in infancy. *Clin Endocrinol (Oxf)* 1999;50:149–55.

7. Haddow JE, Palomaki GE, Allan WC, Williams JR, Knight GJ, Gagnon J, *et al.* Maternal thyroid deficiency during pregnancy and subsequent neuropsychological development of the child. *N Engl J Med* 1999;341:549–55.

8. Man EB, Brown JF, Serunian SA. Maternal hypothyroxinemia: psychoneurological deficits of progeny. *Ann Clin Lab Sci* 1991;21:227–39.

9. Lejeune B, Lemone M, Kinthaert J. The epidemiology of autoimmune and functional thyroid disorders in pregnancy. *J Endocrinol Invest* 1992;15 Suppl 2:77.

10. Klein RZ, Haddow JE, Faix JD, Brown RS, Hermos RJ, Pulkkinen A, *et al.* Prevalence of thyroid deficiency in pregnant women. *Clin Endocrinol (Oxf)* 1991;35:41–6.

11. Kamijo K, Saito T, Sato M, Yachi A, Mukai A, Fukusi M, *et al.* Transient subclinical hypothyroidism in early pregnancy. *Endocrinol Jpn* 1998;37:397–403.

12. Mirabella G, Westall C, Perlman K, Koren G, Rovet J. Visual processing deficits in infancy following maternal hypothyroidism and congenital hypothyroidism. Abstracts of the 74th Annual Meeting of the American Thyroid Association; 2002 Oct 10–14; Los Angeles, (CA). *Thyroid* 2002;19 Suppl:160; abstr. 100.

13. Leneman M, Buchanan L, Rovet J. Where and what visuospatial processing in adolescents with congenital hypothyroidism. *J Int Neuropsychol Soc* 2001;7:556–62.

14. Rovet JF, Hepworth S. Attention problems in adolescents with congenital hypothyroidism: a multicomponential analysis. *J Int Neuropsychol Soc* 2001;7:734–44.

15. Mirabella G, Feig D, Astzalos E, Perlman K, Rovet JF. The effect of abnormal intrauterine thyroid hormone economies on infant cognitive abilities. *J Pediatr Endocrinol Metab* 2000;13:191–4.

16. Song SI, Daneman D, Rovet J. The influence of etiology and treatment factors on intellectual outcome in congenital hypothyroidism. *J Dev Behav Pediatr* 2001;22:376–84.

17. Rovet JF, Ehrlich RM, Sorbara DL. Neurodevelopment in infants and preschool children with congenital hypothyroidism: etiological and treatment factors affecting outcome. *J Pediatr Psychol* 1992;17:187–213.

18. Howdeshell KL. A model of the development of the brain as a construct of the thyroid system. *Environ Health Perspect* 2002;110 Suppl 3:337–48.

19. Zoeller TR, Dowling AL, Herzig CT, Iannacone EA, Gauger KJ, Bansal R. Thyroid hormone, brain development, and the environment. *Environ Health Perspect* 2002;110 Suppl 3:355–61.

20. Shepard TH. Onset of function in the human fetal thyroid: biochemical and radioautographic studies from organ culture. *J Clin Endocrinol Metab* 1967;27:945–58.

21. Fisher DA, Klein AH. Thyroid development and disorders of thyroid function in the newborn. *N Engl J Med* 1981;304:702–12.

22. Porterfield SP, Hendrich CE. The role of thyroid hormones in prenatal and neonatal neurological development – current perspectives. *Endocr Rev* 1993;14:94–106.

23. Sinha AK, Prabakaran D, Godbole M, Chattopadhyay N, Karmarkar M, Pickard MR, *et al.* Thyroid hormone and brain maturation. In: *Recent Research Developments in Neuroendocrinology.* Trivandrum, India: Research Signpost; 1997. p. 1–14.

24. Contempre B, Jauniaux E, Calvo R, Jurkovic D, Campbell S, de Escobar GM. Detection of thyroid hormones in human embryonic cavities during the first trimester of pregnancy. *J Clin Endocrinol Metab* 1993;77:1719–22.

25. Costa A, Arisio R, Benedetto C, Bertino E, Fabris C, Giraudi G, *et al.* Thyroid hormones in tissues from human embryos and fetuses. *J Endocrinol Invest* 1991;14:559–68.

26. Calvo RM, Jauniaux E, Gulbis B, Asuncion M, Gervy C, Contempre B, *et al.* Fetal tissues are exposed to biologically relevant free thyroxine concentrations during early phases of development. *J Clin Endocrinol Metab* 2002;87:1768–77.

27. Vulsma T, Gons MH, de Vijlder JJ. Maternal–fetal transfer of thyroxine in congenital hypothyroidism due to a total organification defect or thyroid agenesis. *N Engl J Med* 1989;321:13–16.

28. Fisher DA. Fetal thyroid function: diagnosis and management of fetal thyroid disorders. *Clin Obstet Gynecol* 1997;40:16–31.

29. Thorpe-Beeston JG, Nicolaides KH, McGregor AM. Fetal thyroid function. *Thyroid* 1992;2:207–17.

30. Thorpe-Beeston JG, Nicolaides KH, Felton CV, Butler J, McGregor AM. Maturation of the secretion of thyroid hormone and thyroid-stimulating hormone in the fetus. *N Engl J Med* 1991;324:532–6.

31. Chan S, Kachilele S, Hobbs E, Bulmer JN, Boelaert K, McCabe CJ, *et al.* Placental iodothyronine deiodinase expression in normal and growth-restricted human pregnancies. *J Clin Endocrinol Metab* 2003;88:4488–95.

32. Santini F, Chiovato L, Ghirri P, Lapi P, Mammoli C, Montanelli L, *et al.* Serum iodothyronines in the human fetus and the newborn: evidence for an important role of placenta in fetal thyroid hormone homeostasis. *J Clin Endocrinol Metab* 1999;84:493–8.

33. Koopdonk-Kool JM, de Vijlder JJ, Veenboer GJ, Ris-Stalpers C, Kok JH, Vulsma T, *et al.* Type II and type III deiodinase activity in human placenta as a function of gestational age. *J Clin Endocrinol Metab* 1996;81:2154–8.

34. Calvo R, Obregon MJ, Ruiz de Ona C, Escobar del Ray F, Morreale de Escobar G. Congenital hypothyroidism, as studied in rats. Crucial role of maternal thyroxine but not of 3,5,3`-triiodothyronine in the protection of the fetal brain. *J Clin Invest* 1990;86:889–99.

35. Karmarkar MG, Prabarkaran D, Godbole MM. 5`-Monodeiodinase activity in developing human cerebral cortex. *Am J Clin Nutr* 1993;57(2 Suppl):291S–4S.

36. Santini F, Cortelazzi D, Baggiani AM, Marconi AM, Beck-Peccoz P, Chopra IJ. A study of the serum 3,5,3`-triiodothyronine sulfate concentration in normal and hypothyroid fetuses at various gestational stages. *J Clin Endocrinol Metab* 1993;76:1583–7.

37. Visser TJ. Role of sulfate in thyroid hormone sulfation. *Eur J Endocrinol* 1996;134:12–14.

38. Richard K, Hume R, Kaptein E, Stanley EL, Visser TJ, Coughtrie MW. Sulfation of thyroid hormone and dopamine during human development: ontogeny of phenol sulfotransferases and arylsulfatase in liver, lung, and brain. *J Clin Endocrinol Metab* 2001;86:2734–42.

39. Kohrle J. The deiodinase family: selenoenzymes regulating thyroid hormone availability and action. *Cell Mol Life Sci* 2000;57:1853–63.

40. Visser TJ, Kaptein E, Terpstra OT, Krenning EP. Deiodination of thyroid hormone by human liver. *J Clin Endocrinol Metab* 1988;67:17–24.

41. Visser TJ, Kaplan MM, Leonard JL, Larsen PR. Evidence for two pathways of iodothyronine 5`-deiodination in rat pituitary that differ in kinetics, propylthiouracil sensitivity, and response to hypothyroidism. *J Clin Invest* 1983;71:992–1002.

42. Visser TJ. Pathways of thyroid hormone metabolism. *Acta Med Austriaca* 1996;23:10–16.

43. Kohrle J. Local activation and inactivation of thyroid hormones: the deiodinase family. *Mol Cell Endocrinol* 1999;151:103–19.

44.   Visser TJ, Leonard JL, Kaplan MM, Larsen PR. Kinetic evidence suggesting two mechanisms for iodothyronine 5`-deiodination in rat cerebral cortex. *Proc Natl Acad Sci U S A* 1982;79:5080–4.

45.   Chan S, Kachilele S, McCabe CJ, Tannahill LA, Boelaert K, Gittoes NJL, *et al.* Early expression of thyroid hormone deiodinases and receptors in human fetal cerebral cortex. *Brain Res Dev Brain Res* 2002;138:109–16.

46.   Campos-Barros A, Hoell T, Musa A, Sampaolo S, Stoltenburg G, Pinna G, *et al.* Phenolic and tyrosyl ring iodothyronine deiodination and thyroid hormone concentrations in the human central nervous system. *J Clin Endocrinol Metab* 1996;81:2179–85.

47.   Salvatore D, Bartha T, Harney JW, Larsen PR. Molecular biological and biochemical characterization of the human type 2 selenodeiodinase. *Endocrinology* 1996;137:3308–15.

48.   Bates JM, St Germain DL, Galton VA. Expression profiles of the three iodothyronine deiodinases, D1, D2, and D3, in the developing rat. *Endocrinology* 1999;140:844–51.

49.   Santini F, Pinchera A, Ceccarini G, Castagna M, Rosellini V, Mammoli C, *et al.* Evidence for a role of the type III-iodothyronine deiodinase in the regulation of 3,5,3`-triiodothyronine content in the human central nervous system. *Eur J Endocrinol* 2001;144:577–83.

50.   Morreale de Escobar G, Calvo R, Obregon MJ, Escobar del Rey F. Homeostasis of brain T3 in rat fetuses and their mothers: effects of thyroid status and iodine deficiency. *Acta Med Austriaca* 1992;19 Suppl 1:110–16.

51.   Tannahill LA, Visser TJ, McCabe CJ, Kachilele S, Boelaert K, Sheppard MC, *et al.* Dysregulation of iodothyronine deiodinase enzyme expression and function in human pituitary tumours. *Clin Endocrinol (Oxf)* 2002;56:735–43.

52.   Rodriguez-Garcia M, Jolin T, Santos A, Perez-Castillo A. Effect of perinatal hypothyroidism on the developmental regulation of rat pituitary growth hormone and thyrotropin genes. *Endocrinology* 1995;136:4339–50.

53.   Hernandez A, Obregon MJ. Presence of growth factors-induced type III iodothyronine 5-deiodinase in cultured rat brown adipocytes. *Endocrinology* 1995;136:4543–50.

54.   de Jesus LA, Carvalho SD, Ribeiro MO, Schneider M, Kim SW, Harney JW, *et al.* The type 2 iodothyronine deiodinase is essential for adaptive thermogenesis in brown adipose tissue. *J Clin Invest* 2001;108:1379–85.

55.   Croteau W, Davey JC, Galton VA, St Germain DL. Cloning of the mammalian type II iodothyronine deiodinase. A selenoprotein differentially expressed and regulated in human and rat brain and other tissues. *J Clin Invest* 1996;98:405–17.

56.   Becker KB, Stephens KC, Davey JC, Schneider MJ, Galton VA. The type 2 and type 3 iodothyronine deiodinases play important roles in coordinating development in Rana catesbeiana tadpoles. *Endocrinology* 1997;138:2989–97.

57.   Crantz FR, Silva JE, Larsen PR. An analysis of the sources and quantity of 3,5,3`-triiodothyronine specifically bound to nuclear receptors in rat cerebral cortex and cerebellum. *Endocrinology* 1982;110:367–75.

58.   Ruiz de Ona C, Morreale de Escobar G, Calvo R, Escobar del Rey F, Obregon MJ. Thyroid hormones and 5`-deiodinase in the rat fetus late in gestation: effects of maternal hypothyroidism. *Endocrinology* 1991;128:422–32.

59.   Silva JE, Matthews PS. Production rates and turnover of triiodothyronine in rat-developing cerebral cortex and cerebellum. Responses to hypothyroidism. *J Clin Invest* 1984;74:1035–49.

60.   Guadano-Ferraz A, Escamez MJ, Rausell E, Bernal J. Expression of type 2 iodothyronine deiodinase in hypothyroid rat brain indicates an important role of thyroid hormone in the development of specific primary sensory systems. *J Neurosci* 1999;19:3430–9.

61. Obregon MJ, Ruiz de Ona C, Calvo R, Escobar del Ray F, Morreale de Escobar G. Outer ring iodothyronine deiodinases and thyroid hormone economy: responses to iodine deficiency in the rat fetus and neonate. *Endocrinology* 1991;129:2663–73.

62. Eravci M, Pinna G, Meinhold H, Baumgartner A. Effects of pharmacological and nonpharmacological treatments on thyroid hormone metabolism and concentrations in rat brain. *Endocrinology* 2000;141:1027–40.

63. Asteria C. Crucial role for type II iodothyronine deiodinase in the metabolic coupling between glial cells and neurons during brain development. *Eur J Endocrinol* 1998;138:370–1.

64. Guadano-Ferraz A, Obregon MJ, St Germain DL, Bernal J. The type 2 iodothyronine deiodinase is expressed primarily in glial cells in the neonatal rat brain. *Proc Natl Acad Sci U S A* 1997;94:10391–6.

65. Oppenheimer JH, Schwartz HL. Molecular basis of thyroid hormone-dependent brain development. *Endocr Rev* 1997;18:462–75.

66. Lazar MA. Thyroid hormone receptors: multiple forms, multiple possibilities. *Endocr Rev* 1993;14:184–93.

67. Farsetti A, Desvergne B, Hallenbeck P, Robbins J, Nikodem VM. Characterization of myelin basic protein thyroid hormone response element and its function in the context of native and heterologous promoter. *J Biol Chem* 1992;267:15784–8.

68. Martinez de Arrieta C, Morte B, Coloma A, Bernal J. The human RC3 gene homolog, NRGN contains a thyroid hormone-responsive element located in the first intron. *Endocrinology* 1999;140:335–43.

69. Lazar MA, Hodin RA, Darling DS, Chin WW. A novel member of the thyroid/steroid hormone receptor family is encoded by the opposite strand of the rat c-erbA alpha transcriptional unit. *Mol Cell Biol* 1989;9:1128–36.

70. Iskaros J, Pickard M, Evans I, Sinha A, Hardiman P, Ekins R. Thyroid hormone receptor gene expression in first trimester human fetal brain. *J Clin Endocrinol Metab* 2000;85:2620–3.

71. Kilby MD, Gittoes N, McCabe C, Verhaeg J, Franklyn JA. Expression of thyroid receptor isoforms in the human fetal central nervous system and the effects of intrauterine growth restriction. *Clin Endocrinol (Oxf)* 2000;53:469–77.

72. Gullo D, Sinha AK, Woods R, Pervin K, Ekins RP. Triiodothyronine binding in adult rat brain: compartmentation of receptor populations in purified neuronal and glial nuclei. *Endocrinology* 1987;120:325–31.

73. Dobbing J, Sands J. Quantitative growth and development of human brain. *Arch Dis Child* 1973;48:757–67.

74. Dobbing J. The later growth of the brain and its vulnerability. *Pediatrics* 1974;53:2–6.

75. Strait KA, Zou L, Oppenheimer JH. Beta 1 isoform-specific regulation of a triiodothyronine-induced gene during cerebellar development. *Mol Endocrinol* 1992;6:1874–80.

76. Bernal J, Pekonen F. Ontogenesis of the nuclear 3,5,3`-triiodothyronine receptor in the human fetal brain. *Endocrinology* 1984;114:677–9.

77. Hodin RA, Lazar MA, Chin WW. Differential and tissue-specific regulation of the multiple rat c-erbA messenger RNA species by thyroid hormone. *J Clin Invest* 1990;85:101–5.

78. Kilby MD, Verhaeg J, Gittoes N, Somerset DA, Clark PM, Franklyn JA. Circulating thyroid hormone concentrations and placental thyroid hormone receptor expression in normal human pregnancy and pregnancy complicated by intrauterine growth restriction (IUGR). *J Clin Endocrinol Metab* 1998;83:2964–71.

79. Lane JT, Godbole M, Strait KA, Schwartz HL, Oppenheimer JH. Prolonged fasting reduces rat hepatic beta 1 thyroid hormone receptor protein without changing the level of its messenger ribonucleic acid. *Endocrinology* 1991;129:2881–5.

80. Strait KA, Schwartz HL, Perez-Castillo A, Oppenheimer JH. Relationship of c-erbA mRNA content to tissue triiodothyronine nuclear binding capacity and function in developing and adult rats. *J Biol Chem* 1990;265:10514–21.

81. Bradley DJ, Young WS, III, Weinberger C. Differential expression of alpha and beta thyroid hormone receptor genes in rat brain and pituitary. *Proc Natl Acad Sci U S A* 1989;86: 7250–4.

82. Sjoberg M, Vennstrom B, Forrest D. Thyroid hormone receptors in chick retinal development: differential expression of mRNAs for alpha and N-terminal variant beta receptors. *Development* 1992;114:39–47.

83. Strait KA, Carlson DJ, Schwartz HL, Oppenheimer JH. Transient stimulation of myelin basic protein gene expression in differentiating cultured oligodendrocytes: a model for 3,5,3`-triiodothyronine-induced brain development. *Endocrinology* 1997;138:635–41.

84. Hagen SG, Larson RJ, Strait KA, Oppenheimer JH. A Purkinje cell protein-2 intronic thyroid hormone response element binds developmentally regulated thyroid hormone receptor-nuclear protein complexes. *J Mol Neurosci* 1996;7:245–55.

85. Ibarrola N, Rodriguez-Pena A. Hypothyroidism coordinately and transiently affects myelin protein gene expression in most rat brain regions during postnatal development. *Brain Res* 1997;752:285–93.

86. Dowling AL, Zoeller RT. Thyroid hormone of maternal origin regulates the expression of RC3/neurogranin mRNA in the fetal rat brain. *Brain Res Mol Brain Res* 2000;82:126–32.

87. Dowling AL, Iannacone EA, Zoeller RT. Maternal hypothyroidism selectively affects the expression of neuroendocrine-specific protein A messenger ribonucleic acid in the proliferative zone of the fetal rat brain cortex. *Endocrinology* 2001;142:390–9.

88. Watson JB, Sutcliffe JG, Fisher RS. Localization of the protein kinase C phosphorylation/calmodulin-binding substrate RC3 in dendritic spines of neostriatal neurons. *Proc Natl Acad Sci U S A* 1992;89:8581–5.

89. Iniguez MA, Rodriguez-Pena A, Ibarrola N, Aguilera M, Munoz A, Bernal J. Thyroid hormone regulation of RC3, a brain-specific gene encoding a protein kinase-C substrate. *Endocrinology* 1993;133:467–73.

90. Dowling AL, Martz GU, Leonard JL, Zoeller RT. Acute changes in maternal thyroid hormone induce rapid and transient changes in gene expression in fetal rat brain. *J Neurosci* 2000;20:2255–65.

91. Eayrs JT. Thyroid and central nervous development. *Sci Basis Med Annu Rev* 1966;317–39.

92. Balazs R, Kovacs S, Teichgraber P, Cocks WA, Eayrs JT. Biochemical effects of thyroid deficiency on the developing brain. *J Neurochem* 1968;15:1335–49.

93. Nicholson JL, Altman J. The effects of early hypo- and hyperthyroidism on the development of rat cerebellar cortex. I. Cell proliferation and differentiation. *Brain Res* 1972;44:13–23.

94. Montoro MN. Management of hypothyroidism during pregnancy. *Clin Obstet Gynecol* 1997;40:65–80.

95. Glinoer D, Soto MF, Bourdoux P, Lejeune B, Delange F, Lemone M, *et al*. Pregnancy in patients with mild thyroid abnormalities: maternal and neonatal repercussions. *J Clin Endocrinol Metab* 1991;73:421–7.

96. Leung AS, Millar LK, Koonings PP, Montoro M, Mestman JH. Perinatal outcome in hypothyroid pregnancies. *Obstet Gynecol* 1993;81:349–53.

97. Davis LE, Leveno KJ, Cunningham FG. Hypothyroidism complicating pregnancy. *Obstet Gynecol* 1988;72:108–12.

98. Stagnaro-Green A. Recognizing, understanding, and treating postpartum thyroiditis. *Endocrinol Metab Clin North Am* 2000;29:417–30,ix.

99.   National Institutes of Health and Human Development USA. Hypothyroidism during pregnancy linked to lower IQ for child: early diagnosis and treatment may help. *Front Fetal Health* 1999;1:16.

100. Morreale de Escober G, Obregon MJ, Escobar del Rey F. Is neuropsychological development related to maternal hypothyroidism or to maternal hypothyroxinemia? *J Clin Endocrinol Metab* 2000;85:3975–87.

101. Pop VJ, Brouwers EP, Vader HL, de Vijlder JJ, Vulsma T. Maternal thyroid function during early pregnancy and neurodevelopment of the offspring. *Clin Endocrinol (Oxf)* 2003;59:282–8.

102. Smith SC, Bold AM. Interpretation of *in-vitro* thyroid function tests during pregnancy. *Br J Obstet Gynaecol* 1983;90:532–4.

103. Girling JC. Thyroid disease and pregnancy. *Br J Hosp Med* 1996;56:316–20.

104. Mandel SJ, Larsen PR, Seely EW, Brent GA. Increased need for thyroxine during pregnancy in women with primary hypothyroidism. *N Engl J Med* 1990;323:91–6.

105. Glinoer D. Pregnancy and iodine. *Thyroid* 2001;11:471–81.

106. Calvo R, Morreale de Escobar G, Escobar del Rey F, Obregon MJ. Maternal diabetes mellitus, a rat model for nonthyroidal illness: correction of hypothyroxinemia with thyroxine treatment does not improve fetal thyroid hormone status. *Thyroid* 1997;7:79–87.

107. Kaplan MM. Monitoring thyroxine treatment during pregnancy. *Thyroid* 1992;2:147–52.

108. Girling JC, de Swiet M. The thyroid and pregnancy. *Br J Obstet Gynaecol* 1994;101:180–1.

109. Chan S, Gittoes N, Franklyn J, Kilby M. Iodine intake in pregnancy. *Lancet* 2001;358:583–4.

7

Antioxidants for pre-eclampsia

Lucy Chappell

INTRODUCTION

The search for an effective preventive therapy for pre-eclampsia is proving to be increasingly complex and challenging. Pre-eclampsia occurs in 4–6% of deliveries, and is an important contributor to maternal and perinatal morbidity[1] and mortality[2] in the UK and the developing world. Worldwide, eclampsia is believed to account for approximately 50 000 maternal deaths per year, with pre-eclampsia probably contributing a similar number.[3] With delivery remaining the only known cure, pre-eclampsia is associated with approximately 40% of all elective preterm deliveries in developed countries[4] and contributes significantly to premature infants with a birth-weight of less than 1500 g.[5] Improved prediction, prevention and treatment of pre-eclampsia and its complications is recognised as essential to the reduction of maternal deaths from this disease.

The disease of theories

Although the discovery of an association between convulsions in pregnancy and albuminuria was made as recently as the 19th century, the disease had been recognised many centuries earlier. One of the first references to eclampsia comes from pre-Hippocratic Greece in the 1st century BC: 'in pregnancy, drowsiness and headache accompanied by heaviness and convulsions, is generally bad'.[6] Management strategies over the centuries have included women being 'blistered, bled, purged, lavaged, irrigated, punctured, starved, sedated, anaesthetised, paralysed, tranquilised'.[7] Although some of these therapeutic regimens may seem illogical today, as Chesley commented in 1975 at the Workshop on Hypertension in Pregnancy: 'We should remember that each of the treatments was rational in the light of some hypothesis as to the cause or nature of eclampsia. That is more than we can say for present day management, which is empiric, too often symptomatic, and in some respects, based upon imitative magic'.[8]

The mainstay of management for pre-eclampsia has, for many years, focused on control of the clinical manifestations (e.g. hypertension), with delivery of the baby as definitive treatment. In the last 20 years, significant breakthroughs in our knowledge of the underlying pathophysiology have led to a shift in emphasis towards preventing or delaying the disease. With evidence accumulating that the disease process in pre-eclampsia is initiated many weeks or months prior to the onset of hypertension and proteinuria, it was increasingly recognised that prophylactic therapies should be started before the clinical manifestations of the established disease. Prevention of a disease is easiest when the aetiology and pathophysiology are fully understood and a screening test exists to identify high-risk individuals who can be targeted for prophylactic therapy. In pre-eclampsia, however, difficulties in elucidating this information and in developing a predictive test for use in clinical practice has led to trials of preventive treatment being undertaken prior to full understanding of the disease mechanisms. In addition, the multifactorial aetiology and the heterogeneous nature of the syndrome could imply that a single therapy would not be effective in all cases of pre-eclampsia. Despite the enormous effort, no one treatment is currently used in widespread clinical practice. The proposal that pre-eclampsia can be considered as the extreme end of the range of maternal adaptation to pregnancy has led some to conclude that a single specific predictive test or single preventive effective measure could not be devised.

Several lines of evidence suggest that pre-eclampsia is associated with a state of oxidative stress, raising the possibility of prevention by antioxidant supplementation. This chapter explores the evidence for oxidative stress in the disease and considers the rationale for prophylactic therapy with antioxidants.

THE PATHOGENESIS OF PRE-ECLAMPSIA

Pre-eclampsia is commonly perceived by clinicians as a syndrome comprising hypertension, proteinuria and oedema in pregnancy. It is now clear that these are the endpoints of an endothelial cell disorder, representing the final clinical manifestations of a disease that may have been developing for weeks.[9] There appear to be a number of potential pathways to the development of pre-eclampsia, contributing to the wide variation in presentation and severity of the clinical disease.

The role of the placenta

One major predisposing factor to pre-eclampsia is abnormal placentation, associated with reduced perfusion of the placenta. In the nonpregnant state, the spiral arteries offer high resistance to flow. In normal pregnancy, extravillous trophoblast cells from the developing placenta invade the spiral arteries of the maternal myometrial and decidual layers.[10] Over the first 20–24 weeks of pregnancy, there is loss of the smooth muscle of the artery wall, leading to dilatation of the spiral arteries. This remodelling enables the establishment of a low-pressure, high-flow system to the intervillous space, the site of oxygen and nutrient exchange to the fetus.

In pre-eclampsia, trophoblast invasion is limited to the most superficial portion of the spiral arteries, with little invasion of the myometrium.[11] Additionally, atherotic changes may be found in the spiral arteries,[12] with lesions similar to those observed in coronary artery disease. The spiral arteries remain high-resistance vessels and this can be detected clinically by the finding of abnormal flow velocity waveforms as assessed by Doppler ultrasound of the uterine arteries.

Although the exact mechanisms of impaired trophoblast invasion and spiral artery remodelling in pre-eclampsia are still to be fully understood, the consequences include impaired blood flow in the intervillous space[13] and microthrombi within vessels.[14] It is believed that there are localised regions of ischaemia and hypoxia in the placenta during the second half of gestation,[15] with the resulting production of reactive oxygen species and free radicals in the placenta.

As abnormal placentation is found in intrauterine growth restriction and is not exclusive to pre-eclampsia, it is now recognised that additional susceptibility factors are involved in the development of pre-eclampsia. These include underlying maternal disorders such as essential hypertension, diabetes or antiphospholipid syndrome, or less well characterised contributions from maternal or paternal genes. This has led to the proposal that pre-eclampsia occurs when placental dysfunction is marked or when the maternal response to placentally derived factors or 'debris' is excessive.[16]

Endothelial cell activation in pre-eclampsia

Involvement of the endothelium in pre-eclampsia largely explains the clinical manifestations of the disease because this cell layer is present in all organ systems involved. A healthy endothelium has many roles, including regulation of vascular tone and inflammatory reactions, and maintenance of the integrity of the vessel wall. Activation of the endothelial cell layer leads to vasoconstriction, increased permeability, and adherence of prothrombotic factors to the vessel wall. This results in hypertension, proteinuria and a procoagulant state, all features of the maternal syndrome of pre-eclampsia.

Recognition of endothelial involvement came initially with the description in 1959 of glomerular capillary endotheliosis in the kidney of women with pre-eclampsia.[17] Further evidence for endothelial cell activation has now been obtained from three main sources: structural changes reported in the placental bed and peripheral vessels; functional disturbances as demonstrated by impaired endothelium dependent vasodilatation; and enhanced expression of circulating cell adhesion molecules and procoagulant factors.[18]

THE ROLE OF OXIDATIVE STRESS

Although there is clear evidence for placental dysfunction and endothelial cell activation in pre-eclampsia, interest has now turned to the possible factors mediating the interaction between the two. It now appears that it is the interaction with maternal constitutional factors (e.g. genetics, obesity, vascular disease) that determines development of the disease.[19] Oxidative stress has been proposed as providing the link between abnormal placentation and maternal manifestations of pre-eclampsia.[20]

Oxidative stress is defined as disequilibrium between antioxidant defence systems and free radical synthesis in favour of the latter.[21] Free radicals, the by-products of many normal physiological processes, are usually contained by the spectrum of water and lipid soluble antioxidants in the body. Although free radicals have important physiological functions in cellular signalling, regulation of blood pressure and many other functions, excess production may lead to cellular damage and dysfunction. Increased synthesis and production of free radicals have now been implicated in a wide variety of diseases, including many characterised by decreased perfusion (e.g. coronary artery disease).

Pro-oxidants: free radicals and reactive oxygen species

Reactive oxygen species is a collective term for oxygen-derived free radicals together with other reactive derivatives of oxygen such as hydrogen peroxide that do not contain unpaired electrons. Table 1 includes the most important reactive oxygen species and antioxidant defences most commonly investigated, particularly in pre-eclampsia.

Excess reactive oxygen species may be deleterious in a number of ways, either directly because of DNA and mitochondrial damage or by catalysing the production of other harmful substances, such as lipid peroxides, which are particularly toxic to the endothelium, by stimulating leucocyte activation,[22] promoting thrombus formation,[23] and increasing endothelial cell permeability.[24] Lipid peroxides can inhibit vasorelaxation,[25] and potentiate the response to vasoconstrictors.[26] Other reactive oxygen species such as superoxide anions may also react with nitric oxide, a vasodilator, to form damaging peroxynitrite anions,[27] which can induce both cell necrosis and apoptosis,[28] promoting leakage of proteins from the intravascular compartment, and are also capable of initiating lipid peroxidation.

Antioxidants

An arsenal of intracellular and extracellular antioxidants exists to protect against free radical damage. Enzymatic antioxidants include superoxide dismutase, catalase and glutathione peroxidase.

Table 1 *Reactive oxygen species and antioxidants in biological systems*

Reactive oxygen species	Antioxidant defences
Radicals	*Nonenzymatic*
Superoxide $O_2^{\cdot-}$	Ascorbate (vitamin C), α-tocopherol (vitamin E), urate
Hydroxyl $OH^{\cdot}$	β-carotene (vitamin A), glutathione
	Plasma proteins (e.g. caeruloplasmin, transferrin)
Nonradicals	*Enzymatic*
Hydrogen peroxide H_2O_2	Superoxide dismutases
Ozone O_3	Catalase
Peroxynitrite $ONOO^-$	Glutathione peroxidases

Superoxide dismutase has a central role in competing with nitric oxide for superoxide anions, thus preventing peroxynitrite formation and promoting the vasorelaxant action of nitric oxide.

Nonenzymatic antioxidants include water-soluble compounds such as vitamin C (ascorbic acid), thiols, uric acid and glutathione. Lipid soluble antioxidants include vitamin E (alpha-tocopherol), which may be found within the cell membrane or lipoproteins. Alpha-tocopherol has an important role in preventing the chain reaction of lipid peroxidation by scavenging lipid peroxyl radicals. As alpha-tocopherol accepts the unpaired electron from the lipid peroxyl radical, it becomes a radical itself, with potentially pro-oxidant properties. However, it can be converted back to its active form by reduced ascorbate.[29] An ascorbyl radical is produced in this reaction, but this is much less reactive than an alpha-tocopherol radical.[30] The ascorbyl radical can be converted back into the ascorbate form by both enzymatic and chemical reduction, thus minimising its pro-oxidant potential. This emphasises the need for adequate concentrations of ascorbate to be present for alpha-tocopherol to function as an antioxidant.

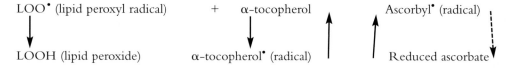

Vitamin C can react with a variety of reactive oxygen species including superoxide and hydroxyl anions and can also scavenge nonradical species such as peroxynitrite. Ascorbate is considered to be the most effective aqueous phase antioxidant in human blood plasma.[31]

Evidence for oxidative stress in pre-eclampsia

A variety of studies have evaluated pro- and antioxidants in the placenta and maternal circulation of women with pre-eclampsia and the evidence for oxidative stress in summarised in Table 2.[32–57] This suggests that oxidative stress in pre-eclampsia is a consequence of increased free radical synthesis coupled with impaired antioxidant capacity. In 2002, decreased dietary intake of anti-oxidants was also proposed as an additional risk factor, with women consuming less than 85 mg of vitamin C daily having double the risk of pre-eclampsia compared with other pregnant women.[57]

Implications for oxidative stress in the placenta

Although there is good evidence for oxidative stress in the placenta, the short half-life of reactive oxygen species necessitates a specific mechanism for the distant activation of endothelial cells in

Table 2 *Evidence for oxidative stress in pre-eclampsia*

Indices of oxidative stress	Placenta	Maternal blood
Pro-oxidants		
Superoxide concentrations	Increased[32]	
Lipid peroxidation products		
Malondialdehyde	Increased[33]	Increased[44]
8-epi-prostaglandin-$F_{2\alpha}$	Increased[34,35]	Increased[45,46]
Protein oxidation products		
Protein carbonyls	Increased[36]	Increased[47]
Nitrotyrosine staining	Increased[37,38]	Increased[48]
Mitochondria	Abnormal in appearance[39]	
	Increased in number[33]	
	Increased malondialdehyde[33]	
LDLs		
Small dense LDLs		Increased[49]
Autoantibodies to oxidized LDLs		Increased[50]
Antioxidants		
Ascorbic acid	Decreased[40]	Decreased[51]
Depletion of endogenous ascorbate		Increased[52]
α-tocopherol	Variable reports[41,42]	Variable reports[51,53]
Uric acid		Increased[54]
β-carotene		Decreased[51]
Glutathione		Decreased[55]
Ratio free: oxidised thiols		Decreased[56]
Superoxide dismutase	Decreased[38,42]	Decreased in RBC[57]
Glutathione peroxidase	Decreased[43]	

LDL = low–density lioproteins; RBC = red blood cells

the maternal circulation. A number of possible factors have been proposed, including oxidised low-density lipoprotein[58] and other lipid peroxidation products, together with cytokines such as tumour necrosis factor-alpha, released under hypoxic conditions from the placenta.[59]

Interest has also focused on activation of neutrophils during passage through the intervillous space, mediated by exposure to locally synthesised lipid peroxides and tumour necrosis factor-alpha.[60] Activated neutrophils produce a variety of substances that are damaging to the endothelium, including superoxide radicals[61] and cytokines. This leads to increased neutrophil adherence and loss of integrity of the endothelium. The systemic inflammatory response has now been characterised in normal pregnancy, with greater activation in pre-eclampsia.[62]

A further candidate for mediating the transfer of oxidative stress from the placental intervillous space to the maternal systemic circulation is microfragments from the syncytiotrophoblast. It has been proposed that the normal deportation of placental debris into the maternal circulation is further enhanced in pre-eclampsia, perhaps as a consequence of oxidative stress in the placenta stimulating excessive apoptosis or necrosis.[16]

Figure 1 shows the proposed pathways linking the synthesis of reactive oxygen species in the placenta to leucocyte and maternal endothelial cell activation.

Potential antioxidant mechanisms of vitamins C and E

With the substantial body of evidence outlined above for placental and maternal oxidative stress in women with pre-eclampsia, attention has turned to the potential use of antioxidants. Vitamins C and E have been studied in some detail both *in vitro* and in a number of disease states, and have

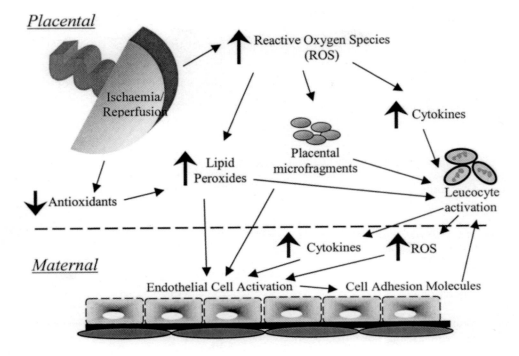

Figure 1 *Consequences of oxidative stress in the placenta*

been shown to exert their antioxidant effects through a wide variety of different mechanisms, as outlined below. *In vitro* studies of vitamin C have demonstrated:

- direct and rapid trapping of free radicals in the aqueous phase[63]

- inhibition of low-density lipoprotein oxidation in vascular endothelial cells[64]

- recycling of alpha-tocopherol in low-density lipoproteins[65]

- inhibition of neutrophil–endothelial cell activation[66]

- lipid peroxides decreased to concentrations similar to those found in normal placentas when infused into the maternal side of placentas from pre-eclamptic women.[67]

In vitro studies of vitamin E have shown:

- scavenging of highly reactive lipid peroxyl and alkoxyl radicals, preventing the propagation of lipid peroxidation[68]

- modulation of apoptosis by alpha-tocopherol in smooth muscle cells[69] and endothelial cells[70]

- decreased production of superoxide radicals and cytokine production[71]

- significant attenuation of lipid-peroxide-induced vascular resistance, using a placental perfusion model.[72]

Evidence is also accumulating from *in vivo* studies of vitamin C supplementation, which have demonstrated:

- decreased concentrations in 8-epi-prostaglandin-$F_{2\alpha}$, held to be the most reliable marker of lipid peroxidation, in smokers[73]

- improvement in brachial artery dilatation in smokers[74] and people with coronary artery disease[75]

- improvement in forearm blood flow in people with type I[76] or type II diabetes[77] or essential hypertension[78]

- markedly reduced plasma concentrations of circulating apoptotic endothelial microparticles.[79]

In vivo studies of vitamin E supplementation have shown:

- decreased platelet aggregation[80]

- improvement in endothelium-dependent vasodilatation in postmenopausal women,[80] smokers,[81] hypercholesterolaemic persons[82] and people with angina,[83] with a parallel fall in markers of lipid oxidation.

Interaction between vitamins C and E

Although both ascorbic acid and alpha-tocopherol have been shown to have powerful antioxidant (and other) properties in isolation, their interaction and potentiation provide a strong argument for co-administration in trials of supplementation. Early *in vitro* studies demonstrated that the combination of antioxidants was much more effective in suppressing membrane lipid peroxidation than the sum of both vitamins alone.[84] The results of work published in 2000 demonstrated a synergistic effect of vitamins C and E in the placenta, with a combination of the antioxidants achieving complete inhibition of lipid peroxidation in human placental mitochondria,[85] an effect more pronounced that that of either vitamin alone.

The Antioxidant Supplementation in Atherosclerosis Prevention study published in 2000[86] provided convincing *in vivo* evidence for the synergistic effect of therapy with vitamins C and E, a combination of which was more effective in decreasing plasma markers of lipid peroxidation than vitamin C alone. In the same study, intima–media thickness of the carotid artery progressed significantly less in those on combination vitamin C and E treatment, while no effect was seen in those taking vitamin C or E alone.[87]

USE OF VITAMINS C AND E IN PREGNANT WOMEN

Before vitamins C and E could be used in pregnant women, data on their safety needed to be examined. Despite 86–92% of women in the USA taking prenatal multivitamin supplementation,[88] knowledge of the individual or collective benefits or disadvantages of this intervention are surprisingly scarce. A decreased risk of preterm delivery and infant low birthweight in women taking prenatal vitamin supplements has been reported.[89] The latter observation was supported by the study by Mathews *et al.*,[90] who reported a 50.8 g (4.6–97.0 g) increase in birthweight for each logarithmic milligram increase in vitamin C among women who did not receive supplements.

The recommended dietary allowance for these vitamins in pregnancy is debatable owing to difficulties in determining requirements. It is defined as 'the average daily dietary intake level that is sufficient to meet the nutrient requirement of nearly all healthy individuals in a group'. Food sources of vitamin C include fruit and vegetables, with citrus fruits, tomatoes and potatoes being major contributors,[91] and some foods also containing added vitamin C as an antioxidant. Growing conditions, season of the year, storage and cooking practices may all affect the vitamin C content of food. The main dietary sources of vitamin E are edible vegetable oils, such as sunflower oil.[92] Vitamin E is also present in unprocessed cereal grains, nuts, fruits, vegetables and fatty portions of meat.

It was argued in 1999 that scientific evidence indicating decreased risk of certain diseases with antioxidant intake in nonpregnant states suggests that the current recommended dietary allowances (70 mg/day for vitamin C and 10 mg/day for vitamin E)[93] are not sufficient to protect against such diseases[94] and that higher allowances may be appropriate. With this in mind, the US National Academy of Sciences introduced in 2000 a new reference intake: the daily tolerable upper intake level.[95] For pregnant women, these are 2000 mg/day of vitamin C and 1515 iu/day of vitamin E. For the mother, adverse effects of these doses of vitamins are rare.

There is no evidence for any teratogenic effect of either vitamin C or E.[96] After reports of a reduction to background rates of congenital malformation occurrence in diabetic animals treated with antioxidants,[97] the use of vitamin C and E has been proposed as a possible antiteratogenic treatment for pregnant women with diabetes mellitus.[98]

Antioxidant trials in established pre-eclampsia

In view of the evidence that decreased antioxidant reserves were a characteristic of pre-eclampsia, some groups have investigated the potential use of antioxidant supplementation in the management of this disease. Stratta et al.[99] reported a nonrandomised trial of varying doses of supplementation with vitamin E. Fourteen women with severe early-onset established pre-eclampsia were treated with 100–300 mg/day of vitamin E and were compared with 22 women managed with conventional therapy alone. While a significant, although small, increase in plasma alpha-tocopherol concentrations was observed one week after commencement of therapy in the treated group, other blood and urine parameters were no different between the two groups. Doppler indices of uteroplacental and fetoplacental waveforms were also similar. The time to delivery was similar in both groups, as was the fetal mortality rate. The high fetal mortality rate (36%) in infants of a mean gestational age of 30 weeks was surprising, questioning the relevance of this study to other groups. The authors concluded that both the dose and the timing of supplementation were crucial, and that the earlier introduction of therapy using possibly higher doses should be tested.

Gulmezoglu et al.[100] reported a randomised, double blind, placebo controlled trial of antioxidants in 56 women with severe established pre-eclampsia, using 800 iu vitamin E, 1000 mg vitamin C and 200 mg allopurinol. They demonstrated a trend towards later delivery in the treated group, together with a significant decrease in the plasma uric acid concentration and a significant increase in plasma vitamin E level. The authors similarly concluded that further randomised trials, with earlier initiation of therapy or different combinations of antioxidants, would be worth while.

Clinical approaches to preventing pre-eclampsia

A wide number of interventions have been tried, including calcium,[101] magnesium,[102] zinc[103] and rhubarb,[104] but the largest trials have focused on the use of aspirin. In a meta-analysis of 42 randomised controlled trials, involving over 32 000 women, low-dose aspirin was associated with a 15% reduction in the occurrence of pre-eclampsia, with a similar reduction in the risk of death of the baby.[105] However, in women identified as being at higher risk of developing pre-eclampsia by abnormal uterine artery Doppler waveforms, a meta-analysis of five randomised controlled trials reported a 45% reduction in pre-eclampsia,[106] demonstrating the benefit of targeting the intervention. Use of this screening method thus enables a reduction in the number needed to treat with aspirin to prevent one case of pre-eclampsia from 89 to 16. However, neither uterine artery Doppler screening nor aspirin for unselected women is currently in widespread use in the UK.

Antioxidants for the prevention of pre-eclampsia

A study published in 1999[107] tested the hypothesis that early supplementation with antioxidants may be effective in decreasing oxidative stress, improving endothelial and placental function, and preventing pre-eclampsia. This was a randomised, double blind placebo controlled trial of vitamins C and E supplementation in women at increased risk of pre-eclampsia, who were recruited if they fulfilled one of two criteria for this increased risk:

- an abnormal uterine artery Doppler waveform at 18–22 weeks of gestation

- pre-eclampsia in the previous pregnancy requiring delivery before 37 weeks of gestation.

The women were randomised to 1000 g vitamin C and 400 iu of vitamin E per day or to two placebo tablets. Those who were identified by abnormal Doppler waveforms were intentionally withdrawn at 24 weeks of gestation if their second Doppler screening at 24 weeks was normal. In total, 283 women formed the 'intention to treat' group, with 160 completing the study to delivery, as shown in the trial profile (Figure 2).

Blood samples were taken every four weeks from recruitment until delivery for assessment of the plasminogen activator inhibitor (PAI)-1/PAI-2 ratio, and for other markers of placental function and oxidative stress. PAI-1 is a marker of endothelial cell activation and is known to be elevated in pre-eclampsia. PAI-2 is synthesised by the placenta and decreases with placental dysfunction. The PAI-1/PAI-2 ratio falls in normal pregnancy, but remains elevated in pre-eclampsia owing to endothelial cell activation and placental insufficiency.[108] This ratio, an index of the disease process, was chosen as the primary outcome measure for the trial because it was anticipated that, if this study demonstrated an improvement in a biochemical marker of the disease, then a much larger multicentre trial would be required to demonstrate a change in clinical outcome.

However, the trial demonstrated that vitamin C and E supplementation was associated with a significantly reduced occurrence of pre-eclampsia in the treated group (Figure 3). By intention-to-treat analysis, 24 of 142 (17%) women in the placebo group developed pre-eclampsia compared with 11 of 141 (8%) in the vitamins C and E group. Analysis by those who completed the study showed a more pronounced effect, with 21 of 81 (26%) women in the placebo group developing pre-eclampsia compared with 6 of 79 (8%) in the supplemented group.

This reduction in pre-eclampsia was mirrored by significant changes in the PAI-1/PAI-2 ratio, with values in the treated group lowered towards those in a low-risk group of pregnant women with normal outcomes who were recruited simultaneously (Figure 4). Similar improvement towards the low-risk cohort values was demonstrated in other biochemical indices of the disease, including markers of oxidative stress and placental function.[109] There were fewer small for gestational age infants in the vitamin group (23%) than in the placebo group (32%) by intention-to-treat analysis, but this difference did not achieve significance ($P = 0.12$), neither was the study powered to do so.

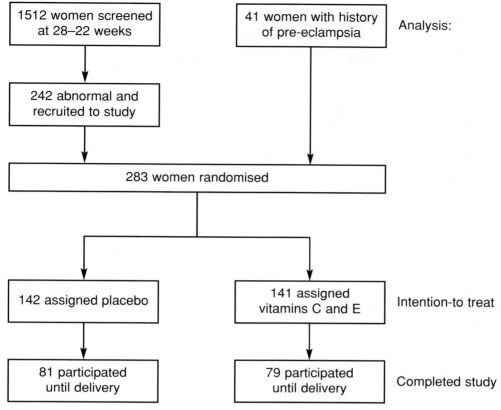

Figure 2 *Trial profile*

THE NEXT STEP

This first report of the benefit of vitamin C and E supplementation in the prevention of pre-eclampsia supports the hypothesis that oxidative stress may play an important role in the pathophysiology of this disease. This study was performed in women principally identified as being at risk by abnormal uteroplacental Doppler waveforms. Multicentre studies are now in progress to determine whether all primiparous women should be offered prophylactic treatment and to assess the potential benefits in other high-risk groups. These will include further evaluation of neonatal morbidity and longer term follow-up of the offspring. In addition, other possible benefits of vitamin C and E supplementation may be explored. Preterm premature rupture of the membranes is the leading identifiable antecedent of preterm birth. With its occurrence being higher in women with low plasma ascorbic acid concentrations[110] and decreased amniotic fluid concentrations of ascorbic acid,[111] there is growing interest in the potential for vitamin C supplementation in the prevention of preterm premature rupture of the membranes and its consequences.

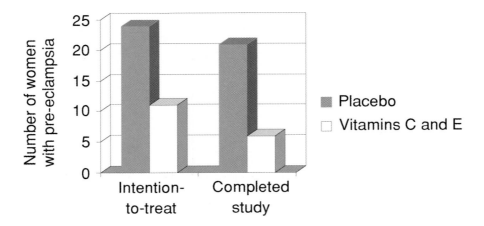

Figure 3 *Clinical outcome in a randomised trial of antioxidants in women at increased risk of pre-eclampsia*

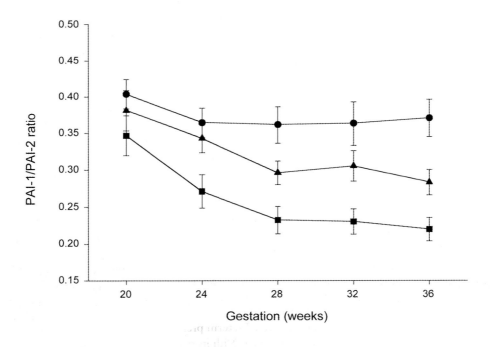

Figure 4 *Longitudinal evaluation of plasminogen activator inhibitor (PAI)-1/PAI-2 ratio in plasma from low-risk women (■) and from women at increased risk of pre-eclampsia in placebo (●) and vitamin supplemented (?) groups; data are given as mean ± standard error of the mean; axes do not include zero (reproduced from: Chappell LC, Seed PT, Kelly FJ, Briley A, Hunt BJ, Charnock-Jones DS, et al. Vitamin C and E supplementation in women at risk of preeclampsia is associated with changes in indices of oxidative stress and placental function. Am J Obstet Gynecol 2002;187:777–84,[109] with permission from Mosby)*

Previous small studies of preventive therapy for pre-eclampsia have shown promise, whereas subsequent multicentre trials have failed to confirm the same degree of benefit. It is therefore essential that the results of the multicentre trials currently being undertaken are awaited before vitamins C and E are introduced into clinical practice. However, the recognition of oxidative stress as the probable convergence point in the pathogenesis of the disease offers a prospect of prophylaxis against pre-eclampsia.

References

1. Waterstone M, Bewley S, Wolfe C. Incidence and predictors of severe obstetric morbidity: case–control study. *BMJ* 2001;322:1089–93.
2. *Confidential Enquiry into Maternal Deaths in the United Kingdom. Why Mothers Die. Report for 1997–1999.* London: RCOG Press 2001.
3. Duley L. Maternal mortality associated with hypertensive disorders of pregnancy in Africa, Asia, Latin America and the Caribbean. *Br J Obstet Gynaecol* 1992;99:547–53.
4. Meis PJ, Goldenberg RL, Mercer BM, Iams JD, Moawad AH, Miodovnik M, *et al.* The preterm prediction study: risk factors for indicated preterm births. *Am J Obstet Gynecol* 1998;178:562–7.
5. Ales KL, Frayer W, Hawks G, Auld PM, Druzin ML. Development and validation of a multivariate predictor of mortality in very low birth weight. *J Clin Epidemiol* 1988;41:1095–103.
6. Chesley LC. A short history of eclampsia. *Obstet Gynecol* 1974;43:599–602.
7. Zuspan FP, Ward MC. Treatment of eclampsia. *South Med J* 1964;57:954–9.
8. Lindheimer MD, Roberts JM, Cunningham FG, Chesley L. *Chesley's Hypertensive Disorders in Pregnancy.* 2nd ed. Stamford: Appleton and Lange; 1999.
9. Roberts JM, Taylor RN, Musci TJ, Rodgers GM, Hubel CA, McLaughlin MK. Preeclampsia: an endothelial cell disorder. *Am J Obstet Gynecol* 1989;161:1200–4.
10. Pijnenborg R, Bland JM, Robertson WB, Brosens I. Uteroplacental arterial changes related to interstitial trophoblast migration in early human pregnancy. *Placenta* 1983;4:397–413.
11. Meekins JW, Pijnenborg R, Hanssens M, McFayden IR, van Assche A. A study of placental bed spiral arteries and trophoblast invasion in normal and severe pre-eclamptic pregnancies. *Br J Obstet Gynaecol* 1994;101:669–74.
12. Pijnenborg R, Anthony J, Davey DA, Rees A, Tiltman A, Vercruysse L, *et al.* Placental bed spiral arteries in the hypertensive disorders of pregnancy. *Br J Obstet Gynaecol* 1991;98:648–55.
13. Kaar K, Jouppila P, Kuikka J, Luotola H, Toivanen J, Rekonen A. Intervillous blood flow in normal and complicated late pregnancy measured by means of an intravenous 133Xe method. *Acta Obstet Gynecol Scand* 1980;59:7–10.
14. Salafia CM, Pezzullo JC, Lopez-Zeno JA, Simmens S, Minior VK, Vintzileos AM. Placental pathologic features of preterm preeclampsia. *Am J Obstet Gynecol* 1995;173:1097–105.
15. Graham CH, Postovit LM, Park H, Canning MT, Fitzpatrick TE. Adriana and Luisa Castellucci award lecture 1999: role of oxygen in the regulation of trophoblast gene expression and invasion. *Placenta* 2000;21:443–50.
16. Redman CW, Sargent IL. Placental debris, oxidative stress and pre-eclampsia. *Placenta* 2000;21:597–602.
17. Spargo BH, McCartney C, Winemiller R. Glomerular capillary endotheliosis in toxaemia of pregnancy. *Arch Pathol* 1959;13:593–9.

18. Roberts JM. Endothelial dysfunction in preeclampsia. *Semin Reprod Endocrinol* 1998;16:5–15.

19. Roberts JM, Cooper DW. Pathogenesis and genetics of pre-eclampsia. *Lancet* 2001;357:53–6.

20. Roberts JM, Hubel CA. Is oxidative stress the link in the two-stage model of pre-eclampsia? *Lancet* 1999;354:788–9.

21. Sies H, editor. *Oxidative Stress II: Oxidants and Antioxidants.* New York: Academic Press; 1991.

22. Gorog P. Activation of human blood monocytes by oxidized polyunsaturated fatty acids: a possible mechanism for the generation of lipid peroxides in the circulation. *Int J Exp Pathol* 1991;72:227–37.

23. Barrowcliffe TW, Gray E, Kerry PJ, Gutteridge JMC. Triglyceride-rich lipoproteins are responsible for thrombin generation induced by lipid peroxides. *Thromb Haemost* 1984;52:7–10.

24. Granger DN, Rutili G, McCord JM. Superoxide radicals in feline intestinal ischaemia. *Gastroenterology* 1981;81:22–9.

25. Hubel CA, Griggs KC, McLaughlin MK. Lipid peroxidation and altered vascular function in vitamin E-deficient rats. *Am J Physiol* 1989;256:H2577–83.

26. Hubel CA, Davidge ST, McLaughlin MK. Lipid hydroperoxides potentiate mesenteric artery vasoconstrictor responses. *Free Radic Biol Med* 1993;14:397–407.

27. Beckman JS, Koppenol WH. Nitric oxide, superoxide, and peroxynitrite: the good, the bad and the ugly. *Am J Physiol* 1996;271:C1424–37.

28. Sandau K, Pfeilschifter J, Brune B. The balance between nitric oxide and superoxide determines apoptotic and necrotic death of rat mesangial cells. *J Immunol* 1997;158:4938–46.

29. Bowry VW, Mohr D, Cleary J, Stocker R. Prevention of tocopherol-mediated peroxidation in ubiquinol 10-free human low-density lipoprotein. *J Biol Chem* 1995;270:5756–63.

30. Buettner GR. The pecking order of free radicals and antioxidants: lipid peroxidation, alpha-tocopherol and ascorbate. *Arch Biochem Biophys* 1993;300:535–43.

31. Frei B, England L, Ames BN. Ascorbate is an outstanding antioxidant in human blood plasma. *Proc Natl Acad Sci U S A* 1989;86:6377–81.

32. Sikkema JM, van Rijn BB, Franx A, Bruinse HW, de Roos R, Stroes ES, et al. Placental superoxide is increased in pre-eclampsia. *Placenta* 2001;22:304–8.

33. Wang Y, Walsh SW. Placental mitochondria as a source of oxidative stress in pre-eclampsia. *Placenta* 1998;19:581–6.

34. Staff AC, Halvorsen B, Ranheim T, Henriksen T. Elevated level of free 8-iso-prostaglandin F2alpha in the decidua basalis of women with preeclampsia. *Am J Obstet Gynecol* 1999;181:1211–15.

35. Walsh SW, Vaughan JE, Wang Y, Roberts LJ 2nd. Placental isoprostane is significantly increased in preeclampsia. *FASEB J* 2000;14:1289–96.

36. Zusterzeel PL, Rutten H, Roelofs HM, Peters WH, Steegers EA. Protein carbonyls in decidua and placenta of pre-eclamptic women as markers for oxidative stress. *Placenta* 2001;22:213–19.

37. Myatt L, Rosenfield RB, Eis ALW, Brockman DE, Greer I, Lyall F. Nitrotyrosine residues in placenta: evidence of peroxynitrite formation and action. *Hypertension* 1996;28:488–93.

38. Many A, Hubel CA, Fisher SJ, Roberts JM, Zhou Y. Invasive cytotrophoblasts manifest evidence of oxidative stress in preeclampsia. *Am J Pathol* 2000;156:321–31.

39. Shanklin DR, Sibai BM. Ultrastructural aspects of preeclampsia II: Mitochondrial changes. *Am J Obstet Gynecol* 1990;163:943–53.

40. Mutlu-Turkoglu U, Ademoglu E, Ibrahimoglu L, Aykac-Toker G, Uysal M. Imbalance between lipid peroxidation and antioxidant status in preeclampsia. *Gynecol Obstet Invest* 1998;46:37–40.

41.   Wang Y, Walsh SW. Antioxidant activities and mRNA expression of superoxide dismutase, catalase, and glutathione peroxidase in normal and preeclamptic placentas. *J Soc Gynecol Investig* 1996;3:179–84.

42.   Poranen A-K, Ekblad U, Uotila P, Ahotupa M. Lipid peroxidation and antioxidants in normal and pre-eclamptic pregnancies. *Placenta* 1996;17:401–5.

43.   Walsh SW, Wang Y. Deficient glutathione peroxidase activity in preeclampsia is associated with increased placental production of thromboxane and lipid peroxides. *Am J Obstet Gynecol* 1993;169:1456–61.

44.   Hubel CA, McLaughlin MK, Evans RW, Hauth BA, Sims CJ, Roberts JM. Fasting serum triglycerides, free fatty acids, and malondialdehyde are increased in preeclampsia, are positively correlated, and decrease within 48 hours post partum. *Am J Obstet Gynecol* 1996;174:975–82.

45.   Barden A, Beilin LJ, Ritchie J, Croft KD, Walters BN, Michael CA. Plasma and urinary 8-isoprostane as an indicator of lipid peroxidation in pre-eclampsia and normal pregnancy. *Clin Sci* 1996;91:711–18.

46.   McKinney ET, Shouri R, Hunt RS, Ahokas RA, Sibai BM. Plasma, urinary, and salivary 8-epi-prostaglandin F2 alpha levels in normotensive and preeclamptic pregnancies *Am J Obstet Gynecol* 2000;183:874–7.

47.   Zusterzeel PL, Mulder TP, Peters WH, Wiseman SA, Steegers EA. Plasma protein carbonyls in nonpregnant, healthy pregnant and preeclamptic women. *Free Radic Res* 2000;33:471–6.

48.   Roggensack AM, Zhang Y, Davidge ST. Evidence for peroxynitrite formation in the vasculature of women with preeclampsia. *Hypertension* 1999;33:83–9.

49.   Sattar N, Bendomir A, Berry C, Shepherd J, Greer IA, Packard CJ. Lipoprotein subfraction concentrations in pre-eclampsia: pathogenic parallels to atherosclerosis. *Obstet Gynaecol* 1997;89:403–8.

50.   Uotila J, Solakivi T, Jaakkola O, Tuimala R, Lehtimaki T. Antibodies against copper-oxidised and malondialdehyde-modified low density lipoproteins in pre-eclampsia pregnancies. *Br J Obstet Gynaecol* 1998;105:1113–17.

51.   Mikhail MS, Anyaegbunam A, Garfinkel D, Palan PR, Basu J, Romney SL. Preeclampsia and antioxidant nutrients: decreased plasma levels of reduced ascorbic acid, alpha-tocopherol, and beta-carotene in women with preeclampsia. *Am J Obstet Gynecol* 1994;171:150–7.

52.   Hubel CA, Kagan VE, Kisin ER, McLaughlin MK, Roberts JM. Increased ascorbate radical formation and ascorbate depletion in plasma from women with preeclampsia: implications for oxidative stress. *Free Radic Biol Med* 1997;23:597–609.

53.   Valsecchi L, Fausto A, Grazioli V. Severe preeclampsia and antioxidant nutrients. *Am J Obstet Gynecol* 1995;173:673–4.

54.   Redman CW, Beilin LJ, Bonnar J, Wilkinson RH. Plasma urate measurements in predicting fetal death in hypertensive pregnancy. *Lancet* 1976;i:1370–3.

55.   Raijmakers MT, Zusterzeel PL, Steegers EA, Hectors MP, Demacker PN, Peters WH. Plasma thiol status in preeclampsia. *Obstet Gynecol* 2000;95:180–4.

56.   Raijmakers MT, Zusterzeel PL, Roes EM, Steegers EA, Mulder TP, Peters WH. Oxidized and free whole blood thiols in preeclampsia. *Obstet Gynecol* 2001;97:272–6.

57.   Zhang C, Williams MA, King IB, Dashow EE, Sorensen TK, Frederick IO, *et al*. Vitamin C and the risk of preeclampsia – results from dietary questionnaire and plasma assay. *Epidemiology* 2002;13:409–16.

58.   Bonet B, Chait A, Gown AM, Knopp RH. Metabolism of modified LDL by cultured human placental cells. *Atherosclerosis* 1995;112:125–36.

59.   Benyo DF, Miles TM, Conrad KP. Hypoxia stimulates cytokine production by villous explants from the human placenta. *J Clin Endocrinol Metab* 1997;82:1582–8.

60. Walsh SW. Maternal–placental interactions of oxidative stress and antioxidants in preeclampsia. *Semin Reprod Endocrinol* 1998;16:93–104.

61. Tsukimori K, Maeda H, Ishida K, Nagata H, Koyanagi T, Nakano H. The superoxide generation of neutrophils in normal and pre-eclamptic pregnancies. *Obstet Gynecol* 1993;81:536–40.

62. Sacks GP, Studena K, Sargent IL, Redman CW. Normal pregnancy and preeclampsia both produce inflammatory changes in peripheral blood leukocytes akin to those of sepsis. *Am J Obstet Gynecol* 1998;179:180–6.

63. Retsky KL, Freeman MW, Frei B. Ascorbic acid oxidation product(s) protect human low density lipoprotein against atherogenic modification. Anti- rather than prooxidant activity of vitamin C in the presence of transition metal ions. *J Biol Chem* 1993;268:1304–9.

64. Martin A, Frei B. Both intracellular and extracellular vitamin C inhibit atherogenic modification of LDL by human vascular endothelial cells. *Arterioscler Thromb Vasc Biol* 1997;17:1583–90.

65. Doba T, Burton GW, Ingold KU. Antioxidant and co-antioxidant activity of vitamin C. The effect of vitamin C, either alone or in the presence of vitamin E or a water-soluble vitamin E analogue, upon the peroxidation of aqueous multilamellar phospholipid liposomes. *Biochim Biophys Acta* 1985;835:298–303.

66. Jonas E, Dwenger A, Hager A. *In vitro* effect of ascorbic acid on neutrophil–endothelial cell interaction. *J Biolumin Chemilumin* 1993;8:15–20.

67. Poranen AK, Ekblad U, Uotila P, Ahotupa M. The effect of vitamin C and E on placental lipid peroxidation and antioxidative enzymes in perfused placenta. *Acta Obstet Gynecol Scand* 1998;77:372–6.

68. Thomas SR, Neuzil J, Mohr D, Stocker R. Restoration of tocopherol by coantioxidants make alpha-tocopherol an efficient antioxidant for low-density lipoprotein. *Am J Clin Nutr* 1995;62:1357S–64S.

69. De Nigris F, Franconi F, Maida I, Palumbo G, Anania V, Napoli C. Modulation by alpha- and gamma-tocopherol and oxidized low-density lipoprotein of apoptotic signaling in human coronary smooth muscle cells. *Biochem Pharmacol* 2000;59:1477–87.

70. Li D, Saldeen T, Mehta JL. Effects of alpha-tocopherol on ox-LDL-mediated degradation of IkappaB and apoptosis in cultured human coronary artery endothelial cells. *J Cardiovasc Pharmacol* 2000;36:297–301.

71. Van Tits LJ, Demacker PN, de Graaf J, Hak-Lemmers HL, Stalenhoef AF. Alpha-tocopherol supplementation decreases production of superoxide and cytokines by leukocytes *ex vivo* in both normolipidemic and hypertriglyceridemic individuals. *Am J Clin Nutr* 2000;71:458–64.

72. Holles SM, Wang Y, Romney A, Walsh SW. Vitamin E attenuates peroxide-induced vasoconstriction in the human placenta. *Hypertens Pregnancy* 1997;16:389–401.

73. Reilly M, Delanty N, Lawson JA, Fitzgerald G. Modulation of oxidative stress *in vivo* in chronic cigarette smokers. *Circulation* 1996;94:19–25.

74. Motoyama T, Kawano H, Kugiyama K, Hirashima O, Ohgushi M, Yoshimura M, *et al.* Endothelium-dependent vasodilation in the brachial artery is impaired in smokers: effect of vitamin C. *Am J Physiol* 1997;273:H1644–50.

75. Gokce N, Keaney JF Jr, Frei B, Holbrook M, Olesiak M, Zachariah BJ, *et al.* Long-term ascorbic acid administration reverses endothelial vasomotor dysfunction in patients with coronary artery disease. *Circulation* 1999;99:3234–40.

76. Timimi FK, Ting HH, Haley EA, Roddy MA, Ganz P, Creager MA. Vitamin C improves endothelium-dependent vasodilation in patients with insulin-dependent diabetes mellitus. *J Am Coll Cardiol* 1998;31:552–7.

77. Ting HH, Timimi FK, Boles KS, Creager SJ, Ganz P, Creager MA. Vitamin C improves endothelium-dependent vasodilation in patients with non-insulin-dependent diabetes mellitus. *J Clin Invest* 1996;97:22–8.

78. Taddei S, Virdis A, Ghiadoni L, Magagna A, Salvetti A. Vitamin C improves endothelium-dependent vasodilation by restoring nitric oxide activity in essential hypertension. *Circulation* 1998;97:2222–9.

79. Rossig L, Hoffmann J, Hugel B, Mallat Z, Haase A, Freyssinet JM, *et al.* Vitamin C inhibits endothelial cell apoptosis in congestive heart failure. *Circulation* 2001;104:2182–7.

80. Calzada C, Bruckdorfer KR, Rice-Evans CA. The influence of antioxidant nutrients on platelet function in healthy volunteers. *Atherosclerosis* 1997;128:97–105.

81. Heitzer T, Yla Herttuala S, Wild E, Luoma J, Drexler H. Effect of vitamin E on endothelial vasodilator function in patients with hypercholesterolemia, chronic smoking or both. *J Am Coll Cardiol* 1999;33:499–505.

82. Green D, O'Driscoll G, Rankin JM, Maiorana AJ, Taylor RR. Beneficial effect of vitamin E administration on nitric oxide function in subjects with hypercholesterolaemia. *Clin Sci* 1998;95:361–7.

83. Motoyama T, Kawano H, Kugiyama K, Hirashima O, Ohgushi M, Tsunoda R, *et al.* Vitamin E administration improves impairment of endothelium-dependent vasodilation in patients with coronary spastic angina. *J Am Coll Cardiol* 1998;32:1672–9.

84. Leung HW, Vang MJ, Mavis RD. The cooperative interaction between vitamin E and vitamin C in suppression of peroxidation of membrane phospholipids. *Biochim Biophys Acta* 1981;664:266–72.

85. Milczarek R, Klimek J, Zelewski L. The effects of ascorbate and alpha-tocopherol on the NADPH-dependent lipid peroxidation in human placental mitochondria. *Mol Cell Biochem* 2000;210:65–73.

86. Porkkala-Sarataho E, Salonen JT, Nyyssonen K, Kaikkonen J, Salonen R, Ristonmaa U, *et al.* Long-term effects of vitamin E, vitamin C, and combined supplementation on urinary 7-hydro-8-oxo-2`-deoxyguanosine, serum cholesterol oxidation products, and oxidation resistance of lipids in nondepleted men. *Arterioscler Thromb Vasc Biol* 2000;20:2087–93.

87. Salonen JT, Nyyssonen K, Salonen R, Lakka HM, Kaikkonen J, Porkkala-Sarataho E, *et al.* Supplementation in Atherosclerosis Prevention (ASAP) study: a randomized trial of the effect of vitamins E and C on 3-year progression of carotid atherosclerosis. *J Intern Med* 2000;248:377–86.

88. Preston-Martin S, Pogoda JM, Mueller BA, Lubin F, Modan B, Holly EA, *et al.* Prenatal vitamin supplementation and pediatric brain tumors: huge international variation in use and possible reduction in risk. *Childs Nerv Syst* 1998;14:551–7.

89. Scholl TO, Hediger ML, Bendich A, Schall JI, Smith WK, Krueger PM. Use of multivitamin/mineral prenatal supplements: influence on the outcome of pregnancy. *Am J Epidemiol* 1997;146:134–41.

90. Mathews F, Yudkin P, Neil A. Influence of maternal nutrition on outcome of pregnancy: prospective cohort study. *BMJ* 1999;319:339–43.

91. Sinha R, Block G, Taylor PR. Problems with estimating vitamin C intakes. *Am J Clin Nutr* 1993;57:547–50.

92. McLaughlin PJ, Weihrauch JL. Vitamin E content of foods. *J Am Diet Assoc* 1979;75:647–65.

93. National Research Council. *Recommended Dietary Allowances.* 10th ed. Washington, DC: National Academy Press; 1989.

94. Carr AC, Frei B. Toward a new recommended dietary allowance for vitamin C based on antioxidant and health effects in humans. *Am J Clin Nutr* 1999;69:1086–107.

95.   Food and Nutrition Board, National Academy of Sciences USA. *Dietary Reference Intakes for Vitamin C, Vitamin E, Selenium and Carotenoids.* Washington DC: National Academy Press; 2000.

96.   Diplock AT. Safety of antioxidant vitamins and beta-carotene. *Am J Clin Nutr* 1995;62:1510S–16S.

97.   Reece EA, Wu YK. Prevention of diabetic embryopathy in offspring of diabetic rats with use of a cocktail of deficient substrates and an antioxidant. *Am J Obstet Gynecol* 1997;176:790–7.

98.   Siman M. Congenital malformations in experimental diabetic pregnancy: aetiology and antioxidative treatment. Minireview based on a doctoral thesis. *Ups J Med Sci* 1997;102:61–98.

99.   Stratta P, Canavese C, Porcu M, Dogliani M, Todros T, Garbo E, *et al.* Vitamin E supplementation in preeclampsia. *Gynecol Obstet Invest* 1994;37:246–9.

100.   Gulmezoglu AM, Hofmeyr GJ, Oosthuisen MM. Antioxidants in the treatment of severe preeclampsia: an explanatory randomised controlled trial. *Br J Obstet Gynaecol* 1997;104:689–96.

101.   Atallah AN, Hofmeyr GJ, Duley L. Calcium supplementation during pregnancy for preventing hypertensive disorders and related problems. *Cochrane Database Syst Rev* 2001;(2).

102.   Sibai BM, Villar MA, Bray E. Magnesium supplementation during pregnancy: a double-blind randomized controlled clinical trial. *Am J Obstet Gynecol* 1989;161:115–19.

103.   Mahomed K, James DK, Golding J, McCabe R. Zinc supplementation during pregnancy: a double blind randomised controlled trial. *BMJ* 1989;299:826-30.

104.   Zhang ZJ, Cheng WW, Yang YM. [Low dose of processed rhubarb in preventing pregnancy induced hypertension.] *Zhonghua Fu Chan Ke Za Zhi* 1994;29:463–4.

105.   Duley L, Henderson-Smart D, Knight M, King J. Antiplatelet drugs for prevention of preeclampsia and its consequences: systematic review. *BMJ* 2001;322:329–33.

106.   Coomarasamy A, Papaioannou S, Gee H, Khan KS. Aspirin for the prevention of preeclampsia in women with abnormal uterine artery Doppler: a meta-analysis. *Obstet Gynecol* 2001;98:861–6.

107.   Chappell LC, Seed PT, Briley AL, Kelly FJ, Lee R, Hunt BJ, *et al.* Effect of antioxidants on the occurrence of pre-eclampsia in women at increased risk: a randomised trial. *Lancet* 1999;354:810–16.

108.   Reith A, Booth NA, Moore NR, Cruickshank DJ, Bennett B. Plasminogen activator inhibitors (PAI-1 and PAI-2) in normal pregnancies, pre-eclampsia and hydatidiform mole. *Br J Obstet Gynaecol* 1993;100:370–4.

109.   Chappell LC, Seed PT, Kelly FJ, Briley A, Hunt BJ, Charnock-Jones DS, *et al.* Vitamin C and E supplementation in women at risk of preeclampsia is associated with changes in indices of oxidative stress and placental function. *Am J Obstet Gynecol* 2002;187:777–84.

110.   Casanueva E, Avila-Rosas H, Polo E, Tejero E, Narcio-Reyes ML, Pfeffer F. Vitamin C status, cervico-vaginal infection and premature rupture of amniotic membranes. *Arch Med Res* 1995;26:S149–52.

111.   Barrett BM, Sowell A, Gunter E, Wang M. Potential role of ascorbic acid and beta-carotene in the prevention of preterm rupture of fetal membranes. *Int J Vitam Nutr Res* 1994;64:192–7.

8

Endometrial endocrinology

Hilary Critchley

INTRODUCTION

Key reproductive events are implantation and, in the absence of pregnancy, menstruation and endometrial repair. The uterus plays a crucial role in sustaining the species. The human endometrium is a dynamic tissue, which, in order to prepare for implantation, undergoes well defined cycles of proliferation, differentiation and degradation in response to the prevailing steroid environment. Pivotal to reproductive events is the ability of the uterine endometrial lining repetitively to shed and regenerate if pregnancy does not occur. Both humoral and local immune responses are intimately involved in the recognition and maintenance of pregnancy. Some 50 years ago Medawar[1] addressed the immunological and endocrinological problems raised by the evolution of viviparity in mammals. On entry of the developing embryo into the uterine cavity a series of complex interactions take place between the endometrium and the trophoblast. In recent years it has become recognised that the endometrium provides a unique environment where the response of the mother to the foreign antigens of the invading trophoblast may be modulated so that a successful pregnancy can be ensured. The adaptive changes in the local immune system are regulated by steroid hormones, which are secreted by the ovary and placenta. In the absence of pregnancy, the same cells are involved in the process of endometrial breakdown and shedding at the time of menstruation.

Since the latter part of the 20th century women have had control over their own fertility.[2] Consequently, nowadays they have fewer pregnancies and menstruate more often. Post-puberty the average woman with access to contraception may expect to menstruate over 400 times in her reproductive lifetime. In contrast, women living in societies without contraceptive choice, spend much of their reproductive lifetime in a state of amenorrhoea owing to later puberty, pregnancy and prolonged lactation.[3] Menstruation is a crucial reproductive process whereby the upper two-thirds of the endometrium (functional layer) is shed and regenerated on a repetitive basis. The endometrium is thus a site of physiological injury and repair. As such, information pertaining to this normal monthly process can provide valuable insights into injury and repair mechanisms (often pathological) elsewhere in the body.

Studies performed some 70 years ago[4,5] established the role for ovarian steroids, oestradiol and progesterone in regulating the changes in endometrial structure across the menstrual cycle. The characteristic features of endometrial proliferation and differentiation are the consequence of the sequential exposure of endometrial cells to oestradiol and progesterone. Menstruation is the response of the endometrium to the withdrawal of progesterone (and oestrogen) that takes place with the demise of the corpus luteum in the absence of pregnancy. The molecular mechanisms by which sex steroids induce these events within the endometrium at the time of menstruation involve complex interactions between the endocrine and immune systems; these were reviewed in 2001.[6]

Progesterone is essential for the transformation of an oestrogen-primed endometrium in preparation for implantation. Much remains poorly understood about the molecular and cellular mechanisms involved by which the sex steroid hormones promote uterine receptivity. It is, however, recognised that sex steroids, acting via their cognate receptors, initiate a pattern of gene expression that is important for implantation and the early stages of pregnancy.

It is essential to have a detailed knowledge of the local mechanisms regulating endometrial events involved in implantation and menstruation if we are to understand the mechanisms responsible for early pregnancy failure and aberrations of menstrual bleeding. Indeed, through a better understanding of the local mechanisms involved in endometrial function, there will be an ability to modulate sex steroid interactions, with far reaching applications for the management of female reproductive health. Examples include endometrial contraception, the medical management of menorrhagia and endometriosis.[7]

STEROIDS AND THEIR RECEPTORS IN THE ENDOMETRIUM

Steroids interact with their target organs via specific nuclear receptors. Members of the nuclear receptor superfamily include progesterone, oestrogen, androgen and glucocorticoid receptors. These receptors share a common structure and functional domains, denoted A/B, C, D, E and F.[8] The A/B region is located at the N-terminal end and is not well conserved. It contains a transactivation domain (AF1). The C domain contains a highly conserved DNA-binding domain consisting of two 'zinc' fingers. Sequences within the C domain determine the specificity of the different receptors for specific hormone response elements. Aberrations in DNA and mutations in this region can result in receptor dysfunction. Next to the DNA-binding domain is the variable hinge region (D). The ligand-binding domain, region E, has a dimerisation region and two transactivation domains (AF-2 and AF-2a). The ligand-binding domain determines whether or not the receptor is activated.

The expression of oestrogen receptor (ER) and progesterone receptor (PR) are under the dual control of oestradiol and progesterone. The expression of endometrial sex steroid receptors (PR, ER, androgen receptor [AR]) varies temporally and spatially across the menstrual cycle. [9–14]

Both endometrial ER and PR are upregulated during the follicular phase by ovarian oestradiol and subsequently downregulated in the luteal phase by progesterone (Figure 1) acting at both the transcriptional and post-transcriptional levels.[15] The presence of PR is considered to be evidence of a functional ER mediated pathway. The administration of an antigestogen, mifepristone (RU486), in the early luteal phase (day LH+2, where LH = day of leuteinising hormone surge) blocks the progesterone-induced downregulation of PR (and ER) in nonpregnant human endometrium.[16,17]

Progesterone receptor

There are two distinct subtypes of the human PR:[18] PRA (Mr 81 000) and PRB (Mr 116 000), which arise from a single gene and function as transcriptional regulators of progestin-responsive genes. PRA is the shorter subtype, missing about 164 amino acids present at the N-terminus of the B subtype. It is otherwise identical to the B subtype.[19] There is a significant decline in PR expression in the glands of the functional layer of the endometrium (the upper two-thirds, which is shed at menstruation) with the transition from the proliferative to the secretory phase of the cycle (Figure 1). In contrast, PR expression persists in the stroma in the upper functional region, being particularly highly expressed in stromal cells in close proximity to the uterine vasculature. The basal layer is differentially regulated in that the glands and stroma of the deeper zones express

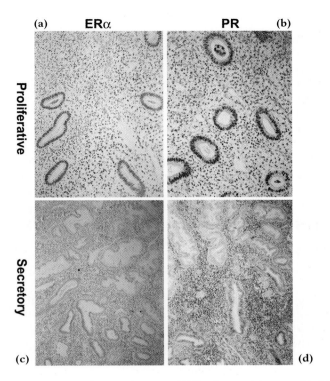

Figure 1 *Sex steroid receptor expression in human endometrium: (a) ERα (brown staining) in nuclei of glandular and stromal cells in proliferative endometrium; (b) PR immunostaining in nuclei of glands and stromal cells in proliferative endometrium; (c) ERα immunostaining in secretory endometrium (superficial and basal layers); in the superficial zone, immunostaining of ERα is downregulated in both the glandular and stromal compartments; (d) PR immunostaining in secretory endometrium; note that the progesterone immunoreactivity is downregulated only in the glandular component of the superficial layer; modest PR immunoreactivity persists in the stroma*

PR throughout the cycle. These differences between the superficial and basal layers of the endometrium are likely to be functionally important, given that only the upper zones are shed at menstruation. Localisation studies utilising antibodies that recognise both PR subtypes have described differential regulation of PR in the endometrial epithelium and stromal cells. For example, during the luteal phase the PRB subtype appears to decline in the stroma and PRA becomes the predominant form.[20,21]

The roles of PR isoforms have been studied by production of PRA and PRB knockout mice.[22] In PRA knockouts, for example, oestrogen treatment induces uterine epithelial hyperplasia, which progesterone treatment cannot suppress. This indicates that the progesterone-mediated suppression of epithelial growth stimulated by oestrogen depends on PRA, not PRB. Moreover, in the PRA+PRB knockout mice, there is a dramatic traffic of inflammatory leucocytes into the uterus, which cannot be prevented by progesterone,[23] suggesting that progesterone suppresses the influx of inflammatory cells into the uterus in wildtype animals. Furthermore, by selective ablation of PRA in mice, it has also been shown that the PRB isoform modulates some reproductive functions of progesterone, by regulation of a subset of progesterone-responsive target genes.[24] Thus, PRA and PRB are functionally distinct mediators of progesterone action *in vivo*. It is important to note, however, that we do not know if these observations in mice can be extrapolated to reproductive function in humans.

Oestrogen receptor

Two structurally related subtypes of ER, commonly known as alpha (ERα) and beta (ERβ) have been identified in humans as well as in other mammals.[25,26] The ERβ gene, like ERα, is encoded by eight exons with maximum levels of homology between ERα and ERβ present in the DNA and ligand-binding domains.[27] The function of ERβ in the uterus is still not fully elucidated. In the functional layer ERα expression increases in both glandular and stromal cells in the proliferative phase and declines in the secretory phase owing to suppression by progesterone (Figure 1). In the basal zone ERα is present in glandular and stromal cells across the cycle.[9,11] In both the human and nonhuman primate endometrium, ERβ, like ERα, is expressed in the nuclei of glandular epithelial and stromal cells and has been reported to decline in the late secretory phase in the functional layer.[12] However, unlike ERα, ERβ has been detected with both polyclonal and monoclonal anti-ERβ antibodies in the nuclei of the vascular endothelial cells. The presence of ERβ in endometrial endothelial cells has indicated for the first time that oestrogen may act directly on endometrial blood vessels.[12,28] Such direct effects of oestrogen may be involved in endometrial angiogenesis and vascular permeability changes during the cycle. In contrast, thus far, PR is reportedly absent from the vascular endothelium[12,29] of the spiral arteries. Thus the effect of progesterone withdrawal on these vessels, which plays a key role in menstrual induction, is likely to be indirectly mediated by the PR positive perivascular stromal cells.

In vitro studies published in 1997 have shown that homodimers (ERα-ERα or ERβ-ERβ) or heterodimers of the oestrogen receptor subtypes (ERα-ERβ) can be formed when both isoforms are expressed in the same cell[30,31] and that the pattern and amount of expression of each isoform is likely to influence gene transcription within that cell. In 1998, two articles reported that mRNAs encoding isoforms of human ERβ formed by alternative splicing of the last (eighth coding) exon were expressed in human tissues.[32,33] Both the mRNA and protein corresponding to one of these splice variants (ERβcx/β2) are expressed in human endometrium.[34] This splice variant lacks the ligand-binding site and may act as a negative inhibitor of ERβ action.[32]

Androgen receptor

The endometrium is also a target for androgen action, either directly via the AR or indirectly via the ER after aromatisation to oestrogen.[35] The circulating concentrations of testosterone show little if any change throughout the menstrual cycle (in contrast to the cyclical variations in oestradiol and progesterone) but are present at levels approximately ten times greater than oestradiol.[36,37] Throughout the menstrual cycle, the AR is expressed predominantly in the endometrial stroma, and there is considerably higher intensity of AR immunostaining during the follicular compared with the luteal phase.[13] Although the physiological role of endometrial AR is not known, androgen treatments can suppress oestrogen action in the endometrium, and this effect is considered to be mediated by endometrial AR.[38,39] The roles, if any, for AR in the implantation and/or menstrual processes remain to be determined.

Glucocorticoid receptor

Glucocorticoids have been shown to exert specific effects on endometrial cells but their role in endometrial physiology is not well understood.[40–43] In 2001 Bamberger *et al.*[44] briefly described the localisation of glucocorticoid receptor (GR) across the menstrual cycle.[44] The GR was almost exclusively expressed in the stromal compartment, including endothelial and lymphoid cells. It has since been demonstrated at both mRNA and protein level that the phenotypically unique uterine natural killer (NK) cells express GR.[45] The role of glucocorticoids in endometrial immune function has as yet not been extensively studied. In other body systems the immunosuppressive effects of glucocorticoids have led to their wide application in the treatment of inflammatory states. Suggested roles for glucocorticoids in reproductive function include effects on implantation,[40] endometrial cellular proliferation,[41] apoptosis[42] and endometrial remodelling.[43] Glucocorticoids have also been shown to repress the decidual prolactin promoter[46] and the corticotrophin-releasing hormone promoter,[47] both of which are markers of decidualisation. This and the expression of GR in the endometrial stroma indicate that glucocorticoids may have a role in the process of decidualisation.[44]

The effects of glucocorticoids are likely to be regulated not only by GR expression but also by the expression of steroid metabolising enzymes (which determine the availability of the ligand). The 11β-hydroxysteroid dehydrogenase (11β HSD) family modulates the action of glucocorticoids by either converting cortisone (inactive) to cortisol (11βHSD1) or cortisol (active) to cortisone (11βHSD2). Smith et al.[48] reported that levels of the glucocorticoid metabolising enzyme 11βHSD2 are higher across the menstrual cycle than 11βHSD1. 11βHSD2 was present in the luminal and glandular epithelium with raised levels in the secretory phase of the cycle. These authors suggested that the expression of 11βHSD2 could facilitate trophoblast invasion by removing the glucocorticoid mediated inhibition of matrix metalloproteinases (MMPs). It is interesting, therefore, that GR-expressing uterine NK cells are found aggregated close to the glandular epithelium and also have proposed roles in controlling trophoblast invasion.

ENDOMETRIAL LEUCOCYTE TRAFFIC

Leucocyte populations within the endometrial stroma vary during the menstrual cycle and throughout pregnancy. Endometrial leucocytes include T and B cells, mast cells, macrophages and neutrophils, but it is the phenotypically unique uterine NK cells that make up the majority of the leucocyte population in the late secretory phase and early pregnancy.[49] In the absence of pregnancy, uterine NK cells may also be important in the initiation of menstruation. They have a unique phenotype (CD56[bright], CD16[-], CD3[-]), which distinguishes them from peripheral blood NK cells (CD56[dim], CD16[bright], CD3[-]).

In the proliferative phase, few cells are apparent but their numbers increase from day LH+3, particularly so in the mid to late secretory phase (day LH+11–13), where they are found in close contact with endometrial glands and spiral vessels.[50,51] It remains to be established whether the increase in cell numbers is solely the result of in situ proliferation or whether there is also de novo migration from the peripheral circulation. However, there is evidence that proliferation of uterine NK cells does occur in the endometrium because the proliferation marker Ki67 has been co-localised with this cell type by immunohistochemistry.[52,53] In the nonpregnant cycle, King et al.[49] have observed changes suggestive of cell death of these cells on day LH+12–13 before any of the more accepted signs of menstruation such as neutrophil infiltration, clumping of stromal cells and interstitial haemorrhage have occurred.

The association of uterine NK cell demise and falling levels of progesterone, as well as the cyclical nature of their appearance, would seem to suggest hormonal regulation of these cells. However, to date, it has not been possible to localise either oestrogen (ERα) or PRs to these cells,[45,54,55] and therefore it has been proposed that oestrogen and progesterone may exert their effects on uterine NK cells indirectly via cytokines such as interleukin (IL)-15 and prolactin or other soluble factors.[56,57]

In support, quantitative real-time reverse transcriptase polymerase chain reaction studies published in 2003 have demonstrated an absence of ERα and PR mRNA in purified uterine NK cells.[45] In contrast, however, mRNA for ERβ and GR have been demonstrated in uterine NK cells.[45] Co-localisation using specific monoclonal antibodies has confirmed that uterine NK cells are immunonegative for ERα and PR protein. These cells are also immunonegative for the ERβcx/β2 isoform but do express ERβ1 and GR proteins. These results have thus raised the possibility that oestrogens and glucocorticoids could in fact be acting directly on uterine NK cells through ERβ and GR respectively, to influence gene transcription in the endometrium and decidua.[45] In this context it is interesting that uterine NK cells, which strongly express GR, have proposed roles in decidualisation[51] and have been shown in 2002 to express the prolactin receptor.[58]

Endometrial differentiation, menstruation and placentation all involve the remodelling of endometrial vasculature. The angiogenic factor, vascular endothelial growth factor-A (VEGF-A), plays an important role in new blood vessel formation, inducing endothelial cell proliferation, migration and differentiation in the endometrium, and also affects vascular permeability. VEGF-A has been shown to be regulated by oestradiol in isolated human endometrial cells, causing increased mRNA and protein levels.[59] It is interesting to note that VEGF-A has also been localised to individual cells, thought to be leucocytes, scattered in the endometrial stroma. These cells have been identified by Mueller *et al.*[60] as neutrophils by dual immunohistochemical staining. VEGF-A has also been reported in uterine macrophages in the secretory phase of the cycle.[61] VEGF-C and other angiogenic factors, placental growth factor and angiopoietin-2 mRNA are expressed in uterine NK cells.[62] VEGF-C was originally characterised as a growth factor for lymphatic vessels but it can also stimulate endothelial cell proliferation and migration.[63] This pattern of growth factor expression and the close spatial association of uterine NK cells with spiral arterioles are suggestive of a role for these cells in endometrial angiogenesis.

PROGESTERONE ACTION IN HUMAN ENDOMETRIUM AND EARLY PREGNANCY DECIDUA: RELEVANCE TO IMPLANTATION

Progesterone is essential for the transformation of an oestrogen-primed endometrium in preparation for implantation. The molecular and cellular mechanisms involved by which the sex steroid hormones promote uterine receptivity are still to be fully defined.

Sex steroids, acting via their cognate receptors, initiate a pattern of gene expression that is important for implantation and the early stages of pregnancy. Thus, if specific steroid-induced molecules are identified there is the potential for their use as markers of uterine receptivity or targets for early pregnancy interruption. Multiple studies have examined the temporal and spatial expression of presumed progesterone regulated genes across the menstrual cycle.

An example is the expression of calcitonin mRNA across the menstrual cycle. Calcitonin mRNA has been demonstrated to be temporally restricted to the mid-secretory phase of the cycle (maximal expression during days 19–21), a period that coincides with the putative window of implantation.[64] The site of postovulatory synthesis of calcitonin mRNA and protein is the glandular epithelium. Evidence for regulation of this gene by progesterone was derived from examination of endometrium collected from women treated with a progesterone antagonist, mifepristone (administered early in the luteal phase: day LH+2). Calcitonin expression was dramatically reduced in women exposed to acute administration of mifepristone in the early luteal phase. Further examples include endometrial enzymes that are regulated by progesterone, the glandular secretion of glycodelin (PP14),[65,66] 15-hydroxyprostaglandin dehydrogenase (PGDH) expression[17,67,68] and 17βHSD2 expression.[16] Other locally produced factors in the endometrium that are regulated by progesterone are: ebaf (i.e. endometrial bleeding associated factor),[69] IGBP-1,[70] integrins,[71,72] Hoxa 10 and Hoxa 11,[73–76] and uteroglobin.[77]

Decidualisation is a crucial step in the initiation and establishment of pregnancy. In humans, decidualisation is independent of the blastocyst and early signs of predecidual changes are first observed in stromal cells close to vascular structures in the mid to late secretory phase. These same stromal cells express PR throughout the luteal phase. *In vivo*, decidualisation is controlled most effectively by progesterone action on an oestrogen–primed uterus. This process can however also be induced as a consequence of administration of exogenous progestogens, such as observed in the endometrium of women using a levonorgestrel-releasing intrauterine system (Figure 2).[78] *In vitro* studies have demonstrated a central role for cyclic adenosine monophosphate as a decidualisation stimulus.[79,80]

Interesting studies in mouse mutants, in which decidualisation does not occur, have facilitated the identification of genes necessary for this process in the endometrial epithelium and/or stromal cells.[81] Examples of key genes include cyclooxygenase 2 (COX-2, the rate-limiting enzyme in prostaglandin [PG] synthesis),[82] and Hoxa 10 and 11.[74,75] The progesterone dependence of the Hoxa 11 gene was demonstrated in 1999.[76]

Valuable insights into requirements for implantation have again been derived from gene ablation studies. The prolactin receptor knockout mouse displays an implantation defect[83] that may be a reflection of a central pituitary defect. Ablation of the PR leads to inappropriate inflammation in the uteri of mice and to defective implantation.[23]

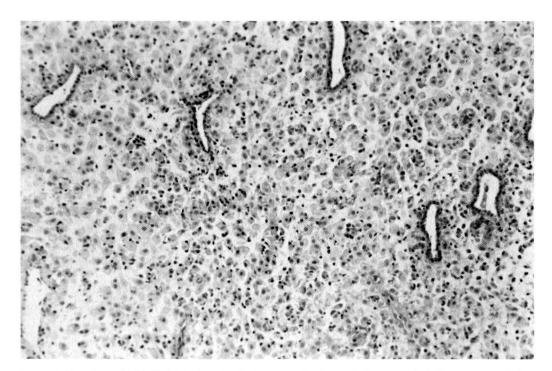

Figure 2 *Photomicrograph of decidualised endometrium in the presence of an intrauterine levonorgestrel releasing system; note the atrophic glands*

The cellular interactions and progesterone target genes involved in decidualisation are thus complex. Multiple growth factors, cytokines and protein hormones have been described as important signals for both the initiation and maintenance of decidualisation.[84–86] Prolactin is a key cytokine secreted by decidualised endometrium and expression is controlled by progesterone.[87] The *in vivo* administration of the antiprogestin, mifepristone significantly reduces prolactin expression in decidualised stromal cells.[88] Although the available evidence indicates that progesterone is important for inducing and maintaining decidualisation, it does not directly induce the prolactin gene. Prolactin mediates its effect on target cells via single-pass transmembrane spanning receptors. Prolactin receptor expression in the human endometrium is temporally regulated throughout the menstrual cycle. There is minimal expression during the proliferative phase and expression is upregulated during the mid to late secretory phase. The prolactin receptor in nonpregnant endometrium is localised predominantly to the glandular epithelial cells. Prolactin receptor expression is maintained during pregnancy and localised to the decidualised stromal cells.[89,90] The prolactin receptor is also expressed by uterine NK cells[58] (and see above).

PHYSIOLOGICAL PROGESTERONE WITHDRAWAL: RELEVANCE TO MENSTRUATION

The classic study reported in 1979 by Csapo and Resch[91] identified that progesterone was indispensable for normal pregnancy. It had earlier been demonstrated in a rabbit model that, regardless of its stage, normal pregnancy could not withstand the withdrawal of progesterone of a critical degree.[5] The pharmacological interruption of progesterone action in early pregnancy interferes with the normal progress of pregnancy and forms the basis for the therapeutic medical termination of pregnancy.[92,93]

In the absence of a pregnancy, owing to the demise of the corpus luteum, the physiological withdrawal of progesterone from an oestrogen-progesterone primed endometrium is the triggering event for the cascade of molecular and cellular interactions that result in menstrual bleeding. A current hypothesis for menstruation is based on lines of evidence derived from studies on local endometrial response to progesterone withdrawal[6] (Figure 3).

The withdrawal of progesterone will initially affect cells expressing the PR. Kelly et al.[94] have proposed that there are two phases of menstruation. The early events in menstruation involve vasoconstriction and cytokine changes; they are initiated by progesterone withdrawal and are likely to be reversible. Subsequent events are probably inevitable and will include the activation of lytic mechanisms that are presumably the consequence of hypoxia. The latter phase of menstruation is thus progesterone independent and consequently involves cells that may not express the PR, for example, luteal phase epithelial cells and uterine leucocytes.[45,54,55] Consistent with the view that early events occurring in PR positive cells may be inhibited by add-back of progesterone, are observations from a study in the rhesus macaque monkey.[95] The 'adding back' of progesterone before 36 hours after progesterone withdrawal prevented menstrual bleeding, whereas add-back of progesterone after 36 hours failed to inhibit the onset of menstruation.

The withdrawal of progesterone upregulates several important inflammatory mediators, these being chemokines (IL-8, monocyte chemotactic peptide-1), and also the inducible enzyme responsible for synthesis of PGs, cyclooxygenase-2 (COX-2).[6] COX-2 is markedly expressed in human menstrual phase endometrium at a time when PG levels have been demonstrated to rise.[96] It is of note that these important local mediators display a perivascular location for their site of expression.[97] IL-8, an alpha chemokine that is chemotactic for neutrophils and monocyte chemotactic peptide-1, a beta chemokine that is chemotactic for monocytes. Both these

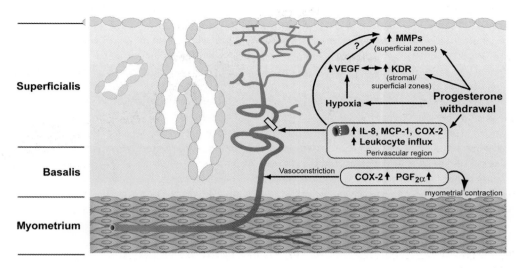

Figure 3 *Menstrual induction hypothesis: progesterone withdrawal results in upregulation of inflammatory mediators, the production of matrix metalloproteinases, a leucocyte influx, and expression of stromal KDR in the upper endometrial zones; menstrual sloughing takes place from the superficial regions of the endometrium; MMPs = matrix metalloproteinases; VEGF = vascular endothelial growth factor; KDR = kinase domain receptor; IL-8 = interleukin-8; MCP-1 = monocyte chemotactic peptide-1; COX-2 = cyclooxygenase-2; PGF$_{2\alpha}$ = prostaglandin F2α (reproduced from: Critchley HOD, Kelly RW, Brenner RM, Baird DT. The endocrinology of menstruation – a role for the immune system. Clin Endocrinol (Oxf) 2001;55:701–10,[6] with permission from Blackwell Science)*

chemokines have been reported to have a perivascular localisation.[96,98,99] PGDH, the enzyme responsible for metabolism of PGs to inactive metabolites, is a progesterone dependent enzyme.[67] Antagonism of progesterone action results in an inhibition of PGDH expression.[100] These early local events in response to progesterone withdrawal result in an elevation of PG concentrations (PGE and PGF2α) and potential synergism with the chemokine, IL-8.[101,102] As a consequence, there is a perimenstrual influx of leucocytes consisting of neutrophils, macrophages and other haemopoietic cells. The endometrial population of leucocytes is a source of cytokines that operates in a positive feedback manner further to augment leucocyte traffic.[6]

The withdrawal of progesterone is also associated with upregulation of MMPs.[103–105] An important observation in this context is the secretion of MMPs by stromal cells in the upper endometrial zones later than 48 hours after progesterone withdrawal[6,106] (Figure 4).

The increased production of PGF2α, with vasoconstrictor action consequent upon progesterone withdrawal, produces myometrial contractions and vasoconstriction[107] together with progesterone withdrawal. There is thus coincident vasoconstriction of the endometrial spiral arteries.[4] The uppermost endometrial zones are presumed to become hypoxic, with resultant distal ischaemia. There is current controversy about the timing and role for hypoxia in the endometrium.[108]

Local mediators that may be stimulated by hypoxia, or indeed progesterone withdrawal from endometrial stromal cells, include the potent angiogenic factor VEGF.[109,110] Progesterone withdrawal has been reported by our group to upregulate the endometrial stromal expression of kinase domain receptor (KDR) in women and nonhuman primates.[111] The stromal but not vascular endothelial expression of KDR can be blocked by adding back progesterone 24 hours after

Mid-secretory phase

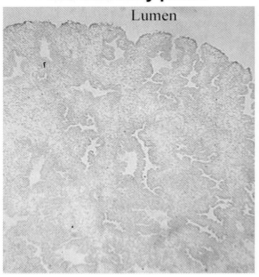

Lumen

Premenstrual phase

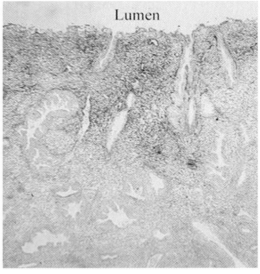

Lumen

Figure 4 *Photomicrographs illustrating (a) the premenstrual upregulation of matrix metalloproteinases (MMP-3) in stromal cells of the upper endometrial zones; and (b) mid-secretory phase showing no immunoreactivity for MMP-3 in contrast to premenstrual phase endometrium, which displays positive immunostaining for MMP-3 in the upper zones only (courtesy of RM Brenner, Oregon National Primate Research Center, Oregon, USA)*

progesterone withdrawal. Pro-MMP-1 is also upregulated in a coordinate manner in the same stromal cell population by withdrawal of progesterone. Hence, as VEGF, KDR and MMPs are coordinately expressed by stromal cells of the upper zones of premenstrual-stage endometrium at the time of progesterone withdrawal, the conclusion is that a VEGF–KDR–MMP link is a component of the premenstrual/menstrual process[6,111] (Figure 3). The consequence of these interactions is breakdown of the endometrium and initiation of menstrual bleeding. Many other factors may of course also operate during the premenstrual phase and are implicated in the complex process of menstruation.[112]

Inevitably, other factors not addressed herein will also operate in the premenstrual/menstrual event. The molecular and cellular mechanisms by which the withdrawal of sex steroids induces breakdown of the endometrium necessarily involves a complex interaction between the endocrine and immune systems.

SUMMARY

In conclusion, the key reproductive events in which the endometrium plays a major role are implantation and, in the absence of pregnancy, menstruation. These processes are regulated by steroids and their interactions with cognate receptors. There is a subsequent cascade of complex downstream events involving both the endocrine and immune systems. Both implantation and menstruation have an inflammatory character.

Progesterone is indispensable in the establishment and maintenance of pregnancy, and there is evidence that many critical factors implicated in endometrial receptivity and implantation are regulated by progesterone. In the absence of pregnancy, the corpus luteum dies and progesterone is withdrawn. Withdrawal of progesterone from an oestrogen-progesterone primed endometrium is the initiating event for the cascade of molecular and cellular interactions that result in menstruation. Menstruation involves sloughing of the superficial layer of endometrium over a period of days, bleeding and subsequent repair, in order that the uterus is receptive to any potential implanting embryo in the next cycle.

In addition to the epithelial, stromal and endothelial cells that share in the cyclic morphological and functional events in the endometrium, there is a dynamic population of leucocytes that play an important role in both implantation and menstruation. The factors responsible for the regulation of this diverse and unique cell population are still to be fully determined. There is no doubt, however, that a complex dialogue exists in the endometrium between the sex steroid hormones and the resident leucocyte population, locally produced cytokines and growth factors. It is likely that endocrine, paracrine, autocrine and even intracrine cellular interactions are involved in implantation and menstruation.

It is essential to have a detailed knowledge of the local mechanisms regulating implantation and menstruation if we are to understand the mechanisms responsible for early pregnancy failure and aberrations of menstrual bleeding.

Acknowledgements

Thanks are due to Ted Pinner (Centre for Reproductive Biology, Edinburgh) for expert assistance with the illustrations and Natasha Mallion for her secretarial help. Some of the data described herein have been derived from studies supported by the Medical Research Council (Grant Nos: G 9620138; G0000066); Wellbeing/RCOG (Grant No. C2/99) and The Wellcome Trust (Grant No. 044744).

References

1. Medawar PB. Some immunological and endocrinological problems raised by the evolution of viviparity in vertebrates. *Symp Soc Exp Biol* 1953;11:320–8.
2. Baird D. A fifth freedom. *BMJ* 1965;ii:1141–8.
3. Short RV. Oestrous and menstrual cycles. In: Austin CR, Short RV, editors. *Hormonal Control of Reproduction*. Cambridge: Cambridge University Press; 1984; p. 115–52.
4. Markee JE. Menstruation in intraocular transplants in the rhesus monkey. *Contrib Embryol Carnegie Inst* 1940;177:211–308.
5. Corner GW, Allen WM. Physiology of corpus luteum – VII. Maintenance of pregnancy in rabbit after early castration, by corpus luteum extracts. *Proc Soc Exp Biol Med* 1930;27:403–5.
6. Critchley HOD, Kelly RW, Brenner RM, Baird DT. The endocrinology of menstruation – a role for the immune system. *Clin Endocrinol (Oxf)* 2001;55:701–10.
7. Brenner RM, Nayak NR, Slayden OD, Critchley HOD, Kelly RW. Premenstrual and menstrual changes in the macaque and human endometrium. *Ann N Y Acad Sci* 2002;955:60–74.
8. Carson-Jurnica MA, Schrader WT, O'Malley BW. Steroid receptor superfamily: structure and functions. *Endocr Rev* 1990;11:209–20.

9.   Garcia E, Bouchard P, DeBrux J, Berdah J, Frydman R, Schaison G, *et al.* Use of immunocytochemistry of progesterone and estrogen receptors for endometrial dating. *J Clin Endocrinol Metab* 1988;67;80–7.

10.   Lessey BA, Killam AP, Metzger DA, Haney AF, Greene, GL, McCarty KS Jr. Immunohistochemical analysis of human uterine estrogen and progesterone receptors throughout the menstrual cycle. *J Clin Endocrinol Metab* 1988;67;334–40.

11.   Snijders MP, de Goeij AFPM, Debets-Te Baerts MJC, Rousch MJ, Koudstaal J, Bosman FT. Immunocytochemical analysis of oestrogen receptors and progesterone receptors in the human uterus throughout the menstrual cycle and after the menopause. *J Reprod Fertil* 1992;94;363–71.

12.   Critchley HOD, Brenner RM, Drudy TA, Williams K, Nayak NR, Slayden OD, *et al.* Estrogen receptor beta, but not estrogen receptor alpha, is present in vascular endothelium of the human and nonhuman primate endometrium. *J Clin Endocrinol Metab* 2001;86;1370–8.

13.   Slayden OD, Nayak NR, Chwalisz K, Cameron ST, Critchley HOD, Baird DT, *et al.* Progesterone antagonists increase the androgen receptor expression in the rhesus macaque and human endometrium. *J Clin Endocrinol Metab* 2001;86:2668–79.

14.   Critchley HOD. Endometrial steroid receptor expression throughout the menstrual cycle. In: O'Brien PMS, Cameron IT, MacLean A, editors. *Disorders of the Menstrual Cycle*. London: RCOG; 2000. p. 56–70.

15.   Chauchereau A, Savouret JF, Milgrom E. Control of biosynthesis and post-transcriptional modification of the progesterone receptor. *Biol Reprod* 1992;6:174–7.

16.   Maentausta O, Svalander P, Gemzell-Danielsson K, Bygdeman M, Vihko R. The effects of an antiprogestin, mifepristone, and an anti-estrogen, tamoxifen, on endometrial 17β hydroxysteroid dehydrogenase and progestin and estrogen receptors during the luteal phase of the menstrual cycle: an immunohistochemical study. *J Clin Endocrinol Metab* 1993;77:913–18.

17.   Cameron ST, Critchley HOD, Buckley CH, Chard T, Baird DT. The effects of post ovulatory administration of onapristone on the development of a secretory endometrium. *Hum Reprod* 1996;11:40–9.

18.   Clarke CL, Sutherland RL. Progestin regulation of cellular proliferation. *Endocr Rev* 1990;11: 266–301.

19.   Tung B, Guller S, Gurpide E. Mechanism of human endometrial stromal cell decidualization. *Ann NY Acad Sci* 1994;734:19–25.

20.   Wang H, Critchley HOD, Kelly RW, Shen D, Baird DT. Progesterone receptor subtype B is differentially regulated in human endometrial stroma. *Mol Hum Reprod* 1998;4:407–12.

21.   Brosens JJ, Hayashi N, White JO. Progesterone receptor regulates decidual prolactin expression in differentiating human endometrial stromal cells. *Endocrinology* 1999;140:4809–20.

22.   Conneely OM, Lydon JP. Progesterone receptors in reproduction: functional impact of the A and B isoforms. *Steroids* 2000;65:571–7.

23.   Lydon JP, Demayo FJ, Funk CR, Mani SK, Hughes AR, Montgomery CA, *et al.* Mice lacking progesterone receptor exhibit pleiotropic reproductive abnormalities. *Genes Dev* 1995;9:2266–78.

24.   Mulac-Jericevic B, Mullinax RA, DeMayo FJ, Lydon, JP, Conneely OM. Subgroup of reproductive functions of progesterone mediated by progesterone receptor-B isoform. *Science* 2000;289:1751–4.

25.   Green S, Walter P, Kumar V, Krust A, Bornert JM, Argos P, *et al.* Human oestrogen receptor cDNA: sequence, expression and homology to v-erb-A. *Nature* 1986;320:134–9.

26.   Kuiper GGJM, Enmark E, Pelto-Hukko M, Nilsson S, Gustafsson JA. Cloning of a novel estrogen receptor expressed in rat prostate and ovary. *Proc Natl Acad Sci U S A* 1996;93:5925–30.

27. Enmark E, Pelto-Huikko M, Grandien K, Lagercrantz S, Lagercrantz J, Fried G, *et al.* Human estrogen receptor beta gene structure, chromosomal localization, and expression pattern. *J Clin Endocrinol Metab* 1997;82:4258–65.

28. Leece G, Meduri G, Ancelin M, Bergeron C, Perrot-Applanat M. Presence of estrogen receptor β in the human endometrium through the cycle: expression in glandular, stromal, and vascular cells. *J Clin Endocrinol Metab* 2001;86:1379–86.

29. Perrot-Applanat M, Deng M, Fernandez H, Lelaidier C, Meduri G, Bouchard P. Immunohistochemical localisation of estradiol and progesterone receptors in human uterus throughout pregnancy: expression in endometrial blood vessels. *J Clin Endocrinol Metab* 1994;78:216–24.

30. Cowley SM, Hoare S, Mosselman S, Parker MG. Estrogen receptors alpha and beta form heterodimers on DNA. *J Biol Chem* 1997;272:19858–62.

31. Pettersson K, Grandien K, Kuiper GG, Gustafsson JA. Mouse estrogen receptor beta forms estrogen response element-binding heterodimers with estrogen receptor alpha. *Mol Endocrinol* 1997;11:1486–96.

32. Ogawa S, Inoue S, Watanabe T, Orimo A, Hosoi T, Ouchi Y, *et al.* Molecular cloning and characterization of human estrogen receptor betacx: a potential inhibitor of estrogen action in human. *Nucleic Acids Res* 1998;26:3505–12.

33. Moore JT, McKee DD, Slentz-Kesler K, Moore LB, Jones SA, Horne EL, *et al.* Cloning and characterization of human estrogen receptor beta isoforms. *Biochem Biophys Res Commun* 1998;247:75–8.

34. Critchley HOD, Henderson TA, Kelly RW, Scobie GS, Evans LR, Groome NP, *et al.* Wild type estrogen receptor β1 and the splice variant (ER βcx/β2) are both expressed within the human endometrium throughout the normal menstrual cycle. *J Clin Endocrinol Metab* 2002;87:5265–73.

35. Horie K, Takakura K, Imai K, Liao S, Mori T. Immunohistochemical localisation of androgen receptor in the human endometrium, decidua, placenta and pathological conditions of the endometrium. *Hum Reprod* 1992;7:1461–6.

36. Ribeiro WO, Mishell DR, Thorneycroft IH. Comparison of the patterns of androstenedione, progesterone, and estradiol during the human menstrual cycle. *Am J Obstet Gynecol* 1974;119,1026–32.

37. Goebelsman U, Arce JJ, Thorneycroft IH, Mishell DR. Serum testosterone concentrations in women throughout the menstrual cycle and following HCG administration. *Am J Obstet Gynecol* 1974;119:445–52.

38. Grody MH. Estrogen-androgen substitution therapy in the aged female. *Obstet Gynecol* 1953;2:36–45.

39. Tuckerman EM, Oxon MA, Li T-C, Laird SM. Do androgens have a direct effect on endometrial function? An *in-vitro* study. *Fertil Steril* 2002;74:771–9.

40. Hoffman LH, Davenport GR, Brash AR. Endometrial prostaglandins and phospholipase activity related to implantation in rabbits: effects of dexamethasone. *Biol Reprod* 1984;30:544–55.

41. Bigsby RM. Progesterone and dexamethasone inhibition of estrogen-induced synthesis of DNA and complement in rat uterine epithelium: effects of antiprogesterone compounds. *J Steroid Biochem Mol Biol* 1993;45:295–301.

42. Jo T, Terada N, Saji F, Tanizawa O. Inhibitory effects of estrogen, progesterone, androgen and glucocorticoid on death of neonatal mouse uterine epithelial cells induced to proliferate by estrogen. *J Steroid Biochem Mol Biol* 1993;46:25–32.

43. Salamonsen LA. Matrix metalloproteinases and their tissue inhibitors in endocrinology. *Trends Endocrinol Metab* 1996;7:28–34.

44. Bamberger AM, Milde-Langosch K, Loning T, Bamberger CM. The glucocorticoid receptor is specifically expressed in the stromal compartment of the human endometrium. *J Clin Endocrinol Metab* 2001;86:5071–4.

45. Henderson TA, Saunders PTK, Moffet-King A, Groome NP, Critchley HOD. Steroid receptor expression in uterine NK cells. *J Clin Endocrinol Metab* 2003;88:440–9.

46. Gellerson B, Kempf R, DeBrux J, Berdah J, Frydman R, Schaison G, *et al.* Use of immunocytochemistry of progesterone and estrogen receptors for endometrial dating. *J Clin Endocrinol Metab* 1998;67:80–7.

47. Makrigiannakis A, Zoumakis E, Margioris AN, Stournaras C, Chrousos GP, Gravanis A. Regulation of the promoter of the human corticotropin-releasing hormone gene in transfected human endometrial cells. *Neuroendocrinology* 1996;64:85–92.

48. Smith RE, Salamonsen LA, Komesaroff PA, Li KX, Myles KM, Lawrence M, *et al.* 11 beta-Hydroxysteroid dehydrogenase type II in the human endometrium: localization and activity during the menstrual cycle. *J Clin Endocrinol Metab* 1997;82:4252–7.

49. King A, Wellings V, Gardner L, Loke YW. Immunocytochemical characterization of the unusual large granular lymphocytes in human endometrium throughout the menstrual cycle. *Hum Immunol* 1989;24:195–205.

50. King A, Burrows T, Verma S, Hiby S, Loke YW. Human uterine lymphocytes. *Hum Reprod Update* 1998;4:480–5.

51. King A. Uterine leukocytes and decidualization. *Hum Reprod Update* 2000;6:28–36.

52. King A, Balendran N, Wooding P, Carter NP, Loke YW. CD3-leukocytes present in the human uterus during early placentation: phenotypic and morphologic characterization of the CD56++ population. *Dev Immunol* 1991;1:169–90.

53. Kammerer U, Marzusch K, Krober S, Ruck P, Handgretinger R, Dietl J. A subset of CD56+ large granular lymphocytes in first-trimester human decidua are proliferating cells. *Fertil Steril* 1999;71:74–9.

54. King A, Gardner L, Loke YW. Evaluation of oestrogen and progesterone receptor expression in uterine mucosal lymphocytes. *Hum Reprod* 1996;11:1079–82.

55. Stewart JA, Bulmer JN, Murdoch AP. Endometrial leucocytes: expression of steroid hormone receptors. *J Clin Pathol* 1998;51:121–6.

56. Verma S, Hiby SE, Loke YW, King A. Human decidual natural killer cells express the receptor for and respond to the cytokine interleukin 15. *Biol Reprod* 2000;62:959–68.

57. Dunn CL, Critchley HOD, Kelly RW. IL-15 regulation in human endometrial stromal cells. *J Clin Endocrinol Metab* 2002;87:1898–901.

58. Gubbay O, Critchley HOD, Bowen JM, King A, Jabbour HN. Prolactin induces ERK phosphorylation in epithelial and CD56+ killer cells of the human endometrium. *J Clin Endocrinol Metabol* 2002;87:2329–35.

59. Shifren JL, Tseng JF, Zaloudek CJ, Ryan IP, Meng YG, Ferrara N, *et al.* Ovarian steroid regulation of vascular endothelial growth factor in the human endometrium: implications for angiogenesis during the menstrual cycle and in the pathogenesis of endometriosis. *J Clin Endocrinol Metab* 1996;81:3112–18.

60. Mueller MD, Lebovic DI, Garrett E, Taylor RN. Neutrophils infiltrating the endometrium express vascular endothelial growth factor: potential role in endometrial angiogenesis. *Fertil Steril* 2000;74:107–12.

61. Charnock-Jones DS, Macpherson AM, Archer DF, Leslie S, Makkink WK, Sharkey AM, *et al.* The effect of progestins on vascular endothelial growth factor, oestrogen receptor and progesterone receptor immunoreactivity and endothelial cell density in human endometrium. *Hum Reprod* 2000;15 Suppl 3:85–95.

62. Li XF, Charnock-Jones DS, Zhang E, Hiby S, Malik S, Day K, *et al.* Angiogenic growth factor messenger ribonucleic acids in uterine natural killer cells. *J Clin Endocrinol Metab* 2001;86:1823–34.

63. Olofsson B, Jeltsch M, Eriksson U, Alitalo K. Current biology of VEGF-B and VEGF-C. *Curr Opin Biotechnol* 1999;10:528–35.

64. Kumar S, Zhu L-J, Polihronis M, Cameron ST, Baird DT, Schatz F, *et al.* Progesterone induces calcitonin gene expression in human endometrium within the putative window of implantation. *J Clin Endocrinol Metab* 1998;83:4443–50.

65. Chard T, Olajide F. Endometrial protein PP14: a new test of endometrial function. *Reprod Med Rev* 1994;3:43–52.

66. Taylor RN, Vigne J-L, Zhang P, Hoang P, Lebovic DI, Mueller MD. Effects of progestins and relaxin on glycodelin gene expression in human endometrial cells. *Am J Obstet Gynecol* 2000;182:841–9.

67. Casey ML, Hemsell DL, MacDonald PC, Johnston JM. NAD+-dependent 15-hydroxyprostaglandin dehydrogenase activity in human endometrium. *Prostaglandins* 1980;19:115–22.

68. Greenland KJ, Jantke I, Jennatschke S, Bracken KE, Vinson C, Gellerson B. The human NAD+ dependent 15-hydroxyprostaglandin dehydrogenase gene promoter is controlled by Ets and activating protein-1 transcription factors and progesterone. *Endocrinology* 2000;141:581–97.

69. Tabibzadeh S, Mason J, Shea W, Yiqiang C, Murray MJ, Lessey B. Dysregulated expression of ebaf, a novel molecular defect in the endometria of patients with infertility. *J Clin Endocrinol Metab* 2000;85:2526–36.

70. Guidance LC. Multifaceted roles for IGFBP-1 in human endometrium during implantation and pregnancy. *Ann N Y Acad Sci* 1997;828:146–56.

71. Lessey BA. Integrins and the endometrium: new markers of uterine receptivity. *Ann N Y Acad Sci* 1997;828:111–22.

72. Illera MJ, Cullinan E, Gui Y, Yuan L, Beyler SA, Lessey BA. Blockade of $\alpha_v\beta_3$ integrin adversely affects implantation in the mouse. *Biol Reprod* 2000;62:1285–90.

73. Bagot CN, Troy PJ, Taylor HS. Alteration of maternal Hoxa 10 expression by *in vivo* gene transfection affects implantation. *Gene Ther* 2000;7:1378–84.

74. Benson GV, Lim H, Paria BC, Satokata I, Dey SK, Maas RL. Mechanisms of reduced fertility in Hoxa-10 mutant mice: uterine homeosis and loss of maternal Hoxa-10 expression. *Development* 1996;122:2687–96.

75. Gendron RL, Paradis H, Hsieh-Li HM, Lee DW, Potter SS, Markoff E. Abnormal uterine stromal and glandular function associated with maternal reproductive defects in Hoxa-11 null mice. *Biol Reprod* 1997;56:1097–105.

76. Taylor HS, Igarashi P, Olive DL, Arici A. Sex steroids mediate HOXA11 expression in the human peri-implantation endometrium. *J Clin Endocrinol Metab* 1999;84:1129–35.

77. Beier HM, Classen-Linke I, Hey S, Herrler A, Müller-Schöttle F, Sterzik K, *et al.* Progesterone and antiprogestin effects on uteroglobin (UGB) expression and secretion in the human endometrium. *Second International Symposium on Progestins, Progesterone Receptor Modulators and Progesterone Antagonists, 20–23 November 2002, Siena, Italy.* p. 30.

78. Critchley HOD, Wang H, Jones RL, Kelly RW, Drudy TA, Gebbie AE, *et al.* Morphological and functional features of endometrial decidualisation following long term intrauterine levonorgestrel delivery. *Hum Reprod* 1998;13:1218–24.

79. Tang B, Guller S, Gurpide E. Mechanism of human endometrial stromal cell decidualization. *Ann N Y Acad Sci* 1994;734:19–25.

80. Brosens JJ, Takeda S, Acevedo CH, Lewis MP, Kirby PL, Symes EK, *et al*. Human endometrial stromal fibroblasts immortalized by simian virus 40 large T antigen differentiate in response to a decidualization stimulus. *Endocrinology* 1996;137:2225–31.

81. Paria BC, Ma W, Tan J, Raja S, Das SK, Dey SK, *et al*. Cellular and molecular responses of the uterus to embryo implantation can be elicited by locally applied growth factors. *Proc Natl Acad Sci U S A* 2001;98:1047–52.

82. Lim H, Gupta RA, Ma WG, Paria BC, Moller DE, Morrow JD, *et al*. Cyclo-oxygenase-2-derived prostacyclin mediates embryo implantation in the mouse via PPAR delta. *Genes Dev* 1999;13:1561–74.

83. Ormandy CJ, Camus A, Barra J, Damotte D, Lucas B, Buteau H, *et al*. Null mutation of the prolactin receptor gene produces multiple reproductive defects in the mouse. *Genes Dev* 1997;11:167–78.

84. Osteen KG. The endocrinology of uterine decidualisation. In: FW Bazer, editor. *Endocrinology of Pregnancy*. Totowa, NJ: Humana Press; 1999. p. 541–53.

85. Jabbour HN, Critchley HOD. Potential roles of decidual prolactin in early pregnancy. *Reproduction* 2001;121:197–205.

86. Jabbour HN, Critchley HOD. Prolactin action and signalling in the human endometrium. *Reprod Med Rev* 2002;10:117–32.

87. Maslar IA, Ansbacher R. Effects of progesterone on decidual prolactin production by organ cultures of human endometrium. *Endocrinology* 1986;118:2102–8.

88. Wang JD, Zhu JB, Shi WL, Zhu PD. Immunocytochemical colocalisation of progesterone receptor and prolactin in individual stromal cells of human decidua. *J Clin Endocrinol Metab* 1994;79:293–7.

89. Jabbour HN, Critchley HO, Boddy SC. Expression of functional prolactin receptors in nonpregnant human endometrium: janus kinase-2, signal transducer and activator of transcription-1 (STAT-1), and STAT 5 proteins are phosphorylated after stimulation with prolactin. *J Clin Endocrinol Metab* 1998;83:2545–53.

90. Jones RL, Critchley HOD, Brooks J, Jabbour HN, McNeilly AS. Localisation and temporal pattern of expression of prolactin receptor in human endometrium. *J Clin Endocrinol Metab* 1998;83:258–62.

91. Csapo AI, Resch BA. Prevention of implantation by antiprogesterone. *J Steroid Biochem* 1979;11:963–9.

92. Rodger MW, Baird DT. Induction of therapeutic abortion in early pregnancy with mifepristone in combination with prostaglandin pessary. *Lancet* 1987;ii:1415–18.

93. Baird DT. Medical abortion in the first trimester. *Best Pract Res Clin Obstet Gynaecol* 2002;16:221–36.

94. Kelly RW, King AE, Critchley HOD. Cytokine control in human endometrium. *Reproduction* 2001;121:3–19.

95. Slayden OD, Mah K, Brenner RM. A critical period of progesterone withdrawal exists for endometrial MMPs and menstruation in macaques. *Biol Reprod* 1999;60 Suppl 1:273;abstr. 579.

96. Jones RL, Kelly RW, Critchley HOD. Chemokine and cyclooxygenase-2 expression in human endometrium coincides with leukocyte accumulation. *Hum Reprod* 1997;12:1300–6.

97. Kelly RW, King AE, Critchley HOD. Inflammatory mediators and endometrial function – focus on the perivascular cell. *J Reprod Immunol* 2002;57:81–93.

98. Critchley HOD, Kelly RW, Kooy J. Perivascular expression of chemokine interleukin-8 in human endometrium. *Hum Reprod* 1994;9:1406–9.

99. Milne SA, Critchley HOD, Drudy TA, Kelly RW, Baird DT. Perivascular interleukin-8 messenger ribonucleic acid expression in human endometrium varies across the menstrual

cycle and in early pregnancy decidua. *J Clin Endocrinol Metab* 1999;84:2563–7.

100. Cheng L, Kelly RW, Thong KJ, Hume R, Baird DT. The effects of mifepristone (RU486) on prostaglandin dehydrogenase in decidual and chorionic tissue in early pregnancy. *Hum Reprod* 1993;8:705–9.

101. Colditz IG. Effect of exogenous prostaglandin E2 and actinomycin D on plasma leakage induced by neutrophil activating peptide-1/interleukin-8. *Immunol Cell Biol* 1990;68:397–403.

102. Rampart M, Van Damme J, Zonnekyn L, Herman AG. Granulocyte chemotactic protein/ interleukin-8 induces plasma leakage and neutrophil accumulation in rabbit skin. *Am J Pathol* 1989;135:21–5.

103. Schatz F, Papp C, Aigner S, Krikun G, Hausknecht V, Lockwood CJ. Biological mechanisms underlying the clinical effects of RU486: modulation of cultured endometrial stromal cell stromelysin-1 and prolactin expression. *J Clin Endocrinol Metab* 1997;82:188–93.

104. Lockwood CJ, Krikun G, Hausknecht VA, Papp C, Schatz F. Matrix metalloproteinase and matrix metalloproteinase inhibitor expression in endometrial stromal cells during progestin-initiated decidualisation and menstruation-related progestin withdrawal. *Endocrinology* 1998;139:4607–13.

105. Salamonsen LA, Woolley DE. Menstruation: induction by matrix metalloproteinases and inflammatory cells. *J Reprod Immunol* 1999;44:1–27.

106. Rudolph-Owen LA, Slayden O, Matrisan LM, Brenner RM. Matrix metalloproteinase expression in *Macaca mulatta* endometrium: evidence for zone-specific regulatory tissue gradients. *Biol Reprod* 1998;59:1349–59.

107. Ducharme DW, Weeks JR, Montgomery RG. Studies on the mechanism of the hypertensive effect of prostaglandin F2-alpha. *J Pharmacol Exp Ther* 1968;160:1–10.

108. Zhang J, Salamonsen LA. Expression of hypoxia-inducible factors in human endometrium and suppression of matrix metalloproteinases under hypoxic conditions do not support a major role for hypoxia in regulating tissue breakdown at menstruation. *Hum Reprod* 2002;17:265–74.

109. Sharkey AM, Day K, McPherson A, Malik S, Licence D, Smith SK, *et al.* Vascular endothelial growth factor expression in human endometrium is regulated by hypoxia. *J Clin Endocrinol Metab* 2000;85:402–9.

110. Nayak NR, Brenner RM. Vascular proliferation and vascular endothelial growth factor expression in the rhesus macaque endometrium. *J Clin Endocrinol Metab* 2002;87:1845–55.

111. Nayak NR, Critchley HOD, Slayden O, Menrad A, Chwalisz K, Baird DT, *et al.* Progesterone withdrawal up-regulates vascular endothelial growth factor receptor type 2 in the superficial zone stroma of the human and macaque endometrium: potential relevance to menstruation. *J Clin Endocrinol Metab* 2000;85:3442–52.

112. Critchley HOD. Antiprogestins as a model for progesterone withdrawal. *Steroids* 2003;68:1061–8.

9

Fetal gene therapy: the present and the prospects

Anna L David, Michael Themis, Charles Coutelle and Charles H Rodeck

INTRODUCTION

Gene therapy uses the intracellular delivery of genetic material for the treatment of disease. A wide range of conditions, including cancer, vascular and neurodegenerative disorders, and inherited genetic diseases, are being considered as targets for this therapy in adults. Application of gene therapy *in utero* has been considered as a strategy for treatment of early-onset genetic disorders such as cystic fibrosis (CF) and Duchenne muscular dystrophy.[1] Gene transfer to the developing fetus, in particular by the use of retroviral vectors, which need cell division for stable integration into the host genome, may be more easily achieved than later in life. Moreover, rapidly expanding stem cell populations that are inaccessible after birth may also be targeted. The functionally immature fetal immune system may permit induction of immune tolerance against vector and transgene, and thereby facilitate repeated treatment after birth. Finally, and most importantly for clinicians, fetal gene therapy would give a third choice to parents after prenatal diagnosis of inherited disease, where, currently, termination of pregnancy or acceptance of an affected child have been the only options. Application of this therapy in the fetus must be safe, reliable and cost effective. Developments over the past three years in the understanding of genetic disease, vector design, and minimal access delivery techniques have brought fetal gene therapy closer to clinical practice. Prenatal studies in animal models are being pursued in parallel with adult studies of gene therapy, but currently they remain at the experimental stage. This chapter reviews the latest developments in the field of gene therapy and explores their implications for its application *in utero*.

THE CANDIDATE DISEASES

Fetal gene therapy has been proposed to be appropriate for life threatening disorders in which *in utero* intervention maintains a clear advantage over transplantation or postnatal gene therapy and for which there are currently no satisfactory treatments available.[2] Table 1 shows some of the diseases that may be suitable for *in utero* treatment. Studies on animal models of human disease such as haemophilia B have improved our understanding of disease processes and shown that gene therapy treatment is possible.[3] Transgenic mouse models, such as for spinal muscular atrophy[4] and sickle cell disease,[5] have been developed and will enable the results of gene transfer to be evaluated. Two diseases, CF and haemophilia B, are discussed in more detail below to illustrate progress.

Table 1 *Examples of candidate diseases for fetal gene therapy*

Disease	Therapeutic gene product	Target cells/organ
Cystic fibrosis (CF)	CF transmembrane conductance regulator	Airway and intestinal epithelial cells
Metabolic disorders: Ornithine transcarbamylase deficiency	Ornithine transcarbamylase	Hepatocytes
Glycogen storage disorders: Pompe disease	α-1,4-glucosidase	Hepatocytes, myocytes, neurons
Sphingolipid storage disorders: Tay–Sachs disease	β-N-acetylhexosaminidase	Fibroblasts, neurons
Mucopolysaccharide storage disorders: Hurler disease	α-L-iduronidase	Haematopoietic stem cells
Muscular dystrophies: Duchenne	Dystrophin	Myocytes
Neurological disorders: Spinal muscular atrophy	Survival motor neuron protein	Motor neurons
Haemophilias: Haemophilia B	Human clotting factor IX	Hepatocytes
Haemoglobinopathies: α^{0}-thalassemia	α-globin chains of hemoglobin	Haematopoietic precursor cells
Immunodeficiency disorders: X-linked severe combined immunodeficiency	γc cytokine receptor	Haematopoietic precursor cells
Noninherited perinatal diseases: Neonatal respiratory distress syndrome	Surfactant	Airway epithelial cells
Infectious diseases: Herpes simplex	Herpes DNA	Oral mucosa
Placental disorders: Severe pre-eclampsia	Nitric oxide synthase	Trophoblasts

Cystic fibrosis

CF appears to be an ideal candidate for treatment with *in utero* gene therapy. First, it is the most common lethal autosomal recessive disorder in white people, with an incidence of 1 in 2000 live births in Western Europe and North America. Several mutations of the CF transmembrane regulator (CFTR) gene encoding the CFTR protein have been identified and the resulting disease is characterised by abnormal electrolyte transport in airway, sweat ductal, intestinal and pancreatic ductal epithelia. The predominant site of CFTR expression in the non-CF human bronchus is the submucosal glands.[6] *In vitro* studies in which normal and CF airway cells were mixed suggest that only 6–10% of cells expressing normal CFTR are required to correct the ion transport defect in all cells of an epithelial monolayer;[7] thus successful gene therapy may require only relatively low-level epithelial airway transduction.

The CFTR gene has also been proposed to play an important physiological role in normal fetal development.[8,9] Furthermore the CF disease process begins during the development of CF fetuses since, by the mid-trimester a pro-inflammatory state exists in fetal CF airways[10] and there are abnormalities of the pancreatic[11] and male genital ducts[12] due to obstruction by fetal secretions.

Phase I gene therapy trials directed towards pulmonary disease in CF have shown equivocal results and highlight the problems of applying this therapy in adults.[13] The lungs may be severely damaged or obstructed even in young adults, limiting delivery of gene therapy to the airway epithelium. Fluorocarbon liquids such as perflubron have been shown to improve distribution of adenoviral vectors and gene expression in normal and diseased adult lungs.[14,15] Pretreatment of airways with detergents[16] or the fatty acid sodium caprate[17] also improves adenoviral mediated airways transduction. Immune responses to the vector, particularly in the case of adenoviral vectors, limit the dose that may safely be administered and reduce the duration of expression.

The early disease manifestation and poor results from gene therapy treatment of adults with CF has led to research on *in utero* treatment for this disease in animal models. Submucosal gland progenitors have been identified in the human lung[18] and results of adenoviral mediated gene transfer to human fetal lung xenografts *in vitro* are encouraging.[19]

Haemophilia B

Haemophilia B is also particularly suitable for gene therapy *in utero*. This X-linked hereditary haemorrhagic disorder occurs in 1 in 25 000 men and is caused by the absence or dysfunction of human factor IX (hFIX) clotting factor.[20] Current treatment uses replacement therapy with hFIX. Unfortunately, a number of patients develop antibodies to therapy, which leads to ineffective treatment and occasional anaphylaxis.[21] Indeed, the complications of haemophilia treatment have been far worse than the disease itself, increasing the morbidity and mortality of the disease.[22] Induction of immune tolerance to the replacement of hFIX is only partly successful. Restoration of the functional hFIX gene by *in utero* gene therapy could provide long-term treatment by using a single injection, avoid immune sensitisation, and also prevent any haemorrhagic complications that could occur at the time of delivery.

Successful delivery and expression of FIX has been achieved after the administration of adenoviral vectors in adult animal models.[23,24] Sustained FIX expression was also observed after intramuscular injection of adult haemophiliac dogs with adeno-associated viral (AAV) vectors expressing canine FIX[2,25] and after intravascular injection of adult haemophiliac mice with AAV vectors containing hFIX.[26] These results have culminated in the first clinical trial in humans that shows promising results, although only low-level hFIX expression has so far been observed.[27]

GENE DELIVERY VECTORS

Vector design is extremely important in the development of this therapy and rapid progress has been made. The ideal vector for fetal somatic gene therapy would introduce a transcriptionally regulated therapeutic gene into all organs relevant to the genetic disorder by a single safe application. Although none of the present vector systems meet all these criteria, many of them have characteristics that may be beneficial to the fetal approach.

Nonviral vectors

Cationic liposome/DNA complexes have the advantage of being relatively nontoxic and nonimmunogenic, but they are somewhat inefficient for gene delivery. One drawback with these gene therapy vehicles is that DNA introduced as plasmid molecules remains episomal in nature and therefore may be lost over time after cell division. This is especially important in the fetus where cell populations are rapidly dividing. Nonviral systems have been developed that integrate into the host genome but these vectors are still at an early stage of experimental design.[28]

Viral vectors

Studies of *in utero* gene therapy have therefore concentrated on viral vectors, many of which have been designed to deliver reporter genes such as the beta-galactosidase gene (*lacZ*). These allow tracking of cells transduced after vector gene transfer and define tissue expression by biochemical staining assays. Alternatively, by using vectors carrying the hFIX gene, analysis of blood may be used to measure levels of therapeutic protein over time and readministration of hFIX protein or the hFIX vector to fetally treated animals can be used to examine whether immune tolerance has been achieved.

Retrovirus

Vectors that are able to integrate into the host genome, such as retroviruses, lentiviruses and adeno-associated viruses, offer the possibility of permanent gene delivery. Retroviruses were used in the first successful gene therapy treatment, where bone marrow stem cells transduced *ex vivo* with retroviral vectors expressing the correct gene were delivered to infants suffering from an X-linked form of severe combined immunodeficiency.[29] The infants were able to leave protective isolation, discontinue treatment and appear to be developing normally.[30]

Figure 1 illustrates the production of attenuated therapeutic retrovirus vectors and demonstrates how these vectors are assembled and packaged in virus producer cells using only vital elements from the wildtype virus. Although only fairly low virus titres can be produced by cell lines

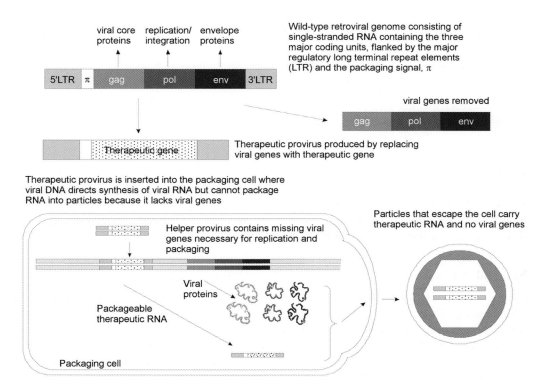

Figure 1 *Safe retrovirus vectors from wildtype retrovirus (reproduced from: David AL, Themis M, Cook T, Coutelle C, Rodeck CH. Fetal gene therapy.* Ultrasound Rev Obstet Gynecol *2001;1:14–27,[128] with permission from Parthenon Publishing)*

generating these particles, virus gene transfer may be improved by complexing vectors with cationic agents,[31] or by the administration of retrovirus producer cells *in vivo* to allow local gene delivery to the desired organs.[32,33]

Retroviruses require dividing cells for gene transfer,[34] which suggests that they may be better suited for use in fetal tissues, where cells are rapidly dividing, rather than in adult tissues. Other problems include reports of premature promoter shutdown,[35,36] leading to transcriptional shutoff. Human serum can almost completely inactivate some retroviral particles,[37] which limits their use *in vivo*, although increased resistance to serum inactivation can be achieved by generating retroviruses from particular human packaging cells[38] or by pseudotyping, which replaces the natural envelope of the retrovirus with a heterologous envelope.[39] A particular problem with *in utero* application is that amniotic fluid has also been shown *in vitro* to have a mild inhibitory effect on retrovirus infection.[40] A further problem is the relatively short half-life of the retroviral particles *in vivo*,[32,41–43] which may hinder transduction because fetal cell division is nonsynchronised and only those cells undergoing cell division at the time of infection will become transduced.

A serious adverse event associated with retroviral gene transfer was reported in 2002.[44] A patient treated for X-linked severe combined immunodeficiency using autologous transplantation of retrovirally transduced bone marrow stem cells was found to have developed leukaemia, which has been shown to involve insertional mutagenesis. An expanded clonal population of T cells was demonstrated to be carrying the transgene inserted at 11p13 in the region of *LMO2*, an oncogene frequently overexpressed in T cell leukaemias. Insertional mutagenesis is an acknowledged potential complication of retroviral mediated gene transfer because gene integration occurs randomly into the genome. This is the first report of malignant change in humans after retroviral gene therapy and only one example has been found in extensive animal studies using this vector.[45] Investigations are continuing to determine whether any other factor contributed to the development of insertional mutagenesis and clonal expansion in this particular patient.

Lentivirus

Progress has been made in the development of lentiviral vectors, a retroviral subgroup based on the HIV or the equine infectious anaemia virus (EIAV).[46] HIV vectors are capable of transferring genes into nondividing cells such as neurons[47] and quiescent haematopoietic progenitor cells,[48] which will be useful for particular tissue targets. Lentiviral vectors also integrate randomly into the genome and are therefore theoretically able to cause insertional mutagenesis.

Lentiviruses can be made more stable by pseudotyping, which allows virus titres to be improved by ultracentrifugation. This offers the opportunity of infecting a greater number of cells *in vivo* and different envelopes allow targeted gene transfer, for example, to the nervous system[49] and airways.[50] The EIAV vector is an alternative vector derived from nonprimate animal lentiviruses,[51] and feline immunodeficiency virus[52] has also been developed in an attempt to create vectors for use in human treatment that are not associated with any human pathology. Currently unpublished work has shown that high-level sustained transgene expression can be achieved using the EAIV vector in fetal mice after intravascular administration.[53]

Adeno-associated viral vectors

AAV is also a promising novel vector system. It is a common human parvovirus that is not associated with any human pathology. AAV naturally requires co-infection with adenovirus as a helper virus, but the latest AAV vectors to have been developed circumvent the need for adenovirus and therefore make the production of pure AAV particles easier.[54] AAV is also able to infect nondividing cells and to achieve long-lasting gene correction *in vitro* and *in vivo*.[3,27,55] The basis for long-term transgene expression is not quite clear. Integration of the wildtype virus is predominantly at a specific functionally unimportant location on human chromosome 19, reducing the theoretical risk of insertional mutagenesis; however, recombinant vector appears to integrate at low levels and nonspecifically.[56] AAV vectors have a limited capacity for the insertion of foreign genes that is about 4.7 kb, although strategies to increase the packaging capacity include hydrid vector systems[57] and heterodimerisation of separate AAV vectors.[58]

Adenovirus

Adenoviral vectors are attractive candidates for proof of principle studies for gene therapy because they have continually achieved highly efficient gene transfer *in vivo*. Adenoviral coding sequences necessary for viral reproduction are deleted, rendering them replication defective. They are relatively stable and can be obtained at high titres, making feasible their systemic administration in humans and large animal models. The adenovirus genome replicates in an extra-chromosome state, which circumvents the risk of insertional mutagenesis but results in only transient gene expression. Another advantage is their broad host range and tropism to most cells of the human body, including the respiratory epithelium. They are therefore particularly useful for exploring different technical approaches to fetal gene therapy, in essence as a 'pathfinder' vector, and have been used extensively in this field.

Factors that determine the kinetics of transgene expression include vector elimination (because adenovirus is not an integrating vector), promoter shutdown and the half-life of the transgenic protein. Adenoviral vectors are also highly immunogenic. Major concerns about the safety of adenoviral vectors were raised after the death of Jesse Gelsinger, an 18-year-old participant in a phase I gene therapy clinical trial, from a systemic inflammatory response to a first generation adenovirus vector used for correction studies of the inherited metabolic disorder, ornithine transcarbamylase deficiency.[59] Even fetal administration has been associated with an immune response,[60] particularly after postnatal repeat exposure to the vector.[61] Attempts to reduce the immunogenicity and toxicity of the vector and to increase its insert capacity have led to the generation of the socalled 'gutless vectors' in which essentially all adenoviral coding sequences have been eliminated.[62,63] Developments since the late 1990s include the production of chimeric vectors, which combine specific biological properties of viruses such as adenoviruses and retroviruses.[64,65]

ULTRASOUND-GUIDED DELIVERY TECHNIQUES

Developments in vectorology must be accompanied by improvements in minimally-invasive methods of delivering vectors to the fetus if this therapy is to be clinically applicable. Well established techniques used clinically in fetal medicine are being investigated and adapted.

Coelocentesis allows access to the extraembryonic coelom in the early first trimester. It has a success rate of >95% at 6–11 weeks of gestation, and has been suggested as a possible technique for stem cell engraftment in early gestation.[2] It may be of little use, however, for *in utero* gene therapy because of the limited transfer from the extraembryonic coelom via the amniotic membrane to the amniotic cavity.[66] In addition, the risk of miscarriage in continuing pregnancies is approximately 25%.[67]

Amniocentesis has been used for intra-amniotic delivery of viral vectors in fetal primates,[68] although this route may be of limited use in fetal gene therapy because of vector dilution by the large volume of amniotic fluid.

Accessing the systemic circulation has greater potential. Fetal blood can be obtained in the second trimester under ultrasound guidance, from the placental cord insertion, the fetal heart or, more safely, from the intrahepatic vein.[69] The procedure has a good success rate, is low risk and is used commonly for rapid karyotyping or fetal blood transfusion.[70] From 12 weeks of gestation, ultrasound-guided intracardiac puncture for fetal blood sampling has been performed on women undergoing surgical termination of pregnancy.[71] Similarly, radiolabelled fetal liver cells were successfully injected into the heart of 13-week-old fetuses under ultrasound guidance[72] prior to prostaglandin termination of pregnancy. No fetal heart rate abnormalities were detected and all fetuses were alive at least six hours after the procedure. Intraperitoneal injection has been used for *in utero* stem cell transplantation from 14 weeks[73] and is an alternative route for blood transfusion before 18 weeks of gestation.[74] Corticosteroid therapy for maturation of preterm infant lungs and also vitamin K have been delivered to the fetus *in utero* by ultrasound-guided intramuscular injection.[75,76]

Fetoscopy was developed in the early 1980s for examination of second trimester fetuses and fetal blood sampling.[77] It is now being used with ultrasound in endoscopic fetal surgery for conditions such as severe feto-fetal transfusion syndrome[78] and congenital diaphragmatic hernia,[79] and could be adapted to apply gene therapy. Our group commenced work in early 2001 and has developed a percutaneous transthoracic route of injection of the fetal trachea in mid-gestation sheep using ultrasound guidance to target the fetal airways as illustrated in Figure 2.[80]

Fetal gene therapy studies

In utero gene therapy has so far been investigated in a broad range of small animals using a variety of techniques. The possible routes of administration are illustrated in Figure 3. Studies in large animals have mainly used sheep because primates are more costly and difficult to maintain. Unfortunately, there are few large-animal models of human genetic disease available for testing of gene therapy. It is for this reason that small animals such as mice are commonly used, although their size precludes the development of minimally invasive techniques of application.

Direct targeting of the fetal circulation

The delivery of vectors to the systemic fetal circulation appears to be a highly effective route for targeting gene therapy to a range of fetal tissues, particularly to the liver.[81] This can be accomplished by injection via the umbilical vein,[81–83] by intracardiac injection,[84,85] or by injection into the yolk sac vessels.[86] Successful local gene transfer to the ductus arteriosus has been achieved using a nonviral vector after surgical exteriorisation of the ductus in fetal sheep at 90 days of gestation.[87] This biological engineering is a promising approach to maintaining a patent ductus arteriosus prior to surgery for congenital heart defects in neonates.

Ultrasound-guided intracardiac injection has been used to deliver adenoviral vectors to the late gestation fetal rabbit.[85] Transgene expression was observed in up to 40% of fetal hepatocytes and was transient, as expected. A fetal immune response to the vector and transgene was detected. Unfortunately, the procedure also had a 25–40% mortality rate, comparable with other studies on fetal blood sampling in rabbits.[88]

Our group has delivered adenoviral vectors containing the *lacZ* or hFIX genes into the umbilical vein of late-gestation fetal sheep using ultrasound-guided percutaneous injection from 102 days of gestation (term = 145 days).[82] Positive *lacZ* expression was seen in 30% of fetal hepatocytes, and hFIX expression in fetal and neonatal plasma by enzyme-linked immunosorbent assay reached therapeutic levels within a week of delivery in two animals. Although vector DNA

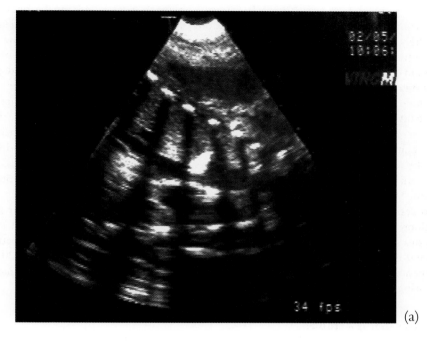

(a)

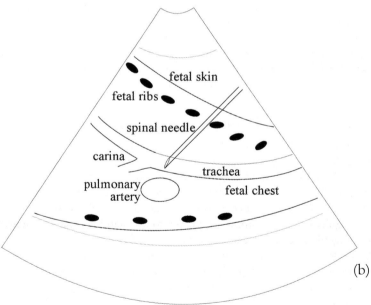

(b)

Figure 2 *(a) Ultrasonogram and (b) diagram of sheep fetus at 114 days of gestation in longitudinal section; a 20 gauge spinal needle is inserted into the fetal thorax between the third and fourth ribs, penetrating the lung parenchyma and entering the fetal trachea just proximal to the carina (reproduced from: David AL, Peebles DM, Gregory L, Themis M, Cook T, Coutelle C, et al. Percutaneous ultrasound-guided injection of the trachea in fetal sheep: a novel technique to target the fetal airways.* Fetal Diagn Ther 2003;18:385–90,[112] *with permission from Karger, Basel)*

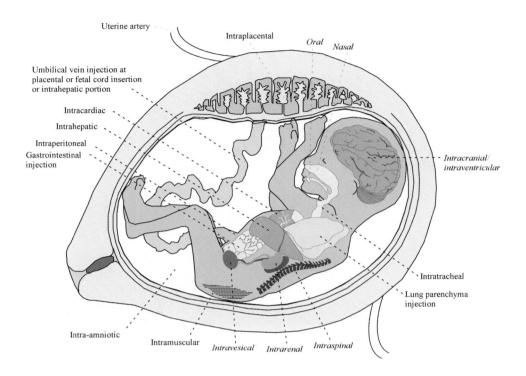

Figure 3 *Routes of administration of gene therapy to the fetus; routes in italics have not yet been applied in a fetal animal model (reproduced from: David AL, Themis M, Waddington SN, Gregory L, Buckley SMK, Nivsarkar M, et al. The current status and future direction of fetal gene therapy. Gen Ther Mol Biol 2003;7:181–209,[129] with permission from Gene Therapy Press)*

was detectable by polymerase chain reaction (PCR) in the gonads, extensive investigation by reverse transcriptase-PCR could not detect any gene expression. Antibodies against the vector and the transgene were observed in some animals.

In early gestation, delivery of adenoviral vectors into the umbilical vein of fetal sheep at 60 days of gestation via hysterotomy resulted in widespread transduction of fetal tissues with no humoral immune response to the adenoviral vector.[83] Our group has attempted ultrasound-guided intracardiac and umbilical vein injection of adenoviral vectors in fetal sheep at the earlier time of 53 days of gestation but this was unsuccessful owing to procedure-related mortality.[80]

Intravascular delivery of adenoviral hFIX vectors to fetal mice was shown in 2002 to result in long-term tolerance of hFIX into adulthood on repeated applications of purified proteins.[89] This provides proof of principle that gene therapy application *in utero* may allow induction of immune tolerance.

Alternative routes for targeting the fetal circulation and liver

Targeting gene therapy to the fetal liver will be important for treatment of many genetic diseases that are amenable to fetal gene therapy. Hepatocytes have been targeted by intrahepatic injection of fetal mice[90–93] and rats.[43] Gene transfer to tissues outside the peritoneal cavity was usually much

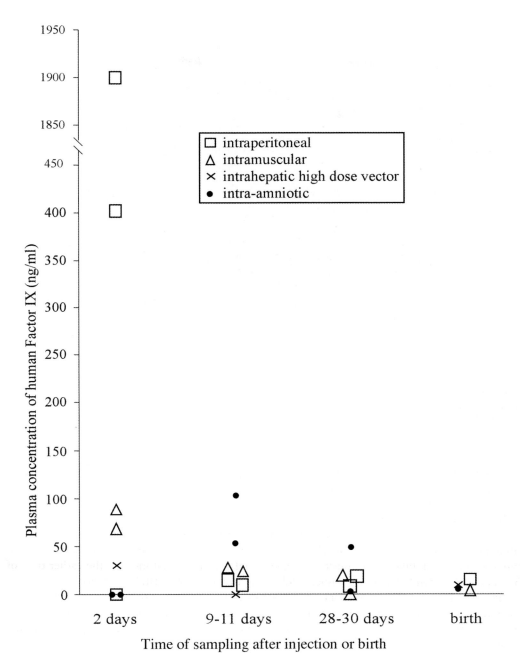

Figure 4 *Time course of transgene expression after ultrasound-guided intraperitoneal, intramuscular, intrahepatic or intra-amniotic delivery of an adenoviral vector containing the human factor IX gene to early gestation sheep fetuses; concentrations of human factor IX in fetal or lamb plasma were determined by enzyme-linked immunosorbent assay; fetal samples were collected at post mortem (reproduced from: David A, Cook T, Waddington S, Peebles D, Nivsarkar M, Knapton H, et al. Ultrasound-guided percutaneous delivery of adenoviral vectors encoding the β-galactosidase and human factor IX genes to early gestation fetal sheep in utero. Hum Gene Ther 2003;14:353–64,[80] with permission from Mary Ann Liebert Inc.)*

higher after intrahepatic delivery when compared with injection of the peritoneal cavity, most likely because the vector was also delivered directly into the systemic circulation during injection of the hepatic parenchyma. Intraperitoneal injection has also been used for successful gene transfer to multiple tissues including the liver in fetal mice,[91] rats[43,94] and sheep.[95] Retroviral vectors have been injected into the peritoneal cavity of fetal sheep at 57–65 days of gestation at laparotomy and long-term transduction of haematopoietic stem cells in the bone marrow and blood could be demonstrated five years later.[41] Gene delivery to the germline through haematogenic spread is a potential risk when using retroviral vectors, but this was not detected by extensive PCR analysis of the sperm derived from rams injected *in utero*. A similar risk of germline transduction occurs with AAV that can integrate into the genome. No AAV sequences were detectable in the germline tissues of fetal mice receiving injection of AAV vectors via the intraperitoneal route nor the tissues of their progeny.[96] Finally, intramuscular injection is an established route for vector administration by which our group and others have successfully achieved *in vivo* expression of hFIX after injection of adenovirus and AAV hFIX vectors in adult and fetal mice.[97,98]

Our group has used ultrasound guidance to deliver adenoviral vectors to early gestation fetal sheep (33–61 days of gestation, term = 145 days) and compared the effect of route of administration on spread and expression of transgenes.[80] Fetal survival was 77%, 81%, 86% and 91% after intraperitoneal, intrahepatic, intra-amniotic and intramuscular injection respectively. We found that intraperitoneal injection was the optimal route of application of adenoviral vectors containing the hFIX gene and therapeutic hFIX production was achieved, albeit transiently (Figure 4). Therapeutic levels of hFIX were also obtained after intramuscular delivery, suggesting that skeletal muscle may be a potential alternative site for therapeutic gene expression. Immunohistochemical analysis showed positive expression of beta-galactosidase on the surface of the umbilical cord, in the fetal small bowel serosa and in the hepatocytes beneath the fetal liver capsule after intraperitoneal injection (Figure 5 A–C) and widespread gene transfer to cells of the fetal skin and nasal cavities after intra-amniotic delivery (Figure 5 D–F). The intraperitoneal route also gave the most comprehensive spread of vector to fetal tissues as determined by PCR analysis. No vector was detectable on sensitive PCR analysis in the germline of lambs born after each route of administration. These results show that ultrasound guidance can be used for *in utero* gene delivery as early as the first trimester of pregnancy.

Targeting the fetal airways

Gene transfer to the fetal airways is important for *in utero* treatment of CF. Intra-amniotic application has been investigated extensively and, in general, transgene expression is maximal in those tissues in contact with the amniotic fluid, namely the amniotic membranes and the fetal skin, with less transduction of the gut and the mucosae.[32,61,68,99–103] Indeed, therapeutic plasma concentrations of hFIX were achieved in fetal mice after intra-amniotic injection of adenoviral vectors carrying the hFIX gene[104] and the transgenic protein remained detectable after birth. This suggests that transduction of keratinocytes *in utero* may be able to deliver proteins to the circulation as well as to treat hereditary skin disease. Ultrasound-guided intra-amniotic injection of adenoviral vectors in mid-trimester rhesus macaque fetuses resulted in significant transgene spread to tissues coming into contact with amniotic fluid but low-level transgene expression in the fetal airways and intestine.[68] Similar findings were observed in fetal rabbits[105] and the low-level airways transduction is probably due to dilution of the vector by the relatively larger volume of the amniotic fluid. In our study of ultrasound-guided intra-amniotic delivery of adenoviral vectors to fetal sheep at early gestation (33–39 days) there was no significant airway or gastrointestinal tissue transduction.[80] This is most likely due to the lack of fetal breathing movements or fetal swallowing

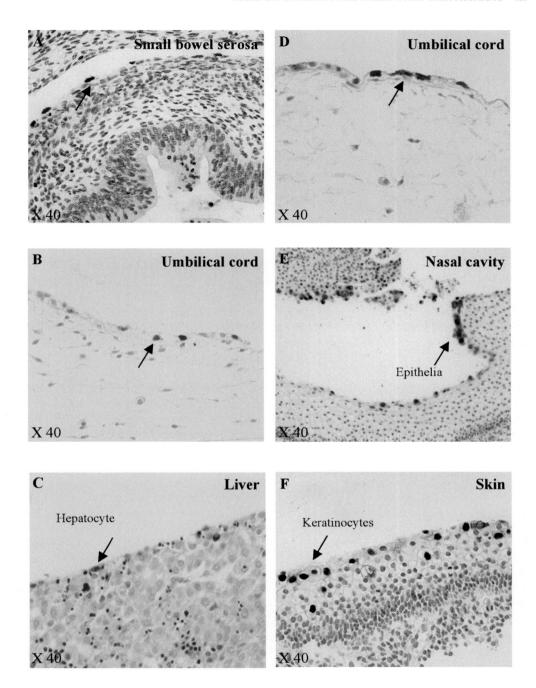

Figure 5 *Expression of β-galactosidase by immunohistochemistry two days after intraperitoneal or intra-amniotic delivery of an adenoviral vector containing the β-galactosidase gene to early gestation fetal sheep. Original magnifications are as indicated; intraperitoneal injection at 52 days of gestation: positive staining is seen in (A) fetal small bowel serosa, (B) surface of umbilical cord and (C) fetal subcapsular hepatocytes; intra-amniotic injection at 33 days of gestation: positive staining is seen in (D) surface of umbilical cord, (E) fetal nasal cavity and (F) fetal skin (reproduced from: David A, Cook T, Waddington S, Peebles D, Nivsarkar M, Knapton H, et al. Ultrasound-guided percutaneous delivery of adenoviral vectors encoding the β-galactosidase and human factor IX genes to early gestation fetal sheep in utero. Hum Gene Ther 2003;14:353–64[80] with permission from Mary Ann Liebert Inc.)*

at this early gestation. It may be possible to enhance fetal breathing movements in later gestation by using agents such as theophylline[106] that lead to an intake of amniotic fluid into the lungs against the continuous outflow of tracheal fluid.[107,108]

Direct injection of the lung parenchyma has been attempted to access the fetal airways but with poor results. In mid-gestation fetal primates, ultrasound-guided injection of lentiviral vectors into the lung resulted in low-level transgene expression in the fetal airways.[109] However, in our hands, ultrasound-guided delivery of an adenoviral vector to the lung parenchyma of a mid-gestation sheep fetus elicited only localised gene transfer and no spread within the airways could be detected.

Direct instillation of vector into the trachea has been more successful. Placement of catheters in the tracheae of fetal sheep can be performed by highly invasive techniques at laparotomy[42,60,110] or fetoscopically.[83,111] Low-level transduction of the proximal airways can be achieved using adenoviral or retroviral vectors, and occlusion of the trachea with a balloon improves distal airway transduction. These techniques, however, carry a significant morbidity and mortality.

Using our recently developed percutaneous ultrasound-guided injection technique,[112] we achieved good transgene expression in the fetal trachea and airways after intratracheal delivery of an adenovirus containing the beta-galactosidase gene.[113] Transgene expression was enhanced by pretreatment of the fetal airways with sodium caprate, a fatty acid that opens the tight junctions between airway epithelial cells. This allows the vector to reach the basolateral surface where the receptor responsible for binding adenovirus is situated. Further enhancement of transgene expression was achieved by complexing the adenoviral vector with diethylaminoethyl dextran, a poly-cation that neutralises the negative charge on the vector, improving vector binding to the coxsackie-adenovirus receptor (Figure 6). Instillation of perflubron, an inert fluorocarbon, resulted in a redistribution of expression from the upper to the peripheral airways, which is most likely due to flushing of the vector solution further down the airways by the water immiscible perflubron.[114] These results show proof of principle for the relatively safe and minimally invasive *in utero* delivery of a gene therapy vector to the fetal airways that resulted in levels of transgene expression in the airway epithelia relevant to a therapeutic application in CF gene therapy.

Development of the fetal immune system

One of the main caveats in adult gene therapy is the immune response to vector and/or transgene. *In utero* application, on the other hand, aims to circumvent this by treatment before maturity of the functional immune system and this depends critically on the time at which fetal tolerance can be induced. The human immune system develops progressively through the first trimester and is not fully functional until 1–2 years after birth.[115] Lymphoid cells appear first in the fetal liver from eight weeks of gestation with B lymphocytes and natural killer cells predominating over T cells.[116] T lymphocytes increase in number in the fetal liver and circulation from 12 weeks of gestation. Although they are not capable of producing a definitive cytotoxic response until 18 weeks of gestation,[117] natural killer cells and some T cell lines may provide a limited immune response earlier in gestation.[118,119] The fetal lamb is able to produce detectable circulating antibody in response to some antigenic stimuli from 66 days of gestation[120] and reject skin grafts after 77 days of gestation.[121] This would suggest a 'window of opportunity' in the first third to half of pregnancy, during which time the introduction of foreign genetic material may not produce an immune response. In our early gestation ultrasound-guided injection experiments we observed no humoral immune response to the transgene, although antibodies to the adenoviral vector were detected for each route of injection.[80]

Expression of a foreign antigen during early fetal development may also result in its recognition as 'self' where exposure of the fetus to foreign antigen is maintained,[122,123] thus allowing the

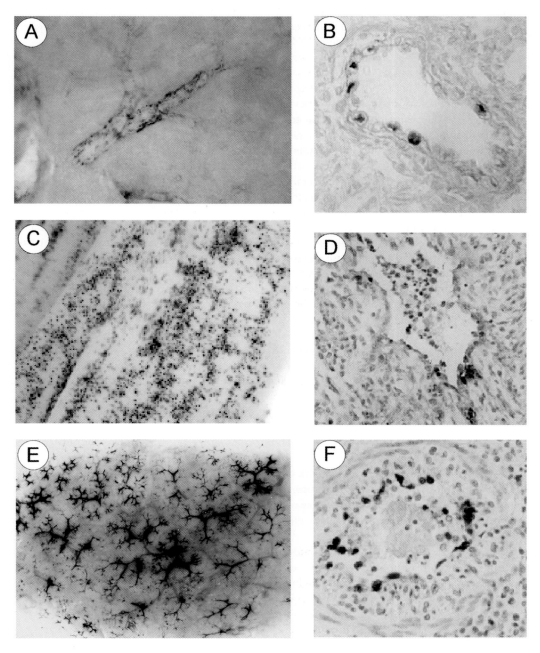

Figure 6 *Adenovirus mediated β-galactosidase expression in the airways of mid-gestation fetal sheep after ultrasound-guided injection of an adenoviral vector containing the lacZ gene into the fetal trachea; the airways were pretreated with the fatty acid sodium caprate, and the adenoviral vector was complexed with the poly-cation diethylaminoethyl dextran to improve transduction of airways epithelium; widespread gene expression on X-gal staining can be seen in the small airways (A) and (B) and the trachea (C); there is also widespread immunohistochemical localisation of β-galactosidase expression in the distal airway epithelium (D); instillation of perflubron, an inert fluorocarbon, after delivery of sodium caprate and diethylaminoethyl dextran complexed adenoviral vectors to the trachea, resulted in enhanced transduction of the distal airways (E) and (F) (photographs courtesy of L Gregory, Gene Therapy Research Group, Imperial College, London)*

development of tolerance. Evidence to support induced tolerance has been reported after *in utero* intraperitoneal delivery of retroviral vectors in fetal sheep[124] and intravascular delivery of adenoviral vectors in fetal mice.[89]

ETHICAL ISSUES

There are some serious ethical issues in relation to *in utero* gene therapy that need to be addressed.[125,126] One major concern is that fetal gene therapy has potential adverse effects on the fetus as well as on the mother, such as injury, infection, severe immune reactions or preterm labour. Furthermore, many parents decide to terminate an affected pregnancy, and therefore the option of *in utero* treatment must be at least as safe as this, and should also reliably treat the disease.

Fetal somatic gene therapy does not aim to modify the genetic content of the germline but inadvertent gene transfer to the germline is a risk that raises ethical concerns. Compartment-alisation of the primordial germ cells in the gonads is complete by seven weeks of gestation in humans and it is unlikely, therefore, that any therapy applied after this time would result in germline transduction. Examination of germ cells in some studies,[41] and in our early gestation injection experiments, has shown no detectable transmission.[80,95] Many of these issues are not confined to *in utero* gene therapy[2] and can be raised for other treatments such as adult gene therapy and chemotherapy.

The general public, however, remain concerned that ethical discussion about issues such as gene therapy, cloning and the Human Genome Project is falling behind the technology.[127] It is therefore important to provide adequate information that will allow the public to understand the risks and benefits of these novel techniques and to enable an educated involvement in the decision-making process together with health professionals. This will also help individuals to give fully informed consent as these procedures become used in clinical practice.

CONCLUSIONS

Fetal gene therapy offers the potential for obstetricians not only to diagnose but also to treat inherited genetic disease. However, for the treatment to be acceptable, it must offer advantages over postnatal gene therapy, be safe for both mother and fetus, and preferably avoid germline transmission. Currently, *in utero* gene therapy remains an experimental procedure but, in the future, better understanding of the development of genetic disease in the fetus, and improvements in vector design and targeting of fetal tissues should allow this technology to move into clinical practice.

References

1. Coutelle C, Douar A-M, Colledge WH, Froster U. The challenge of fetal gene therapy. *Nat Med* 1995;1:864–6.
2. Wilson JM, Wivel NA. Report on the potential use of gene therapy *in utero*. Gene Therapy Advisory Committee. *Hum Gene Ther* 1999;10:689–92.
3. Herzog RW, Yang EY, Couto LB, Hagstrom JN, Elwell D, Fields PA, *et al*. Long-term correction of canine hemophilia B by gene transfer of blood coagulation factor IX mediated by adeno-associated viral vector. *Nat Med* 1999;5:56–63.
4. Hsieh-Li HM, Chang J, Jong Y, Wu M, Wang NM, Tsai CH, *et al*. A mouse model for spinal muscular atrophy. *Nat Genet* 2000;24:66–70.

5.   Blouin M, Beauchemin H, Wight A, De Paepe M, Sorette M, Bleau A, *et al*. Genetic correction of sickle cell disease: insights using transgenic mouse models. *Nat Med* 2000;6:177–82.

6.   Engelhardt JF, Yankaskas JR, Ernst SA, Yang Y, Marino CR, Boucher RC, *et al*. Submucosal glands are the predominant site of CFTR expression in the human bronchus. *Nat Genet* 1992;2:240–8.

7.   Johnson LG, Olsen JC, Sarkadi B, Moore KL, Swanstrom R, Boucher RC. Efficiency of gene transfer for restoration of normal airway epithelial function in cystic fibrosis. *Nat Genet* 1992;2:21–5.

8.   Gaillard D, Ruocco S, Lallemand A, Dalemans W, Hinnrasky J, Puchelle E. Immunohistochemical localization of cystic fibrosis transmembrane conductance regulator in human fetal airway and digestive mucosa. *Pediatr Res* 1994;36:137–43.

9.   Tizzano EF, O'Brodovich H, Chitayat D, Benichou JC, Buchwald M. Regional expression of CFTR in developing human respiratory tissues. *Am J Respir Cell Mol Biol* 1994;10:355–62.

10.   Hubeau C, Puchelle E, Gaillard D. Distinct pattern of immune cell population in the lung of human fetuses with cystic fibrosis. *J Allergy Clin Immunol* 2001;108:524–29.

11.   Boué A, Muller F, Nezolod C, Oury JF, Duchatel F, Dumez Y, *et al*. Prenatal diagnosis in 200 pregnancies with a 1-in-4 risk of cystic fibrosis. *Hum Genet* 1986;74:288–97.

12.   Harris A, Coleman L. Ductal epithelial cells cultured from human foetal epididymis and vas deferens: relevance to sterility in cystic fibrosis. *J Cell Sci* 1989;92:687–90.

13.   Bigger B, Coutelle C. Perspectives on gene therapy for cystic fibrosis airway disease. *BioDrugs* 2001;15:615–34.

14.   Weiss DJ, Bonneau L, Liggitt D. Use of perfluorochemical liquid allows earlier detection of gene expression and use of less vector in normal lung and enhances gene expression in acutely injured lung. *Mol Ther* 2001;3:734–45.

15.   Weiss DJ, Strandflord TP, Liggitt D, Clark JG. Perflubron enhances adenovirus-mediated gene expression in lungs of transgenic mice with chronic alveolar filling. *Hum Gene Ther* 1999;10:2287–93.

16.   Parsons DW, Grubb BR, Johnson LG, Boucher RC. Enhanced *in vivo* airway gene transfer via transient modification of host barrier properties with a surface-active agent. *Hum Gene Ther* 1998;9:2661–72.

17.   Gregory LG, Harbottle RP, Lawrence L, Knapton HJ, Themis M, CoutelleC. Enhancement of adenovirus-mediated gene transfer to the airways by DEAE dextran and sodium caprate *in vivo*. *Mol Ther* 2003;7:19–26.

18.   Engelhardt JF, Schlossberg H, Yankaskas JR, Dudus L. Progenitor cells of the adult human airway involved in submucosal gland development. *Development* 1995;121:2031–46.

19.   Peault B, Tirouvanziam R, Sombardier MN, Chen S, Perricaudet M, Gaillard D. Gene transfer to human fetal pulmonary tissue developed in immunodeficient SCID mice. *Hum Gene Ther* 1994;5:1131–7.

20.   Furie B, Limentani SA, Rosenfield CG. A practical guide to the evaluation and treatment of hemophilia. *Blood* 1994;84:3–9.

21.   Lusher JM. Inhibitors in young boys with haemophilia. *Baillieres Best Pract Res Clin Haematol* 2000;13:457–68.

22.   Soucie JM, Nuss R, Evatt B, Abdelhak A, Cowan L, Jill H, *et al*. Mortality among males with hemophilia: relations with source of medical care. The Hemophilia Surveillance System Project Investigators. *Blood* 2000;96:437–42.

23.   Yei SP. *In vivo* evaluation of the safety of adenovirus-mediated transfer of the human cystic fibrosis transmembrane conductance regulator cDNA to the lung. *Hum Gene Ther* 1994;5:731–44.

24. Fields PA, Armstrong E, Hagstrom JN. Intravenous administration of an E1/E3-deleted adenoviral vector induces tolerance to factor IX in C57BL/6 mice. *Gene Ther* 2001;8:354–61.

25. Chao H, Samulski RJ, Bellinger D, Monahan PE, Nichols T, Walsh CE. Persistent expression of canine factor IX in hemophilia B canines. *Gene Ther* 1999;6:1695–704.

26. Snyder RO, Miao C, Meuse L, Tubb J, Donahue BA, Lin H-F, *et al*. Correction of hemophilia B in canine and murine models using recombinant adeno-associated viral vectors. *Nat Med* 1999;5:64–70.

27. Kay MA, Manno CS, Ragni MV, Larson PJ, Couto LB, McClelland A, *et al*. Evidence for gene transfer and expression of factor IX in haemophilia B patients treated with an AAV vector. *Nat Genet* 2000;24:257–61.

28. Olivares EC, Hollis RP, Chalberg TW, Meuse L, Kay MA, Calos MP. Site specific genomic integration produces therapeutic factor IX levels in mice. *Nat Biotechnol* 2002;20:1124–8.

29. Cavazzana-Calvo M, Hacein-Bey S, de Saint Basile G, Gross F, Yvon E, Nusbaum P, *et al*. Gene therapy of human severe combined immunodeficiency (SCID)-X1 disease. *Science* 2000;288:669–72.

30. Hacein-Bey-Abina S, Le Deist F, Carlier F, Bouneaud C, Hue C, De Villartay JP, *et al*. Sustained correction of X-linked severe combined immunodeficiency by *ex vivo* gene therapy. *N Engl J Med* 2002;346:1185–93.

31. Themis M. Enhanced *in vitro* and *in vivo* gene delivery using cationic agent complexed retrovirus vectors. *Gene Ther* 1998;5:1180–6.

32. Douar A-M, Adebakin S, Themis M, Pavirani A, Cook T, Coutelle C. Foetal gene delivery in mice by intra-amniotic administration of retroviral producer cells and adenovirus. *Gene Ther* 1997;4:883–90.

33. Russel DW, Berger MS, Miller AD. The effects of human serum and cerebrospinal fluid on retroviral vectors and packaging cell lines. *Hum Gene Ther* 1995;6:635–41.

34. Miller DG, Adam MA, Miller AD. Gene transfer by retrovirus vectors occurs only in cells that are actively replicating at the time of infection. *Mol Cell Biol* 1990;10:4239–42.

35. Palmer TD, Rosman GJ, Osborne WRA, Miller D. Genetically modified skin fibroblasts persist long after transplantation but gradually inactivate introduced genes. *Proc Natl Acad Sci U S A* 1991;88:1330–4.

36. Challita PM, Kohn DB. Lack of expression from a retroviral vector after transduction of murine hematopoietic stem cells is associated with methylation *in vivo*. *Proc Natl Acad Sci U S A* 1994;91:2567–71.

37. Welsh RJ, Cooper NR, Jensen FC, Oldstone MB. Human serum lyses RNA tumor viruses. *Nature* 1975;257:612–14.

38. Cosset F-L. High-titer packaging cells producing recombinant retroviruses resistant to human serum. *J Virol* 1995;69:7430–6.

39. Engelstädter M, Buchholz CJ, Bobkova M, Steidl S, Merget-Millitzer H, Willemsen RA, *et al*. Targeted gene transfer to lymphocytes using murine leukaemia virus vectors pseudotyped with spleen necrosis virus envelope proteins. *Gene Ther* 2001;8:1202–6.

40. Douar A-M. Effect of amniotic fluid on cationic lipid mediated transfection and viral infection. *Gene Ther* 1996;3:789–96.

41. Porada CD, Tran N, Eglitis M, Moen RC, Troutman L, Flake AW, *et al. In utero* gene therapy: transfer and long-term expression of the bacterial neo® gene in sheep after direct injection of retroviral vectors into preimmune fetuses. *Hum Gene Ther* 1998;9:1571–85.

42. Pitt BR, Schwarz MA, Pilewski JM, Nakayama D, Mueller GM, Robbins PD, *et al*. Retrovirus-mediated gene transfer in lungs of living fetal sheep. *Gene Ther* 1995;2:344–50.

43. Hatzoglou M, Moorman A, Lamers W. Persistent expression of genes transferred in the fetal rat liver via retroviruses. *Somat Cell Mol Genet* 1995;21:265–78.

44. Marshall E. Gene therapy a suspect in leukemia-like disease. *Science* 2002;298:34–5.

45. Li Z, Düllmann J, Schiedlmeier B, Schmidt M, von Kalle C, Meyer J, *et al*. Murine leukemia induced by retroviral gene marking. *Science* 2002;296:497.

46. Trono D. Lentiviral vectors: turning a deadly foe into a therapeutic agent. *Gene Ther* 2000;7:20–3.

47. Naldini L. *In vivo* gene delivery and stable transduction of nondividing cells by a lentiviral vector. *Science* 1996;272:263–7.

48. Case SS, Price MA, Jordan CT, Yu XJ, Wang L, Bauer G, *et al*. Stable transduction of quiescent CD34(+)CD38(–) human hematopoietic cells by HIV-1-based lentiviral vectors. *Proc Natl Acad Sci U S A* 1999;96:2988–93.

49. Mazarakis ND, Azzouz M, Rohll JB, Ellard FM, Wilkes FJ, Olsen AL, *et al*. Rabies virus glycoprotein pseudotyping of lentiviral vectors enables retrograde axonal transport and access to the nervous system after peripheral delivery. *Hum Mol Genet* 2001;10:2109–21.

50. Kobinger GP, Weiner DJ, Yu QC, Wilson JM. Filovirus-pseudotyped lentiviral vector can efficiently and stably transduce airway epithelia *in vivo*. *Nat Biotechnol* 2001;19:225–30.

51. Mitrophanous K, Yoon S, Rohll J, Patil D, Wilkes F, Kim V, *et al*. Stable gene transfer to the nervous system using a non-primate lentiviral vector. *Gene Ther* 1999;6:1808–18.

52. Wang G, Slepushkin V, Zabner J, Keshavjee S, Johnston JC, Sauter SL, *et al*. Feline immunodeficiency virus vectors persistently transduce nondividing airway epithelia and correct the cystic fibrosis defect. *J Clin Invest* 1999;104:R55–62.

53. Waddington SN, Mitrophanous KA, Ellard F, Buckley SMK, Nivsarkar M, Lawrence L, *et al*. Long-term transgene expression by administration of a lentivirus-based vector to the fetal circulation of immuno-competent mice. *Gene Ther* 2003;10:1234–40.

54. Xiao X, Li J, Samulski RJ. Production of high-titer recombinant adeno-associated virus vectors in the absence of helper adenovirus. *J Virol* 1998;72:2224–32.

55. Wang L, Takabe K, Bidlingmaier SM, Ill CR, Verma IM. Sustained correction of bleeding disorder in hemophilia B mice by gene therapy. *Proc Natl Acad Sci U S A* 1999;96:3906–10.

56. Monahan PE, Samulski RJ. Adeno-associated virus vectors for gene therapy: more pros than cons? *Mol Med Today* 2000;6:433–40.

57. Ponnazhagan S, Weigel KA, Raikwar SP, Mukherjee P, Yoder MC, Srivastava A. Recombinant human parvovirus B19 vectors: erythroid cell-specific delivery and expression of transduced genes. *J Virol* 1998;72:5224–30.

58. Sun L, Li J, Xiao X. Overcoming adeno-associated virus vector size limitation through viral DNA heterodimerization. *Nat Med* 2000;6:599–602.

59. Lehrman S. Virus treatment questioned after gene therapy death. *Nature* 1999;401:517–18.

60. McCray PB, Armstrong K, Zabner J, Miller DW, Koretzky GA, Couture L, *et al*. Adenoviral-mediated gene transfer to fetal pulmonary epithelia *in vitro* and *in vivo*. *J Clin Invest* 1995;95:2620–32.

61. Iwamoto HS, Trapnell BC, McConnell CJ, Daugherty C, Whitsett JA. Pulmonary inflammation associated with repeated, prenatal exposure to an E1, E3-deleted adenoviral vector in sheep. *Gene Ther* 1999;6:98–106.

62. Chen HH, Mack LM, Kelly R, Ontell M, Kochanek S, Clemens PR. Persistence in muscle of an adenoviral vector that lacks all viral genes. *Proc Natl Acad Sci U S A* 1997;94:1645–50.

63. Schiedner G, Morral N, Parks RJ, Wu Y, Koopmans SC, Langston C, *et al*. Genomic DNA transfer with a high-capacity adenovirus vector results in improved *in vivo* gene expression and decreased toxicity. *Nat Genet* 1998;18:180–3.

64. Feng M, Jackson WH, Goldman CK, Rancourt C, Wang M, Dusing SK, et al. Stable in vivo gene transduction via a novel adenoviral/retroviral chimeric vector. Nat Biotechnol 1997;15:866–70.

65. Caplen NJ, Higginbotham JN, Scheel JR, Vahanian N, Yoshida Y, Hamada H, et al. Adeno-retroviral chimeric viruses as in vivo transducing agents. Gene Ther 1999;6:454–9.

66. Jauniaux E, Gulbis B. Fluid compartments of the embryonic environment. Hum Reprod Update 2000;6:268–78.

67. Ross J, Jurkovic D, Nicolaides KH. Coelocentesis: a study of short-term safety. Prenat Diagn 1997;17:913–17.

68. Larson JE, Morrow SL, Delcarpio JB, Bohm RP, Ratterree MS, Blanchard JL, et al. Gene transfer into the fetal primate: evidence for the secretion of transgene product. Mol Ther 2000;2:631–9.

69. Chinnaiya A, Venkat A, Dawn C, Chee WY, Choo KB, Gole LA, et al. Intrahepatic vein fetal blood sampling: current role in prenatal diagnosis. J Obstet Gynaecol Res 1998;24:239–46.

70. Nicolini U, Nicolaidis P, Fisk NM, Tannirandorn Y, Rodeck CH. Fetal blood sampling from the intrahepatic vein: analysis of safety and clinical experience with 214 procedures. Obstet Gynecol 1990;76:47–53.

71. Jauniaux E, Gulbis B, Gerloo E. Free amino acids in human fetal liver and fluids at 12–17 weeks of gestation. Hum Reprod 1999;14:1638–41.

72. Westgren M, Ek S, Bui T, Jansson B, Kjaeldgaard A, Markling L, et al. Tissue distribution of transplanted fetal liver cells in the human fetal recipient. Am J Obstet Gynecol 1997;176:49–53.

73. Touraine JL. Induction of transplantation tolerance in humans using stem cell transplants prenatally or postnatally. Transplant Proc 1999;31:2735–7.

74. Rodeck CH, Deans A. Red cell alloimmunisation. In: Rodeck CH, Whittle MJ, editors. Fetal Medicine: Basic Science and Clinical Practice. London: Churchill Livingstone; 1999. p. 785-804.

75. Larsen JF, Jacobsen B, Holm HH, Pedersen JF, Mantoni M. Intrauterine injection of vitamin K before the delivery during anticoagulant therapy of the mother. Acta Obstet Gynecol Scand 1978;57:227–30.

76. Ljubic A, Cvetkovic M, Sulovic V, Radunovic N, Antonovic O, Vukolic D, et al. New technique for artificial lung maturation. Direct intramuscular fetal corticosteroid therapy. Clin Exp Obstet Gynecol 1999;26:16–19.

77. Rodeck C. Fetoscopy guided by real-time ultrasound for pure fetal blood samples, fetal skin samples, and examination of the fetus in utero. Br J Obstet Gynaecol 1980;87:449–56.

78. Ville Y, Van Peborgh P, Gagnon A, Frydman R, Fernandez H. Surgical treatment of twin-to-twin transfusion syndrome: coagulation of anastomoses with a Nd:YAG laser, under endosonographic control. Forty four cases. J Gynecol Obstet Biol Reprod (Paris) 1997;26:175–81.

79. Harrison MR, Mychaliska GB, Albanese CT, Jennings RW, Farrell JA, Hawgood S, et al. Correction of congenital diaphragmatic hernia in utero IX: fetuses with poor prognosis (liver herniation and low lung-to-head ratio) can be saved by fetoscopic temporary tracheal occlusion. J Pediatr Surg 1998;33:1017–22.

80. David A, Cook T, Waddington S, Peebles D, Nivsarkar M, Knapton H, et al. Ultrasound-guided percutaneous delivery of adenoviral vectors encoding the β-galactosidase and human factor IX genes to early gestation fetal sheep in utero. Hum Gene Ther 2003;14:353–64.

81. Senoo M, Matsubara Y, Fujii K, Nagasaki Y, Hiratsuka M, Kure S, et al. Adenovirus-mediated in utero gene transfer in mice and guinea pigs: tissue distribution of recombinant adenovirus determined by quantitative TaqMan-polymerase chain reaction assay. Mol Genet Metab 2000;69:269–76.

82. Themis M, Schneider H, Kiserud T, Cook T, Adebakin S, Jezzard S, et al. Successful expression of β-galactosidase and factor IX transgenes in fetal and neonatal sheep after ultrasound-guided percutaneous adenovirus vector administration into the umbilical vein. Gene Ther 1999;6:1239–48.

83. Yang EY, Cass DL, Sylvester KG, Wilson JM, Adzick NS. Fetal gene therapy: efficacy, toxicity, and immunologic effects of early gestation recombinant adenovirus. J Pediatr Surg 1999;34:235–41.

84. Christensen G, Minamisawa S, Gruber PJ, Wang Y, Chien KR. High-efficiency, long-term cardiac expression of foreign genes in living mouse embryos and neonates. Circulation 2000;101:178–84.

85. Wang G. Ultrasound-guided gene therapy to hepatocytes in utero. Fetal Diagn Ther 1998;13:197–205.

86. Schachtner SK, Buck CA, Bergelson JM, Baldwin HS. Temporally regulated expression patterns following in utero adenovirus-mediated gene transfer. Gene Ther 1996;6:1249–57.

87. Mason CA. Gene transfer in utero biologically engineers a patent ductus arteriosus in lambs by arresting fibronectin-dependent neointimal formation. Nat Med 1999;5:176–82.

88. Moise KJ, Hesketh DE, Belfort MM, Saade G, Van den Veyer IB, Hudson KM, et al. Ultrasound-guided blood sampling of rabbit fetuses. Lab Anim Sci 1992;42:398–401.

89. Waddington SN, Buckley SMK, Nivsarkar M, Jezzard S, Schneider H, Dahse T, et al. In utero gene transfer of human factor IX to fetal mice can induce postnatal tolerance of the exogenous clotting factor. Blood 2003101:1359–66.

90. Lipshutz GS, Flebbe-Rehwaldt L, Gaensler KML. Adenovirus-mediated gene transfer in the midgestation fetal mouse. J Surg Res 1999;84:150–6.

91. Lipshutz GS, Flebbe-Rehwaldt L, Gaensler KML. Adenovirus-mediated gene transfer to the peritoneum and hepatic parenchyma of fetal mice in utero. Surgery 1999;126:171–7.

92. Lipshutz GS, Flebbe-Rehwaldt L, Gaensler KML. Reexpression following readministration of an adenoviral vector in adult mice after initial in utero adenoviral administration. Mol Ther 2000;2:374–80.

93. Mitchell M, Jerebtsova M, Batshaw ML, Newman K, Ye X. Long-term gene transfer to mouse fetuses with recombinant adenovirus and adeno-associated virus (AAV) vectors. Gene Ther 2000;7:1986–92.

94. Hatzoglou M, Lamers W, Bosch F, Wynshaw-Boris A, Clapp DW, Hanson RW. Hepatic gene transfer in animals using retrovirus containing the promoter from the gene for phosphoenolpyruvate carboxykinase. J Biol Chem 1990;265:17285–93.

95. Tran ND, Porada CD, Zhao Y, Almeida-Porada G, Anderson WF, Zanjani ED. In utero transfer and expression of exogenous genes in sheep. Exp Hematol 2000;28:17–30.

96. Lipshutz GS, Gruber CA, Cao Y, Hardy J, Contag CH, Gaensler KML. In utero delivery of adeno-associated viral vectors: intraperitoneal gene transfer produces long-term expression. Mol Ther 2001;3:284–92.

97. Schneider H, Mühle C, Douar A-M, Waddington S, Jiang Q-J, von der Mark K, et al. Sustained delivery of therapeutic concentrations of human clotting factor IX – a comparison of adenoviral and AAV vectors administered in utero. J Gene Med 2002;4:46–53.

98. Yang EY, Kim HB, Shaaban AF, Milner R, Adzick NS, Flake AW. Persistent postnatal transgene expression in both muscle and liver after fetal injection of recombinant adenovirus. J Pediatr Surg 1999;34:766–72.

99. Larson JE, Morrow SL, Happel L, Sharp JF, Cohen JC. Reversal of cystic fibrosis phenotype in mice by gene therapy in utero. Lancet 1997;349:619–20.

100. Holzinger A, Trapnell BC, Weaver TE, Whitsett JA, Iwamoto HS. Intraamniotic

administration of an adenoviral vector for gene transfer to fetal sheep and mouse tissues. *Pediatr Res* 1995;38:844–50.

101. Sekhon HS, Larson JE. *In utero* gene transfer into the pulmonary epithelium. *Nat Med* 1995;1:1201–3.

102. Papaioannou VE. *In utero* manipulations. In: Copp AJ, Cockroft DL, editors. *Postimplantation Mammalian Embryos. A Practical Approach.* Oxford: JRL Press; 1990. p. 61–80.

103. Bennett M, Galan H, Owens G, Dewey R, Banks R, Hobbins J, et al. *In utero* gene delivery by intraamniotic injection of a retroviral vector producer cell line in a nonhuman primate model. *Hum Gene Ther* 2001;12:1857–65.

104. Schneider H, Adebakin S, Themis M, Cook T, Douar A-M, Pavirani A, et al. Therapeutic plasma concentrations of human factor IX in mice after gene delivery into the amniotic cavity: a model for the prenatal treatment of haemophilia B. *J Gene Med* 1999;1:424–32.

105. Boyle MP, Enke RA, Adams RJ, Guggino WB, Zeitlin PL. *In utero* AAV-mediated gene transfer to rabbit pulmonary epithelium. *Mol Ther* 2001;4:115–21.

106. Moss IR, Scarpelli EM. Stimulatory effect of theophylline on regulation of fetal breathing movements. *Pediatr Res* 1981;15:870–3.

107. Kalache KD, Chaoui R, Marcks B, Nguyen-Dobinsky TN, Wernicke KD, Wauer R, et al. Differentiation between human fetal breathing patterns by investigation of breathing-related tracheal fluid flow velocity using Doppler sonography. *Prenat Diagn* 2000;20:45–50.

108. Badalian SS, Chao CR, Fox HE, Timor TI. Fetal breathing-related nasal fluid flow velocity in uncomplicated pregnancies. *Am J Obstet Gynecol* 1993;169:563–7.

109. Tarantal AF, Lee CI, Ekert JE, McDonald R, Kohn DB, Plopper CG, et al. Lentiviral vector gene transfer into fetal rhesus monkeys (*Macaca mulatta*): lung-targeting approaches. *Mol Ther* 2001;4:614–21.

110. Vincent MC, Trapnell BC, Baughman RP, Wert SE, Whitsett JA, Iwamoto HS. Adenovirus-mediated gene transfer to the respiratory tract of fetal sheep *in utero*. *Hum Gene Ther* 1995;6:1019–28.

111. Sylvester KG, Yang EY, Cass DL, Crombleholme TM, Scott Adzick N. Fetoscopic gene therapy for congenital lung disease. *J Pediatr Surg* 1997;7:964–9.

112. David AL, Peebles DM, Gregory L, Themis M, Cook T, Coutelle C, et al. Percutaneous ultrasound-guided injection of the trachea in fetal sheep: a novel technique to target the fetal airways. *Fetal Diagn Ther* 2003;18:385–90.

113. Peebles D, Gregory LG, David A, Themis M, Waddington S, Knapton HJ. et al. Widespread and efficient marker gene expression in the airway epithelia of fetal sheep after minimally invasive tracheal application of recombinant adenovirus *in utero*. *Gene Ther* 2003;11:70–8.

114. Weiss DJ, Strandjord TP, Jackson JC, Clark JG, Liggitt D. Perfluorochemical liquid-enhanced adenoviral vector distribution and expression in lungs of spontaneously breathing rodents. *Exp Lung Res* 1999;25:317–33.

115. Riley RL. Neonatal immune response. In: Delves PJ, Roitt IM, editors. *Encyclopedia of Immunology.* London: Academic Press; 1998. p. 1818–21.

116. Pahal GS, Jauniaux E, Kinnon C, Thrasher AJ, Rodeck C. Normal development of human fetal hematopoiesis between eight and seventeen weeks' gestation. *Am J Obstet Gynecol* 2000;183:1029–34.

117. Mackenzie IZ, Maclean DA. Pure fetal blood from the umbilical cord obtained at fetoscopy: experience with 125 consecutive cases. *Am J Obstet Gynecol* 1980;138:1214–18.

118. Phillips JH, Hori T, Nagler A, Bhat N, Spits H, Lanier LL. Ontogeny of human natural killer (NK) cells: fetal NK cells mediate cytolytic function and express cytoplasmic CD3 epsilon, delta proteins. *J Exp Med* 1992;175:1055–66.

119. Miyagawa Y, Matsuoka T, Baba A, Nakamura T, Tsuno T, Tamura A, *et al*. Fetal liver T cell receptor gamma/delta+ T cells as cytotoxic T lymphocytes specific for maternal alloantigens. *J Exp Med* 1992;176:1–7.

120. Silverstein AM, Uhr JW, Lukes RJ. Fetal response to antigenic stimulus II. Antibody production by the fetal lamb. *J Exp Med* 1963;117:799–812.

121. Silverstein AM, Prendergast RA, Kraner KL. Fetal response to antigenic stimulus IV. Rejection of skin homografts by the fetal lamb. *J Exp Med* 1964;119:955–64.

122. Billingham RE, Brent L, Medawar PB. Quantitative studies on tissue transplantation immunity III: Actively acquired tolerance. *Phil Trans R Soc (Lond) B Biol Sci* 1956;B239:357–69.

123. Binns R. Bone marrow and lymphoid cell injection of the pig fetus resulting in transplantation tolerance or immunity, and immunoglobulin production. *Nature* 1967;214:179–80.

124. Tran ND, Porada CD, Almeida-Porada G, Glimp HA, Anderson WF, Zanjani ED. Induction of stable prenatal tolerance to beta-galactosidase by *in utero* gene transfer into preimmune sheep fetuses. *Blood* 2001;97:3417–23.

125. Fletcher JC, Richter G. Human fetal gene therapy: moral and ethical questions. *Human Gene Ther* 1996;7:1605–14.

126. Coutelle C, Rodeck C. On the scientific and ethical issues of fetal somatic gene therapy. *Gene Ther* 2002;9:670–3.

127. Brown P. Regulations not keeping up with developments in genetics, says poll. *BMJ* 2000;321:1369.

128. David AL, Themis M, Cook T, Coutelle C, Rodeck CH. Fetal gene therapy. *Ultrasound Rev Obstet Gynecol* 2001;1:14–27.

129. David AL, Themis M, Waddington SN, Gregory L, Buckley SMK, Nivsarkar M, *et al*. The current status and future direction of fetal gene therapy. *Gene Ther Mol Biol* 2003;7:181–209.

10

Repair of perineal trauma

Kara Dent, Christine Kettle and Shaughn O'Brien

INTRODUCTION

Under-reporting of perineal damage was recognised even as early as 1897, when Jellet described it as 'one of the most common accidents occurring in midwifery... it occurs far more frequently than is supposed; as, unless it be looked for with care, it may not be noticed.'[1]

Over 85% of women undergoing a vaginal delivery will experience some degree of perineal trauma. Of these, two-thirds will need suturing,[2] a significant number will suffer short-term complications, with one in five of these resulting in long-term difficulties.[3] Despite the size of the problem, there has been relatively little research in this area and modern day obstetricians have a notable lack of training and experience.

Perineal trauma is defined as any damage occurring to the lower genital tract during delivery. This can be either a consequence of the birth itself or iatrogenic (an episiotomy) in order to facilitate delivery. It is divided into anterior or posterior perineal trauma. Anterior perineal injury is that involving the labia, anterior vagina, urethra or clitoris. Posterior injury affects the posterior vaginal wall, perineal muscles or anal sphincters. The latter leads to the more serious complications and maternal morbidity.

This is a sensitive but important area for newly delivered mothers. Less than a third of those women who do suffer from some of the more serious complications, such as anal incontinence, ever consult with a physician or seek medical help.[4] Unfortunately, nonconsultation perpetuates our lack of awareness and conceals the magnitude of problems that affect such a large number of women.

CLASSIFICATION

Until a few years ago, there has been little consensus in how the different degrees of perineal tears should be classified. A survey of consultants and trainees in obstetrics and gynaecology showed that a third of the current consultants and a fifth of the trainees incorrectly classified a partial or complete tear of the external anal sphincter as a second degree tear.[5] If tears are not being properly identified then they are almost certainly not being sutured appropriately. The blame for this confusion may be the inconsistency found in medical texts, including some of the more popular reference books used for training and examination purposes. Out of 65 popular texts examined in one study, a sixth did not address the issue of classification of perineal tears at all, while a fifth incorrectly defined a sphincter defect as a second degree tear.[6] The Royal College of Obstetricians and Gynaecologists guidelines have been updated suggesting a more explicit classification for perineal tears:[7]

- **first degree tears:** involve only skin

- **second degree tears:** injury to perineum involving perineal muscles but not involving the anal sphincter

- **third-degree tears:** injury to perineum involving the anal sphincter complex: external anal sphincter and internal anal sphincter
  - 3a: less than 50% of external anal sphincter thickness torn
  - 3b: more than 50% of external anal sphincter thickness torn
  - 3c: internal anal sphincter torn

- **fourth-degree tears:** injury to perineum involving the anal sphincter complex (external and internal anal sphincters) and rectal mucosa.

This differentiates between third and fourth-degree tears on whether the rectal mucosa is involved, while subclassifying third-degree tears depending on whether the internal and external anal sphincters are torn. It is important to reach international consensus on the classification of perineal tears for comparative research purposes.

RISK FACTORS FOR PERINEAL TRAUMA

Recognising the risk factors for perineal trauma provides the opportunity to practise preventive obstetrics. Studies have consistently shown forceps deliveries to result in a higher percentage of perineal damage when compared with ventouse deliveries.[4,6,8–10] On studying third-degree tears, Sultan et al.[4] reported an incidence of 50% in primiparous women undergoing a forceps delivery (compared with 7% of normal vaginal deliveries in the control group), with no third-degree tears reported in the ventouse deliveries. In a separate study (n = 43), the use of anal endosonography identified subclinical sphincter defects in 81% of the primiparous women delivered by forceps and in only 24% of those delivered by ventouse.[8] Forceps are therefore a recognised risk factor for perineal damage.

The group at greatest risk of perineal trauma are primiparous women. The aetiology is uncertain but it has been suggested that it may be due to the relative 'inelasticity of their perineum'.[11] Other known risk factors for third-degree tears are:

- primiparity

- persistent occipito–posterior positions

- babies weighing > 4 kg

- prolonged second stage

- precipitate birth

- instrumental delivery.

It has been postulated that instrumental deliveries and a prolonged second stage are particular risk factors for anal sphincter damage in primiparous women,[1,12] whereas macrosomia is a more specific risk factor in multiparous women.[10,13]

Other maternal factors that may influence the extent of injury include ethnicity, maternal age and nutritional state of the mother prepregnancy.

METHODS OF REPAIR

First and second degree tears

Nonsuturing

Practice varies on whether midwives and obstetricians suture first and second degree tears or whether they leave them to heal by primary intention. A survey in the West Midlands showed that 50% of first and second degree tears were left unsutured by midwives with the argument that this results in less pain, less infection and faster healing.[14] Conversely, other professionals argue that this method is less aesthetic, decreases the strength of the pelvic floor and predisposes to prolapse. There is no strong evidence to refute either of these points of view. A randomised controlled trial (RCT) from Sweden comparing nonsuturing (*n* = 40) to suturing (*n* = 38) of minor perineal tears concluded that there was no difference in short-term discomfort or long-term healing complications. This was a small trial and the results must be interpreted with care.[15]

Suturing

Perineal trauma is conventionally repaired in three stages. First, a continuous 'locking' stitch is used for the vaginal tissue, starting at the apex of the wound and finishing at the level of the fourchette with a loop knot. It is traditional to use a 'locking' stitch to repair the vagina because a continuous 'running' stitch may cause shortening of the vagina if it is pulled too tight. No controlled studies have been carried out to investigate this theory. Next, the perineal muscles are re-approximated with three or four interrupted sutures or a continuous 'running' stitch. Finally, the skin is closed using either continuous subcutaneous or interrupted transcutaneous sutures.

A meta-analysis, carried out in 2001, reviewed the RCTs that compared the techniques of continuous subcuticular versus interrupted transcutaneous sutures for perineal skin closure.[16] The authors found only four RCTs suitable for inclusion and judged only one of these to be of high quality in terms of method (randomisation, adequate blinding and with good documentation). Surprisingly, all of these trials were carried out between 1978 and 1989, with nothing more current published at the time of the meta-analysis. This included 1864 women (primiparous and multiparous) and used short-term and long-term morbidity as outcomes, in terms of pain, analgesia, superficial dyspareunia, removal of sutures, the need for resuturing and resumption of intercourse. The authors concluded that the only significant outcomes were a decrease in perineal pain at ten days and a reduction in suture removal up to three months postpartum in the subcuticular suturing group. They noted that these results should be interpreted with caution because only one of the four trials was able to prove a significant difference in postpartum pain and therefore further research was necessary.

Subsequently, the results of a large RCT were published in the *Lancet*.[17] A total of 1542 women were randomised to the two techniques, when there was conclusive evidence that the continuous suturing technique for all layers resulted in significantly less perineal pain at 10 days (26.5% versus 44%) with no significant difference at 3 and 12 months. This means that, by using the continuous suturing technique, one in six women are prevented from experiencing pain in the immediate postpartum period. The advantage of the continuous technique may be due to the tension being transferred equally throughout the suture[18] or because the sutures are in the subcutaneous tissue, thus avoiding the plethora of nerve endings in the skin surface.[19]

Third and fourth-degree tears

The incidence of third and fourth-degree tears reported in the literature varies between 0.55 and 3%,[4,5] which means that, in the UK, as many as 15 000 women a year may be affected.[5] The complications associated with these tears are so serious and debilitating that it is recommended that only trained personnel should undertake the repair procedure under optimum conditions. This involves performing the procedure in theatre with the appropriate instruments, good lighting and adequate assistance.[7,20] Access to regional or general anaesthesia means that the woman is pain free and that the anal sphincter is relaxed. This allows the torn areas to be retrieved properly and then approximated without tension.[21]

Controversy exists regarding the suturing of these tears concerning whether the technique of overlapping the external anal sphincter is superior to the end-to-end (approximation) method. The most recent literature search[7] on this subject identified only one RCT that directly compared the two methods.[22] A total of 112 women were recruited and randomised to a method of repair. Although fewer women complained of faecal urgency with the overlap method (20% versus 30%), the results were not significant. Equally, no significant differences were shown in the incontinence scores between the two groups. Further research is needed to determine conclusively which is the superior method. Follow-up of the data needs to be adequate. Observational data have suggested that there may be an initial benefit to using the overlap method, which then deteriorates over time.[23] It is argued that dissection of the torn sphincter to allow overlap may impair the nerve supply to this region and lead to long-term deterioration. Information will subsequently become available from a larger RCT that includes a five-year follow-up of both methods of suturing.

Postoperative management

Antibiotic cover is advocated; both anaerobic and aerobic agents are necessary. Stool softeners will prevent faecal impaction and possible damage to the recently repaired sphincter.[20]

These women need education in good hygiene and pelvic floor exercises, and would benefit from open access to a specific perineal clinic where multidisciplinary (physiotherapy, colorectal, obstetric and midwifery) staff are available.[22]

Despite immediate primary repair of third and fourth-degree tears, anal incontinence is reported to be 29–48% up to three years post-delivery.[4] This could be due to breakdown of the initial surgical repair, a pudendal nerve neuropathy, or incorrect surgical technique. The latter highlights the importance of having adequately trained personnel and also being able to identify the sphincter sufficiently at the time of repair and to reapproximate it along its entire length.[4]

Subsequent pregnancies

There are no available data from randomised controlled trials or systematic reviews addressing the management in subsequent deliveries of women who have sustained third and fourth-degree tears. Nonrandomised data show that 17–24% of these women may develop faecal symptoms, which may become worse after a second vaginal delivery when there has been sphincter damage in the first delivery.[7] The morbidity and mortality of a caesarean section needs to be weighed against possible further damage to the anal sphincter, with a vaginal delivery possibly resulting in incontinence as a consequence. It is not clear what role the pregnancy itself plays in sphincter damage when considering the hormonal effects and the growing fetus.

An elective section may be justified in those women who have had a previous sphincter repair for incontinence after childbirth; a previous third degree tear with minor incontinence that may be made worse by another vaginal delivery, previous anal surgery, or even a successful repair of a third degree tear that is asymptomatic.[20] What is clear is that medical staff have an obligation to counsel these women carefully and that there is a necessity for all women, nulliparous and multiparous, to be informed antenatally about possible perineal trauma at delivery.[20]

SUTURE MATERIALS

The aim when suturing perineal tears is to promote healing by primary or first intention, with good haemostasis and minimal scarring. Generally, healing occurs rapidly within two weeks, aided by the optimal conditions naturally present during parturition. These include the increased vascularity of the area with reduced exposure, moisture, warmth and a favourable pH of around 4.5 in which organisms are generally unable to grow.[24]

The ideal suture material is one that opposes the tissue for the necessary healing time but is not present long enough to be recognised by the body as a foreign body (and thus excite an inflammatory response) or be a nidus for infection.

First and second degree tears

Standard Vicryl® (standard polyglactin 910; Ethicon, Brussels, Belgium) and Dexon® (polyglycolic acid; Davis and Geck, Gosport, UK) are synthetic absorbable sutures that have been available since the 1970s. They are broken down by hydrolysis and are thought to cause less tissue reaction than nonabsorbable sutures. Catgut is a collagen based substance that is broken down by a different process, namely phagocytosis and proteolytic enzymes.[25] The absorption time of Vicryl and Dexon is significantly shorter than that of chromic catgut (60–90 days versus 90–120 days).[26]

A meta-analysis published in 2000,[16] comparing the effects of absorbable synthetic suture materials with catgut, identified eight RCTs that varied in suture materials and methods used. The authors of this review admitted to adopting broad inclusion criteria because there were only a small number of RCTs available for comparison. Six of the trials compared Dexon with catgut, one compared chromic with plain catgut, and only one compared Vicryl with catgut. Methods of suturing varied between the continuous and interrupted methods. One study omitted to describe the method of suturing used. Conclusions drawn from the review were that the absorbable synthetic suture, when compared with catgut, resulted in less pain at three days, less analgesia being required in the first seven days, and less suture dehiscence. There were no significant differences in long-term pain. The main disadvantage of absorbable sutures was that they were twice as likely to need removal during the first three months.[27]

Vicryl Rapide® (Ethicon, Brussels, Belgium) has been licensed for use in the UK since 1996. Changes in the sterilisation process mean that it has a lower molecular weight than standard Vicryl and is therefore absorbed in less time (35–42 days).[25] There have been two small RCTs comparing standard Vicryl with Vicryl Rapide. One of the studies demonstrated no discernible difference in the short- or long-term pain suffered in either group, but there was a significant disparity in 'pain' when walking at day 14 assessment with Vicryl Rapide compared with standard Vicryl (33.3% versus 48.5%).[28] The significant outcome from the other RCT was a reduction in dyspareunia in the Vicryl Rapide group at 6 and 12 weeks, as well as a lower level of wound complications (dehiscence, pain or removal of sutures).[29] A larger, more robust, trial has now been completed that compares Vicryl Rapide with standard Vicryl.[17] With cooperation from the suppliers, these researchers were able to obtain undyed Vicryl so that true blinding could be achieved in the use of sutures (standard Vicryl is usually dyed purple for identification purposes while Vicryl Rapide is undyed). This study provided convincing evidence that one in ten women avoided suture removal during the first three months with Vicryl Rapide compared with standard Vicryl.

Third and fourth-degree tears

In the absence of a Cochrane Review or an RCT on the best suture materials to use for repair of the anal sphincter, PDS® (polydioxanone; Ethicon, Brussels, Belgium) has been recommended as good practice.[7] This has the advantage over Vicryl and catgut of having a longer half-life and a decreased risk of infection. Warning is given about the possibility of knot migration with this suture.[7]

TRAINING ISSUES

Four main components are necessary for a successful perineal repair: good technique, accurate diagnosis and classification, the correct suturing material, and operator skill.[30] When asked, 80% of trainees, at the time of carrying out their first perineal repair, believed that their training had been inadequate.[31] There has been little research into the training issues or into which is the best method of training, be it with simulators, videos or apprenticeship.[16] Proposals from a consensus meeting held in 2001 on obstetric perineal injury and incontinence included: 'Obstetric training should ensure an adequate knowledge of anatomy and suturing techniques…' for trainees in order to 'focus greater interest on the prevention and treatment of post-obstetric injuries'.[20]

It is interesting to note that units undertaking trials in perineal trauma have seen a rise in the incidence of sphincter damage reported during the time of their study. In a study at Queen Charlotte's Hospital (London),[32] additional perineal assessment by trained personnel resulted in an increased reporting of third-degree tears (14.9%). A further study carried out in Ireland[33] noted an increase in the incidence of documented perineal injury from 0.6% before the study to 1% during the time of the study. It would be reasonable to assume that this apparent increase in third and fourth-degree tears was due to heightened awareness and better recognition of this condition.[33]

Risk management

Failure to recognise a sphincter injury and suture it appropriately has led to successful negligence cases.[20] In this current climate of increasing litigation it is essential that accurate documentation should be available on any form of perineal repair.[7] This should include the following points:

- anatomical structures involved
- method of repair
- suture materials used
- a count of swabs and sharps used
- outline of information given to the woman
- plan for adequate follow-up
- instruction for advice on hygiene, exercises and diet
- prescription of antibiotics and laxatives.

Documentation may be improved by including a diagram to illustrate clearly both the trauma and the repair technique used.

COMPLICATIONS AFTER PERINEAL TRAUMA

Perineal pain

Perineal pain affects between 21% and 42% of women in the first ten days postpartum.[2,34] Contributing factors are oedema and bruising from delivery, sutures that are too tight, infection, and wound dehiscence. The few studies that have followed up these women to 12–18 months show that 8–10% continue to have pain long term.[2,35]

Dyspareunia

Dyspareunia is defined as any pain that occurs during sexual intercourse. It may present as deep or superficial dyspareunia. The latter is more common after perineal trauma and repair. It affects a significant number of women following childbirth (23% in the first three months[25]) and can have a major effect on these women's intimate relationships.

Urinary incontinence

Genuine stress incontinence (involuntary loss of urine in the absence of detrusor contraction) is one of the major complications of pregnancy and childbirth. Its pathophysiology is not entirely clear but it is probably multifactorial: a combination of mechanical strain on the pelvic floor muscles by a gravid uterus during the pregnancy, damage to the pelvic floor muscles, and pudendal nerve damage (this nerve supplies the distal urethral sphincter). It can affect up to 24% of women after childbirth and appears more prevalent with increasing parity, thereby having a cumulative effect.[36] A study of 937 women showed the prevalence of stress incontinence to increase from 17% in nulliparous women to around 50% in parous women.[37]

We know that, during pregnancy, the primary function of the pelvic floor is to support the pelvic organs, and the chorionic cytotrophoblast cells produce relaxin, which softens the pelvic muscles and ligaments, allowing them to stretch during childbirth. This effect is reversed after delivery because of the elasticity of the pelvic floor muscles. However, prolonged or extreme stretching, trauma, or compression of the pelvic floor muscles and nerves may cause permanent damage, resulting in urinary incontinence.

As well as parity, other obstetric influences reported to increase the risk of urinary incontinence are prolonged labour, large babies weighing over 4 kg, and forceps delivery.[37–40] Prepregnancy factors include maternal age over 30 years and a body mass index of over 30. Together, these can lead to a 7% increased risk of incontinence at three months postpartum.[39]

Anal incontinence

Anal incontinence is described as any involuntary loss of solid or liquid stool per rectum or incontinence of flatus. After childbirth, it is estimated that between 2% and 16% of women exhibit faecal incontinence with 4–23% describing incontinence of flatus.[34,41–43] The aetiology is again probably multifactorial, with sphincter injury, pelvic floor trauma, perineal trauma and pudendal nerve neuropathy (the pudendal nerves supply S2–4) contributing. Some women with no demonstrated sphincter or pudendal nerve damage are asymptomatic, whereas only a third of those with anal sphincter defects confirmed on anal endosonography have clinical bowel symptoms.[10] Conversely, although pudendal nerve latency has been confirmed after delivery, there is no apparent association with early faecal incontinence. Neuropathy is suggested as a cause for incontinence that presents later in life and is thought to be a progressive condition.

With the introduction of anal endosonography, we are now able to recognise asymptomatic sphincter damage, otherwise known as an occult defect. This differs from overt defects, which are seen and recognised at the time of delivery. Published reports note the incidence of third/fourth-degree tears to be between 0.5% and 3%.[4,5] With the aid of ultrasound, these figures increase to show that occult damage is much more frequent, affecting 35% of primiparous women and 44% of multiparous women. Predelivery, 40% of the multiparous group already had confirmed occult defects, so only 4% suffered new damage.[10] Apart from primiparity, babies weighing over 4 kg, forceps deliveries and persistent occipito-posterior position are other risk factors for third-degree tears.[4] It has been shown that 94% of women with sphincter damage after a vaginal delivery have at least one of these risk factors.[4]

CONCLUSION

Current evidence shows that each year approximately 350 000 women sustain some form of perineal trauma in the UK.[17] If we hope to decrease the complications that result from these tears, we need to focus on training to ensure that the right sutures are being used and the best techniques employed.

There is evidence of a lack of adequate training in this area.[31] Without training, third- and fourth-degree tears are not identified correctly and are therefore not treated appropriately. The consequences are debilitating and involve long-term management. This has cost and economic implications for the health service. Failure to recognise a sphincter injury is a principal cause of successful court cases, alongside poor technique and failure to perform an appropriate caesarean section, for postobstetric incontinence.[20]

Absorbable synthetic sutures are associated with less perineal pain, analgesic requirement, dehiscence and resuturing when compared with catgut (Grade A evidence: i.e. requires at least one RCT as part of a body of literature of overall good quality and consistency addressing the specific recommendation[25]). Of these, Vicryl Rapide results in one in ten fewer women needing suture removal in the first three months and therefore avoiding further unnecessary discomfort (Grade A evidence).[17]

There is now Grade A evidence that the continuous technique for suturing the perineum results in less short-term pain when compared with the interrupted method.[25] Less suture material is used in this method, so this also has cost implications.

FUTURE RESEARCH

Conclusive evidence is still required before recommendations on the optimum technique and suturing methods for third and fourth-degree tears can be made. This research is currently being developed so results are awaited.

Follow-up of women who have suffered perineal trauma remains inadequate and is an area that needs addressing. There is a call for further research to investigate preventive measures to avoid unnecessary perineal trauma and to identify how best to educate trainees to manage it correctly.

It is hoped that by highlighting this topic we can serve to improve our current standards and training in an area of obstetrics that concerns a huge percentage of the women undergoing vaginal delivery nationally and worldwide.

Acknowledgement

Ethicon provided the sutures (to CK) and partially funded a part-time clerk for the RCT conducted.[17]

References

1. Jellet H. *A Short Practice of Midwifery, Embodying the Treatment Adopted in the Rotunda Hospital, Dublin*. London: J&A Churchill; 1897. p. 282–6.

2. Sleep J, Grant A, Garcia J, Elbourne D, Spencer J, Chalmers I. West Berkshire perineal management trial. *BMJ* 1984;289:587–90.

3. Enkin M, Keirse M, Renfrew M, Neilson J, editors. *A Guide to Effective Care in Pregnancy and Childbirth*. Oxford: Oxford University Press; 1995. p. 273.

4. Sultan AH, Kamm MA, Hudson CN, Bartram CI. Third degree obstetric anal sphincter tears: risk factors and outcome of primary repair. *BMJ* 1994;308:887–91.

5. Fernando RJ, Sultan AH, Radley S, Jones PW, Johanson RB. Management of obstetric anal sphincter injury: a systematic review and national practice survey. *BMC Health Serv Res* 2002;2:9.

6. Sultan AH, Thaker R. Lower genital tract and anal sphincter trauma. *Best Pract Res Clin Obstet Gynaecol* 2002;16:99–115.

7. Royal College of Obstetricians and Gynaecologists. *Management of Third and Fourth Degree Perineal Tears Following Vaginal Delivery*. Guideline No. 29. RCOG Press: London; 2001.

8. Sultan AH, Kamm MA, Bartram CI, Hudson CN. Anal sphincter trauma during instrumental delivery. *Int J Gynaecol Obstet* 1993;43:263–70.

9. Johanson RB, Rice C, Doyle M, Arthur M, Anyanwu L, Ibrahim J, *et al.* A randomised prospective study comparing the new vacuum extractor policy with forceps delivery. *Br J Obstet Gynaecol* 1993;100:524–30.

10. Sultan AH, Kamm MA, Hudson CN, Thomas JM, Bartram CI. Anal sphincter disruption during vaginal delivery. *N Engl J Med* 1993;329:1905–11.

11. Sultan AH, Monga AK, Stanton SL. The pelvic floor sequelae of childbirth. *Br J Hosp Med* 1996;55:575–9.

12. Donnelly V, Fynes M, Campbell D, Johnson H, O'Connell PR, O'Herlihy C. Obstetric events leading to anal sphincter damage. *Obstet Gynecol* 1998;92:955–61.

13. Snooks SL, Setchell M, Swash M, Henry MM. Injury to innervation of pelvic floor sphincter musculature in childbirth. *Lancet* 1984;ii:546–50.

14. Metcalfe A, Tohill S, Williams A, Haldon V, Brown L, Henry L. A pragmatic tool for the measurement of perineal tears. *Br J Midwifery* 2002;10:412–17.

15. Lundquist M, Olsson A, Nissen E, Norman M. Is it necessary to suture all lacerations after a vaginal delivery? *Birth* 2000;27:79–85.

16. Kettle C, Johanson RB. Continuous versus interrupted sutures for perineal repair. *Cochrane Database Syst Rev* 2000;(2):CD000947.

17. Kettle C, Hills RK, Jones P, Darby L, Gray R, Johanson R. Continuous versus interrupted perineal repair with standard or rapidly absorbed sutures after spontaneous vaginal birth: a randomised controlled trial. *Lancet* 2002;359:2217–23.

18. Rucker MP. Immediate perineorrhaphy with knotless sutures. *Am J Obstet Gynecol* 1939;38:703–7.

19. Fleming N. Can the suturing method make a difference in postpartum perineal pain? *J Nurse Midwifery* 1990;35:19–25.

20. Keighley MRB, Radley S, Johanson R. Consensus on prevention and management of post-obstetric bowel incontinence and third degree tear. *Clinical Risk* 2000;6:231–7.

21. Sultan AH, Monga AK, Kumar D, Stanton SL. Primary repair of obstetric anal sphincter

rupture using the overlap technique. *Br J Obstet Gynaecol* 1999;106:318–23.

22. Fitzpatrick M, Behan M, O'Connell PR, O'Herlihy C. A randomised trial comparing primary overlap with approximation repair of third-degree obstetric tears. *Am J Obstet Gynecol* 2000;183:1220–4.

23. Malouf AJ, Norton CS, Engel AF, Nicholls RJ, Kamm MA. Long-term results of overlapping anterior anal-sphincter repair for obstetric trauma. *Lancet* 2000;355:260–5.

24. Quick C, Thomas P. *Principles of Surgical Management.* Oxford: Oxford University Press; 2000.

25. Irvin TT. *Wound Healing – Principles and Practices.* London: Chapman & Hall; 1981.

26. Royal College of Obstetricians and Gynaecologists. *Methods and Materials Used in Perineal Repair.* Guideline No. 23. London: RCOG Press; 2000.

27. Mahomed K, Grant A, Ashurst H, James D. The Southmead perineal suture study. A randomised comparison of suture materials and suturing techniques for repair of perineal trauma. *Br J Obstet Gynaecol* 1989;96:1272–80.

28. Gemynthe A, Langhoff-Roos J, Sahl S, Knudsen J. New Vicryl formulation: an improved method of perineal repair? *Br J Midwifery* 1996;4:230–4.

29. McElhinney BR, Glenn DRJ, Harper MA. Episiotomy repair. Vicryl versus Vicryl rapide. *Ulster Med J* 2000;69:27–9.

30. Grant A. Repair of perineal trauma after childbirth. In: Chalmers I, Enkin MW, Keirse MJNC, editors. *Effective Care in Pregnancy and Childbirth.* Oxford: Oxford University Press; 1989. p. 1173–5.

31. Sultan AH, Kamm MA, Hudson CN. Obstetric perineal trauma: an audit of training. *J Obstet Gynaecol* 1995;15:19–23.

32. Groom K, Paterson-Brown S. Can we improve on the diagnosis of third-degree tears? *Eur J Obstet Gynecol Reprod Biol* 2002;101:19–21.

33. Fitzpatrick M, Fynes M, Cassidy M, Behan M, O'Connell PR, O'Herlihy C. Prospective study of the influence of parity and operative technique on the outcome of primary anal sphincter repair following obstetrical injury. *Eur J Obstet Gynecol Reprod Biol* 2000;89:159–63.

34. Sleep J, Grant A. Pelvic floor exercises in postnatal care. *Midwifery* 1987;3:158–64.

35. Carroli G, Belizan J, Stamp G. Episiotomy for vaginal birth. *Cochrane Database Syst Rev* 2000;(2)CD000081.

36. Thomas TM, Plymat KR, Blannin J, Meade TW. Prevalence of urinary incontinence. *BMJ* 1980;281:1243–5.

37. Jolleys J. Reported prevalence of urinary incontinence in women in a general practice. *BMJ* 1988;296:1330–2.

38. MacArthur C, Lewis M, Knox EG. *Health After Childbirth.* London: HMSO; 1991.

39. Wilson PD, Herbison RM, Herbison GP. Obstetric practice and the prevalence of urinary incontinence three months after delivery. *Br J Obstet Gynaecol* 1996;103:154–61.

40. Yarnell JWG, Voyle GJ, Sweetnam PM, Millbank J, Richards CJ, Stephenson TP. Factors associated with urinary incontinence in women. *J Epidemiol Community Health* 1982;36:58–63.

41. Read NW, Harford WV, Schmulen AC, Read MG, Santa Ana C, Fordtran JS. A clinical study of patients with faecal incontinence and diarrhoea. *Gastroenterology* 1979;76:747–56.

42. Kamm MA. Obstetric damage and faecal incontinence. *Lancet* 1994;344:730–3.

43. Varma A, Gunn J, Gardiner A, Lindow SW, Duthie GS. Obstetric anal sphincter injury: prospective evaluation of incidence. *Dis Colon Rectum* 1999;42:1537–43.

44. Kettle C. Perineal Repair: a Randomised Controlled Trial of Suturing Techniques and Materials Following Spontaneous Vaginal Birth [thesis]. North Staffs: Keele University; 2002.

11

The menopausal management of breast cancer survivors and those at increased risk of the disease

Andrew J Drakeley, Charles R Kingsland and Margaret CP Rees

INTRODUCTION

Breast disease is a common indication for women to be referred to a specialist menopause clinic. This may be owing to a past history of either benign or malignant disease, concurrent treatment for breast cancer in the presence of severe menopausal symptoms, or anticipated future concerns.[1]

This chapter attempts to address the effects of hormone replacement therapy (HRT) on breast tissue, outline a practical management strategy based on current best evidence and note research advances occurring within the past few years. The appropriate use of a clinical geneticist is clarified, as is the use of complementary medicines in a patient group that is sometimes reluctant to take conventional drugs.

CELLULAR EFFECTS OF HRT ON BREAST TISSUE

Ovarian steroids are known to be essential for the development, proliferation and differentiation of the normal human breast. There is long-standing epidemiological evidence that ovarian hormones affect the risk of breast cancer. The greater risk from an increased reproductive lifespan is thought to relate to the total number of times that the breast epithelium undergoes cyclical proliferation in response to ovarian hormones, which increases the likelihood of cancer initiation and promotion.[2] In the premenopausal adult, nonpregnant, nonlactating breast, epithelial proliferation is maximal during the luteal phase of the menstrual cycle when both oestrogen and progesterone are being secreted by the corpus luteum.[3-11] Data obtained from cell cultures are of limited use because both oestrogen and progesterone receptors may be lost and the concentrations of steroid may be higher than those reached physiologically.[12] In the one study where receptors were demonstrated to be expressed, oestrogen, but not progesterone, was demonstrated to be mitogenic.[13] Many studies have therefore been carried out on implantation of normal breast tissue into mice, where steroid receptors are expressed and tissue architecture is maintained. In these studies, steroid levels were modulated to mimic human premenopausal physiological levels and oestrogen was demonstrated to have a dose–dependent effect on epithelial cell proliferation, but no significant effect of progesterone was seen alone or in combination with oestrogen.[14-19]

Epidemiological data published since 1999[20-22] on the risk of breast cancer in relation to HRT suggest that it is the combination of oestrogen and progesterone in long-term HRT that is most associated with an increased risk of breast cancer, while oestrogen alone with HRT has a lesser risk. Where analysed, there is conflicting evidence on the question of whether sequential or continuous combined HRT is worse for breast cancer risk. The Swedish study[21] also reported that the use of testosterone-derived progestogen (such as the 19-norprogestogen) increased breast cancer risk when compared with progesterone-derived progestogen. However, the use of testosterone-derived progestogen in the USA is uncommon but the combined HRT risk for breast cancer is similar to the Swedish study. Two groups have investigated further the effects of HRT on breast tissue by looking at the proliferation rates of normal breast epithelium removed from women on oestrogen only, or oestrogen plus progesterone HRT, and comparing them with untreated women. A clear effect of the length of HRT administration was observed, with less than five years' use of HRT of any type having no effect on proliferation. In contrast, more than five years on combined oestrogen plus progesterone HRT significantly increased breast epithelial proliferation rates compared with those in untreated women.[23,24] The increased proliferation seen in normal breast epithelium taken from postmenopausal women being treated with combination oestrogen plus progesterone HRT concurs with increased breast cancer risk. These data suggest that long-term progesterone treatment has an effect on the breast that has not been observed in experimental models of short-term treatment. It seems that either progesterone has a different effect in the postmenopausal breast, especially when given as a long-term treatment, or, alternatively, that the form of progesterone may be important. For example, it has been shown that 19-norprogestins, which are more commonly used in European formulations of HRT, can induce proliferation in breast cell lines by directly activating the oestrogen receptor.[25–27] Secondly, it has been reported that the endogenous enzyme 5alpha-reductase can convert progesterone to a 5alpha-metabolite that stimulates the growth of breast cancer cells in culture.[28] The effects of alternative forms of HRT that are available are somewhat unclear. Tibolone, a steroid with mixed oestrogenic, progestogenic and androgenic activity, has been proposed to be an alternative to conventional HRT, but its effects at the cellular level are not so well described as for oestrogen and progesterone. In steroid receptor positive breast cells in culture, tibolone has been shown to be antiproliferative and to increase cell death.[29] However, its mechanism of action in the breast remains to be clearly demonstrated.[30,31]

Data regarding the selective oestrogen receptor modulator, raloxifene, used to maintain bone density, are strongly suggestive that it reduces the incidence of breast cancer.[32] In the short term this effect may be due to prevention of the growth of nonpalpable breast tumours that are oestrogen dependent, but in the longer term, inhibitory effects on the normal epithelium may prevent the initiation of new tumours. Further studies are continuing.

MANAGEMENT STRATEGY

There are two main categories of women who consult a gynaecologist: those with a personal history and those at risk of breast disease. The reasons for consultation are control of menopausal symptoms or concerns about long-term risks of the menopause, such as osteoporosis. Some women will have undergone an early menopause owing to their chemotherapy. Some may be taking tamoxifen, which *per se* induces hot flushes.

Although systemic hormone replacement therapy is not contraindicated in women with a personal or family history of breast cancer, alternatives may be sought.[33]

Control of menopausal symptoms

Systemic hormone replacement therapy

Breast cancer survivors who request HRT pose a management problem because conventional advice is to stop medication at the time of diagnosis and avoid future use of exogenous systemic oestrogens.

The various clinical studies of women with breast cancer who have been prescribed HRT have not shown an adverse effect on survival in either tamoxifen users or nonusers.[34,35] However, these involved small numbers with short-term follow-up. The results of randomised trials are awaited. Systemic oestrogen may ultimately be used in women whose symptoms are not controlled by other strategies.

There is little evidence that the use of HRT in women with a family history of breast cancer will further increase their risk, but for the most part studies have failed accurately to document a family history. In *BRCA1* carriers limited data suggest that the use of HRT does not negate the reduction in breast cancer risk after surgery.[36] Benign breast disease encompasses a diverse range of conditions, not all of which are associated with an increased risk of breast cancer. Of these changes, only those of ductal or lobular atypical hyperplasia are associated with a significant increase in risk.[37] Although HRT may be associated with mastalgia and promotion of breast cysts, there is no convincing evidence that breast cancer risk is increased in women with benign disease.[38] The failure accurately to categorise benign disease, however, prevents determination of whether women involved in these studies were at a significantly increased risk of breast cancer or not.

Vaginal oestrogens

Low-dose vaginal oestradiol and oestriol are not absorbed to any significant degree and can be used long term for urogenital symptoms.

Alternative therapies

The progestogen megestrol acetate and the selective serotonin re-uptake inhibitors, venlafaxine, paroxetine and fluoxetine, are effective in dealing with hot flushes. Although it will reduce the risk of vertebral fracture, the selective oestrogen receptor modulator, raloxifene, does not alleviate hot flushes. Furthermore, data are limited in breast cancer survivors. The evidence regarding the benefit of clonidine is conflicting.[39] Alternative therapies may also be sought, such as phyto-oestrogens, vitamins and herbalism (e.g. black cohosh).[40] However, there are concerns about efficacy and safety especially for the last mentioned because some herbal compounds have oestrogenic activity. Vaginal lubricants are not contraindicated.[41]

Prevention of osteoporosis

In women in whom there is concern about osteoporosis and who are at risk of the disease, it would be prudent to measure bone mineral density to evaluate whether therapy is required. Systemic oestrogen will conserve bone mass and significantly reduce the risk of fracture at both the spine and the hip. Anti-osteoporotic agents such as the bisphosphonates, alendronate, risedronate and etidronate, are effective agents. All have been given (in 2000) an A grade of recommendation for antifracture efficacy at the spine; and alendronate and risedronate A and etidronate B grade at the hip, by the Royal College of Physicians of London, UK.[42]

It is important to maintain an adequate calcium intake and most studies show that about 1.5 g of elemental calcium daily is necessary to preserve bone health in postmenopausal women not taking oestrogen.[43]

ALTERNATIVE MANAGEMENT STRATEGIES

Women who have had breast cancer experience menopausal difficulties for a number of reasons, some of which are due to a normal menopause and some to the breast cancer treatment. Each woman will also experience a different cluster of problems, which need to be assessed to determine the appropriate approach to management. However, it is still the case that this group of women see the menopause as a natural event and many will seek natural methods of coping with their difficulties. They require information about what to expect from the menopause and how they can adjust their lifestyle to maximise the benefit to their health. They need to be informed about the increased risk of osteoporosis and cardiovascular disease and relevant advice given with regard to diet and exercise. Much of this advice will also help to relieve some of the symptoms of the menopause, such as hot flushes.

Many women go on to seek further alternatives to build into their diet or lifestyle, and evidence is beginning to be available regarding their use. Cessation of smoking, managing weight, and reduction in alcohol and caffeine consumption may reduce hot flushes. Stress has been shown to increase the frequency and intensity of flushing. Early studies have supported the use of relaxation training in reducing flushes.[44-46] Women who exercise regularly have less flushes and so an exercise programme may help.[47,48]

There is much debate about the use of phyto-oestrogens in the alleviation of hot flushes. If they have a beneficial effect on flushing, then what other oestrogenic effects may they exert in the body? Some epidemiological studies suggest that phyto-oestrogens may be protective against breast cancer,[49] but this is not yet clear and, on the contrary, it is possible that some may have proliferative effects on the breast or endometrium.

There are many food products that contain phyto-oestrogens, such as soya, flax, linseed, and a variety of beans and herbal remedies. Evidence for the safety or efficacy of most of these is lacking, but studies are now emerging regarding the most commonly used products.[41]

Several studies have shown that the addition of soya powder to the diet can reduce the incidence of hot flushes,[50-52] although this has not been supported by all others.[53,54] There may be difficulties with standardisation of products and variations in amounts consumed, which may account for these differences. Currently, adverse effects of phyto-oestrogens have not been noted[51,55] and so the increase of soya in the diet may be a possible alternative for some women.

Black cohosh (*Cimicifuga racemosa*), also known as Remifemin® (Schaper and Brummer, Salzgitter, Germany) is used extensively in Germany at a dose of 40 mg daily. Studies vary concerning the reported effect on hot flushes. Some noncontrolled studies have shown up to a 70% reduction in flushes,[56,57] but again this has not been repeated in all studies.[58] None of these was able to demonstrate unwanted oestrogenic effects of black cohosh in the body and so again it may be a suitable alternative.

Red clover (*Trifolium pratense*) has not been shown to have a beneficial effect on hot flushes, nor have the potential oestrogenic effects on breast and endometrium been adequately assessed.[59] The evidence is conflicting. With the exception of a study published in 2002,[60] most have shown no effect. Because of the presence of coumarins there is some concern about the effect of red clover on clotting, although this has not yet been established. Dong quai (*Angelica sinensis*) does not reduce hot flushes,[61] nor has it been shown to have any oestrogenic effect, but it may affect blood clotting.

There is a current trend for women to take natural progesterone, or wild yam (*Dioscorea villosa*), as a topical application for hot flushes. This contains a number of substances that are further metabolised in the body and so it is uncertain which ingredients play any active role.[62] However, it is unlikely that enough progesterone is absorbed to have any significant effect after application to the skin. If taken with oestrogen, care should be taken to confirm endometrial protection. Work done by Komesaroff et al.[63] showed that wild yam cream (BioGest®, WildMedicine, Australia) did not help hot flushes, nor did it have any effect on other hormones. Blood progesterone levels were not significantly raised.

Vitamin E (800 iu daily) has been shown slightly to reduce the incidence of hot flushes.[64] Other vitamins or supplements, including evening primrose oil, have not been shown to be helpful.[65]

Many other complementary therapies are proposed for the relief of menopausal difficulties. Some small, uncontrolled studies have shown a reduction in hot flushes with acupuncture,[66,67] but there is little to support the use of any other complementary therapies.

APPROPRIATE USE OF A CLINICAL GENETICIST

Laboratory advances in cancer genetics have been well publicised, and the identification of *BRCA1* and *BRCA2*, in particular, is well known. In primary care, health professionals often raise the question of whether enquiring about a family history of breast cancer is important if women have arranged an appointment primarily to discuss other matters, including use of HRT.[68] Although the number of women asking these questions in one practice may be small, overall there is a significant need for accurate information in both primary and secondary care.

Over the last few years all departments of clinical genetics across the UK have had to deal with an increasing number of cancer genetics referrals. The number of consultants with a major interest in clinical cancer genetics is small,[69] therefore a model of service delivery has gradually evolved in which the scarce resources of the cancer genetics service are reserved for high-risk women who are most likely to benefit:[70]

- four family members with breast or ovarian cancer at any age

- three family members with breast cancer diagnosed under the age of 60 years, or ovarian cancer at any age

- two family members with breast cancer diagnosed under the age of 40 years

- one family member with both breast and ovarian cancer as two separate primaries.

Referral criteria used are not intended to be completely exclusive and there will undoubtedly be some clinical circumstances where a referral for expert discussion rather than testing is appropriate. In the Ashkenazi Jewish population, for example, the presence of three founder mutations at a population frequency of around 1% means that many services will offer testing with a much weaker family history.[71]

The theory behind this model of service delivery is sound, but there are considerable difficulties in putting it into practice. Central to the model is the concept that scarce services must be limited to 'appropriate' groups, which is radically different from the current model where funding is dependent on maximising the number of patients seen irrespective of 'appropriateness'. The development of this model of clinical service delivery in the management of familial breast cancer forms a central plank of one of the four paradigm projects of the London Genetics Knowledge Park (IDEAS: innovation, dissemination, evaluation and application strategy for genetics across the community).[72] Within the London Park, several innovative methods of delivering consultant-led clinical care and advice are being explored, including the use of direct teleconferencing facilities to connect up the consultant with patients and nursing staff at a remote location.

ADVANCES IN THE ENDOCRINE MANAGEMENT OF POSTMENOPAUSAL WOMEN WITH EARLY BREAST CANCER

Breast cancers, in company with prostate cancers, are almost unique in their sensitivity to endocrine manipulation. Consequently, the endocrine therapy of breast cancer has been a remarkable success story. Over the past 15 years there has been a dramatic fall in mortality from

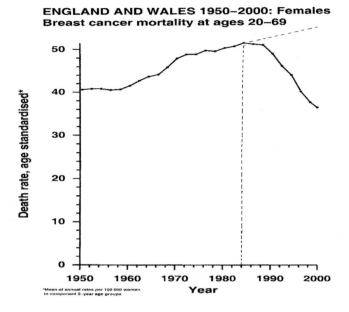

Figure 1 *Trends in age adjusted mortality for breast cancer in England and Wales 1950–2000: women – breast cancer mortality at ages 20–69 years; *mean of annual rates per 100 000 women in component 5-year age groups*

the disease in both the UK and the USA (Figure 1). Most commentators attribute this to the direct or indirect effect of adjuvant hormonal manipulation.

Thus the cycle continues, from Beatson in 1896,[73] to the 'Arimidex', Tamoxifen Alone or in Combination (ATAC) trial in 2002.[74] Approximately 50 years after Beatson's landmark series of cases of surgical castration for the treatment of advanced breast cancer, Huggins *et al.*[75] first described surgical adrenalectomy as second-line endocrine therapy. Both these remarkable studies were in fact empirical observations, with either little or a misguided understanding of the biological rationale underlying the responses. The past 50 years have seen a concerted effort by endocrinologists and clinicians alike to understand and exploit these mechanisms for full clinical benefit.

Although adrenalectomy may have been effective in the management of breast cancer, many women with metastatic disease are poor operative risks. A medical ablation of adrenal function would have wider application. Aminoglutethimide, the first of such drugs, blocks adrenal steroidogenesis high in the biosynthetic pathway. 'Medical adrenalectomy' induced by the interruption of steroidogenesis at the level of the conversion of cholesterol to pregnenolone can achieve an objective response in metastatic breast cancer among women without ovarian function, to a similar extent as a surgical adrenalectomy. Medical adrenalectomy may, therefore, be more widely applicable to women who are a poor operative risk.

Tamoxifen has been considered the gold standard for the treatment of breast cancer for the past 25 years, despite some tolerability and resistance issues.[74] The newer generation of aromatase inhibitors, anastrozole, letrozole and exemestane, work by reducing the biosynthesis of oestrogen.

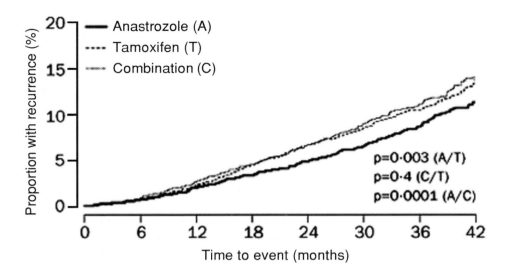

Figure 2 *Results of the ATAC trial: breast cancer events in the oestrogen receptor positive subgroup; including new contralateral tumours, but censoring women who had died from non-breast cancer causes before recurrence: HR = hazard ratio (redrawn from: Beral V, Hermon C, Reeves G, Peto R. Sudden fall in breast cancer death rates in England and Wales.* Lancet *1995;345:1642–3,[87] with permission from Elsevier)*

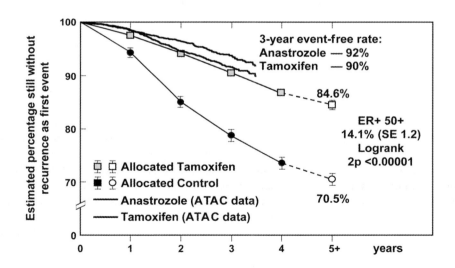

*ATAC data truncated at 42 months   ¹EBCTCG. *The Lancet* **1998; 351: 1451–1467**

Figure 3 *Comparison of ATAC results with the tamoxifen and control arms of the most recent published overview (reproduced from: Early Breast Cancer Trialists' Collaborative Group. Tamoxifen for early breast cancer: an overview of the randomised trials.* Lancet *1998;351:1451–67,[74] with permission from Elsevier)*

The results of phase III studies have shown that anastrozole and letrozole have resulted in superior time-to-disease progression compared with tamoxifen as first-line treatment in postmenopausal women with hormone sensitive advanced breast cancer. As second-line treatment after tamoxifen, both anastrozole and exemestane have shown superior survival compared with megestrol acetate. Anastrozole is the only aromatase inhibitor to have reported in the adjuvant setting and the first results of the ATAC study have shown anastrozole to be superior to tamoxifen with respect to disease-free survival, time to recurrence, the incidence of contralateral breast primary tumours as first events, and a number of important tolerability parameters. Figure 2 demonstrates breast cancer events in the oestrogen receptor positive subgroup for anastrozole, for tamoxifen and for a combination of the two, whereas Figure 3 refers to the Kaplan–Meier survival curve for the event-free rate.[76]

In the treatment of postmenopausal advanced breast cancer the aromatase inhibitors should be considered as the first treatment option; in the adjuvant setting, anastrozole now offers a choice for postmenopausal women with hormone-responsive tumours, although a longer follow-up will enable a more definitive benefit/risk assessment to be made. From the point of view of the gynaecologist, anastrozole has the advantage of lacking the agonist effect on the endometrium. As a result there were significantly fewer cases of gynaecological symptoms and endometrial cancers in the anastrozole group compared with tamoxifen. Against that, an accelerated loss in bone mineral density suggests that long-term treatment with anastrozole will have to be monitored carefully by bone density scans, with perhaps the introduction of bisphosphonates before osteoporosis develops.[76]

CONTINUING RESEARCH: THE UK NATIONAL RANDOMISED TRIAL OF HRT IN SYMPTOMATIC WOMEN WITH EARLY STAGE BREAST CANCER

Women with breast cancer may experience iatrogenic oestrogen deficiency symptoms as a direct consequence of their treatment (i.e. surgical, radiation induced or chemical ovarian ablation, the anti-oestrogen effects of tamoxifen, or chemotherapy induced ovarian suppression), but symptoms occurring subsequent to a natural menopause may be just as debilitating. Cross-sectional studies have demonstrated that, at any one time, oestrogen deficiency symptoms are the most common adverse effect of adjuvant therapy, occurring in up to 66% of patients aged less than 65 years. They may be more bothersome and persist for longer in breast cancer survivors compared with healthy postmenopausal women and have a significant, negative impact on quality of life.[77–80] Chemical castration with chemotherapy and gonadotrophin-releasing agonists can produce vaginal dryness, which, together with decreased wellbeing are important predictors of sexual health in breast cancer survivors.[81] Although vaginal dryness and dyspareunia are less frequent in women taking tamoxifen, problems with sexual interest, arousal and orgasm are reported with its use.[82] Since the clear survival benefits shown in worldwide overviews of adjuvant breast cancer therapy trials published since the late 1990s, its more widespread use is anticipated to increase the prevalence of oestrogen deficiency symptoms and premature menopause.[74,83–85] Currently, HRT is the most effective treatment available for symptom relief but it is contraindicated for fear of stimulating disease recurrence or a secondary primary breast cancer. Observational data have failed to show any adverse effect of HRT in breast cancer survivors, irrespective of whether unopposed oestrogen or oestrogen combined with progestin have been prescribed.[34,85,86] However, in the absence of randomised data, clinicians will be left in the unsatisfactory position of having to make decisions about the costs and benefits of HRT against a background of clinical uncertainty and increasing patient demand to prescribe it.

The UK randomised trial of HRT in symptomatic women with early stage breast cancer was planned, as were two further randomised trials in Scandinavia, after the successful implementation of a pilot study that was conducted between The Royal Marsden, and St George's and King's College Hospital Trusts in London.[80] The pilot study investigated the feasibility of conducting such a randomised trial (Figure 4). One hundred postmenopausal women experiencing vasomotor symptoms and/or vaginal dryness were randomised to receive either HRT or no HRT for six months. The main endpoints were to determine: (1) study acceptance; (2) the reasons why eligible women declined study entry; and (3) continuance rates at six months. Despite detailed informed consent with specific emphasis on the uncertainty associated with HRT and potential recurrence, the acceptance rate was encouraging (38.3%, 100/261 eligible women), as were continuance rates in both arms of the trial (>80%). Feedback from 90% of the women declining to participate demonstrated that, although fear of recurrence was an important factor influencing their decision, previous inadequate explanations about the potential adverse effects of their cancer treatments resulted in an unwillingness to be exposed to further drugs that could cause adverse effects, those of HRT being perceived as particularly unpleasant (i.e. weight gain and withdrawal bleeding). In parallel with the pilot study, an NHS Research and Development funded project was undertaken in which the views of women with breast cancer about the menopause and the use of HRT were elicited in nationwide focus groups. Relevant issues were debated at a joint meeting between patient representatives and the clinicians designing the national UK trial to ensure that the priorities of both groups were accounted for in the trial design.

The design of the national UK HRT trial is similar to that of the pilot study except that the treatment duration is longer at two years and nonhormonal alternatives to HRT for the control of symptoms are being offered in the opposing trial arm (Figure 5). It is intended to recruit 3000 postmenopausal women with stage I/II breast cancer who are experiencing vasomotor symptoms. The main outcomes of the trial are disease-free and overall survival, and quality of life. However, recruiting this number of women would provide sufficient statistical power to determine whether tumour receptor status or other prognostic factors should be considered when prescribing HRT in this group, and if any antagonism exists between HRT and endocrine therapies such as tamoxifen. Recruitment for this trial commenced in March 2002 and is anticipated to complete within three to five years.

SUMMARY

Breast cancer survivors are an increasingly common group who are often afflicted by severe menopausal symptoms, due in part to the adjuvant therapy they receive. Newer adjuvant therapies for hormonal tumours seem promising. These women are often reluctant to take hormone replacement therapy regardless of oestrogen receptor status. This can pose a management dilemma for the menopause clinic doctor. Alternative therapies should be sought that help to alleviate vasomotor symptoms and provide long-term benefit to often young women who have been rendered prematurely menopausal. These should be nonhormonal in the first instance wherever possible. A good working knowledge of complementary medicines is important because these women frequently enquire about their benefit. The genetics service in the UK is under-resourced at present and so its appropriate use is helpful to expedite patient care.

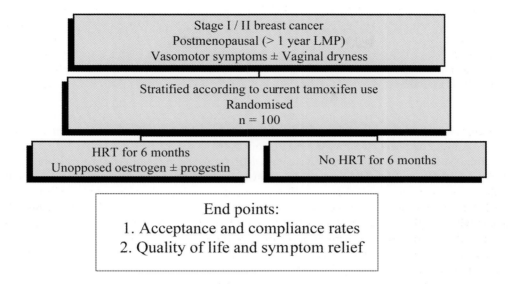

Figure 4 *UK pilot randomised study of HRT in women with early stage breast cancer: LMP = last menstrual period*

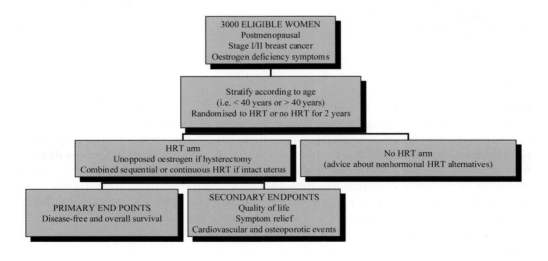

Figure 5 *The national UK randomised trial of HRT in symptomatic women with early stage breast cancer*

Acknowledgements

The authors would like to acknowledge the contributions made to this chapter by: Prof. M Baum, London; Dr R Clarke, Manchester; Miss D Fenlon, London; Dr J Mackay, London; and Jo Marsden, London.

References

1. Drakeley AJ, Marsden J, Kingsland CR. Management of breast cancer survivors and those at risk of the disease. *J Br Menopause Soc* 2001;7:182–3.
2. Pike MC, Spicer DV, Dahmoush L, Press MF. Estrogens, progestogens, normal breast cell proliferation, and breast cancer risk. *Epidemiol Rev* 1993;15:17–35.
3. Anderson TJ, Ferguson DJ, Raab GM. Cell turnover in the 'resting' human breast: influence of parity, contraceptive pill, age and laterality. *Br J Cancer* 1982;46:376–82.
4. Battersby S, Robertson BJ, Anderson TJ, King RJ, McPherson K. Influence of menstrual cycle, parity and oral contraceptive use on steroid hormone receptors in normal breast. *Br J Cancer* 1992;65:601–7.
5. Ferguson DJ, Anderson TJ. Morphological evaluation of cell turnover in relation to the menstrual cycle in the 'resting' human breast. *Br J Cancer* 1981;44:177–81.
6. Going JJ, Anderson TJ, Battersby S, MacIntyre CC. Proliferative and secretory activity in human breast during natural and artificial menstrual cycles. *Am J Pathol* 1988;130:193–204.
7. Masters JR, Drife JO, Scarisbrick JJ. Cyclic variation of DNA synthesis in human breast epithelium. *J Natl Cancer Inst* 1977;58:1263–5.
8. Meyer JS. Cell proliferation in normal human breast ducts, fibroadenomas, and other ductal hyperplasias measured by nuclear labeling with tritiated thymidine. Effects of menstrual phase, age, and oral contraceptive hormones. *Hum Pathol* 1977;8:67–81.
9. Potten CS, Watson RJ, Williams GT, Tickle S, Roberts SA, Harris M, *et al*. The effect of age and menstrual cycle upon proliferative activity of the normal human breast. *Br J Cancer* 1998;58:163–70.
10. Soderqvist G, Isaksson E, von Schoultz B, Carlstrom K, Tani E, Skoog L. Proliferation of breast epithelial cells in healthy women during the menstrual cycle. *Am J Obstet Gynecol* 1997;176:123–8.
11. Williams G, Anderson E, Howell A, Watson R, Coyne J, Roberts SA, *et al*. Oral contraceptive (OCP) use increases proliferation and decreases oestrogen receptor content of epithelial cells in the normal human breast. *Int J Cancer* 1991;48:206–10.
12. Anderson E, Clarke RB, Howell A. Estrogen responsiveness and control of normal human breast proliferation. *J Mammary Gland Biol Neoplasia* 1998;3:23–35.
13. Malet C, Gompel A, Yaneva H, Cren H, Fidji N, Mowszowicz I, *et al*. Estradiol and progesterone receptors in cultured normal human breast epithelial cells and fibroblasts: immunocytochemical studies. *J Clin Endocrinol Metab* 1991;73:8–17.
14. Clarke RB, Howell A, Anderson E. Estrogen sensitivity of normal human breast tissue *in vivo* and implanted into athymic nude mice: analysis of the relationship between estrogen-induced proliferation and progesterone receptor expression. *Breast Cancer Res Treat* 1997;45:121–33.
15. Laidlaw J, Clarke RB, Howell A, Owen AW, Potten CS, Anderson E. The proliferation of normal human breast tissue implanted into athymic nude mice is stimulated by estrogen but not progesterone. *Endocrinology* 1995;136:164–71.

16. McManus MJ, Welsch CW. The effect of estrogen, progesterone, thyroxine, and human placental lactogen on DNA synthesis of human breast ductal epithelium maintained in athymic nude mice. *Cancer* 1984;54:1920–7.

17. Popnikolov N, Yang J, Liu A, Guzman R, Nandi S. Reconstituted normal human breast in nude mice: effect of host pregnancy environment and human chorionic gonadotropin on proliferation. *J Endocrinol* 2001;168:487–96.

18. Popnikolov NK, Yang J, Guzman RC, Swanson SM, Thordarson G, Collins G, et al. In vivo growth stimulation of collagen gel embedded normal human and mouse primary mammary epithelial cells. *J Cell Physiol* 1995;163:51–60.

19. Sheffield LG, Welsch CW. Transplantation of human breast epithelia to mammary-gland-free fat-pads of athymic nude mice: influence of mammotrophic hormones on growth of breast epithelia. *Int J Cancer* 1988;41:713–19.

20. Rossouw JE, Andersen GL, Prentice RL, LaCroix AZ, Kooperberg C, Stefanick ML, et al. Risks and benefits of estrogen plus progestin in healthy postmenopausal women: principal results from the Women's Health Initiative randomized controlled trial. *JAMA* 2002;288:321–33.

21. Magnusson C, Baron JA, Correia N, Bergstrom R, Adami HO, Persson I. Breast-cancer risk following long-term oestrogen- and oestrogen-progestin-replacement therapy. *Int J Cancer* 1999;81:339–44.

22. Ross RK, Paganini-Hill A, Wan PC, Pike MC. Effect of hormone replacement therapy on breast cancer risk: estrogen versus estrogen plus progestin. *J Natl Cancer* Inst 2000;92:328–32.

23. Hargreaves DF, Knox F, Swindell R, Potten CS, Bundred NJ. Epithelial proliferation and hormone receptor status in the normal post-menopausal breast and the effects of hormone replacement therapy. *Br J Cancer* 1998;78:945–9.

24. Hofseth LJ, Raafat AM, Osuch JR, Pathak DR, Slomski CA, Haslam SZ. Hormone replacement therapy with estrogen or estrogen plus medroxyprogesterone acetate is associated with increased epithelial proliferation in the normal postmenopausal breast. *J Clin Endocrinol Metab* 1999;84:4559–65.

25. Catherino WH, Jeng MH, Jordan VC. Norgestrel and gestodene stimulate breast cancer cell growth through an oestrogen receptor mediated mechanism. *Br J Cancer* 1993;67:945–52.

26. Jeng MH, Parker CJ, Jordan VC. Estrogenic potential of progestins in oral contraceptives to stimulate human breast cancer cell proliferation. *Cancer Res* 1992;52:6539–46.

27. Jordan VC, Jeng MH, Catherino WH, Parker CJ. The estrogenic activity of synthetic progestins used in oral contraceptives. *Cancer* 1993;71:1501–5.

28. Wiebe JP, Muzia D, Hu J, Szwajcer D, Hill SA, Seachrist JL. The 4-pregnene and 5alpha-pregnane progesterone metabolites formed in nontumorous and tumorous breast tissue have opposite effects on breast cell proliferation and adhesion. *Cancer Res* 2000;60:936–43.

29. Gompel A, Chaouat M, Jacob D, Perrot JY, Kloosterboer HJ, Rostene W. In vitro studies of tibolone in breast cells. *Fertil Steril* 2002;78:351–9.

30. Valdivia I, Ortega D. Mammographic density in post-menopausal women treated with tibolone, estriol or conventional hormone replacement therapy. *Clin Drug Invest* 2000;20:101–7.

31. Kloosterboer HJ. Tibolone: a steroid with a tissue-specific mode of action. *J Steroid Biochem Mol Biol* 2001;76:231–8.

32. Cummings SR, Eckert S, Krueger KA, Grady D, Powles TJ, Cauley JA, et al. The effect of raloxifene on risk of breast cancer in postmenopausal women: results from the MORE randomized trial: Multiple Outcomes of Raloxifene Evaluation. *JAMA* 1999;281:2189–97.

33. Rees M, Purdie DW, editors. *Management of the Menopause*. 3rd ed. Marlow: BMS Publications; 2002.

34. O'Meara ES, Rossing MA, Daling JR, Elmore JG, Barlow WE, Weiss NS. Hormone replacement therapy after a diagnosis of breast cancer in relation to recurrence and mortality. *J Natl Cancer Inst* 2001;93:754–61.

35. Vassilopoulou-Sellin R. Hormone replacement therapy in breast cancer survivors. *J Br Menopause Soc* 1999;5:99–101.

36. Rebbeck TR, Levin AM, Eisen A, Snyder C, Watson P, Cannon-Albright L, *et al.* Breast cancer risk after bilateral prophylactic oophorectomy in *BRCA1* mutation carriers. *J Natl Cancer Inst* 1999:91:1475–9.

37. Dupont WD, Page DL, Parl FF, Plummer WD Jr, Schuyler PA, Kasami M, *et al.* Estrogen replacement therapy in women with a history of proliferative breast disease. *Cancer* 1999;85:1277–83.

38. Stearns V, Hayes DF. Approach to menopausal symptoms in women with breast cancer. *Curr Treat Options Oncol* 2002;3:179–90.

39. Bertelli G, Venturini M, Del Mastro L, Bergaglio M, Sismondi P, Biglia N, *et al.* Intramuscular depot medroxyprogesterone versus oral megestrol for the control of postmenopausal hot flashes in breast cancer patients: a randomized study. *Ann Oncol* 2002 13:883-8.

40. Ernst E. Herbalism and the menopause. *J Br Menopause Soc* 2002;8:72–4.

41. Kronenberg F, Fugh-Berman A. Complementary and alternative medicine for menopausal symptoms: a review of randomised controlled trials. *Ann Intern Med* 2002;137:805-13.

42. Royal College of Physicians. *Osteoporosis: Clinical Guidelines for Prevention and Treatment. Update on Pharmacological Interventions and an Alogorithm for Management.* London: Royal College of Physicians; 2000 [http://www.rcplondon.ac.uk/pubs/wp_osteo_update.htm].

43. National Institutes of Health. Consensus conference: Optimal calcium intake. *JAMA* 1994;272:1942–8.

44. Fenlon D. Relaxation therapy as an intervention for hot flushes in women with breast cancer. *Eur J Oncol Nurs* 1999;3:223–31.

45. Irvin JH, Domar AD, Clark C, Zuttermeister PC, Friedman R. The effects of relaxation response training on menopausal symptoms. *J Psychosom Obstet Gynaecol* 1996;17:202–7.

46. Wijma K, Melin A, Nedstrand E, Hammar M. Treatment of menopausal symptoms with applied relaxation: a pilot study. *J Behav Ther Exp Psychiatry* 1997;28:251–61.

47. Hammar M, Berg G, Lindgren R. Does physical exercise influence the frequency of postmenopausal hot flushes? *Acta Obstet Gynecol Scand* 1990;69:409–12.

48. Ivarsson T, Spetz AC, Hammar M. Physical exercise and vasomotor symptoms in postmenopausal women. *Maturitas* 1998;29:139–46.

49. Ingram D, Sanders K, Kolybaba M, Lopez D. Case–control study of phyto-oestrogens and breast cancer. *Lancet* 1997;350:990–4.

50. Murkies AL, Lombard C, Strauss BJ, Wilcox G, Burger HG, Morton MS. Dietary flour supplementation decreases post-menopausal hot flushes: effect of soy and wheat. *Maturitas* 1995;21:189–95.

51. Vincent A, Fitzpatrick LA. Soy isoflavones: are they useful in menopause? *Mayo Clin Proc* 2000;75:1174–84.

52. Albertazzi P, Pansini F, Bonaccorsi G, Zanotti L, Forini E, De Aloysio D. The effect of dietary soy supplementation on hot flushes. *Obstet Gynecol* 1998;91:6–11.

53. Quella SK, Loprinzi CL, Barton DL, Knost JA, Sloan JA, LaVasseur BI, *et al.* Evaluation of soy phytoestrogens for the treatment of hot flashes in breast cancer survivors: a North Central Cancer Treatment Group Trial. *J Clin Oncol* 2000;18:1068–74.

54. Van Patten CL, Olivotto IA, Chambers GK, Gelmon KA, Hislop TG, Templeton E, *et al.* Effect of soy phytoestrogens on hot flashes in postmenopausal women with breast cancer: a randomized, controlled clinical trial. *J Clin Oncol* 2002;20:1449–55.

55. Whitten PL, Naftolin F. Reproductive actions of phytoestrogens. *Baillieres Clin Endocrinol Metab* 1998;12:667–90.

56. Lieberman S. A review of the effectiveness of *Cimicifuga racemosa* (black cohosh) for the symptoms of menopause. *J Womens Health* 1998;7:525–9.

57. Liske E, Hanggi W, Henneicke-von Zepelin HH, Boblitz N, Wustenberg P, Rahlfs VW. Physiological investigation of a unique extract of black cohosh (*Cimicifugae racemosae rhizoma*): a 6-month clinical study demonstrates no systemic estrogenic effect. *J Womens Health Gend Based Med* 2002;11:163–74.

58. Jacobson JS, Troxel AB, Evans J, Klaus L, Vahdat L, Kinne D, *et al.* Randomized trial of black cohosh for the treatment of hot flashes among women with a history of breast cancer. *J Clin Oncol* 2001;19:2739–45.

59. Fugh-Berman A, Kronenberg F. Red clover (*Trifolium pratense*) for menopausal women: current state of knowledge. *Menopause* 2001;8:333–7.

60. van de Weijer PH, Barentsen R. Isoflavones from red clover (Promensil) significantly reduce menopausal hot flush symptoms compared with placebo. *Maturitas* 2002;42:187–93.

61. Hirata JD, Swiersz LM, Zell B, Small R, Ettinger B. Does dong quai have estrogenic effects in postmenopausal women? A double-blind, placebo-controlled trial. *Fertil Steril* 1997;68:981–6.

62. National Center for Complementary and Alternative Medicine [http://nccam.nih.gov/health/alerts/menopause/].

63. Komesaroff PA, Black CV, Cable V, Sudhir K. Effects of wild yam extract on menopausal symptoms, lipids and sex hormones in healthy menopausal women. *Climacteric* 2001;4:144–50.

64. Barton DL, Loprinzi CL, Quella SK, Sloan JA, Veeder MH, Egner JR, *et al.* Prospective evaluation of vitamin E for hot flashes in breast cancer survivors. *J Clin Oncol* 1998;16:495–500.

65. Chenoy R, Hussain S, Tayob Y, O'Brien P, Moss M, Morse P. The effect of oral gamolenic acid from evening primrose oil on menopausal flushing. *BMJ* 1994;308:501–3.

66. Dong H, Ludicke F, Comte I, Campana A, Graff P, Bischof P. An exploratory pilot study of acupuncture on the quality of life and reproductive hormone secretion in menopausal women. *J Altern Complement Med* 2001;7:651–8.

67. Porzio G, Trapasso T, Martelli S, Sallusti E, Piccone C, Mattei A, *et al.* Acupuncture in the treatment of menopause-related symptoms in women taking tamoxifen *Tumori* 2002;88:128–30.

68. Hyland F, Kinmonth AL, Marteau TM, Griffin S, Murrell P, Spiegelhalter D, *et al.* Raising concerns about family history of breast cancer in primary care consultations: prospective, population based study. Women's Concerns Study Group. *BMJ* 2001;322:27–8.

69. Wonderling D, Hopwood P, Cull A, Douglas F, Watson M, Burn J, *et al.* A descriptive study of UK cancer genetics services: an emergency clinical response to the new genetics. *Br J Cancer* 2001;85:166–70.

70. Pharoah P, Mackay J. Medical genetics and breast cancer: current thinking on the utility of genetic screening in the determination of clinical risk. In: Mansel R, Smith IE, Kunkler I, Miles A, editors. *The Effective Management of Breast Cancer.* (UK Key Advances in Clinical Practice series.) London: Aesculapius; 2000. p. 13–28.

71. Tonin P, Weber B, Offit K, Couch F, Rebbeck TR, Neuhausens S, *et al.* Frequency of recurrent *BRCA1* and *BRCA2* mutations in Ashkenazi Jewish breast cancer families. *Nat Med* 1996;2:1179–83.

72. The London Genetics Knowledge Park (IDEAS) [www.gene.ucl.ac.uk/ideas].

73. Beatson JT. On the treatment of inoperable cases of carcinoma of the mamma: suggestions for a new method of treatment, with illustrative cases. *Lancet* 1896;ii:104–7,162–5.

74. Early Breast Cancer Trialists' Collaborative Group. Tamoxifen for early breast cancer: an overview of the randomised trials. *Lancet* 1998;351:1451–67.

75. Huggins CB. Current cancer concepts: adrenalectomy as palliative treatment. *JAMA* 1967;200:973.

76. Baum M, Budzar AU, Cujick J, Forbes J, Houghton JH, Kliijn JG, *et al.* Anastrozole alone or in combination with tamoxifen versus tamoxifen alone for adjuvant treatment of postmenopausal woman with early breast cancer: first results of the ATAC randomized trial. *Lancet* 2002;359:2131-9.

77. Canney PA, Hatton MQF. The prevalence of menopausal symptoms in patients treated for breast cancer. *Clin Oncol* 1994;6:297–9.

78. Carpenter JS, Andykowski MA, Cordova M, Cunningham L, Studts J, McGrath P, *et al.* Hot flashes in postmenopausal women treated for breast carcinoma. *Cancer* 1998;82:1682–91.

79. Couzi RJ, Helzlsouer KJ, Fetting JH. Prevalence of menopausal symptoms among women with a history of breast cancer and attitudes toward estrogen replacement therapy. *J Clin Oncol* 1995;13:2737–44.

80. Marsden J, Sacks NPM, Baum M, A'Hern R, Whitehead MI. Are randomised trials of hormone replacement therapy in symptomatic breast cancer patients feasible? *Fertil Steril* 2000;73:292–9.

81. Ganz PA, Desmond K, Belin TR, Meyerowitz BE, Rowland JH. Predictors of sexual health in women after a breast cancer diagnosis. *J Clin Oncol* 1999;17:2371–80.

82. Day R, Ganz PA, Costantino JP, Cronin WM, Wickerham L, Fisher B. Health-related quality of life and tamoxifen in breast cancer prevention: a report form the National Surgical Adjuvant Breast and Bowel Project P-1 Study. *J Clin Oncol* 1999;17:2659–69.

83. Early Breast Cancer Trialists' Collaborative Group. Ovarian ablation in early breast cancer: overview of the randomised trials. *Lancet* 1996;348:1189–96.

84. Goodwin PJ, Ennis M, Pritchard KI, Trudeau M, Hood N. Risk of menopause during the first year after breast cancer diagnosis. *J Clin Oncol* 1999;17:2365–70.

84. Col NF, Kirota LK, Orr RK, Erban JK, Wong JB, Lau J. Hormone replacement therapy after breast cancer: a systematic review and quantitative assessment of risk. *J Clin Oncol* 2001;19:2357–63.

86. Marttunen MB, Hietanen P, Pyrhonen S, Tiitinen A, Ylikorkala O. A prospective study on women with a history of breast cancer with or without estrogen replacement therapy. *Maturitas* 2001;39:217–25.

87. Beral V, Hermon C, Reeves G, Peto R. Sudden fall in breast cancer death rates in England and Wales. *Lancet* 1995;345:1642–3,

12

Genetic testing for gynaecological and breast cancers

Diana M Eccles

INTRODUCTION

In general terms all cancers arise as a result of mutations in genes that control cell proliferation. In the majority of common adult cancers these mutations are all acquired (somatic) and arise in the cell destined to become the malignant clone only. These mutations are not transmitted to the individual's offspring and would not be detectable in normal tissue. Some cancers have precursor lesions. Mutations that occur early in the development of a malignant clone can be found frequently in precursor lesions, thus helping to map out the genes of importance in contributing to early carcinogenesis. This has been well documented for colorectal cancer because of the well recognised pathological progression from adenoma through degrees of dysplasia, to carcinoma *in situ*, invasive and finally metastatic cancer. Somatic mutations are acquired as a tumour progresses and malignant cells in general have disordered genes and chromosomes. Families with inherited high-risk cancer predisposition are relatively uncommon and represent probably less than 5% of all common adult cancer cases. Nevertheless, for a common cancer site, most oncologists will, in their working lives, certainly treat many women who fall into this category, and genetic predisposition may impact on how they are managed clinically. For an overview published in 2002, see Knudson.[1]

In this chapter some general principles and basic genetic terms relevant to cancer genetics are outlined, but the emphasis is on genetic assessment of breast cancer and gynaecological cancers, a proportion of which can be accounted for by hereditary factors.

HEREDITARY CANCER

Terminology

Autosomal inheritance

Humans have 23 pairs of chromosomes: 22 pairs of autosomes and a pair of sex chromosomes. For each pair of chromosomes, one or other of a pair of genes will be transmitted to an offspring with equal probability. Thus, if an individual is carrying a mutated copy of a gene on one chromosome and a normal copy on the other, either the normal or the abnormal gene sequence will be passed on to each offspring with a 50:50 chance. Most cancer predisposition genes are dominantly inherited, which means that only one copy of an abnormal gene is required before cancer predisposition is conferred. Rare cancer predisposing genes exert their main effect only when a faulty copy is transmitted from both parents and no normal copy exists. Here, the mode of inheritance is autosomal recessive, an example of which is Bloom's syndrome, a devastating and rare condition associated with premature ageing and an increase in haematological and other tumours from childhood.[2] In 2002, recessively inherited colonic polyposis and cancer due to mutations in the *MYH* gene were described.[3]

Expression

The particular clinical manifestations that are associated with a specific gene may be quite variable. For example, a woman who carries a faulty copy of the *BRCA1* gene may develop either ovarian or breast cancer, or sometimes both. Expression may be influenced by the precise site or type of gene mutation, or potentially by environmental carcinogenic exposure. For example, in *BRCA1* gene carriers, limited evidence points to a reduction in ovarian cancer risk for users of the oral contraceptive pill but an increase in breast cancer risk.[4]

Penetrance

This term is used frequently in relation to cancer predisposing genes. The chance of any relevant disease manifesting itself in a gene carrier depends on a variety of factors. Some gene mutations are fully penetrant from birth; for example, in achondroplasia a single point mutation in the fibroblast growth factor type 3 gene (*FGFR3*) leads to classic short-limbed dwarfism in all cases.[5] In contrast, *BRCA1* penetrance is incomplete (not all carriers of a *BRCA1* mutation develop cancer, although the cumulative risk increases with age). The chance that a female gene carrier will develop breast cancer is between 45% and 87%; for ovarian cancer it is between 36% and 66%.[6] The higher risks are estimates based on the observed incidence in families with multiple cancers, collected for the purpose of identifying breast (and ovarian) cancer predisposition genes. However, some families may have a lower penetrance owing to factors that modify the penetrance of the high-risk gene[7] and this is reflected when population based series are used for penetrance estimates.[8] These may be environmental factors (e.g. oral contraceptive pill use, pregnancy, breastfeeding, and diet) or other genetic factors (e.g. the avidity of androgen receptor binding, which varies according to the length of a repetitive sequence within the gene and has been extensively investigated, is a plausible candidate modifier gene).[9] Population based assessment of the penetrance of specific mutations for *BRCA1* and *BRCA2* give lower penetrance estimates than those estimated from multiplex families.[8,10,11]

Sex-limited penetrance

This indicates that a gene mutation is associated with a disease that is more likely to be manifest in one sex than the other; for example, in *BRCA1* families, women are at high risk of breast and ovarian cancer but men clearly have no risk of ovarian cancer and little increase in breast cancer risk. This term must be distinguished from X-linked inheritance where the disease gene is transmitted on the X chromosome.

Frequency

This refers to the estimated population frequency of a mutated gene. Ethnicity can affect the frequency of certain gene mutations; for example, in the Ashkenazi Jewish population a specific fault in the *BRCA1* gene (185delAG) is found in up to 1% of the population, often making genetic testing for *BRCA1* mutation more straightforward in this group. The frequency of *BRCA1* mutations in more genetically diverse populations is less easily tested.

High-penetrance genes

Features of families with an inherited cancer predisposition include:

- multiple cases of the same (or associated) cancers

- more than one affected generation

- average age at onset is younger than that in the general population.

Figure 1 illustrates a typical *BRCA1* related family history.

When assessing the likelihood of a faulty gene being responsible for the pattern of cancers in a family, it is important to have all the relevant information to hand and to have some verification of the information given by an individual. A three-generation pedigree is usually necessary, with information about both maternal and paternal family history being important. Faulty breast and gynaecological predisposition genes may be transmitted by the father with a good probability of no adverse effect in the transmitting male. Questions aimed at assessing how likely a given history is to be medically correct are valuable; for example, a history of an ovarian cancer found on screening in a 24-year-old cousin is more likely in reality to be an abnormal cervical smear with information passed between family members in the context of some other event (such as an ovarian cancer in a mother) and distorted in the process. Such diagnoses, if critical to the assessment or unlikely, must be verified from medical records. When taking the family history, information about the sex and age of relatives unaffected by cancer is also important because this modifies the likelihood of a cancer being due to a high-risk gene, especially when only one or two family members are reported to be affected (Figure 2).

FAMILIAL CANCER

Many family clusters are, however, rather less striking than the example in Figure 1. Possible explanations for one or two cancers of the same sort in a family are:

- chance

- shared environmental risks

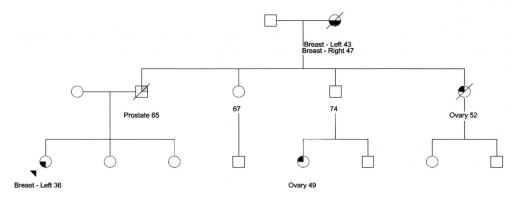

Figure 1 *A typical family history where a* BRCA1 *mutation was detected in the index case (arrowed)*

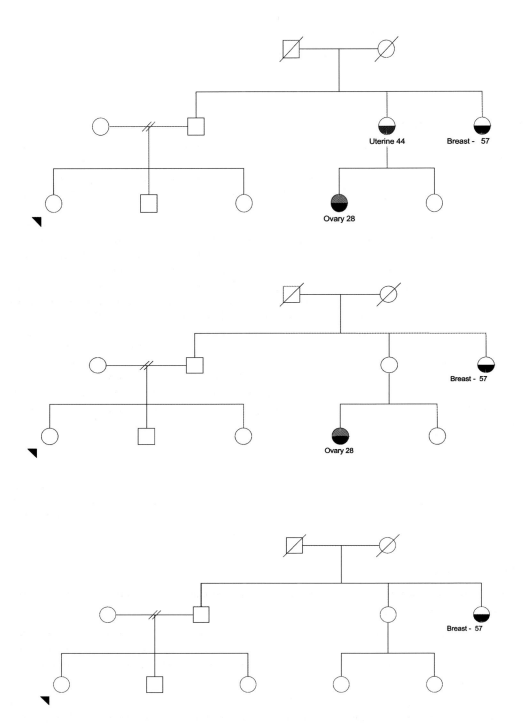

Figure 2 *(a) Initial family history from referral letter (the consultand is the individual consulting the genetics service and is indicated by an arrow); (b) family history taken by genetic counsellor; (c) family history after verification sought from medical records*

- low-penetrance, high-frequency genes

- high-penetrance, low-frequency genes with, for example, a small family, unknown family history (adopted), or perhaps paternal transmission with few paternal female relatives to manifest disease.

Low-penetrance genes

Current understanding of inherited cancer predisposition genes suggests that, in addition to the small proportion of high-risk hereditary cancers, there is a much larger proportion, perhaps a quarter to a third of some common adult cancers, which have some genetic component (termed familial cancer predisposition).[12] Much genetic predisposition is likely to be due to common genetic variants within the population. Such variation may, for example, affect enzymatic metabolism of environmental carcinogens.[13] Genetic variants leading to cancer susceptibility may be common in the population at large but they will also be inherited and will therefore lead to cancers being more likely to cluster in families. On an individual basis the increased cancer risk is marginal (i.e. the associated excess risk is small but in a large population study the effect may be measurable, claims of association are frequently refuted in subsequent studies, publication bias in favour of positive findings is likely, and many associations will be population dependent). In general, the interpretation of results from association studies should be cautious.[14]

Genetic risk profiling using data from association studies to predict susceptibility to complex disease is now being offered commercially via the internet or various alternative therapy outlets. It is unlikely to be clinically useful in the short term for the individual as it is still unclear how the various factors being examined interact with each other and with the environment. However, in the future, a better understanding of how genes work together and how environmental manipulation may ameliorate risks may eventually allow such genetic profiling to be medically useful.

Molecular genetics

If there is a clinical suspicion of an underlying genetic predisposition to cancer it is important to involve the regional clinical genetics service to ensure optimum use of molecular genetic testing and interpretation of results. There are several important steps involved in attempting to clarify a molecular culprit in a suspected case of hereditary cancer predisposition.

Mutation searching

This is used when an underlying genetic predisposition to cancer is suspected. Prerequisites to a mutation search are:

- A DNA sample from an affected family member: For choice, this would be the youngest affected relative but, often because of early death, the choice is compromised. Testing in more than one family member may be ideal, but may double the cost and would not routinely be contemplated.

- Informed consent: This would normally involve at least a telephone consultation with a member of the genetics team, but more commonly the affected family member has the opportunity for a genetics consultation when the possible outcomes of such a test can be discussed in detail.

- An experienced geneticist should review the family history and additional information to assess which gene or genes need to be examined.

Interpretation of results

There are a number of possible outcomes when the mutation search result is returned (often six months after blood has been taken because of the size of the genes being examined; commercial testing is available in the USA with a turn around time of about four weeks, but this is expensive and the outcome still needs careful interpretation). The types of results that can be reported are summarized in Table 1.

Cost of mutation searching

Although compared with many cancer treatments and high tech imaging investigations, a cost of around £2000 to look for mutations in *BRCA1* and *BRCA2* may seem reasonable, the cost of finding one mutation would be enormous if this test were applied indiscriminately in situations where the probability of finding a high-risk gene mutation is low (e.g. Figure 2c). In addition, a negative outcome from testing is often of no real value in terms of refining risk estimates.

HEREDITARY BREAST CANCER

BRCA1 and BRCA2

An inherited component responsible for cancer predisposition has long been recognised in the medical literature, with accounts as far back as the 19th century. Familial clustering was, for example, noted by Sir James Paget in 1853 and contemporaneously by a French Physician, Paul Broca, who, it is thought, was probably describing the family history of his wife in his account of a striking breast (and possibly ovarian) cancer family.[15,16]

Table 1 *Genetic test results and interpretation*

Mutation type	Interpretation
No mutation found	This may mean that the method used for detection has failed to pick up the mutation in the genes examined (false negative result), that the wrong gene has been examined, or that there is no genetic predisposition (unlikely if the family history is very strong). A negative result from this type of test when there is a significant family history is therefore essentially uninformative
Mutation of uncertain pathogenicity (unclassified variant)	This type of mutation usually, but not always, is predicted to cause an amino acid substitution. However, the consequence of this for protein function is difficult to predict: some of these unclassified variants may prove to have a low level of pathogenicity but at results are present these very difficult to interpret
Clearly pathogenic mutation	This is an alteration in the DNA sequence that is predicted to lead to either a shortened or an absent protein product that will not function normally and is very likely therefore to be the underlying cause of the family predisposition to cancer
Two pathogenic mutations	It is possible to have a mutation in both *BRCA1* and *BRCA2*, for example, and have no worse a phenotype than for a single mutation; inheritance would usually (but not always) be from both parents. This situation is rare. In reality many UK laboratories stop screening once one pathogenic mutation is detected. If the family history involves breast and ovarian cancer in both parental lines, this possibility should be considered

Segregation analysis is a method of mathematically modelling inheritance in a population using a variety of computer algorithms and family history information. Several such analyses have been carried out in breast cancer cohorts and similar solutions from all studies suggested clearly the likely presence of one or more relatively uncommon (3/1000) highly penetrant, dominantly inherited predisposition genes.[17,18]

The search for the genes predisposing to cancer was greatly facilitated by the development of the powerful polymerase chain reaction, a molecular technique that allows million-fold replication of short pieces of DNA, making the use of small amounts of poor quality DNA amenable to molecular investigation (such as that which can be extracted from paraffin embedded tissue). Thus, living affected relatives were no longer essential for whole-family analysis looking for an area in the genome consistently linked with the observed disease predisposition (linkage analysis). In 1990 an American group located the first breast cancer gene (termed *BRCA1*) to the long arm of chromosome 17 (Figure 3) in families with multiple breast cancers of unusually young average age at onset.[19] It was not until four years later that the correct gene was identified and the sequence could be determined.[20]

It rapidly became apparent that ovarian cancer was a common feature of *BRCA1* families. By looking for a distinguishing feature in families with a high incidence of breast cancer, but where the cancers did not seem to be linked to an abnormal gene on chromosome 17q, a British group

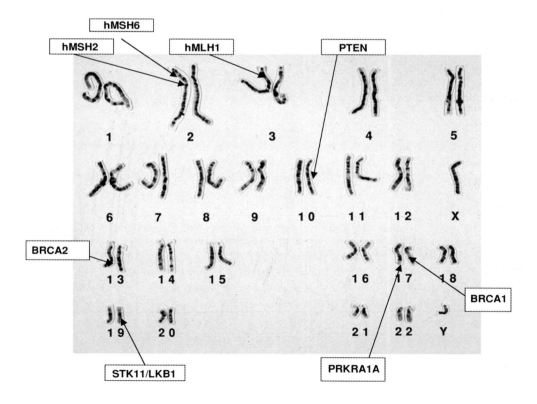

Figure 3 *Chromosomal locations of some cancer predisposition genes*

found the location of *BRCA2* and, soon after, the sequence.[21] The distinguishing feature in question was the presence of male as well as female breast cancer cases. In common with most cancer predisposition genes, the mutations that cause the predisposition are scattered throughout the gene and, since both *BRCA1* and *BRCA2* are large genes with thousands of bases wherein the mutation may lie, searching for causative mutations is not simple. As outlined above, in most practical settings a negative result when a mutation search is initiated may not be too helpful; it certainly cannot exclude the possibility that another gene (even an as yet unidentified gene) could be responsible. However, since the vast majority of breast cancers in families in which ovarian cancer has also occurred are due to either *BRCA1* or *BRCA2,* it is reasonable to assume that, in a family with only breast cancer, a negative outcome from mutation testing for *BRCA1* and *BRCA2* makes it less likely that there would be any significant increase in ovarian cancer risk. This assumes that a sensitive strategy for mutation detection has been used on appropriate DNA sample from a family member likely to carry the breast cancer predisposition gene. Ovarian cancer risk is often overlooked in families with only breast cancer but it may be a risk where the features of the family and the tumours suggest possible *BRCA1* in particular (see below).

Breast cancer risk in a *BRCA1* gene carrier is high. The figures used most commonly to estimate risk are derived from families selected for a high incidence of cancer and are possibly an overestimate, as outlined above.

In *BRCA2* gene carriers the onset of breast cancer is on average 5–10 years later than for *BRCA1,* but it can occur at any age from the early twenties onwards. Ovarian cancer risk is dealt with later. Because of the difficulties associated with finding a gene mutation in an individual, population based studies to determine penetrance are impossible to carry out except where there is a specific founder mutation known to be common in a given population.[22–24] Estimates of penetrance in these population studies are invariably lower than in the family based studies, but figures vary quite widely. Where there have been many cases of cancer in a family, then a higher penetrance should be used to estimate risk.

Other genes

Less than 50% of familial clusters of three or more breast cancer only cases are accounted for by mutations in *BRCA1* and *BRCA2*, so it is likely that other rare high-penetrance genes may still be discovered. Mutations in *CHK2* and *ATM* have been implicated in familial breast cancer.[25,26]

Some rare genetic conditions with striking features have been found to be associated with an increased risk of both benign and malignant breast disease. These include the Peutz–Jegher syndrome (lentigenes including lips and mucous membranes, gastrointestinal hamartomas with predisposition to intussusception in childhood, and gastrointestinal malignancy in adulthood). The increase in breast cancer risk is at least three times the population risk, but may be higher.[27] The Peutz–Jegher syndrome is due to mutations in the *STK11* gene on chromosome 19, but in some affected families it seems to be due to other genes.[28] Cowden syndrome is associated with trichilemmomas, macrocephaly, mucosal neuromas, and an increased risk of benign and malignant tumours of the breast and thyroid in particular.[29]

MANAGEMENT OF WOMEN AT INCREASED BREAST CANCER RISK

Management strategies come with varying degrees of evidence base and varying degrees of patient acceptability.

Early detection

Most of these women want to be screened. Mammography is the conventional tool used for early breast cancer detection. A small but significant reduction in mortality is observed in population based studies of screening in women aged 50 years and older.[30,31] The evidence for a reduction in mortality before 50 years of age is less clear. There is no evidence of a mortality reduction in younger women screened because of a family history of breast cancer, although there is good evidence for detection at earlier stages than in a nonscreened population, including *in situ* cancer, which has been taken as a surrogate indicator of a likely long-term mortality reduction. The appropriate studies to determine this have not yet been done. In the absence of gold standard evidence the policy in most centres is to offer screening mammography yearly from age 35 years to women either known to carry or at risk of carrying a high-risk breast cancer predisposition gene. In many centres this is also extended to women with a less striking family history, depending on the available resources and locally negotiated arrangements. A number of guidelines are published aimed at assisting the triage process. Some knowledge of genetic and epidemiological risk assessment is helpful for those carrying out the triage process.[32,33] A committee for the National Institute for Clinical Excellence is currently examining evidence for management strategies in familial breast cancer and should report in 2004.

Prevention

Medical

Oestrogen exposure is clearly a risk factor for breast cancer: men have a much smaller risk of developing breast cancer than women and many other epidemiological risk altering factors can be explained, perhaps simplistically, by a reduction or prolongation of oestrogen exposure (e.g. late menopause and early menarche reduce risk; hormone replacement therapy at the menopause increases risk). Over the last decade of the 20th century there has been an interest in chemoprevention and a number of large well conducted trials have looked at whether tamoxifen (an oestrogen receptor antagonist) may reduce breast cancer risk in women who have not yet had the disease.[34] In the USA, tamoxifen is licensed for chemoprevention; in the UK, there are still concerns about the overall benefit to risk ratio, and longer term follow-up from the European International Breast Cancer Intervention Study (IBIS) is awaited. IBIS2 will look at the effect of anastrozole, an aromatase inhibitor also used for breast cancer treatment in postmenopausal women. Meanwhile, in the high-risk group of women who either have a proven high-risk gene mutation or are at risk of having one, a pilot study is examining the acceptability of a more dramatic intervention at younger ages using a gonadotrophin-releasing hormone agonist, goserelin, with raloxifene (a more selective oestrogen receptor modulator than tamoxifen, licensed for prevention of osteoporosis in postmenopausal women).[35] The rationale for this approach is the observation that breast cancer risk is reduced by 50% in women who carry a *BRCA1* gene mutation and elect to have bilateral salpingo-oophorectomy before the menopause.[36,37]

Surgical

Prophylactic mastectomy has been proven to reduce the risk of breast cancer in high-risk gene carriers. In some centres take-up rates for proven gene carriers is 50%; uptake is more common in younger women and in women with young children.[38] The procedure seems to be well tolerated, in particular when the woman is properly prepared and has made the decision for herself rather than being coerced into undergoing the surgery.[39] A high incidence of occult malignant and premalignant lesions of the breast has been reported, particularly with increasing age.[40] Risk reduction can also be shown in women who are at lower risk, although the data on satisfaction are less clear in this group.[41]

HEREDITARY OVARIAN CANCER

BRCA1 and BRCA2

Most families featuring ovarian cancer in a dominantly inherited pattern will turn out to have mutations in either BRCA1 or BRCA2, although rare ovarian site-specific ovarian cancer genes cannot be ruled out. In a family with a dominant pattern of ovarian cancer inheritance (three cases, two generations) the risk for breast cancer in female family members is likely to be at least as high, and probably higher, than the risk for ovarian cancer. On average (from families with mutations and multiple cancer cases), the chance of a female gene carrier developing ovarian cancer in her lifetime is about 40% for BRCA1 and around 27% for BRCA2, but this varies somewhat between families.[42,43] The risk of ovarian malignancy in hereditary predisposition is small before 40 years of age, but rises steadily after this.[43,44] It is important to remember that fallopian tube cancer is also a feature of BRCA1 and BRCA2 carriers, which has serious implications when considering the procedure for prophylactic surgery in these women.[45,46] There is a suggestion for both BRCA1 and BRCA2 that the position of the mutation causing the cancer predisposition is important in determining the likelihood of ovarian cancer developing.[47,48] Ovarian tumours are usually epithelial carcinomas with under-representation of the mucinous type. Tumours of borderline malignant potential are not thought to be associated with inherited BRCA1 mutations.[49]

The outlook after diagnosis is poor, as for most ovarian cancers, although there is a suggestion that BRCA1 and BRCA2 ovarian cancers may respond better to adjuvant therapies, giving a slightly prolonged survival compared with sporadic cases.[50] This observation in a large cohort has not been confirmed in a subsequent study and the study methods for examining this question are difficult.[51]

Hereditary nonpolyposis colorectal cancer or Lynch syndrome

The predominant cancer in most families with hereditary nonpolyposis colorectal cancer (HNPCC) is colorectal cancer. However, endometrial cancer is common in this condition and will be discussed later. Ovarian cancer is included among the tumours accepted as more frequent in HNPCC. HNPCC-associated extracolonic tumours include tumours of the endometrium, ovary, stomach and small intestine, and transitional cell tumours of the renal pelvis, ureter, bladder and hepatobiliary tract. Ovarian tumours are usually epithelial ovarian carcinomas, but endometrioid and mucinous carcinomas do occur. As for the colorectal cancers in HNPCC, ovarian cancers may have a better prognosis than sporadic tumours.[52]

Management of women at increased risk of ovarian cancer

Screening for ovarian cancer by using any of the available methods is currently of unproven value. There is no evidence yet that mortality can be reduced and the propensity for harm, given the high rate of false positive results when ovarian ultrasound scans and serum CA125 levels are combined, makes new approaches necessary for population screening.[53] Two large UK trials are currently recruiting to try to address the question of how best to screen for ovarian cancer in the older population (UK Collaborative Trial of Ovarian Cancer screening: UKTOCSS) and in those with a family history of ovarian cancer (UK Familial Ovarian Cancer Screening Study: UKFOCCS) [www.ncrn.org].

Surgery to remove ovaries and fallopian tubes (with or without hysterectomy) does reduce ovarian cancer risk. In *BRCA1* gene carriers, uptake of prophylactic oophorectomy is high and data published in 2002 suggest that, in this group of gene carriers who have not had breast cancer at the time of oophorectomy, the risk of developing a subsequent breast cancer is reduced by approximately 50%.[36,37] Hormone replacement therapy may be useful for control of menopausal symptoms without causing an elevation in breast cancer risk above the level of the gene carrier who chooses to retain the ovaries.[54] Cases of primary peritoneal carcinoma are well described in *BRCA1* and oophorectomy will not prevent these. Peritoneal carcinoma may occur in up to 5% of *BRCA1* gene carriers. The precise incidence is unknown. After prophylactic oophorectomy, careful pathological review of ovaries and fallopian tubes is mandatory; peritoneal washing for cytology is also important.[45] A number of past case reports of peritoneal carcinomatosis that have been published may relate to unrecognised and untreated occult tumours of ovaries or fallopian tubes at the time of prophylactic surgery.

Rare genetic conditions associated with ovarian tumours (Figure 3)

- Gorlin syndrome (naevoid basal cell carcinoma syndrome) is due to mutations in the *PTCH* gene on chromosome 9q and is associated with predominantly multiple basal cell carcinomas (often of early-onset), odontogenic keratocysts of the jaw, and palmar and plantar pits. Other features include medulloblastoma and ovarian fibromas.[55]

- Carney complex, due to mutations in the *PKAR1A* gene on chromosome 17q, is a condition recognised by the variable intensity lentigenes and, in some cases, mucosal pigmentation. The external appearance can be confused with Peutz–Jegher syndrome. The predominant tumour type is myxoma, which can occur in the skin or the breast, but the principal and life-threatening lesion is cardiac myxoma. Endocrine anomalies also arise and ovarian carcinoma has occasionally been described, although it is still unclear whether there is a significant risk for epithelial ovarian carcinoma.[56]

- Peutz–Jegher syndrome, due to mutations in the *STK11* gene on chromosome 19p, is characterised by freckling similar to that seen in Carney complex and mucosal pigmentation. The key feature in Peutz–Jegher syndrome is gastrointestinal hamartomas, without which the diagnosis should not be made. There is an increased incidence of malignancy of the gastrointestinal tract and of the breast. Other rare malignancies have been described, including ovarian tumours and sex cord tumours with annular tubules, which are typically multifocal, bilateral and benign in contrast to sporadic tumours of this type.[56] Both men and women with Peutz–Jegher syndrome can develop Sertoli cell tumours of the gonad, which can be hormonally active and cause precocious puberty. Rarely, adenocarcinoma of the cervix (adenoma malignum) occurs in this syndrome.

- Swyer syndrome, or 46XY gonadal dysgenesis, displays sexual infantilism, a normal vagina and uterus, and streak gonads. The retention of male gonadal tissue inside the abdomen predisposes to the development of gonadoblastoma. Removal of the nonfunctioning gonads is usually advisable to avert this complication.[57]

HEREDITARY ENDOMETRIAL CANCER

Endometrial carcinoma is a key feature of HNPCC. In some series the incidence of endometrial cancer in women who are HNPCC gene carriers exceeds the colorectal cancer incidence.[58] The chance of a female gene carrier developing endometrial cancer in her lifetime is estimated at around 60%, with 20% of cases occurring before the menopause.[59] The majority of HNPCC is caused by mutations in the mismatch repair genes *hMLH1* and *hMSH2*. A third gene has been described (*hMSH6*), in the presence of which there appears to be a high incidence of endometrial cancer with a later onset and fewer cases of colon cancer.[60] Atypical endometrial hyperplasia in young women with possible HNPCC should be treated medically with great caution because carcinoma commonly ensues. When premenopausal endometrial cancer and colon cancer occur in a family, referral for further genetic investigation should be made (Table 2).

Management of hereditary endometrial cancer

Prophylactic hysterectomy may be warranted in HNPCC after childbearing, although, in common with sporadic endometrial cancer, symptoms usually lead to early diagnosis, perhaps with the exception of premenopausal women, although this has not been systematically examined. Screening with an ultrasound scan and endometrial biopsy has not been studied in relevant trials, although a high index of suspicion should encourage full evaluation, with hysteroscopy and biopsy for any menstrual disturbance and certainly for postmenopausal bleeding. Trials of screening in this high-risk group are needed. Some gene carriers elect to undergo prophylactic hysterectomy (usually with bilateral salpingo-oophorectomy) once their families are complete.

SUMMARY

Our understanding of the genetic predisposition to gynaecological and breast cancer has grown rapidly over the last decade. Over the coming decade it is hoped that our understanding of the factors that influence gene penetrance and expression in high-risk gene carriers may become clearer. Better methods for screening and prevention are needed and will become available through continuing laboratory and clinical research endeavours.

Table 2 *Clinical criteria used for selecting families with increased likelihood of being due to one of the HNPCC mismatch repair gene mutations*

Classic Amsterdam	Modified Amsterdam (small families)	Bethesda
• 3 directly related (first degree) relatives affected by colorectal cancer • 2 generations affected • 1 case diagnosed at <50 years • familial polyposis excluded	as for Amsterdam criteria, but can substitute HNPCC associated tumours; these include cancer of the endometrium, ovary, hepatobiliary tract, urothelial tract, skin (keratoacanthoma) and sebaceous glands	• as for Amsterdam criteria • 2 HNPCC associated tumours in 1 person • colorectal cancer in 1 individual + a first degree relative with colorectal cancer or HNPCC associated cancer diagnosed at < 45 years; or an adenoma diagnosed at < 40 years • colorectal cancer or endometrial cancer diagnosed at <45 years • proximal undifferentiated colorectal cancer diagnosed at <45 years • signet ring colorectal cancer diagnosed at < 45 years • adenomas diagnosed at < 40 years

References

1. Knudson AG. Cancer genetics. *Am J Med Genet* 2002;111:96–102.

2. Thompson LH, Schild D. Recombinational DNA repair and human disease. *Mutat Res* 2002;509:49–78.

3. Al Tassan N, Chmiel NH, Maynard J, Fleming N, Livingston AL, Williams GT, *et al*. Inherited variants of MYH associated with somatic G:C?T:A mutations in colorectal tumors. *Nat Genet* 2002;30:227–32.

4. Narod SA, Sun P, Risch HA; Hereditary Ovarian Cancer Clinical Study Group. Ovarian cancer, oral contraceptives, and BRCA mutations. *N Engl J Med* 2001;345:1706–7.

5. Shiang R, Thompson LM, Zhu YZ, Church DM, Fielder TJ, Bocian M, *et al*. Mutations in the transmembrane domain of FGFR3 cause the most common genetic form of dwarfism, achondroplasia. *Cell* 1994;78:335–42.

6. Thompson D, Easton DF, Breast Cancer Linkage Consortium. Cancer incidence in *BRCA1* mutation carriers. *J Natl Cancer Inst* 2002;94:1358–65.

7. Begg CB. On the use of familial aggregation in population-based case probands for calculating penetrance. *J Natl Cancer Inst* 2002;94:1221–6.

8. Antoniou A, Pharoah P, Narod S, Risch HA, Eyfjord J, Hopper J, *et al*. Average risks of breast and ovarian cancer associated with mutations in *BRCA1* or *BRCA2* detected in case series unselected for family history: a combined analysis of 22 studies. *Am J Hum Genet* 2003;72:1117–30.

9. Dagan E, Friedman E, Paperna T, Carmi N, Gershoni-Baruch R. Androgen receptor CAG repeat length in Jewish Israeli women who are *BRCA1/2* mutation carriers: association with breast/ovarian cancer phenotype. *Eur J Hum Genet* 2002;10:724–8.

10. Anglian Breast Cancer Study Group. Prevalence and penetrance of *BRCA1* and *BRCA2* mutations in a population-based series of breast cancer cases. *Br J Cancer* 2000;83:1301–8.

11. Levy-Lahad E, Catane R, Eisenberg S, Kaufman B, Hornreich G, Lishinsky E, *et al*. Founder *BRCA1* and *BRCA2* mutations in Ashkenazi Jews in Israel: frequency and differential penetrance in ovarian cancer and in breast-ovarian cancer families. *Am J Hum Genet* 1997;60:1059–67.

12. Antoniou AC, Pharoah PD, McMullan G, Day NE, Ponder BA, Easton D. Evidence for further breast cancer susceptibility genes in addition to *BRCA1* and *BRCA2* in a population-based study. *Genet Epidemiol* 2001;21:1–18.

13. de Jong MM, Nolte IM, te Meerman GJ, van der Graaf WT, Oosterwijk JC, Kleibeuker JH, *et al*. Genes other than *BRCA1* and *BRCA2* involved in breast cancer susceptibility. *J Med Genet* 2002;39: 225–42.

14. Ioannidis JP, Trikalinos TA, Ntzani EE, Contopoulos-Ioannidis DG. Genetic associations in large versus small studies: an empirical assessment. *Lancet* 2003;361:567–71.

15. Paget J. *Lectures on Surgical Pathology*. Volume II: *Tumours*. London: Longman; 1853.

16. Broca P. *Trait des Tumeurs. Des Tumeurs en General*. Paris: Becket et Labe; 1886.

17. Claus EB, Risch N, Thompson WD. Genetic analysis of breast cancer in the cancer and steroid hormone study. *Am J Hum Genet* 1991;48:232–42.

18. Eccles D, Marlow A, Royle G, Collins A, Morton NE. Genetic epidemiology of early onset breast cancer. *J Med Genet* 1994;31:944–9.

19. Hall JM, Lee MK, Newman B, Morrow JE, Anderson LA, Huey B, *et al*. Linkage of early-onset familial breast cancer to chromosome 17q21. *Science* 1990;250:1684–9.

20. Miki Y, Swensen J, Shattuck-Eidens D, Futreal FA, Harshman K, Tavtigian S, *et al.* A strong candidate gene for the breast and ovarian cancer susceptibility gene *BRCA1*. *Science* 1994;266:66–71.

21. Wooster R, Bignell G, Lancaster J, Swift S, Seal S, Mangion J, *et al.* Identification of the breast cancer susceptibility gene *BRCA2*. *Nature* 1995;378:789–92.

22. Struewing J, Abeliovich D, Peretz T, Avishai N, Kaback MM, Collins FS, *et al.* The carrier frequency of the *BRCA1* 185delAG mutation is approximately 1 percent in Ashkenazi Jewish individuals. *Nat Genet* 1995;11:198–200.

23. Thorlacius S, Olafsdottir G, Tryggvadottir L, Neuhausen S, Jonasson JG, Tavtigian SV, *et al.* A single *BRCA2* mutation in male and female breast cancer families from Iceland with varied cancer phenotypes. *Nat Genet* 1996;13:117–19.

24. Johannsson O, Ostermeyer EA, Hakansson S, Friedman LS, Johansson U, Sellberg G, *et al.* Founding *BRCA1* mutations in hereditary breast and ovarian cancer in Southern Sweden. *Am J Hum Genet* 1996;58:441–50.

25. Meijers-Heijboer H, van den OA, Klijn J, Wasielewski M, de Snoo A, Oldenburg R, *et al.* Low-penetrance susceptibility to breast cancer due to CHEK2(★)1100delC in noncarriers of *BRCA1* or *BRCA2* mutations. *Nat Genet* 2002;31:55–9.

26. Chenevix-Trench G, Spurdle AB, Gatei M, Kelly H, Marsh A, Chen X, *et al.* Dominant negative ATM mutations in breast cancer families. *J Natl Cancer Inst* 2002;94:205–15.

27. Hemminki A. The molecular basis and clinical aspects of Peutz–Jeghers syndrome. *Cell Mol Life Sci* 1999;55:735–50.

28. Olschwang S, Boisson C, Thomas G. Peutz–Jeghers families unlinked to STK11/LKB1 gene mutations are highly predisposed to primitive biliary adenocarcinoma. *J Med Genet* 2001;38:356–60.

29. Eng C. Genetics of Cowden syndrome: through the looking glass of oncology. *Int J Oncol* 1998;12:701–10.

30. Duffy SW, Tabar L, Chen HH, Holmqvist M, Yen MF, Abdsalah S, *et al.* The impact of organized mammography service screening on breast carcinoma mortality in seven Swedish counties. *Cancer* 2002;95:458–69.

31. Lee CH. Screening mammography: proven benefit, continued controversy. *Radiol Clin North Am* 2002;40:395–407.

32. Eccles DM, Evans DG, Mackay J. Guidelines for a genetic risk based approach to advising women with a family history of breast cancer. UK Cancer Family Study Group (UKCFSG). *J Med Genet* 2000;37:203–9.

33. The British Association of Surgical Oncology guidelines for surgeons on the management of symptomatic breast disease in the UK (1998 revision). BASO Breast Speciality Group. *Eur J Surg Oncol* 1998;24:464–76.

34. Cuzick J, Powles T, Veronesi U, Forbes J, Edwards R, Ashley S, *et al.* Overview of the main outcomes in breast-cancer prevention trials. *Lancet* 2003;361:296–300.

35. Eccles DM, Dowsett M, Howell A, Evans DGR, Chapman K, Eeles, R, *et al.* The raloxifene plus Zoladex (RAZOR) trial for breast cancer risk reduction. *Proceedings of the AACR, Frontiers in Chemoprevention Research, 14–18 October 2002, Boston MA, USA.* Abstract 10032.

36. Rebbeck TR, Lynch HT, Neuhausen SL, Narod SA, Van't Veer L, Garber JE, *et al.* Prophylactic oophorectomy in carriers of *BRCA1* or *BRCA2* mutations. *N Engl J Med* 2002;346:1616–22.

37. Kauff ND, Satagopan JM, Robson ME, Scheuer L, Hensley M, Hudis CA, *et al.* Risk-reducing salpingo-oophorectomy in women with a *BRCA1* or *BRCA2* mutation. *N Engl J Med* 2002;346:1609–15.

38. Meijers-Heijboer EJ, Verhoog LC, Brekelmans CT, Seynaeve C, Tilanus-Linthorst MM, Wagner A, et al. Presymptomatic DNA testing and prophylactic surgery in families with a BRCA1 or BRCA2 mutation. Lancet 2000;355:2015–20.

39. Contant CM, Menke-Pluijmers MB, Seynaeve C, Meijers-Heijboer EJ, Klijn JG, Verhoog LC, et al. Clinical experience of prophylactic mastectomy followed by immediate breast reconstruction in women at hereditary risk of breast cancer (HB(O)C) or a proven BRCA1 and BRCA2 germ-line mutation. Eur J Surg Oncol 2002;28:627–32.

40. Hoogerbrugge N, Bult P, Widt-Levert LM, Beex LV, Kiemeney LA, Ligtenberg MJ, et al. High prevalence of premalignant lesions in prophylactically removed breasts from women at hereditary risk for breast cancer. J Clin Oncol 2003;21:41–5.

41. Hartmann LC, Schaid DJ, Woods JE, Crotty TP, Myers JL, Arnold PG, et al. Efficacy of bilateral prophylactic mastectomy in women with a family history of breast cancer. N Engl J Med 1999;340:77–84.

42. Brose M, Rebbeck TR, Calzone KA, Stopfer JE, Nathanson K, Weber BL. Cancer risk estimates for BRCA1 mutation carriers identified in a risk evaluation program. J Natl Cancer Inst 2002;94:1365–72.

43. Ford D, Easton D, Stratton M, Godgar D, Devilee P, Bishop DT, et al. Genetic heterogeneity and penetrance analysis of the BRCA1 and BRCA2 genes in breast cancer families. Am J Hum Genet 1998;62:676–89.

44. Eccles DM, Forabosco P, Williams A, Dunn B, Williams C, Bishop DT, et al. Segregation analysis of ovarian cancer using diathesis to include other cancers. Ann Hum Genet 1997;61:243–52.

45. Agoff SN, Mendelin JE, Grieco VS, Garcia RL. Unexpected gynecologic neoplasms in patients with proven or suspected BRCA-1 or -2 mutations: implications for gross examination, cytology, and clinical follow-up. Am J Surg Pathol 2002;26:171–8.

46. Lu KH, Garber JE, Cramer DW, Welch WR, Niloff J, Schrag D, et al. Occult ovarian tumors in women with BRCA1 or BRCA2 mutations undergoing prophylactic oophorectomy. J Clin Oncol 2000;18:2728–32.

47. Gayther SA, Warren W, Mazoyer S, Russell PA, Harrington PA, Chiano M, et al. Germline mutations of the BRCA1 gene in breast and ovarian cancer families provide evidence for a genotype-phenotype correlation. Nat Genet 1995;11:428–33.

48. Gayther SA, Mangion J, Russell PA, Seal S, Barfoot R, Ponder BAJ, et al. Variation of risks of breast and ovarian cancer associated with different germline mutations of the BRCA2 gene. Nat Genet 1997;15:103–5.

49. Shaw PA, McLaughlin JR, Zweemer RP, Narod SA, Risch H, Verheijen RH, et al. Histopathologic features of genetically determined ovarian cancer. Int J Gynecol Pathol 2002;21:407–11.

50. Ben David Y, Chetrit A, Hirsh-Yechezkel G, Friedman E, Beck BD, Beller U, et al. Effect of BRCA mutations on the length of survival in epithelial ovarian tumors. J Clin Oncol 2002;20:463–6.

51. Buller RE, Shahin MS, Geisler JP, Zogg M, De Young BR, Davis CS. Failure of BRCA1 dysfunction to alter ovarian cancer survival. Clin Cancer Res 2002;8:1196–202.

52. Watson P, Butzow R, Lynch HT, Mecklin JP, Jarvinen HJ, Vasen HF, et al. The clinical features of ovarian cancer in hereditary nonpolyposis colorectal cancer. Gynecol Oncol 2001;82:223–8.

53. Jacobs IJ, Skates SJ, MacDonald N, Menon U, Rosenthal AN, Prys-Davies A, et al. Screening for ovarian cancer: a pilot randomised controlled trial. Lancet 1999;353:1207–10.

54. Rebbeck TR, Levin AM, Eisen A, Snyder C, Watson P, Cannon-Albright L, et al. Breast cancer risk after bilateral prophylactic oophorectomy in BRCA1 mutation carriers. J Natl Cancer Inst 1999;91:1475–9.

55. Kimonis VE, Goldstein AM, Pastakia B, Yang ML, Kase R, DiGiovanna JJ, *et al.* Clinical manifestations in 105 persons with nevoid basal cell carcinoma syndrome. *Am J Med Genet* 1997;69:299–308.

56. Papageorgiou T, Stratakis CA. Ovarian tumors associated with multiple endocrine neoplasias and related syndromes (Carney complex, Peutz–Jeghers syndrome, von Hippel–Lindau disease, Cowden's disease). *Int J Gynecol Cancer* 2002;12:337–47.

57. Kempe A, Engels H, Schubert R, Meindl A, van der Ven K, Plath H, *et al.* Familial ovarian dysgerminomas (Swyer syndrome) in females associated with 46 XY-karyotype. *Gynecol Endocrinol* 2002;16:107–11.

58. Dunlop M, Farrington SM, Carothers AD, Wyllie A, Sharp L, Burn J, *et al.* Cancer risk associated with germline DNA mismatch repair gene mutations. *Hum Mol Genet* 1997;6:105–10.

59. Vasen HFA, Wijnen JT, Menko FH, Kleibeuker JH, Taal BG, Griffioen G, *et al.* Cancer risk in families with hereditary nonpolyposis colorectal cancer diagnosed by mutation analysis. *Gastroenterology* 1996;110:1020–7.

60. Wagner A, Hendriks Y, Meijers-Heijboer EJ, de Leeuw WJ, Morreau H, Hofstra R, *et al.* Atypical HNPCC owing to MSH6 germline mutations: analysis of a large Dutch pedigree. *J Med Genet* 2001;38:318–22.

13

Childbirth and subsequent faecal continence

Maeve Eogan and Colm O'Herlihy

INTRODUCTION

Faecal incontinence is a common but often unreported symptom, which can become a serious and debilitating social handicap. It is accepted that a significant proportion (up to 25%) of women experience transient altered continence after vaginal delivery[1] and a smaller percentage suffer long-term symptoms.[2] Exact prevalence in different age groups is, however, unknown, not least because perceived embarrassment and uncertainty about possible therapies seem to discourage many women from seeking medical advice. Nevertheless, Kok *et al.*,[3] in a large community based study, identified symptoms of altered faecal continence in 4.2% of women under 85 years of age; even at age 45, symptoms occur much more frequently in women than in men, with an eightfold female preponderance, implicating childbirth as the principal causative factor.[4]

Until about 10 years ago, obstetricians devoted relatively little attention to altered faecal continence after childbirth. Since then, the spectrum of symptoms ranging from faecal urgency to frank faecal incontinence has been widely investigated in the obstetric context. It is now possible to paint a relatively clear picture of the circumstances in which damage to the anal sphincter is more likely to occur. What remains less clear are the factors that influence why many parous women may develop incontinence symptoms only in later life, and it is clear that further long-term research will be required to clarify this pathogenesis.

This review focuses on the physiological mechanism of faecal continence and its assessment, as well as on obstetric factors that increase the risk of damage to continence control. Potential alterations in practice that may reduce the incidence of obstetric injury to the anal sphincter mechanism are outlined, as are therapeutic options to alleviate resulting morbidity.

MECHANISMS OF CONTINENCE

Faecal incontinence is defined as the involuntary loss of flatus, liquid or solid faeces.[5] Continence is maintained by the coordinated action of the anatomical elements of the pelvic floor. The anal canal is a tubular structure measuring 3–4 cm in length. It extends from the perineal skin to the lower end of the rectum and is surrounded by two distinct muscles: the internal and external anal sphincters. An intact, innervated anal sphincter complex is vital to the maintenance of continence.

Internal anal sphincter

This involuntary muscle is a continuation of the circular smooth muscle of the rectum. It receives its sympathetic supply from nerves from the fifth lumbar segment and its parasympathetic supply via the pelvic plexus arising from the sacral nerve roots. This sphincter is about 3 cm long and 2–3 mm thick.[6] Because it maintains anal sphincter tone at rest, disruption of the internal sphincter leads to passive faecal incontinence (loss of faeces without awareness).

External anal sphincter

This striated muscle encircles the internal sphincter and is subdivided into three layers: subcutaneous, superficial and deep. The subcutaneous component is represented by a ring of muscle with no distinct dorsal or ventral attachments; the superficial portion is an elliptical muscle ring attached posteriorly to the coccyx; and the deep external sphincter extends superiorly to blend with the puborectalis muscle.

The external anal sphincter, puborectalis and other components of the levator ani constitute a muscle complex that contributes further to the resting tone of the anal canal, but which can also be contracted or relaxed voluntarily to assist passage of flatus or faeces. External anal sphincter dysfunction leads to faecal urgency and incontinence, resulting from an inability to delay defaecation.

Pudendal nerve

Pudendal nerve integrity is essential for faecal continence. This nerve arises in the pelvis from the second, third and fourth sacral nerve roots, passes through the greater sciatic foramen close to the ischial spine, re-enters the pelvis through the lesser sciatic foramen and enters the perineum through the pudendal canal (Alcock's canal) in the obturator fascia on the lateral wall of the ischiorectal fossa. At this point it terminates in three branches: the inferior rectal nerve (supplying the external anal sphincter), the perineal nerve (supplying vulval skin and subcutaneous tissues), and the dorsal nerve to the clitoris (innervating the anterior pelvic compartment). Injury may occur at any point along the length of the nerve and have significant effects on faecal continence.

Anorectal angle

The rectum and anal canal lie above and below the pelvic floor respectively. Thus, the anorectal junction lies at the level of the puborectalis portion of the levator ani muscles, at which point there is normally a sharp 'anorectal angle'. This angle is also important in the maintenance of continence.[7]

Sensory and motor interplay forms the basis for continence and defaecation. The rectum usually functions as a low-pressure reservoir to accommodate faecal contents. However, a sensation of rectal fullness is mediated by sensory stretch receptors when a volume of about 200 ml is reached. The internal anal sphincter relaxes to permit the faecal bolus to descend towards the anal canal, where voluntary contraction of the anal sphincter prevents it from passing any further. For defaecation to occur, the external sphincter and puborectalis complex must relax and intra-abdominal pressure increase, thus straightening the anorectal angle. To defer defaecation, the external sphincter complex remains contracted, which returns the luminal contents to the rectum.

EFFECTS OF PREGNANCY AND CHILDBIRTH ON FAECAL CONTINENCE

Although altered faecal continence may follow vaginal delivery, pregnancy itself does not appear directly to influence anal sphincter or pudendal nerve function.[8,9] Antepartum faecal incontinence is thus infrequently seen in nulliparous women, except in the presence of co-morbid conditions (e.g. Crohn's disease or neurological disorders). This contrasts with urinary incontinence, which may present for the first time in the antenatal period. Viktrup et al.[10] carried out repeated interviews about stress urinary incontinence before and after delivery with a single cohort of antenatal patients. While 32% reported the symptom during pregnancy, this resolved in the majority and only 3% had persistent symptoms one year postpartum.

Mechanisms of injury

Childbirth is the most important aetiological factor in the pathogenesis of faecal incontinence in women; symptoms are thus more common in the parous female population. MacArthur et al.[11] found that 4% of women admitted to new symptoms of altered faecal continence when questioned at a mean interval of ten months after delivery and Sultan et al.[2] identified altered faecal continence in 13% of primigravid and 23% of multiparous women six weeks after vaginal delivery. Excluding obstetric fistulas, which may lead to incontinence, there are essentially three mechanisms of injury to the anal canal that can occur during childbirth:

- direct anal sphincter muscle disruption by third or fourth degree perineal tears, most commonly at first vaginal delivery[8]

- neuropathy of the pudendal nerve(s), which is often transient but may be cumulative with successive deliveries and over time[12]

- combined mechanical and neurological trauma.

Direct anal sphincter disruption

Primary sphincter injury most commonly follows deep perineal lacerations. First and second degree perineal tears are confined to the skin, superficial perineal muscles and vaginal epithelium only; there is little evidence that these tears have any long-term consequences.[13] Anal sphincter disruption, either partial or complete, constitutes a third degree tear, and the less common fourth degree tear refers to extension through the sphincter into the anal mucosa. Clinically detected third or fourth degree tears occur in up to 3% of deliveries.[14] Obstetric damage to the anal sphincter is usually repaired at the time of diagnosis after delivery (primary repair).

Despite appropriate identification and repair of anal sphincter tears, the outcome of primary repair may be suboptimal, at least when judged by anal ultrasonography, which has documented residual sphincter defects in up to 50% of women who have undergone apparently satisfactory primary repair procedures.[15–17] Only a minority of these women, however, experience symptoms. Nevertheless, in a series of 84 such women interviewed by Wood et al.,[18] faecal incontinence was reported by up to 25%; flatal incontinence seems to be even more prevalent.[19] These observations suggest that current surgical practices for the repair of third and fourth degree perineal tears require improvement. Repair techniques need to be standardised and audited, and formal training of obstetric staff is necessary if long-term sequelae are to be minimised.[20] As with surgery for stress urinary incontinence, the first attempt at repair is most likely to lead to long-term success.

Not all anal sphincter disruptions are recognised at delivery; some become apparent only when the woman later develops altered faecal continence. In its worst form, an injury may present for the first time as a rectovaginal fistula, which can be associated with unrecognised third and fourth degree tears. Fistulas usually present with recurring perineal sepsis, persistent foul smelling discharge, or passage of flatus or faeces per vaginum. Expert surgical repair offers good results in over 90% of women,[21] provided the external anal sphincter has remained innervated.

Another management problem relates to asymptomatic occult anal sphincter injury. As we have come to realise that the natural process of childbirth carries inherent risks to the perineum, it has become evident that anal sphincter defects may be overdiagnosed by postpartum endosonography. Not all defects result in symptoms; indeed, two prospective studies in women undergoing vaginal delivery showed that, while as many as one in three women may sustain some degree of occult anal sphincter injury,[1,2] only one-third of these develop symptoms. The true clinical significance and natural history of most of these minor sphincter deformities is uncertain and may become apparent only after many years of follow-up, but a proportion may become symptomatic after subsequent deliveries[22,23]or in later life.[24]

Pudendal nerve injury

Because the pudendal nerves are fixed at the ischial spines they are predisposed to traction injury during the late first and second stages of labour as the fetal head reaches the pelvic floor; neural disruption may also occur at traumatic instrumental delivery.[5] Although disruption of the anal sphincter is more likely at the first vaginal delivery, pudendal nerve injury is reported to be more common with successive deliveries, so neuropathy can be cumulative over time.[24]

ASSESSMENT OF CONTINENCE

Ideally, all women who have sustained a recognised or suspected obstetric injury to the anal sphincter mechanism, or who complain of altered faecal continence in the postnatal period, should be assessed in a dedicated, suitably equipped clinic.[25] Women may be reluctant to discuss symptoms that they perceive as embarrassing[4] and such a 'perineal' clinic provides an ideal environment for full and frank discussion of symptoms, their aetiologies and prognosis, as well as providing the opportunity to carry out examination, neurophysiological assessment, endoanal ultrasound and ultimately to arrange further referral for physiotherapy or colorectal surgery. Timely referral for specialist assessment reduces the time to recovery and symptomatic improvement, and thus minimises patient dissatisfaction and complaints.

Clinical evaluation

History and examination alone cannot adequately assess anal sphincter function, but they are essential components of a continence assessment. Direct questioning using a detailed bowel function questionnaire is essential to document the severity and progress of incontinence, and permits a continence score to be calculated[26] (Table 1); it also enables reliable serial comparisons to be made.

Clinical signs that should be sought include perineal soiling, absence of the cutaneous anal reflex, a patulous anus, local signs of scarring or fistula, or palpable defects in the levator muscles.[27]

Anal manometry

By providing a pressure profile of the anal canal, manometry assesses sphincter tone and contractile function.[28,29] Three resting and three squeeze anal canal pressure readings are obtained to calculate the mean maximum resting and squeeze pressures, reflecting internal and external anal sphincter activity respectively. Anal canal vector symmetry can then be derived from these measurements.[29,30] Manometry assesses anal sphincter function but does not identify whether the underlying cause of dysfunction is muscular or neurological; further tests of anal sphincter morphology and neurology are required to elucidate this.

Table 1 *Faecal continence scoring system (modified from Jorge and Wexner[26])*[a]

	Never	Rarely	Sometimes	Usually	Always
Incontinence for solid stool	0	1	2	3	4
Incontinence for liquid stool	0	1	2	3	4
Incontinence for flatus	0	1	2	3	4
Wears pad	0	1	2	3	4
Faecal urgency	0	1	2	3	4

[a] Add together one score from each row; a score of 0 implies complete continence; a score of 20 implies complete incontinence

Endoanal ultrasound

A high-resolution rotating endosonographic probe can provide a remarkably clear image of internal and external anal sphincter structure and integrity.[6] In selected women with complex injury or suspected rectovaginal fistula, magnetic resonance imaging provides valuable additional anatomical information.

Pudendal nerve assessment

Neurophysiological assessment of the pelvic floor has been pioneered using measurements of the pudendal nerve terminal motor latency.[31] This technique, however, assesses only the short distal segment of the nerve extending from the ischial spine to the perineum. Diagnostic accuracy is improved by evaluating the full length of the pudendal nerve using a combination of concentric needle electromyography of the external anal sphincter with pudendal nerve conduction assessment, using the clitoral–anal reflex. This diagnostic procedure can identify a range of neurophysiological abnormalities that have different aetiologies, symptoms and prognoses.[32,33] In particular, it is possible to differentiate demyelinating (transient) injury from axonal disruption, which is likely to lead to chronic symptoms. The assessment of neural integrity is an essential prerequisite to successful secondary anal sphincter repair, which is compromised by an irreversible pudendal neuropathy.

OBSTETRIC RISK FACTORS FOR FAECAL INCONTINENCE

Obstetric risk factors for anal sphincter injury and postpartum faecal incontinence are:

- primiparity

- age >30 years

- Asian race

- vaginal delivery

- epidural anaesthesia

- prolonged second stage of labour (>1 hour)

- episiotomy (especially midline incision)

- fetal macrosomia (>4 kg) and shoulder dystocia

- persistent occipitoposterior position

- instrumental vaginal delivery (forceps > vacuum)

- previous third degree tear.

Anal sphincter injury at vaginal delivery poses the single greatest threat to faecal continence; significant perineal injury is a potential consequence of childbirth and in most cases is unavoidable. Nevertheless, it is important to evaluate the management of labour and delivery to determine whether modifications in practice could reduce the incidence of altered faecal continence.

Some risk factors cannot be modified, such as maternal age, parity and ethnicity; anal sphincter injury is more common in primiparous women over 30 years, and among those of Asian origin.[34]

Epidural anaesthesia

Epidural anaesthesia is a safe and effective form of intrapartum pain relief. Its use has become increasingly widespread and had been assumed to have a beneficial effect on the risk of perineal injury, owing to associated pelvic floor relaxation and presumably to greater control over delivery of the fetal head, and consequently fewer perineal lacerations.[35] Conflicting data have emerged, which indicate a higher rate of significant perineal injury with epidural analgesia (16.1% versus 9.7%),[36] thought to result from a more frequent need for instrumental delivery and episiotomy in women in the epidural group. As well as potentially compromising the anal sphincter mechanism, epidural analgesia facilitates pudendal nerve compression by prolonging the second stage of labour.[1] These causal relationships may explain why increasing institutional rates of perineal injury parallel local increases in epidural usage.[37]

Episiotomy

There is a long-held belief that episiotomy protects the anal sphincter. Ould, in 1742, proposed 'surgical opening of the perineum in difficult deliveries to prevent severe perineal tears'.[38] Proponents of episiotomy have suggested that it reduces the duration of the second stage of labour and the incidence of third and fourth degree perineal tears and urinary and faecal incontinence.[39] These claims are unsubstantiated by meta-analysis. The only consistent advantage is a reduction in the incidence of anterior perineal lacerations, which are associated with minimal morbidity, and do not lead to postpartum urinary incontinence.[40]

Furthermore, midline, when compared with mediolateral, episiotomy is associated with significantly higher rates of third and fourth degree perineal tears.[41,42] This predisposition is further compounded by instrumental delivery, with anal sphincter injury rates of 50% reported when forceps delivery and midline episiotomy coexist.[43]

Episiotomy does have a role in obstetrics, in the management of shoulder dystocia, to expedite delivery in cases of fetal distress, or to minimise perineal trauma in the presence of a thick, inelastic perineum. Its use, however, should be restrictive rather than liberal[44] and be carefully audited, with midline episiotomies being avoided completely. It is interesting that when episiotomy is used restrictively it may be protective against pelvic floor injury.[45]

Intrapartum factors

Delivery of a macrosomic infant (weight >4 kg) is associated with an increased risk of anal sphincter disruption.[17] Similarly, and often associated with macrosomia, shoulder dystocia and interventions used to resolve this emergency also predispose to injury.[45] Prolongation of the second stage of labour confers an increased risk of perineal injury,[46,47] often associated with pudendal neuropathy. Vaginal delivery in a persistent occipitoposterior position also leads to a greatly increased incidence of anal sphincter trauma.[48]

Instrumental vaginal delivery

Both forceps and vacuum deliveries increase the risk of anal sphincter damage.[11] Although just 4% of women who undergo forceps delivery sustain a recognised third degree tear, up to 50% of those who do tear have had an instrumental delivery.[2] It is a widely held belief that forceps assisted vaginal delivery is more traumatic to the continence mechanism than vacuum extraction,[43,49] and the impact of mode of vaginal delivery on faecal continence has been evaluated in a number of studies. A prospective evaluation of primiparas before and after delivery showed an eight-fold increase in anal sphincter disruption with instrumental delivery,[1] and assisted delivery emerged as the obstetric intervention with the greatest risk of anal sphincter injury and altered faecal continence. A number of other observational studies have supported this finding, particularly showing that forceps delivery is associated with the greatest risks to the anal sphincter;[2,11,45,50] the evidence implicating vacuum extraction is less conclusive.

It was expected that randomised controlled trials would help to clarify the relative contribution of vacuum extraction and forceps delivery to the causation of faecal incontinence and anal sphincter disruption, and thus provide a useful guideline for obstetric practice. Several of these trials, however, have concentrated on immediate perineal outcome, followed by ultrasonographic findings in the postnatal period (which may be clinically occult), rather than on symptoms of faecal incontinence.[51,52] One study showed no difference between the two methods,[53] while others reported a greater incidence of perineal damage with forceps delivery.[49,52] Results from a further randomised trial comparing forceps and vacuum delivery suggest that, although both techniques increase the risk of altered faecal continence, symptoms are more likely in women who were delivered with forceps (59% versus 33% in those who had vacuum extraction)[54] and the sphincter seems to be at greatest risk when attempted vacuum extraction ends in a forceps delivery. It is interesting that, although current evidence suggests that forceps seem to be more traumatic to the mother at the time of delivery, a review of women who had participated in a randomised trial of the two instruments five years previously failed to show any long-term differences in maternal morbidity.[55] Undoubtedly, the skill of the obstetrician plays as important a role as the choice of the instrument but, in terms of continence outcome, when circumstances and facilities allow, vacuum should be the instrument of first choice in assisted delivery.[56]

Caesarean section

Universal prelabour caesarean section would avoid anal sphincter injury related to childbirth,[1,2] but would be impractical and unjustifiable in terms of logistics and perioperative morbidity and mortality.[57,58] In addition, hundreds of women would need to undergo abdominal delivery to prevent a single injury.[59] Nevertheless, elective caesarean delivery may be appropriate for women who have previously sustained pelvic floor injury or experienced altered continence after vaginal delivery.[9]

In primiparous women delivered by caesarean section without attempted vaginal delivery, anorectal physiology and faecal continence are unchanged.[9] On the other hand, caesarean section performed late in labour does not protect against abnormal postpartum manometry, an important consideration when managing multiparous women with pre-existing anal sphincter dysfunction.

Prelabour caesarean delivery is preferable in this cohort because caesareans late in labour may not protect against cumulative pudendal neuropathy and faecal incontinence.

PREVENTION AND TREATMENT OF POSTNATAL FAECAL INCONTINENCE

Suggested interventions for the prevention and treatment of postnatal faecal incontinence include:

- **primary prevention:**
  - antenatal pelvic floor exercises (unproven but safe)
  - oxytocin augmentation of primigravid labour if indicated
  - vacuum extraction as instrument of first choice

- **perineal repair:**
  - thorough postpartum perineal inspection
  - obstetric training in technique of perineal repair
  - slowly absorbable suture material
  - prophylactic antibiotic therapy
  - postnatal laxative use

- **postnatal review:**
  - routine postnatal enquiry about symptoms of altered faecal continence
  - dedicated perineal clinic review including anorectal physiology tests
  - symptomatic therapy (such as dietary modification and antidiarrhoeal medication)
  - augmented biofeedback physiotherapy
  - selected secondary anal sphincter repair

- **antenatal identification of high-risk multiparous women:**
  - previous primary or secondary anal sphincter repair
  - persistent symptoms of faecal incontinence.

Avoiding primary injury

Kegel[60] proposed that antenatal muscle exercises could strengthen the pelvic floor and thus reduce subsequent damage from childbirth. These exercises have been shown to increase muscle strength in nonpregnant, incontinent women[61,62] and to reduce the frequency of symptoms of urinary incontinence in late pregnancy and during the postnatal period,[63] but a prophylactic effect on the symptoms of faecal incontinence has not been demonstrated.

During labour, judicious use of oxytocin in primiparous women may shorten the later stages of labour and reduce the incidence of persistent occipitoposterior position. Vacuum extraction should be used, where possible, if instrumental delivery is indicated, and mediolateral episiotomy should be used appropriately.

Appropriate anal sphincter repair

To minimise the sequelae of anal sphincter disruption, it is essential that all injuries are recognised and appropriately repaired. This can be achieved by thorough examination of the vagina, perineum and rectum after each vaginal delivery to assess the degree of damage. Increased vigilance concerning anal sphincter injury does increase its detection rate.[64]

Sphincter repair should be carried out in optimal operative circumstances, with appropriate instruments, adequate lighting and either regional or general anaesthesia.[64] Primary repair performed by end-to-end approximation of the torn anal sphincter segments using slowly absorbable synthetic monofilament suture material (polydioxone or polyglyconate) appears to be as effective as the overlapping technique favoured by colorectal surgeons for secondary repair procedures.[65,66] Broad spectrum antibiotics should be administered intraoperatively and during the early postpartum period. The use of a stool softener and a bulking agent is recommended for about ten days after repair.[64]

Postnatal evaluation and management

Routine outpatient review and assessment of all high-risk or symptomatic women is recommended and should be carried out three months after delivery, when perineal healing and genital involution have occurred. Women who have sustained a documented third or fourth degree perineal tear or a traumatic vaginal delivery are considered 'high risk'. Appropriate investigations are performed and results are explained.

Asymptomatic women with satisfactory results are discharged with advice to return for antenatal assessment regarding mode of delivery in their next pregnancy. Women who are symptomatic, or who have abnormal neurophysiological results, can be selectively referred for the most effective and appropriate course of treatment.

Conservative treatment

Because postpartum incontinence symptoms are often transient, dietary advice will help many women with minor degrees of faecal incontinence.[67] A low residue diet reduces the fluidity of the stool, which can then be controlled more easily. Antidiarrhoeal medication, such as codeine phosphate or loperamide, can reduce faecal urgency,[68] and is also useful for those with neurogenic injury. Regular use of suppositories and enemas keep the rectum empty and improve continence in more severe cases.

Physiotherapy

Pelvic floor exercises have been shown to increase muscle strength in women with incontinence[60] and can be carried out by the woman at home and at her convenience, without need for specialist equipment or facilities. Sensory biofeedback is a behavioural technique that combines pelvic floor exercises with a sensory feedback signal, through use of a perineometer or vaginal cones. This has been shown subjectively to improve faecal continence symptoms, although manometry pressures may not alter significantly.[69]

Augmented biofeedback describes a combination of conventional biofeedback with electrical stimulation, using an endo-anal probe to initiate and coordinate voluntary contraction of the pelvic floor muscles. This leads to a subjective reduction of symptoms, as well as an improved manometry profile by enhancing the woman's ability to target the damaged muscle and to initiate its contraction.[69] This treatment is frequently employed in women with demyelinating pudendal nerve injury to maintain sphincter muscle bulk during the neurological recovery period. It is also used to increase residual muscle tone, as an adjunct to surgery, in women with significant muscle damage.[70]

Surgical treatment

Women with persistent faecal incontinence symptoms consequent on large anal sphincter defects should be referred to a colorectal surgeon for delayed overlapping anal sphincter repair. This procedure offers an improved functional outcome in more than 80% of these women.[71] A coexisting pudendal nerve injury greatly reduces the success rate and should be excluded before surgery. The functional result of an initially successful repair may deteriorate with age and menopausal status.[72]

Other surgical options exist to deal with severe or recurrent faecal incontinence. Gracilis muscle transposition and artificial sphincter implantation have been described, but these represent major surgical undertakings and should be carried out only after standard treatments have proved unsuccessful. Since the late 1990s, techniques such as implantation of sacral nerve stimulators, collagen injections into the anal mucosa,[73] and trans-sphincteric injection of silicone biomaterial[74] have been described, although these all remain under evaluation.

ASSESSMENT PRIOR TO SUBSEQUENT DELIVERY

Women with a previous third degree tear may be at risk of cumulative pelvic floor injury and will benefit from antenatal assessment in subsequent pregnancies to discuss the most appropriate mode of delivery on an individual basis. This consultation is best conducted between 28 and 34 weeks of gestation. A full history is taken and a continence score is computed. Previous hospital records are evaluated if necessary, and examination is followed by endo-anal ultrasonography and anal manometry.

Most women who sustain a recognised third degree tear are symptomatically well after a primary repair and remain so throughout subsequent deliveries, irrespective of endo-anal ultrasound findings. A policy of routine caesarean section is, therefore, inappropriate for these women; indeed, such a policy would increase caesarean section rates by up to 15%. It is prudent, however, to avoid a prolonged second stage of labour and instrumental delivery in this cohort, events that are, in any case, less likely to arise in multiparous labour.

In contrast, specific consideration is required for pregnant women who have symptoms of incontinence after anal sphincter injury, or those who have undergone a successful secondary sphincter repair. Women with impaired faecal continence as a consequence of vaginal delivery may experience deterioration in their symptoms after a further vaginal birth,[22] because a tear during the next delivery can damage a previously intact sphincter, increase the severity of a previous tear, or cause further traction injury to the pudendal nerve, with adverse consequences for the continence mechanism. In addition, a proportion of continent women with low antenatal anal manometry pressures who deliver vaginally after a previous third degree tear may develop incontinence symptoms postpartum.[22]

It should be noted that the correlation between symptoms of incontinence and ultrasound defects, particularly those that involve only one quadrant of the external anal sphincter ring, is poor. Endosonographic evidence of a sphincter defect in the presence of normal manometry does not appear to constitute a risk for subsequent postnatal faecal incontinence, so that prophylactic caesarean delivery is not justified in these women. It is likely that, as increasing evidence accrues from prospective investigations of the natural history of anal sphincter trauma, the algorithms for management in subsequent pregnancies will become clearer.

In general, women who have had a previous third degree tear and have persistent symptoms of faecal incontinence or significantly abnormal manometry results are best delivered by prelabour caesarean section, as are those who have undergone previous successful incontinence surgery. These indications would not be expected to add significantly to the overall caesarean section incidence. On the other hand, women who have had a previous sphincter tear who are asymptomatic and have satisfactory manometry pressures should be counselled towards vaginal delivery. These women have a somewhat increased risk of repeat third degree tear compared with the general multiparous population,[75-77] so additional risk factors (such as prolonged second stage of labour and forceps delivery) should be avoided where feasible. This management is summarised in Table 2.

Table 2 *A suggested classification for the subsequent obstetric management of multiparous women with a history of anal sphincter injury*

History	Symptoms (faecal incontinence)	Endoanal ultrasound and anal manometry	Management of delivery
Previous third degree tear (repaired)	No	Normal	Trial of vaginal delivery
Previous third degree tear (repaired)	Yes	Abnormal	Elective caesarean section
Successful secondary sphincter repair	No	Normal/abnormal	Elective caesarean section
Previous third degree tear or occult injury	No	Borderline/abnormal	Discuss vaginal delivery or caesarean section

CONCLUSION

Faecal incontinence affects a proportion of women after vaginal delivery but in the majority these symptoms are mild and transient, and do not recur after subsequent deliveries. Although a universal policy of elective prelabour caesarean section would avoid the problem, such a practice is unjustified on several grounds, not least those of maternal morbidity and healthcare costs.

Instead, obstetric energies should be directed towards avoiding or minimising the impact of known risk factors for anal sphincter injury and pudendal neuropathy. With regard to preventing injury, there is certainly little justification for continued use of midline episiotomy, or for vaginal delivery of women who have undergone a successful secondary anal sphincter repair. Other preventive measures include careful perineal inspection after every delivery to ensure that anal sphincter injury is recognised and repaired, and postnatal outpatient evaluation of high-risk or symptomatic women so as to facilitate the institution of appropriate dietary, physiotherapy or surgical treatment as required. It must be remembered, however, that it is impossible to predict sphincter injury and faecal incontinence, in primiparous women in particular; even in high-risk circumstances, the actual incidence of symptomatic injury is low.

Although the obstetric events surrounding anal sphincter injury are now well documented, the precise mechanisms of damage to the sphincter muscles and particularly to the pudendal nerve remain to be elucidated. In addition, uncertainty surrounds the reasons why a cohort of women will first develop symptoms of incontinence many years after childbirth, which cannot always be temporally related to the loss of trophic oestrogen at the menopause. This late onset of symptoms may represent neural degeneration in a proportion of women, but our understanding of the pathophysiology of faecal incontinence in older women is still largely speculative.

References

1. Donnelly VS, Fynes M, Campbell DM, Johnson H, O'Connell PR, O'Herlihy C. Obstetric events leading to anal sphincter damage. *Obstet Gynecol* 1998;92:955–61.
2. Sultan AH, Kamm MA, Hudson CN, Thomas JM, Bartram CI. Anal-sphincter disruption during vaginal delivery. *N Engl J Med* 1993;329:1905–11.
3. Kok AL, Voorhorst FJ, Burger CW, van Houten P, Kenemans P, Janssens J. Urinary and faecal incontinence in community-residing elderly women. *Age Ageing* 1992;21:211–15.

4.   Leigh RJ, Turnberg LA. Faecal incontinence: the unvoiced symptom. *Lancet* 1982;i:1349–51.

5.   Kamm MA. Obstetric damage and faecal incontinence. *Lancet* 1994;344:730–3.

6.   Bartram CI, Burnett SJD. *Atlas of Anal Endosonography*. Oxford: Butterworth-Heinemann; 1997. p. 7–16.

7.   Parks AG. Anorectal incontinence. *Proc R Soc Med* 1975;68:681–90.

8.   Sultan AH, Kamm MA, Hudson CN, Bartram CI. Effect of pregnancy on anal sphincter morphology and function. *Int J Colorectal Dis* 1993;8:206–9.

9.   Fynes M, Donnelly VS, O'Connell PR, O'Herlihy C. Cesarean delivery and anal sphincter injury. *Obstet Gynecol* 1998;92:496–500.

10.   Viktrup L, Lose G, Rolff M, Barfoed K. The symptom of stress incontinence caused by pregnancy or delivery in primiparas. *Obstet Gynecol* 1992;79:945–9.

11.   MacArthur C, Bick DE, Keighley MR. Faecal incontinence after childbirth. *Br J Obstet Gynaecol* 1997;104:46–50.

12.   Snooks SJ, Setchell M, Swash M, Henry MM. Injury to innervation of pelvic floor musculature in childbirth. *Lancet* 1984;ii:546–50.

13.   Lede R, Belizan J, Carroli G. Is routine use of episiotomy justified? *Am J Obstet Gynecol* 1996;174:1399–402.

14.   Swash M. Faecal incontinence: childbirth is responsible for most cases. *BMJ* 1993;307:636–7.

15.   Fitzpatrick M, Fynes M, Cassidy M, Behan M, O'Connell PR, O'Herlihy C. Prospective study of the influence of parity and operative technique on the outcome of primary anal sphincter repair following obstetrical injury. *Eur J Obstet Gynecol Reprod Biol* 2000;89:159–63.

16.   Kammerer-Doak DN, Wessol AB, Rogers RG, Domonguez CE, Dorin MH. A prospective cohort study of women after primary repair of obstetric anal sphincter laceration. *Am J Obstet Gynecol* 1999;181:1317–23.

17.   Sultan AH, Kamm MA, Hudson CN, Bartram CI. Third degree obstetric anal sphincter tears: risk factors and outcome of primary repair. *BMJ* 1994;308:887–91.

18.   Wood J, Amos L, Rieger N. Third degree anal sphincter tears: risk factors and outcome. *Aust N Z J Obstet Gynaecol* 1998;38:414–17.

19.   Crawford LA, Quint EH, Pearl ML, DeLancey JO. Incontinence following rupture of the anal sphincter during delivery. *Obstet Gynecol* 1993;82:527–31.

20.   Fitzpatrick M, O'Herlihy C. Vaginal birth and perineal trauma. *Curr Opin Obstet Gynecol* 2000;12:487–90.

21.   Venkatesh KS, Ramanujam PS, Larson DM, Haywood MA. Anorectal complications of vaginal delivery. *Dis Colon Rectum* 1989;32:1039–41.

22.   Fynes M, Donnelly V, O'Connell PR, O'Herlihy C. The effect of a second vaginal delivery on anorectal physiology and faecal continence: a prospective study. *Lancet* 1999;354:983–6.

23.   Faltin DL, Sangalli MR, Roche B, Floris L, Boulvain M, Weil A. Does a second delivery increase the risk of anal incontinence? *Br J Obstet Gynaecol* 2001;108:684–8.

24.   Snooks SJ, Swash M, Mathers SE, Henry MM. Effect of vaginal delivery on the pelvic floor: a 5-year follow-up. *Br J Surg* 1990;77:1358–60.

25.   Fitzpatrick M, Cassidy M, O'Connell PR, O'Herlihy C. Experience with an obstetric perineal clinic. *Eur J Obstet Gynecol Reprod Biol* 2002;100:199–203.

26.   Jorge JM, Wexner SD. Etiology and management of fecal incontinence. *Dis Colon Rectum* 1993;36:77–97.

27.   DeLancey JO, Kearney R, Chou Q, Speights S, Binno S. The appearance of levator ani muscle abnormalities in magnetic resonance images after vaginal delivery. *Obstet Gynecol* 2002;101:46–53.

28.   Williams N, Barlow J, Hobson A, Scott N, Irving M. Manometric asymmetry in the anal canal in controls and patients with fecal incontinence. *Dis Colon Rectum* 1995;38:1275–80.

29.   Fynes MM, Behan M, O'Herlihy C, O'Connell PR. Anal vector volume analysis complements endoanal ultrasonographic assessment of postpartum anal sphincter injury. *Br J Surg* 2000;87:1209–14.

30.   Perry RE, Blatchford GJ, Christensen MA, Thorson AG, Attwood SE. Manometric diagnosis of anal sphincter injuries. *Am J Surg* 1990;159:112–16.

31.   Rogers J, Henry MM, Misiewicz JJ. Disposable pudendal nerve stimulation: evaluation of the standard instrument and new device. *Gut* 1988;29:1131–3.

32.   Wexner SD, Marchetti F, Salanga VD, Corredor C, Jagelman DG. Neurophysiologic assessment of the anal sphincters. *Dis Colon Rectum* 1991;34:606–12.

33.   Fitzpatrick M, O'Brien C, O'Connell PR, O'Herlihy C. Patterns of abnormal pudendal nerve conduction associated with postpartum fecal incontinence. *Am J Obstet Gynecol* 2003;189:730–5.

34.   MacArthur C, Glazener CM, Wilson PD, Herbison GP, Gee H, Lang GD, *et al*. Obstetric practice and faecal incontinence three months after delivery. *BJOG* 2001;108:678–83.

35.   Walker MP, Farine D, Rolbin SH, Ritchie JW. Epidural anesthesia, episiotomy and obstetric laceration. *Obstet Gynecol* 1991;77:668–71.

36.   Robinson JN, Norwitz ER, Cohen AA, McElrath TF, Lieberman ES. Epidural analgesia and third- or fourth-degree lacerations in nulliparas. *Obstet Gynecol* 1999;94:259–62.

37.   Buchhave P, Flatlow L, Rydhstroem H, Thorbert G. Risk factors for rupture of the anal sphincter. *Eur J Obstet Gynecol Reprod Med* 1999;87:129–32.

38.   Ould F. *A Treatise of Midwifery*. Dublin: Nelson and Connor; 1742.

39.   Woolley RJ. Benefits and risks of episiotomy: a review of the English language literature since 1980; Parts I and II. *Obstet Gynecol Surv* 1991;50:806–35.

40.   Sleep J, Grant A. West Berkshire perineal management trial: three year follow up. *BMJ* 1987;295:749–51.

41.   Signorello LB, Harlow BL, Chekos AK, Repke JT. Midline episiotomy and anal incontinence: retrospective cohort study. *BMJ* 2000;320:86–90.

42.   Coats PM, Chan KK, Wilkins M, Beard RJ. A comparison between midline and mediolateral episiotomies. *Br J Obstet Gynaecol* 1980;87:408–12.

43.   Robinson JN, Norwitz ER, Cohen A, McElrath TF, Lieberman ES. Episiotomy, operative vaginal delivery and significant perineal trauma in nulliparous women. *Am J Obstet Gynecol* 1999;181:1180–4.

44.   Carroli G, Belizan J. Episiotomy for vaginal birth. *Cochrane Database Syst Rev* 2000;(2):CD000081.

45.   de Leeuw JW, Struijk PC, Vierhout ME, Wallenburg HC. Risk factors for third degree perineal ruptures during delivery. *BJOG* 2001;108:383–7.

46.   Moller Bek KM, Laurberg S. Intervention during labor: risk factors associated with complete tear of the anal sphincter. *Acta Obstet Gynecol Scand* 1992;71:520–4.

47.   Samuelsson E, Ladfors L, Wennerholm UB, Gareberg B, Nyberg K, Hagberg H. Anal sphincter tears: prospective study of obstetric risk factors. *BJOG* 2000;107:926–31.

48.   Fitzpatrick M, McQuillan K, O'Herlihy C. Influence of persistent occiput posterior position on delivery outcome. *Obstet Gynecol* 2001;98:1027–31.

49.   Johanson R, Pusey J, Livera N, Jones P. North Staffordshire/Wigan assisted delivery trial. *Br J Obstet Gynaecol* 1989;96:537–44.

50.   Sultan AH, Kamm MA, Bartram CI, Hudson CN. Anal sphincter trauma during instrumental delivery. *Int J Gynaecol Obstet* 1993;43:263–70.

51. Sultan AH, Johannson RB, Carter JE. Occult anal sphincter trauma following randomised forceps and vacuum delivery. *Int J Gynaecol Obstet* 1998;61:113–19.

52. Johanson RB, Rice C, Doyle M, Arthur J, Anyanwu L, Ibrahim J, *et al.* A randomised prospective study comparing the new vacuum extractor policy with forceps delivery. *Br J Obstet Gynaecol* 1993;100:524–30.

53. Williams MC, Knuppel RA, O'Brien WF, Weiss A, Kanarek KS. A randomised comparison of assisted vaginal delivery by obstetric forceps and polyethylene vacuum cup. *Obstet Gynecol* 1991;78:789–94.

54. Fitzpatrick M, Behan M, O'Connell PR, O'Herlihy C. Randomised clinical trial to assess anal sphincter function following forceps or vacuum delivery. *BJOG* 2003;110:424–9.

55. Johanson RB, Heycock E, Carter J, Sultan AH, Walklate K, Jones PW. Maternal and child health after assisted vaginal delivery: five-year follow up of a randomised controlled study comparing forceps and ventouse. *Br J Obstet Gynaecol* 1999;106:544–9.

56. Johanson RB, Menon BK. Vacuum extraction versus forceps for assisted vaginal delivery. *Cochrane Database Syst Rev* 2000;(2):CD00024.

57. Sultan AH, Stanton SL. Preserving the pelvic floor and perineum during childbirth – elective caesarean section? *Br J Obstet Gynaecol* 1996;103:731–4.

58. Bewley S, Cockburn J. The unfacts of 'request' caesarean section. *BJOG* 2002;109:597–605.

59. Connolly AM, Thorp JM Jr. Childbirth related perineal trauma: clinical significance and prevention. *Clin Obstet Gynecol* 42;4:820–35.

60. Kegel AH. Progressive resistance exercise in the functional restoration of the perineal muscles. *Am J Obstet Gynecol* 1948;56:238–48.

61. Dougherty M, Bishop K, Mooney R, Gimotty P, Williams B. Graded pelvic muscle exercise. Effect on stress urinary incontinence. *J Reprod Med* 1993;39:684–91.

62. Burns PA, Pranikoff K, Nochajski TH, Hadley EC, Levy KJ, Ory MG. A comparison of effectiveness of biofeedback and pelvic muscle exercise treatment of stress incontinence in older community-dwelling women. *J Gerontol* 1993;48:M167–74.

63. Thorp JM, Stephenson H, Jones LH, Cooper G. Pelvic floor (Kegel) exercises – a pilot study in nulliparous women. *Int Urogynecol J* 1994;5:86–9.

64. Royal College of Obstetricians and Gynaecologists. *Management of Third and Fourth Degree Tears Following Vaginal Delivery*. Guideline no. 29. London: RCOG Press; 2002.

65. Parks AG, McPartlin JF. Late repair of injuries of the anal sphincter. *Proc R Soc Med* 1971;64:1187–9.

66. Fitzpatrick M, Behan M, O'Connell PR, O'Herlihy C. A randomised clinical trial comparing primary overlap with approximation repair of third-degree obstetric tears. *Am J Obstet Gynecol* 2000;183:1220–4.

67. Fitzpatrick M, O'Herlihy C. Postpartum anal sphincter dysfunction. *Curr Obstet Gynaecol* 1999;9:210–15.

68. Read M, Read NW, Barber DC, Duthrie H. The effect of loperamide on anal sphincter function in patients complaining of chronic diarrhoea with faecal incontinence. *Dig Dis Sci* 1982;27:807–14.

69. Fynes MM, Marshall K, Cassidy M, Behan M, Walsh D, O'Connell PR, *et al.* A prospective, randomised study comparing the effect of augmented biofeedback with sensory biofeedback alone and on fecal incontinence after obstetric trauma. *Dis Colon Rectum* 1999;42:753–8.

70. Fynes M, O'Herlihy C, O'Connell PR. Childbirth and pelvic floor injury. In: Pemberton JH, Swash M, Henry MM, editors. *The Pelvic Floor*. London: Saunders; 2002. p. 46–59.

71. Oliviera L, Pfeifer J, Wexner SD. Physiological and clinical outcome of anterior sphincteroplasty. *Br J Surg* 1996;83:502–5.

72.   Malouf AJ, Norton CS, Engel AF, Nicholls RJ, Kamm MA. Long-term results of overlapping anterior anal-sphincter repair for obstetric trauma. *Lancet* 2000;355:260–5.

73.   Vaizey CJ, Kamm MA, Nichols RJ. Recent advances in the surgical treatment of faecal incontinence. *Br J Surg* 1998;85:596–603.

74.   Kenefick NJ, Vaisey CJ, Malouf AJ, Norton CS, Marshall M, Kamm MA. Injectable silicone biomaterial for faecal incontinence due to internal anal sphincter dysfunction. *Gut* 2002;51:225–8.

75.   Peleg D, Kennedy CM, Merrill D, Zlatnik FJ. Risk of repetition of a severe perineal laceration. *Obstet Gynecol* 1999;93:1021–4.

76.   Payne TN, Carey JC, Rayburn WF. Prior third- and fourth-degree perineal tears and recurrence risks. *Int J Gynecol Obstet* 1999;64:55–7.

77.   Hawkin R, Fitzpatrick M, O'Connell PR, O'Herlihy C. Anal sphincter disruption at vaginal delivery is recurrence predictable? *Eur J Obstet Gynecol Reprod Biol* 2003;15:149–52.

14

Complementary medicine in obstetrics and gynaecology

Zita West

INTRODUCTION

We should perhaps start by considering the aims of medicine, both complementary and traditional. For me, it is simple: it is about health, not illness. If there is illness, then it is about healing, and healing is the vocation of the healer. We can then consider what we mean by complementary medicine. In this context, 'complementary' is applied to a therapy that adds to techniques for achieving wellbeing and health. 'Alternative medicine' is an inappropriate term because complementary techniques are used in combination with others, not instead of them. The complementary approach is not just about different techniques and systems of treatment. It includes anything relevant to health and wellbeing, such as nutrition, lifestyle and mental state.

There is a popular perception of medicine as primarily a specialist, technical science. I take from medical science what I need to advance a person's health, and add to that a range of techniques and observations from complementary fields. Above all, I look and listen: the person to person interrelationship between practitioner and client gives me the most reliable affirmation of a person's particular needs.

This is one of the strongest aspects of complementary medicine in general. Most techniques, deriving from prescientific cultures, relied on the power of incisive observation. The people who discovered them did not have at their disposal analytical methods based on technology or anatomical dissection to inform their diagnoses. They were forced to use approaches that involved making associations between all aspects of a person's condition, and matching them to the experience of generations. There is much value in this empirical approach, and it surely parallels the pioneering work of early Western medical practice.

Complementary practice requires close engagement with the client. There is much less scope for a detached approach that views the sick person as the unfortunate owner of a faulty mechanism that may or may not be repaired by surgery or pharmaceuticals. Since it is time consuming, it is interesting to consider what the effects of spending that time are. It is morale boosting, supportive and educative. In addition, it helps the woman to understand her condition and to manage it. All of these positive influences place her in a better position to enhance her body's own remarkable healing abilities.

The positiveness of this approach to health and illness is reflected in the business arrangement that ancient Chinese doctors would have with their patients. The principle was that the doctor should keep the person healthy, and the patient would visit him at the change of each season for advice and treatment if necessary. Payment would be made for this service but, if illness occurred, the payment ceased until recovery took place. There was no question of waiting for the illness to occur and then paying for specialised cures. These Chinese doctors were the first to apply preventive medicine.

Of all the human conditions that doctors experience, this positive approach to a person's health is most obviously appropriate to pregnancy. Pregnancy itself is not an illness, although for some women the stress it causes can lead to illness. Healthy women are more likely than unhealthy women to have successful pregnancies, so much of the work is concerned with comparing women's health prior to and during pregnancy. The role of the obstetrician is to look after women who are considered at high risk and Western medicine is excellently equipped to do this.

Personal experience has kindled the desire to promote health and wellbeing for pregnant women generally. Since so many women find minor ailments extremely distressing, the debilitation caused by constant minor assaults may affect physical, emotional and mental health. This increases the likelihood of postnatal depression.

The condition of pregnancy is different from illness because, as almost all pregnant women are aware, drug treatments, which might otherwise be used safely to quell symptoms, are contraindicated. Even the sceptical have resorted to complementary treatments in desperation, and found that many of them work. The different approaches of complementary medicine to analysis and diagnosis offer solutions where conventional medical techniques fail or are unavailable. Acupuncture is particularly effective in this area.

Studies are beginning to show statistically that acupuncture and other techniques offer measurable benefits. Much more research needs to be done to understand the mechanisms of the effects that are observed. The fact that these techniques can offer relief to common ailments of pregnancy at least challenges conventional and popular wisdom that women just have to put up with these problems. To the acupuncturist the discomfort indicates some kind of imbalance in the body's systems; this must be investigated, not tolerated. It is the case that medical research is uncovering a range of small factors (nutritional and hormonal, for example) that can define what some of these imbalances are.

ACUPUNCTURE

Philosophy

Acupuncture is a system of healing that has been known for at least 4000 years. During that time an enormous body of experience has grown up, establishing tried and tested treatments for every aspect of human mental, emotional and physical health. One of the main barriers that the discipline presents to Western medical practitioners is the language and terminology, which expresses well the philosophical and physiological basis of acupuncture but may sound fanciful and unscientific. On the other hand, what could be more descriptive than 'palace of weariness' or 'door of infants', the names the Chinese give to acupuncture points treating fatigue and fertility problems respectively?

The principles of acupuncture (and other related oriental techniques such as shiatsu) are founded in Chinese philosophy. At its heart is the goal of balance and harmony, manifesting itself in, for example, good health. The concept of 'yin' and 'yang' is now familiar in the West to define opposing and complementary qualities: yin signifies cold, damp, dark and passivity, while yang is heat, dryness, light and activity. The universal nature of Chinese philosophy extends such concepts to all aspects of our environment: nature, human relationships, health, and so on. It is embodied in the concept of resonance between people, objects and the world in which they exist, with parallels in the seasons, colours, odours, emotions and substances of which things are made. The same idea of resonance attuned Chinese practitioners to links and associations between different areas and systems of the body and their effects on the state of a person's health.

Although yin and yang may be relatively familiar, the concept of '*qi*' (pronounced 'chee') is less so. *Qi* is energy, a life force, and is fundamental to all living things. The ancient Chinese saw its behaviour in terms of flow. It should perhaps be an easier concept for us to understand, now that we can appreciate unseen forces such as electricity and magnetism, but it is misleading to see it as either of those things. Health is determined by the flow of *qi*. Disruption in its flow, due to imbalances of yin and yang, will create illness. The principle of treatment is to restore balance, having identified the causes of the imbalance.

Techniques and approach

In defining the way that qi flows through the body, the Chinese identified 12 channels, known as meridians, plus two further channels. They observed that stimulating points on the channels had effects on the body's systems, and indeed that certain meridians could be related to particular systems. This phenomenon is in keeping with the concept of resonance. The names of most of the meridians reflect the main organs of the body system with which they are associated (e.g. heart, stomach, lung, spleen, liver, kidney), but there are others, such as 'triple burner' (which relates to the body's control systems) that remind us that we are dealing not with organs but with systems and the relationships between body functions. Of particular significance to obstetrics and gynaecology is the channel known as the 'conception vessel', which runs up the middle of the body and relates to the regulation of the menstrual cycle and fertility. Figure 1 is a diagrammatic representation of the meridian system of the body, showing acupuncture points that should not be used in pregnancy.

As in any system of medicine, the key in complementary practice is thorough diagnosis. For the acupuncturist this entails close observation of the person's appearance, colour, voice and odour. At the first appointment, a full case history is taken; a session may last up to 90 minutes. Everything about that person is relevant (age, lifestyle, emotional and physical traits), not just the condition that the individual has come to have treated. All body systems are taken into account (appetite, digestion, bowel movements, sleep, energy levels), plus emotional issues (relationships, stress, worries). This gives a full picture of the person and treatment can be specifically tailored to suit.

The tongue can be a useful indicator by taking note of its colour, shape, coating, etc. Such techniques should not, in principle, appear strange to the practitioner of Western medicine; this is everyday practice for many doctors. The tongue is a pillar of diagnosis and treatment planning; it is, for example, a good indicator of excessive heat and cold in the body's systems, to which pregnancy is particularly sensitive.

A further diagnostic procedure for the acupuncturist is the taking of pulses. It is not only the pulse rate that is recorded, but also its quality and strength. The character of the pulse varies with different positions on the wrist. On each wrist there are three pairs of pulses, relating to the 12 meridians. Comparisons between them give an indication of the balance of the body systems. With experience, pulses can give very specific information.

Since a traditional Chinese diagnosis can often be more specific about a problem than a Western diagnosis, it can often be matched by a more specific treatment plan. In morning sickness, for example, frequently dismissed as 'par for the course', Chinese diagnosis looks closely at the particular characteristics of the sickness in an individual in the search for a remedy. The time of day and associated symptoms will be related to imbalances in particular body systems. Sickness accompanied by the bringing up of bile may suggest liver disharmony; sickness without bile may suggest stomach disharmony. In each case different acupuncture points would be used to alleviate the sickness.

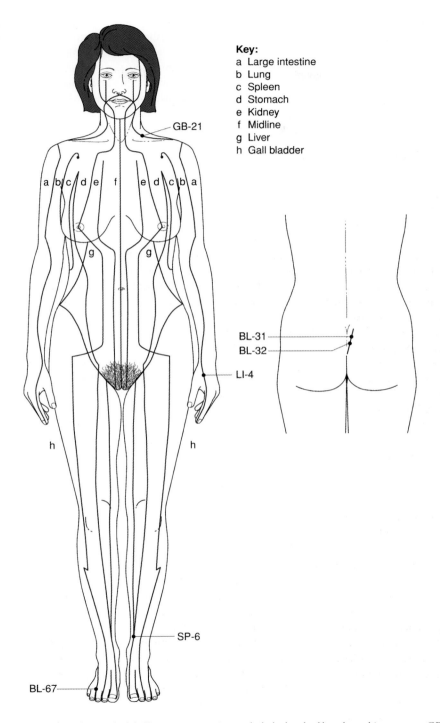

Key:
a Large intestine
b Lung
c Spleen
d Stomach
e Kidney
f Midline
g Liver
h Gall bladder

GB-21

a b c d e f e d c b a

g   g

BL-31
BL-32

LI-4

h   h

SP-6

BL-67

Figure 1 *The meridian system, showing the forbidden acupuncture points on the body that should not be used in pregnancy: GB21 = gallbladder 21; LI4 = large intestine 4; SP6 = spleen 6; BL67 = bladder 67 (reproduced from: West Z. Acupuncture in Pregnancy and Childbirth. Amsterdam: Elsevier; 2000. p. 000,[16] with permission from the publisher)*

The essence of treatment by acupuncture and associated complementary therapies is the stimulation of the meridians at key points to rebalance the body systems they represent and the flow of qi. Acupuncture needling is a precise and very controllable technique, allowing variation in depth, movement and duration. More general stimulation can be given by the application of heat and pressure. A technique used by many acupuncturists to provide local heat is the burning of moxa, a Chinese herb rolled into cigar-like sticks, which smoulder when lit to emit a steady, gentle heat. Needling can be enhanced by electrical stimulus – electro-acupuncture – not to be confused with methods of pain relief such as transcutaneous electrical nerve stimulation, which do not necessarily use acupuncture principles.

The process of treatment is rather like adjusting any kind of system: balancing, testing and rebalancing. In order to approach the underlying causes of the disorder, this process normally goes on through a series of treatments over a period of weeks. Throughout a pregnancy this coincides with fetal development and the changing demands on the mother. Consequently, the flexibility of diagnosis and treatment offered by acupuncture is particularly valuable. At the same time, the common ailments of pregnancy require immediate relief, and acupuncture can be used effectively to target and allay even severe symptoms. It may be used on the maternity ward to treat hyperemesis in conjunction with more usual hospital therapies.

ACUPUNCTURE IN PREGNANCY

The NHS acupuncture clinic for pregnant women at Warwick Hospital was set up as an extension to routine practice in 1993.[1] Women came from all walks of life, but they shared concerns that acupuncture was able to address, in particular the issue of taking drugs during pregnancy to alleviate simple ailments. They perceived other advantages, especially that treatments were orientated towards them personally (rather than the abstract notion of their symptoms) during a time of anxiety. They could talk though their fears with practitioners, and found it comforting that acupuncture provided a continuing basis for management of their pregnancy through to the birth and postnatally.

On the other hand there was scepticism. A common question was: 'Do I have to believe in acupuncture for it to work?' as if an act of faith was involved. Although there is a psychological dimension to a person's capacity to heal, there is a growing body of research and evidence that demonstrates the efficacy of acupuncture. The other major handicap to the use of acupuncture in pregnancy is its availability. The benefit of the clinic at Warwick is that acupuncture and the hospital's facilities are available side by side, each system working to its strengths with the other. This truly complementary way of working with different medical traditions provides women with the best of all worlds, by being mutually effective and mutually respectful.

Acupuncture and other complementary therapies can be effective for the whole range of ailments and conditions seen in pregnancy, which can be placed in four main groups: minor ailments, serious obstetric conditions, labour and birth, and postnatal treatments.

Minor ailments

Most women come for their first visit with a discomfort that may or may not indicate a more serious or complex problem. Acupuncture can be used to treat morning sickness, carpal tunnel syndrome, headaches, migraine, backache, sciatica, sinus discomfort, varicose veins, haemorrhoids and heartburn.[2] Some ailments respond better than others. The principles of Chinese diagnosis are applied to establish treatments on the indicated acupuncture channels, aiming at the underlying cause and not just the presenting symptoms. There are reports that treatments are very effective, but until focused research is carried out they must be considered anecdotal.

Serious obstetric conditions

Although a complementary consultation may identify an issue in advance of a conventional diagnosis, it may not be appropriate to follow a complementary treatment for more serious obstetric problems. In the second category of pregnancy related conditions that complementary medicine can help (i.e. more serious conditions such as hypertension), complementary therapy must be given alongside Western medicine. Practitioners should always keep general practitioners and hospital staff informed of their findings to allow standard interventions to be implemented as required. If a condition does not respond, this may suggest a more significant cause. Backache may be indication of a urinary tract infection or the start of a premature labour, and headache may be a sign of pre-eclampsia.

Labour and birth

The third area of pregnancy in which acupuncture and other complementary practices can make a contribution is the management of labour and birth. The use of electro-acupuncture to achieve pain relief in labour is now well documented. A study by Martoudis and Christofides[3] of 166 women in the first and second stages of labour showed beneficial effects in 86%. Other studies have shown that acupuncture can reduce the need for other methods of analgesia in childbirth.

Excellent results can be achieved in restimulating and maintaining contractions in labour. The points used relate in Chinese terms to the sacral plexus (bladder 31 bladder 32) and are also useful for induction. These can thus contribute to a shorter labour and appear to help with dilatation and softening of the cervix.[4,5] Some research has been done to back up this observation.[5]

Pain relief treatment,[6] especially using auricular points, both diminish discomfort and help to control anxiety and distress. The points used include 'Shenmen', which is also used in other treatments for relaxation and stress relief. Its effectiveness may be associated with endorphin release. With the use of acupuncture, the frequency of epidural analgesia use has been greatly reduced.

An area of obstetric treatment that has recently attracted much interest has been the turning of breech presentation.[7] Traditionally, heat is applied to stimulation acupuncture points related to the bladder meridian by using moxa sticks (moxibustion). The sticks are used bilaterally, close to the acupuncture points on the outside edge of the little toes. Almost all recipients report an increase in fetal movement and trials have shown that this treatment can work. It is important to apply the technique gradually over a number of treatments until cephalic version is achieved. The woman can easily be instructed to carry it out herself with the help of a partner.

The Co-operative Research Group on Moxibustion[8] reported that 1841 of 2041 women with a breech presentation had spontaneous cephalic version with this treatment. The success rate in the 880 women who were given the treatment after 34 weeks of gestation was 84.6%. Eighty-six percent of the versions were achieved after one to four applications of moxibustion and the remaining 14% after five to ten applications. There was no significant difference in the rates of success between primigravidae and multigravidae. The rate of version was higher in women with average tension of the abdominal wall than in those with high or low tension.[8] It is still unknown what mechanism is at work, but it is suggested that moxibustion is associated with increased adrenocortical activity,[3] oestriol production in the placenta and the ratio of prostaglandin $F_{2\alpha}$ to prostaglandin E_2. These changes would raise uterine basal tone and increase contractility, consequently stimulating fetal movement.

Postnatal treatments

The fourth main grouping of treatments in pregnancy and childbirth is for ailments occurring in the postnatal period. Typically, a mother is expected to recover during the six-week puerperium period, at the end of which she will undergo a physical check. However, many women have difficulties for four to six months, or longer, after giving birth, which can be a significant shock to a new mother's system and can affect every part of her life.

There are many common ailments that complementary medicine can help to alleviate, including poor lactation, perineal pain and dyspareunia. Basic assistance in recovery is available, which should include advice on good nutrition. Many traditional programmes of recovery concentrate on remedies that warm the mother, sometimes referred to in oriental cultures as 'mother roasting'! Moxa and acupuncture treatments that enhance heat in the mother's system can be effective and tend to focus on the blood system after childbirth.

Complementary medicine can contribute greatly to the wellbeing of the new mother; the one to one contact of practitioner and woman is a key aspect of treatments at this stage. The clearest benefits are perhaps in connection with postnatal depression. Nevertheless, acupuncture treatments reflect Chinese viewpoints that such emotional problems are bound up with physical issues, and that severe demands on the blood system, for example, are very likely to create imbalances, which treatments aim to correct. There is increasing recognition that depletion of elemental nutrients in a new mother's system will affect hormonal balance and wellbeing on an emotional and physical level.

USE OF OTHER COMPLEMENTARY THERAPIES IN PREGNANCY

So far, this chapter has concentrated on the use acupuncture in pregnancy, although other techniques that follow similar principles are available. Those most commonly used in maternity units are aromatherapy and reflexology because these are most accessible to midwives in terms of training and facilities. Homeopathy, chiropractic and osteopathy are also available.

An antenatal reflexology clinic for treating similar conditions to acupuncture has been set up at the University of Greenwich. This deals with morning sickness and other common ailments and may allow observation of changes in women that typically presage significant developments in their pregnancy. For example, changes in sensitivities of pituitary zones on women's feet[9] are a very good indicator that the onset of labour will occur within a few days. Stimulation of the same area can induce labour contractions.

A study at Oxford Brooks University[10] in conjunction with the John Radcliffe Hospital on the use of aromatherapy during childbirth and labour demonstrated a positive impact on practice and outcomes in the environment of a busy delivery suite. In a sample of 8059 mothers, measurable benefits were a reduction in anxiety and fear, the alleviation of pain and vomiting, an improvement in the strength and regularity of contractions, and an enhancement of maternal wellbeing. The majority (61%) chose aromatherapy to help them to alleviate fear and 50% of these found it helpful. Only 7% chose it for pain relief, but 61% of these found it helpful (12% not helpful).

FERTILITY

The all-embracing philosophy of balance and harmony that is the foundation of most established complementary medicine applies perfectly to the subject of fertility. Prepregnancy and pregnancy states should be seen as a continuum, not as opposites.

The increase in problems of fertility is due to many factors, including environmental and nutritional problems, stressful lifestyles and, often, choices to leave pregnancy until relatively late in life. Such a broad spectrum of issues has to be addressed by a very wide range of medical tools, from very easily manageable changes in personal lifestyle to the most advanced assisted fertility techniques. Complementary medicine has a major part to play in its own right, particularly in helping women to cultivate and maintain optimum health conditions.

Nutritional advice is important. Optimum nutrition may not be widely regarded as a complementary medicine, but it is certainly essential to complement the medical attention that a woman seeking to become pregnant will receive. An alternative lifestyle, excluding alcohol, tobacco, caffeine, processed food, etc. and promoting natural organic products may be advised. Pregnancy is arguably a 15-month commitment: three months to prepare, nine months' pregnancy, and three months to recover. In particular, research published in 1989 on the importance of essential fatty acids including docosahexaenoic acid[11] has shown how building up reserves can benefit fetal development during key growth spurts.

Treatment patterns for fertility

Treatment patterns tend to reflect the strong views that ancient Chinese physicians had about fertility. They placed great importance on the blood and the obvious balances and resonances that a regular menstrual cycle suggests. One of the acupuncture channels, the 'conception vessel', is named for self-evident reasons and it has acupuncture points with evocative names such as 'door of infants', 'sea of qi' and 'gate of life'. The kidney meridian is also of great significance. It represents not just the organ but the whole genitourinary system. Heat is the key concept. The Chinese considered that growth could not take place in a cold yin environment and that it was vital to foster warmth in the lower abdominal region to achieve pregnancy; hence the term 'cold womb'.

Treatments may aim initially at regulating the woman's cycle.[12] Depending on the underlying problem, different points can deal with heavy blood loss, oligomenorrhoea, post-pill amenorrhoea, and other conditions that indicate an imbalance in the cycle. Almost invariably there are kidney deficiencies and disharmonies that require rebalancing. This kind of kidney function declines with age, which is another reason why older women find it hard to become pregnant.

Weekly treatments are usually required for the first month, to achieve a better balance of the woman's systems. This may then decrease to monthly, depending on the problem to be treated. For example, for a woman with a shortened cycle, the treatment will take place in the luteal phase; for high follicle-stimulating hormone levels, different times in the latter part of the cycle are used.

Heat is such a key issue, so moxibustion is usually employed. Auricular acupuncture also seems to be particularly effective for fertility problems. Although the techniques originated in China,[13] they have really been redeveloped in Europe, especially in France and Germany. The ancient Egyptians even used earrings to treat fertility problems.

In vitro fertilisation

Increasing numbers of women who are undergoing or considering *in vitro* fertilisation undergo acupuncture. Again, complementary medicine, and acupuncture in particular, is valuable in boosting the body's natural functions to support the process of *in vitro* fertilisation.[14] Research results are beginning to reveal some statistical benefits for pregnancy outcomes from treatments both before and after egg transfer. Studies have also indicated benefits from acupuncture in improving pelvic blood flow, which could be linked to better follicle production. The measurement of blood flow impedance in the uterine arteries has shown that a pulsatility index

≥ 3.0 at the time of transfer could predict 35% of pregnancy failures.[15] The same US study, published in 1996, showed that electro-acupuncture was able to reduce high artery blood flow impedance in 10 infertile healthy women.

CONCLUSION

The aim of complementary medicine is to promote good health. Despite regard for the scientific rigour on which current Western medical practice is based, it is not necessarily providing all the answers, especially to the everyday issues of managing, helping and comforting patients. Complementary medicine can fill some of the gaps because of its different approaches rather than its different techniques.

A major recent landmark for those who wish to see better mutual understanding and 'complementarity' between different medical approaches, has been the House of Lords Report on Complementary and Alternative Medicine, produced by the Select Committee for Science and Technology in December 2000. A key recommendation was that there should be more research into complementary and alternative medicine. Complementary practitioners welcomed this proposal, although there is still some resistance from those with traditional beliefs. Although the Select Committee ranked acupuncture as a first grade treatment, traditional Chinese medicine, which underpins philosophically all that acupuncture achieves, was rated as third grade. This could suggest that the Committee may have been swayed more by easily measurable criteria that can duplicate conventional medical results than by a deeper understanding of different medical approaches.

Part of the problem is the unfamiliarity of terms and attitudes in complementary medical fields that require traditional terminology. Thus, when describing Chinese understanding of diagnosis and analysis in this chapter, wording such as 'associated with' and 'related to', rather than 'causes' or 'due to', are used because they better represent the holistic approach of the Chinese system.[17] With more research it may become possible to make more categorical statements as preferred by the western scientific process and pronounce that a particular treatment causes a particular effect, or that certain effects are due to a particular physical process.

For clients and practitioners, a major attraction of complementary medicine is that it is mostly founded in a philosophy that remains evident in its everyday practice. This was true in the West; what better understanding is there of the human condition than through the analysis and examination of the body's workings and dysfunctions? Some doctors still swear to observe the principles set out by the philosopher Hippocrates. Much of our basic understanding in medical and other science has come from observation of the natural world, the noting of coincidences and relationships, the postulation of connective theories, and the testing and examination of ideas. We need to extend the same approach to observations and relationships already noted by complementary medicine to provide it with the research it deserves. Complementary practitioners, as the House of Lords recommends, should have a clear understanding of the principles of evidence based medicine and health care. These are the things that complementary and alternative medicine should take from conventional practice.

Acupuncture and other complementary medicine modalities are becoming more readily available in maternity units. Their use alongside traditional hospital practice in treating pregnant and postnatal women is invaluable. For many years, obstetricians and midwives have felt frustration at not being able to offer women relief for the minor ailments of pregnancy. It is now time to start implementing the use of acupuncture in maternity units.

References

1. West Z. Acupuncture within the National Health Service: a personal perspective. *Complement Ther Nurs Midwifery* 1997;3:83–6.

2. Beal MW. Acupuncture and related treatment modalities. Part II: Applications to antepartal and intrapartal care. *J Nurs Midwifery* 1992;37:260–8.

3. Martoudis SG, Christofides K. Electro-acupuncture for pain relief in labour. *Acupunct Med* 1990;8:851–3.

4. Tsuei JJ, Lai YF. Induction of labor by acupuncture and electrical stimulation. *Obstet Gynecol* 1974;43:337–42.

5. Tremeau ML, Fontaine-Ravier P, Teurnier F, Demouzon J. [Protocol of cervical maturation by acupuncture.] *J Gynecol Obstet Biol Reprod (Paris)* 1992;21:375–80 (Fre).

6. Ternov K, NilssonM, Lofberg L, Algotsson L, Akeson J. Acupuncture for pain relief during labour *Acupunct Electrother Res* 1998;23:19–26.

7. Cardini F, Marcolongo A. Moxibustion for correction of breech presentation; a clinical study with retrospective control. *Am J Chin Med* 1993;21:133–8.

8. Cardini F, Weixin H. Moxibustion for correction of breech presentation; a randomised controlled trial. *JAMA* 1998;280:1580–4.

9. Tiran D, Mack S. *Complementary therapies for pregnancy and childbirth.* London: Baillière Tindall, 2001.

10. Burns E, Blamey C Ersser SJ, Lloyd AJ, Barnetson L. *The Use of Aromatherapy in Interpartum Midwifery Practice.* Oxford: Oxford Centre for Health Care Research and Development; 1999.

11. Crawford MA, Doyle W, Drury P, Lennon P, Costeloe K, Leighfield M. n-6 and n-3 fatty acids during early human development. *J Intern Med Suppl* 1989;225:159–69.

12. Andersson S, Lundeberg T. Acupuncture – from empiricism to science: functional background to acupuncture effects in pain and disease. *Med Hypotheses* 1995;45:271–81.

13. Gerhard I, Postneek F. Auricular acupuncture in the treatment of female infertility. *Gynecol Endocrinol* 1992;6:171–81.

14. Paulus WE, Zhang M, Strehler E, El-Danasouri I, Sterzik K. Influence of acupuncture on the pregnancy rate in patients who undergo assisted reproduction therapy. *Fertil Steril* 2002;77:721–4.

15. Stener-Victorin E, Waldenstrom U, Andersson SA, Wikland M. Reduction of blood flow impedance in the uterine arteries of infertile women with electro-acupuncture. *Hum Reprod* 1996;11:1314–17.

16. West Z. *Acupuncture in Pregnancy and Childbirth.* London: Elsevier; 2000.

17. Maciocia G. *Foundations of Chinese Medicine.* London: Elsevier; 1989.

15

Anthropology of the menopause

Laurence Shaw

THE MENOPAUSE

The menopause is the date of the last menstruation. In Western society (both today and in the past few millennia) it occurs around the age of 51 years[1-3] and marks the end of the reproductive phase of a woman's life. In human females, this is characterised by a gradually declining fecundity;[4] the rate of decline increases with time. The hormonal picture is one of primary ovarian failure, a loss of fertility due to lack of oocytes. The store of primordial follicles becomes exhausted. With the absence of follicular development there is a dramatic reduction in the circulating oestrogen and progesterone and a resultant increase in the follicle-stimulating hormone and luteinising hormone. There is a measurable deterioration in quality of life after the menopause.[5] This, and suggestions that there is acceleration in the development of osteoporosis,[6] bowel cancer,[7] Alzheimer's disease,[8] adverse lipid profile,[9] *inter alia*, raise the question of why there could have been any advantage to this in our evolutionary development.

NATURAL LIFE EXPECTANCY

Anatomically modern *Homo sapiens* is said to have developed between 150 000 and 120 000 years ago.[10] Since that time, there have been many milestones with varying effect on our biology and evolutionary direction. Few would argue that, to take a profound example, the adoption of farming approximately 10 000 years ago altered survival skills from the previous hunter-gatherer cultures. Nevertheless it is observed that overall life expectancy is unlikely to have changed significantly as a result of agriculture.[11] Not until the 20th century has there been, as a result of social and scientific progress, a radical alteration in the age distribution in the industrialised world. Population pyramids, tables that show the distribution of age in the population, demonstrate that these changes are modern phenomena. Figure 1 allows comparison of industrialised with nonindustrialised nations and, for the USA, further compares the former with its own recent (half century) history. The observed increase in the proportion of the population living beyond 70 years, while being a source of financial anxiety for governments that provide some form of social security, is a clear demonstration that many more of us exceed the life expectancy of the more natural, less artificial environment of the nonindustrialised world. The pyramid of, say, Ethiopia, a country that is at the cradle of human origins, gives a more realistic appearance of the likely proportion of the premodern population that would have reached the menopause and beyond. It may, therefore, be proposed that menopause is merely a feature of a lifespan that has been increased by developments in the 20th century. This simple explanation, that we have a menopause because we now live longer, fails to address all the observed physiological phenomena, including the increasingly declining reproductive success throughout the female reproductive lifespan and the climacteric events before and after the menopause. If, after all, it were merely senescence, a part of ageing, then

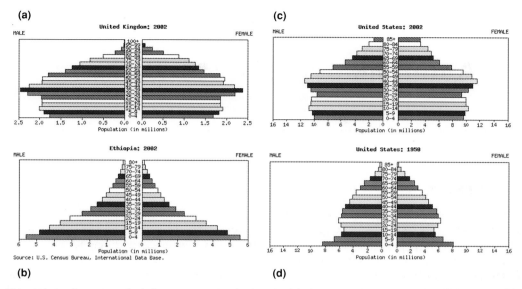

Figure 1 *Population pyramids: (a,b) note comparison of industrialised (UK 2002) with nonindustrialised (Ethiopia 2002) life expectancy; (c,d) note change in one industrialised country (USA) in the last half century (source: US Census Bureau, International Data Base)*

fertility and hormonal support would continue, albeit reducing gradually, until the end of our extended lives. The accelerated decline of the climacteric characterises the human female compared with other primates. Human males, by contrast, have the expected gradual reduction in both libido and fertility well into the post-20th century life extension.[12–15] For men, therefore, reproductive capacity declines in parallel with other body functions as a continuum of senescence. The question that needs to be addressed, then, is why women run out of oocytes but men have lifelong, albeit diminishing, sperm supplies. The first step in understanding this requires comparisons between human and other ape life and reproductive expectancies.

HOMO SAPIENS AS AN APE

Among the primates, it is the great apes (pongids) to whom we are most closely related. They consist of orang-utans (*Pongo*), gorillas (*Gorilla*), chimpanzees (*Pan troglodytes*) and bonobos (*Pan paniscus*). There is a remarkable similarity in the genomes of humans and all of these apes but there is more genetic similarity with *Pan* than any of the others.[16,17] Moreover, these are borne out as somatic similarities in terms of behaviour and appearance.[18]

Total life expectancy is a difficult concept to quantify reliably. Average lifespan, as a parameter, is distorted by infant mortalities, whereas maximum life span is unrepresentative. Moreover, it is important to make fair comparisons between humans and apes. Great apes in captivity live significantly longer than those in the wild; just as humans in industrialised countries have greater longevity than those in nonindustrialised countries. Nevertheless, none of the pongids demonstrate a post-reproductive phase (a menopause), so it is reasonably likely that this developed after our closest relatives, *Pan*, separated from what was to become *Homo*.

There are, around the world, hunter-gatherer societies who have persistently rejected inter-ference from outside. Examples of these still living close to their traditional ways are the Ache of

South America, and the !Kung and Hadza of Africa. Such groups live a nomadic life in small and highly mobile bands (10–100), comprising clusters of nuclear families, dependent on hunted animal and gathered plant foods. The cultures of these groups differ from each other in many respects and none may be representative of the habits of our hunter-gatherer ancestors, whose cultures also would surely have varied from place to place. However, studies on them do allow us to understand better some of the pressures that influenced our gene pool over what was the majority of human existence. Lifespan studies on these groups have suggested that average life expectancy at birth is only 33 years for Hadza, 38 for Ache, and 31 for !Kung. Nevertheless, on reaching maturity, the probability of surviving past 45 is surprisingly high (Hadza 0.71, Ache 0.79, and !Kung 0.66). Moreover, the proportion of adult females over 45 years is 29% in Hadza, 36% in Ache, and 31% in !Kung, so survival to maturity brings a significant chance of longevity. Indeed, individuals of 77 years among the Ache and 88 years among the !Kung have been observed.[19–21]

It is clear that longevity can be recorded in a number of ways. In order to compare the life expectancy of humans with pongids, similar parameters should be used. Verifiable life tables of pongids are not available because close work has not been achieved over long enough periods. However, studies of chimpanzees, gorillas and orang-utans have yielded some data that have been used to produce Figure 2 comparing differences in average lifespan between great apes and humans.[22] Figure 3, by contrast, compares oldest known individuals in protected environments;[23] that is, pongids in captivity and humans in industrialised countries. In both sets of data there appears to be a higher than expected longevity in humans compared with pongids. Furthermore, there is a well known mammalian trend associating body mass and longevity; humans lie above the expected longevity for their mass,[24] so, as apes, humans are characterised by late maturity and naturally enhanced longevity. However, the reproductive lifespan is not increased. This results in a post-reproductive phase. Even in hunter-gatherer societies up to a third of the adult female population lives long enough to experience this.

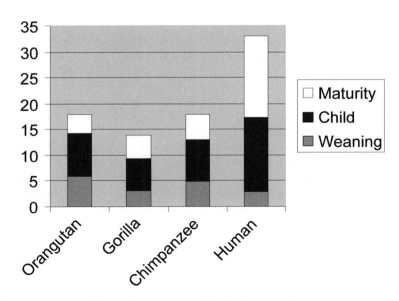

Figure 2 *Average lifespan – great apes and human (from data extracted form Hawkes et al. 1998[22])*

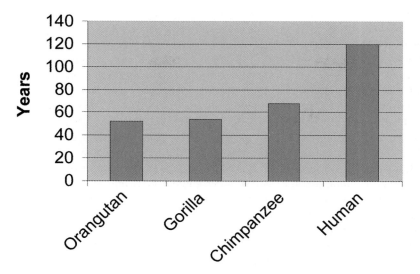

Figure 3 *Maximum longevity in protected environment (from data obtained from: C Furley, personal communication[23])*

Thus, we lived longer than pongids, even before the effects of the 20th century. Has there been evolutionary pressure on our ancestors that gave advantage to later maturity and greater longevity? Are these characteristics that evolved separately or could they be linked and perhaps be related to the uniqueness of a post-reproductive phase to *Homo sapiens*? What evolutionary pressures could have selected for this and when?

HUMAN ORIGINS

There is a public awareness of bipedal ape discoveries. The well known hominid, *Australopithecus afarensis*, attracted attention after the find of a virtually whole skeleton in 1974 in the Hadar Valley, Ethiopia. She was named 'Lucy' by Don Johanson's team as the camp tape recorder was repeatedly playing the Beatles' song 'Lucy in the Sky with Diamonds' out of exuberance on the evening of the day they found the first fossil. She was dated at 3.2 million years ago (Mya) and subsequent study has shown her to be a four-foot tall, largely frugivorous ape that perhaps also scavenged insects and remnants of carnivorous predators' kills.[25]

In 2002 there was much publicity over the discovery in Chad of the 6-million-year-old fossil skull of *Sahelanthropus tchadensis*, strongly suspected from the anatomy to have been bipedal.[26] Reasons for the evolution of bipedalism are not within the scope of this chapter. However, the commonly held misunderstanding that apes became intelligent, so decided to walk on their hind legs to free up limbs for other functions, is not borne out by the fossil evidence. The skull seen in Figure 4 (*Sahelanthropus tchadensis*) shows a small cranial cavity. Bipedal apes developed in different forms and study of their cranial size shows a gradual increase subsequent to the development of bipedal locomotion. This trend markedly increased over the past 2 million years.[27]

In general terms, one of the most profound drivers of evolutionary development is climatic change. Between 2 and 3 Mya there was a global cooling, which is markedly demonstrable in what is now the area of East Africa that includes the highlands of Kenya and Ethiopia.[28] The result was

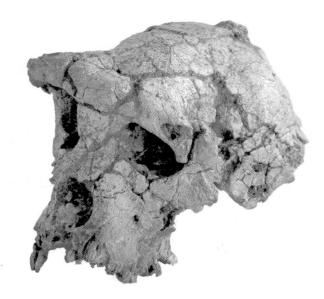

Figure 4 *Cranium of* Sahelanthropus tchadensis *(© MPFT (Mission Paléoanthropologique Franco Tchadienne (Professor Michel Brunet): scientific collaboration between University of Poitiers, University of N'Djamena and Centre National d'Appui à la Recherche)*

that the green plains of the rift valley slowly turned into dry savannah. The increasingly arid and seasonal climate favoured vegetation that stores its starches in tubers underground rather than on branches. Lucy's descendants in this time bracket, *Homo erectus*, found a largely vegetarian diet harder to sustain. At the same time the meat left by predators, who were also under pressure from the changing environment, might have been in shorter supply. Such were the drivers for *Homo erectus* to explore different food sources. These individuals would have been small and ineffectual predators; their bipedalism, an advantage millions of years earlier, now became a disadvantage as it made them slower in the chase than their quadruped rivals and prey such as the big cats and deer, respectively. Nevertheless erect posture still had the benefits of improved thermoregulation[29] and, perhaps, stamina.[30] It is at this stage when cranial size appears to have increased and coincided with the development by *Homo erectus* of hunting to supplement diet rather than merely relying on scavenging from carnivores. The evidence for this lies in the selection of game, as found in the refuse at *Homo erectus* settlements, and also the development of weaponry found at these sites.[31,32] *Homo* lacked the morphological specifications of a predatory carnivore (sharp teeth, claws) and turned to alternative strategies. The ability of *Homo erectus*, a small, slow, relatively weak mammal, to outwit prey compensated for the inability to outrun or simply overpower herbivores of considerably greater size and speed. Those that were 'fitter' in Darwinian terms[33] survived to reproduce. Although brain size may in itself be an important factor in outwitting prey, surely the ability to pass down skills from one generation to another would magnify that value? Those individuals who can spend more time with their parents will have enhanced their skills on reaching maturity. Their parents' longevity therefore has an advantage, as does a longer period of dependency as marked by a later puberty. This characteristic, while having a positive effect on 'fitness' in the way described also has a negative feature in terms of vulnerability to predation. The negative effects of this package of characteristics do not end there as can be seen in Figure 5. The

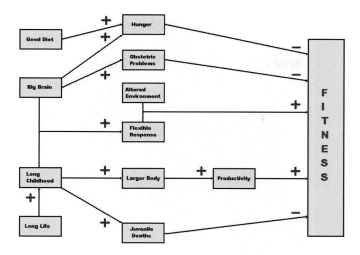

Figure 5 *The trade off: a compromise of adaptation*

larger cranial size produces inevitable obstetric pressures and further vulnerability of large headed babies. Moreover, brains of larger size, while contributing in adulthood to improved food provision, are, in childhood, demanding better quality nutrition for growth, so the means of obtaining food in these hard times, itself, has a cost in food. There are clearly trade offs that the evolutionary process equilibrates. However, the longer childhood allows for a larger body at maturity and a resultant increase in productivity, but primarily it enables more time to learn, allowing flexible responses, enhancing 'fitness' and therefore survival.

The longer lifespan and delayed onset of reproduction has a clear advantage to *Homo erectus* and his successor, who has an even larger brain, *Homo sapiens*. Natural selection may, therefore, have influenced our development to prolong our pre-reproductive time and lengthen our life expectancy. The question therefore remains about the declining reproductive capacity in females towards a post-reproductive life. What has in the past been the apparent advantage to this?

POST-REPRODUCTIVE LIFE

Much of the story so far has been hypothetical conjecture based on fossil evidence and primate behaviour patterns. Indeed, anthropological science is based much more on circumstantial evidence compared with that of medicine. This is not to say that palaeobiology is not methodologically rigorous in using scientific method in hypothesis driven research. Different facets of evidence from varying perspectives knit together to give strength to a hypothesis. In this case there is the hypothesis that longevity has a learning advantage for an organism that is investing in intelligence as a survival strategy. Studies of hunter-gatherer societies existing in isolation today help in the understanding of the complex trade off between the positive and negative characteristics contributing to an overall benefit to a post-reproductive life. Although it is accepted that these are marginalised populations and may not be typical of historic hunter-gatherer groups, there is much to be learnt from them about the behavioural trade offs.

I have already referred to the Hadza, a group of about 750 people living in the Eyasi basin of the rift valley in northern Tanzania. They are bound together by a common language unlike any other and live as hunter-gatherers in small groups of about 35–75. They attracted the particular attention of Kristen Hawkes, now the Professor of Anthropology at University of Utah. Hawkes' team lived with such a group of Hadzabe for seven seasons and kept activity diaries so that account could be taken of seasonal variation in activity. These diaries were collated by means of instantaneous camp scans and focal person follows, with a particular focus on time allocation, foraging and food sharing.

This work[34] observed relationships between foraging times and children's weight gain. A weaned toddler's nutritional welfare is demonstrably proportional to its mother's foraging times. Her effect on that welfare is reduced by the arrival of a new infant. Although there is a statistically significant reduction in the foraging times of the nursing mothers, there can be seen to be an association between the weaned children's weight and their grandmothers' foraging time, which, in turn, demonstrates an increase when their daughters are nursing a new infant. The endpoint of a positive effect on the children's weight is also demonstrated with a statistically significant relationship to the grandmothers' foraging efforts (Figure 6).

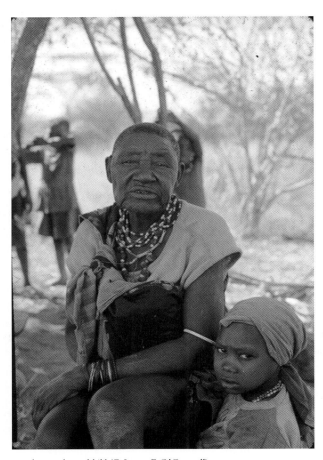

Figure 6 *Hazda woman and weaned grandchild* (© James F O'Connell)

Thus, covariant analyses have demonstrated that:

- A child's nutritional welfare is directly dependent on its mother's foraging time.

- The arrival of a newborn sibling reduces the mother's nutritional contribution to her weaned children.

- A woman's foraging time increases with her baby's age as he/she becomes less demanding.

- Grandmothers forage more with the arrival of a new grandchild.

- The weight of the weaned children of nursing mothers increases in relation to the increase in foraging time of their grandmothers.

Every Hadzabe woman who was observed nursing had an older, childless, related female helper. The amount of foraging support appeared to be mathematically related to kinship. Nevertheless, the weaned children can themselves contribute to their own welfare in some seasons when, for example, easily harvested berries are available; they are less capable in other seasons when only deeply buried tubers are available. The older women therefore support their grandchildren by freeing their daughters to care for the subsequent baby.

No other primate demonstrates this characteristic of extending the mother–offspring sharing to the weaned but not yet mature individuals. There is also no other consistent support from older females in this way. In fact, in chimpanzees, offspring born to older females often fail to survive after their mother's death.[35] The female chimpanzee's fertility deteriorates synchronously with other ageing processes; she remains fertile to the end of her life. The price of this is the high infant mortality of those born to older females whose death precedes the independence of their last offspring. This 'somatic wastage' is the trade off enabling some, albeit a reduced number, of the offspring produced right through to the end of the female's life to survive.

The human grandmothering model is supported by the observation[36] that, in traditional Gambian population groups, women start reproducing earlier if their mother is still alive and that infant survival is significantly higher if the grandmother is still alive. By contrast, the relationship seen between foraging yields of Hadzabe women and the weight gains of their children and grandchildren are not demonstrated in the Ache, the South American group of hunter-gatherers mentioned earlier. They live in forests of eastern Paraguay and have also been studied extensively.[20] Like the Hadza, they live in nuclear families and grandmothers are seen to help, for example, with 'baby sitting'. Why is there not a demonstrable nutritional contribution as with the Hadza?

Hawkes et al.[37] have studied the Hadza men and their hunting habits. It seems that, while women forage almost exclusively for their families and offspring, the hunting men do not control the distribution of their prey. The families of good hunters receive no more than other families unless there has, unusually, been a big kill. Infant nutrition gained from the hunters is therefore relatively constant across the population. Moreover, Kaplan et al.[38] have compared nutritional provisioning sources of these and other hunter-gatherers and, indeed, compared them with chimpanzees. The Hadzabe diet is 52% foraged, 48% hunted, whereas the Ache is 25% foraged, 75% hunted. The Ache men share the food they obtain with all. Again, for slightly different reasons, there is no preferential paternal provisioning. However, the proportion of meat and honey that the males provide is greater than in the Hadza. It may reasonably be surmised, then, that the larger communal contribution of the Ache men is merely concealing the differential effect of grandmother care on weight gain; the food provisioning by the women is a lesser proportion of the total infant nutrition. The smaller hunted complement of the Hadza diet has exposed the effects of the contribution of the women and their dynamics within the family.

The 'grandmother hypothesis' is far from unassailable. There is, after all, no direct evidence and certainly no prospective randomised controlled trials with which we are so familiar in medicine. However, the grandmother hypothesis seems at present to be the most robust theory to explain the post-reproductive life that characterises *Homo sapiens* among the primates.

DISCUSSION

It is clear that, even in premodern cultures, *Homo* has a greater longevity than would be expected by our morphology. Linked to this is the longer period of vulnerability prior to maturity. This is compounded by subsequent pregnancies and the arrival of new sucklings before the independence of the previous child. The nutritional and other help afforded by the older women to their grandchildren at these times enhances survival of their own gene contribution through their grandchildren. Superficially, the human trade off is that, grandmothers' fertility deteriorates at a rate faster than expected, resulting in a personal reduction in their late life pregnancies. This ensures a supply of older women with no current mothering responsibilities. The trade off has an added value, as the traded pregnancies would have been blighted with inherent age-related obstetric problems, not least maternal mortality. Early humans developing this particular trade off strategy might preferentially have survived in habitats that are marginal for pongids.[39] There is no doubt that infant mortality is a vulnerability[38] and that an adaptation that enhances survival to maturity would be of profound benefit, particularly in times of hardship. There are therefore two aspects to the adaptation. The first is the need for the longevity and the second is the accelerated decline in reproductive capability so as to free the surviving older women for foraging. Hawkes *et al.*[34] argue that the human fertile span is not greater or shorter than that expected when comparing with primates in general.

Although she argues that the primary adaptation is longevity, there is the matter of the fact that the menopause does not just arrive out of the blue. It is preceded by a progressive decline in fertility from the end of the second decade of life. The declining fertility and the tradition of elder kin support imbues advantage to progressively diminishing fecundity. This and longevity would ensure that the younger women have access to an adequate cohort of older women without infants of their own. We know there are hazards to long-term oestrogen deficiency and it is likely that the latter years of premodern life are characterised by paucity rather than a total absence of ovarian activity. The Family Planning Association in the UK, after all, advises that contraception should continue to be used until a woman has not had any menstrual loss for two years if aged under 50 years and for one year if over 50. This is because ovulation may occur during that time. The adaptation to fertility to enable grandmothering may therefore have a multiple mechanism, including declining frequency of ovulation, implantation rates and increased miscarriage rates related to nondysjunctional chromosomal errors. Although live birth is possible in these women's latter years, it is not likely, even in the face of ovulation and a possible fertilisation.

The herd 'post-reproductive life' may therefore be characterised by a time of rapidly declining personal reproductive potential rather than an abrupt menopause. Nevertheless, the declining ovulation rate does grind to a halt in a number of longer living individuals. Even among the Hazda and other similar groups, a small number of individuals survive through their seventh decade. As has been seen in Figure 1, the 20th century has seen a greater incidence and duration of this, so that there is an increase in the number of people surviving longer into the anovulatory post-reproductive phase. This demands that we address the enormous length of time that we now spend with no ovulatory activity at the end of our lives. Prior to the last century, the bulk of post-reproductive survivors would have endured this for a matter of only a few months or years, not for decades. Hence we are now vulnerable in the long term to the resultant protracted hormone deficiency and to the associated quality of life and disease implications. This results in discussion about hormone replacement.

The survival benefit from grandmothers is when their daughters are reproducing. The peak reproductive potential in human females is in the late teens and early twenties. Post-20th century society does not seem to encourage teenage pregnancy, so the adaptations that have served us well for millennia are now a source of conflict with 'modern life'.

Moreover, the current trend to delay the first pregnancy by a decade or more results in difficulties with conceiving. The success rate for treatment of couples with fertility problems is inversely proportional to their age, so, again, 20th century pressures are in conflict with our nature.

A greater understanding of why our bodies have developed certain characteristics enables us to address those characteristics in the 21st century, in which we live our lives with the evolutionary baggage of our past, men and women alike, foraging at supermarkets. Some of that baggage remains useful, but some requires new adaptation. Perhaps the development of safer hormone replacement agents, safer contraception and better fertility treatments will be the adaptations of the 21st century.

Acknowledgements

Thanks to Sarah Elton (Lecturer in Biological Anthropology, Eliot College, University of Kent at Canterbury) and Adam Balen (Consultant Gynaecologist, General Infirmary, Leeds) for reading the original manuscript.

References

1. Amundsen DW, Diers CJ. The age of the menopause in classical Greece and Rome. *Hum Biol* 1970;42:79–86.
2. World Health Organization. *Research on the menopause.* (WHO Technical Report Series, No. 670.) Geneva: WHO; 1981.
3. Gold EB, Bromberger J, Crawford S, Samuels S, Greendale GA, Harlow SD, *et al.* Factors associated with age at natural menopause in a multiethnic sample of midlife women. *Am J Epidemiol* 2001;153:865–74.
4. Schwartz D, Mayoux NJ. Female fecundity as a function of age: results of artificial insemination in 2193 nulliparous women with azospermic husbands. Federation CECOS. *N Engl J Med* 1982;306:404–6.
5. Limouzin-Lamothe MA, Mairon N, Joyce CR, Le Gal M. Quality of life after the menopause: influence of hormonal replacement therapy. *Am J Obstet Gynecol* 1994;170:618–24.
6. Hui SL, Slemenda CW, Johnston CC, Appledorn CR. Effects of age and menopause on vertebral bone density. *Bone Miner* 1987;2:141–6.
7. Rossouw JE, Anderson GL, Prentice RL, *et al.*, Writing Group for the Women's Health Initiative Investigators. Risks and benefits of estrogen plus progestin in healthy postmenopausal women: principal results from the Women's Health Initiative randomized controlled trial. *JAMA* 2002;288:321–3.
8. LeBlanc ES, Janowsky J, Chan BKS, Nelson HD. Hormone replacement therapy and cognition – systematic review and meta-analysis. *JAMA* 2001;285:1489–99.
9. Matthews KA, Meilahn E, Kuller LH, Kelsey SF, Caggiula AW, Wing RR. Menopause and risk factors for coronary heart disease *N Engl J Med* 1989;321:641–6.

10. Brauer G. Africa's place in the evolution of *Homo sapiens*. In: Brauer G, Smith FH, editors. *Continuity or Replacement: Controversies in* Homo sapiens *Evolution*. Rotterdam: Balkema; 1992. p. 83–98.

11. Cassidy CM. Nutrition and health in agriculturalists and hunter-gatherers: a case study of two prehistoric populations. In: Jerome NW, Kandel RF, Pelto GH, editors. *Nutritional Anthropology: Contemporary Approaches to Diet and Culture*. New York: Redgrave; 1980. p. 117–45.

12. Silber SJ. *The Male*. New York: Charles Scribner; 1981. p. 11–14, 66–9.

13. Johnson L, Petty CS, Neaves WB. Influence of age on sperm production and testicular weights in men. *J Reprod Fertil* 1984;70:211–18.

14. Johnson L. Spermatogenesis and aging in the human. *J Androl* 1986;7:331–54.

15. Seymour FL, Duffy C, Koerner A. A case of authenticated fertility in a man of 94. *JAMA* 1935;105:1423–4.

16. Jones S. *Almost Like a Whale: The Origin of Species Updated*. London: Transworld; 1999.

17. Gagneux P, Varki A. Genetic differences between humans and great apes. *Mol Phylogenet Evol* 2001;18:2–13.

18. Furuichi T. Social interactions and the life history of female *Pan paniscus* in Wamba, Zaire. *Int J Primatol* 1989;10:173–97.

19. Blurton Jones NG, Smith LC, O'Connell JF, Hawkes K, Kamuzora C. Demography of the Hadza, an increasing and high density population of savanna foragers. *Am J Phys Anthropol* 1992;89:159–81.

20. Hill K, Hurtado AM. *Ache Life History: the Ecology and Demography of a Foraging People*. New York: Aldine de Gruyter; 1996.

21. Howell N. *Demography of the Dobe !Kung*. New York: Academic Press; 1979.

22. Hawkes K, O'Connell JF, Jones NG, Alvarez H, Charnov EL. Grandmothering, menopause, and the evolution of human life histories. *Proc Natl Acad Sci U S A* 1998;95:1336–9.

23. C Furley, personal communication.

24. Charnov EL. *Life History Invariants: Some Explorations of Symmetry in Evolutionary Ecology*. Oxford: Oxford University Press; 1993.

25. Johanson DC, Edey MA. *Lucy – the Beginnings of Humankind*. London: Penguin; 1981. p. 22.

26. Brunet M, Guy F, Pilbeam D, Mackaye HT, Likius A, Ahounta D, *et al*. A new hominid from the Upper Miocene of Chad, Central Africa. *Nature* 2002;418:145–51.

27. Elton S, Bishop LC, Wood B. Comparative context of Plio-Pleistocene hominin brain evolution. *J Hum Evol* 2001;41:1–27.

28. de Menocal PB. Plio-Pleistocene African climate. *Science* 1995;270:53–9.

29. Wheeler PE. The thermoregulatory advantages of hominid bipedalism in open equatorial environments: the contribution of increased convective heat loss and cutaneous evaporative cooling. *J Hum Evol* 1991;21:107–15.

30. Ulijaszek SJ. *Human Energetics in Biological Anthropology*. Cambridge: Cambridge University Press; 1995.

31. Spoonheimer M, Lee-Thorp JA. Isotopic evidence for the diet of an early hominid, *Australopithecus africanus*. *Science* 1999;283:368–70.

32. Bunn HT, Kroll EM. Systematic butchery by Plio-Pleisticene hominids at Olduvai Gorge, Tanzania. *Curr Anthropol* 1986;5:431–52.

33. Darwin C. *On the Origin of Species by Means of Natural Selection or the Preservation of Favoured Races in the Struggle for Life*. London: John Murray; 1859.

34. Hawkes K, O'Connell JF, Blurton Jones NG. Hadza women's time allocation, offspring provisioning, and the evolution of long postmenopausal life spans. *Curr Anthropol* 1997;38:551–77.

35.   Goodall J. *The Chimpanzees of Gombe: Patterns of Behavior.* Cambridge, MA: Harvard University Press; 1986.

36.   Mace R. Evolutionary ecology of human life history. *Anim Behav* 2000;59:1–10.

37.   Hawkes K, O'Connell JF, Blurton Jones NG. Hunting and nuclear families – some lessons from the Hadza about men's work. *Curr Anthropol* 2001;42:681–709.

38.   Kaplan H, Hill K, Lancaster J, Hurtado AM. A theory of human life history evolution: diet, intelligence and longevity. *Evol Anthropol* 2000;9:156–85.

39.   Moore J. Savannah chimpanzees. In: Nishida T, McGrew W, Marler P, Pickford M, de Waal F, editors. *Topics in Primatology,* Vol. 1. *Human Origins.* Tokyo: University of Tokyo Press; 1992. p. 99–118.

16

Obstetric fistula in the 21st century

E Catherine Hamlin, Ambaye Woldemicheal, Mulu Muleta, Biruk Tafesse,
Hailegiorgis Aytenfesu and Andrew Browning

INTRODUCTION

Obstructed labour is a universal problem. Fortunately, in developed countries with good intrapartum care, the sequelae have long been forgotten. However, for the vast majority of the world's population, obstructed labour is a terrifying prospect. Many women, miles from any qualified medical help, labour for days, even sometimes over a week, with no pain relief, little help of any use and certainly no one who can expedite the delivery. After some days the unborn child dies and, in time, collapses, and the women expels a stillborn child. She will lie on the floor of her hut exhausted, frail and weak, hoping that the worst of it is over. Unfortunately, another misery is just beginning. Days of pressure exerted by the presenting part on the soft tissues around the bladder, vagina, pelvic bones, and sometimes the rectum as well, have resulted in ischaemic necrosis. Between three and ten days later,[1] these dead tissues come away in a mass of slough and the often young girl is left with devastating injuries, a vesicovaginal fistula (VVF). She will leak urine continually through this defect day and night. What often follows are stories more tragic for the woman than that of her long labour. She will be ashamed of her offensiveness, continually wet and malodorous. Her husband often abandons her, perhaps for fear of what has happened to her, but mainly because she can no longer perform the duties of a woman. She lives a wretched life of ostracism and misery.

This is not a problem of antiquity, although the first documentation of VVF is probably to be found on an Egyptian papyrus dating from 1550 BC.[2,3] However, it continues to be a major health issue in the 21st century and will surely be so for the foreseeable future. The first institution to deal with the problem was built by Dr James Marion Sims in 1855, the Women's Hospital on Madison Avenue, New York, where up to 270 women with fistula were treated in one year, with about 74% being totally cured.[2] The treatment of women with VVF has become an uncommon practice in the West owing to improvements in obstetric care. In contrast, in the developing world, facilities to manage these conditions are desperately needed; thus the second Fistula Hospital was opened in 1975 by Reginald and Catherine Hamlin in Addis Ababa, Ethiopia. This couple arrived in Ethiopia in 1959 on a three-year contract to start a midwifery school and have been there ever since, with Dr Catherine Hamlin continuing the work after the death of her husband in 1993. They first encountered the misery of these women in the government hospital where they were working and they devoted much time and energy to developing a way of restoring these women's health and dignity. Word spread that these women do have a hope of being cured and more and more women came to them, desperate for help. The numbers increased so much that it became evident that a separate institution would have to be built, and the Fistula Hospital was opened. It now operates on up to 1200 women a year, with a success rate for closure of VVF being 92%.

PATHOPHYSIOLOGY

By performing autopsies on women who had died from obstructed labour, Mafouz,[4] in 1929, estimated that 66% of VVFs were caused by cephalopelvic disproportion and 33% by malpresentation. Whatever the cause of obstructed labour, VVFs can best be described as 'field injuries'.[5] Pressure necrosis not only involves the tissues of the bladder, rectum and vagina but also the adjacent structures, the nerves, bony structures, blood vessels, muscles and soft tissues. The resultant injury also depends on the level at which the obstruction occurs. If it occurs at the pelvic brim, the uterus or the cervix can be involved, especially if the cervix is incompletely dilated, thus resulting in a uterovaginal or cervicovaginal fistula. If the cervix is fully dilated, then the anterior vaginal fornix can be impinged upon, resulting in a high VVF. The posterior vaginal wall can similarly be crushed against the sacrum, resulting an a high rectovaginal fistula.[6] The ureters traverse the lower part of the broad ligament, and extensive trauma also destroys the lower part of the ureters as they enter the bladder anteriorly to the cervix. They are left draining straight into the vagina some distance from the bladder edge. If the impaction occurs in the mid-vagina, the trigone is usually involved. The urethra may be pinched off by the presenting part, and the bladder, grossly distended, rises up into the abdomen, dragging the urethra and bladder neck with it. Large fistulas may involve the ureters, trigone, bladder neck and upper part of the urethra. The nerves of the inferior hypogastric plexus containing the greater part of the nerve supply to the bladder can be injured as they traverse the side of the rectum, uterine cervix, lateral vaginal fornix and posterior bladder,[7,8] resulting in nerve injury to the organ and a high proportion of voiding disorders post-repair.[9] If impaction occurs at the outlet, the whole urethra may be destroyed as well as the bladder neck and the trigone. The lower rectum can also sustain injury. In the worst cases, the vaginal mucosa has completely sloughed away, as has the bladder. Remnant bladder capacity of only 50 ml, or even less, making functional repair impossible, is seen quite often at the Addis Ababa Fistula Hospital. The rectum may also be affected so severely that there is complete detachment of the anus from the rectum. A temporary diverting colostomy is initially needed and later, an end-to-end anastomosis of the rectum to the anus has to be performed.

ASSOCIATED CONDITIONS

After the dead tissue has come away, tissue of dubious viability remains at the edge of the injured area. This results in scarring, which is sometimes so severe that there is complete closure of the vagina.

Conditions that are often seen in association with the fistula include bladder stones because the woman tries to drink less in an attempt to pass less but more concentrated urine. She may even insert a rag into the vagina and bladder and a stone forms around it. The upper ureter, renal pelvis and kidneys themselves can be damaged. Informally reviewing intravenous pyelograms carried out for complicated fistulas at the Addis Ababa Fistula Hospital revealed almost 100% upper renal tract damage, ranging from ureteric dilatation to gross hydronephrosis to nonfunctioning kidneys. Urine continually soiling the perineum results in an uncomfortable urinary dermatitis and sometimes secondary infection. Amenorrhoea is estimated to occur in 64.2% of these women after the first six months.[5] It is assumed that a number will have Asherman's syndrome as a consequence of urine contamination of the endometrium or repeated infection.[10] Amenorrhoea can also result from higher centre involvement owing to the social stresses that the woman sustains and anorexia. Some will have hypothalamic and pituitary dysfunction;[11] a few may have cervical stenosis or a vagina closed by scar tissue, resulting in severe and painful haematometra. Malnutrition, weakness and anaemia are also commonplace.[12] The nerve roots of the sacral plexus can be injured posteriorly during the obstructed labour, resulting in foot drop, hamstring compartment weakness and immobility. Up to 20% of these women may have some degree of foot drop,[5,13] which, together with sacral plexus involvement, may also be attributed to prolonged squatting while in labour and injury to the peroneal nerve.[14] The woman sometimes lies on the floor of a hut for months, even years, in the vain hope that the flow of urine will cease. This results in severe contractures of the lower limbs from disuse. Up to 32% will have some bony abnormalities, including osteopenia, perhaps due to lack of sunlight, renal impairment, malnutrition or a combination of all these factors. Other bony abnormalities include spurs and obliteration or even separation of the symphysis pubis.[15]

DEMOGRAPHICS

Obstetric fistulas are found in areas of poverty. The women affected were often malnourished as children, resulting in stunted growth and poor pelvic development. Repeated or chronic disease, such as malaria, tuberculosis and parasitic infestation, adds to this. Fistulas are also associated with poor infrastructure, poor or absent roads and transport systems, limited means of communication, and absent or inadequate health care, all of which make impossible access to facilities for a woman in need of safe delivery.

Women with these injuries are typically young (mean age 18.9 years, median age 16 years) and 62.7% are primiparous.[16–18] The usual length of labour is 3.9 days.[5] They are often of short stature, commonly less than 150 cm.[19] The average size of a VVF in the hospital in Addis Ababa is 2.3–2.8 cm; the size can range from 0.1 × 0.1 cm to 8 × 10 cm.[5] Of these women, 28.6% have some sort of urethral damage and 5% have total urethral loss. A rectovaginal fistula is also present in 17.4%,[5] but this seems to have some geographical variation. From small personal surveys of 90 women in Sierra Leone, 3.3% had a rectovaginal fistula (T Biruk, personal communication) and, for 72 women in Chad, this was 6.9% (A Browning, personal communication).

Sixty percent have been divorced or separated and 97% have had a stillborn delivery.[18] There are also reports of suicide and suicide attempts.

THE SCOPE OF THE PROBLEM

The World Health Organization estimates that 0.3% of all labours in the developing world will end with a VVF. Although this proportion may sound small, in a country the size of Ethiopia this creates around 8900 new cases of fistula a year. Considering that most women receive these injuries at the age of 16 and have a life expectancy of 55 years,[20] this would mean that in Ethiopia alone they may be over 250 000 women suffering from VVF in the countryside. The communiqué from the international workshop on VVF, Nigeria, 1998 stated that 'VVF affects 2 million women in Africa and Asia, with Nigeria accounting for 200 000 and that it would take between 30–40 years to clear the backlog without attending any new cases' (J Kelly, personal communication). International estimates report an annual incidence of VVF of between 50 000 and 100 000, with possibly many millions of women suffering around the world.[21]

The United Nations Fund for Population Activities and the International Federation for Gynecology and Obstetrics have chartered that they will target the care and treatment of VVF sufferers. Other individuals are doing what they can to help. Nigeria has a busy network caring for these women, treating 1464 in 1998.[22] Kenya has a programme, as does Tanzania and also many other countries around the world but on a smaller scale. However, another problem with treating these women is again the trap of poverty; they are desperately poor and cannot afford to pay hospital fees. Treatment relies on funding from governments or philanthropic organisations, but it can be difficult to raise sufficient money to meet the need.

THE TECHNIQUE OF FISTULA REPAIR

Three factors contribute to the successful outcome of fistula surgery: the experience and skill of the surgeon; the quality of the nursing care; and the extent of the damage to the fistula woman herself.

Treatment can be conservative or surgical. Conservative management involves just leaving the bladder on free drainage for up to six weeks. This can be an option for newly formed fistulas where the edges of the defect come together when the bladder is empty. This can result in spontaneous closure in up to 60% of selected women.[23] However, the vast majority will need surgical management.

Many aspects of fistula surgery are controversial, including its timing. Most centres advocate waiting for at least 10–12 weeks after the delivery, giving the tissues that are left adequate time to heal after the slough has come away.[21,24] The surgical approach is also controversial; urologists prefer the abdominal route, while gynaecologists favour the vaginal route.[25] In expert hands the vaginal route affords a 92–95% success rate for fistula closure, with less morbidity than the abdominal approach. Controversy also surrounds the use of antibiotics; that is, whether to use either induction or postoperative antibiotics. However, one small trial from West Africa reported no benefit from antibiotics.[26] We await the results of a randomised trial currently proceeding at the Addis Ababa Fistula Hospital.

The basic principles of fistula surgery are adequate exposure and correct technique. At the Fistula Hospital all patients have spinal anaesthesia and are placed in the exaggerated lithotomy position with use of a high Trendelenburg position.

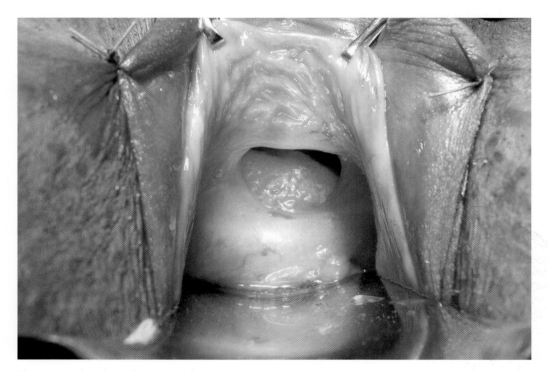

Figure 1 *Simple mid-vaginal vesicovaginal fistula*

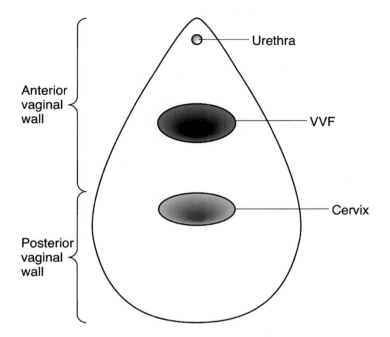

Figure 2 *Simple mid-vaginal vesicovaginal fistula*

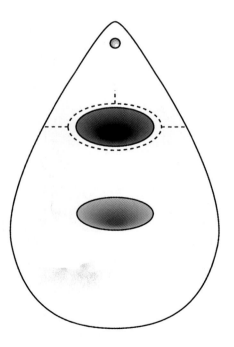

Figure 3 *Incisions for the dissection; VVF = vesicovaginal fistula*

The basic technique is wide mobilisation of the vaginal mucosa off the bladder wall, so that repair of the fistula itself can be performed without any tension.[2,23] Infiltration is routinely used to help with dissection. The fistula margin is incised and the incision extended laterally from the edge of the fistula along the lateral vaginal wall (Figures 1–3). This allows ease of access for dissection as well as space laterally for the introduction of a Martius graft, usually from the right labia. In any large fistula, particularly those near or in the cervix, the ureters should always be identified and catheterised, with the catheters threaded through the fistula and out via the urethra. This is essential because, if this step is omitted, the ureters may be inadvertently sutured during the repair, oedema after the operation may obstruct outflow, or worse, the ureter that was actually draining into the vagina, outside the fistula, may be left unnoticed and the woman will be left as wet after the operation as she was before. Dissection is carried out quite extensively posteriorly to maximise mobility, as well as laterally into the paravesical space and even into the cave of Retzius, but one should not be overambitious in the dissection as to interrupt the blood and nerve supply of the bladder more than is necessary (Figure 4).[21] The repair is undertaken in two layers: we use 2-0 chromic for the first and 3-0 chromic for the second. Care is taken to invert the bladder mucosa and exclude it from the suture line, and successful closure is demonstrated by the performance of a dye test. The next step is the inclusion of the Martius fibrofatty graft from the right labia (Figure 5). This has been shown to increase the success of closure from 70% to 90% at the Fistula Hospital (EC Hamlin, personal communication). It brings in more tissue and blood supply to the repair site as well giving extra strength to the site during the next delivery.[27,28] Other materials have been used as grafts, including the gracilus muscle, peritoneum and omentum. The ease, success and low morbidity of the Marius graft procedure makes it an attractive option.

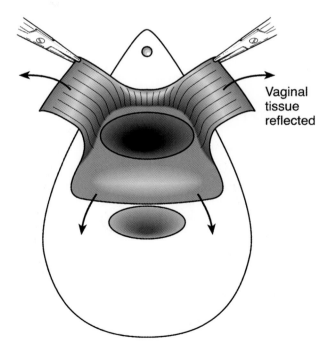

Vaginal tissue reflected

Figure 4 *Vaginal wall reflected off the bladder*

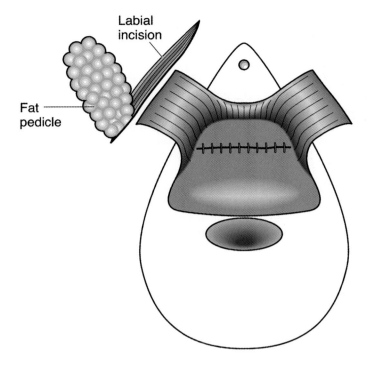

Figure 5 *Bladder repaired with no tension; incision on the right labia majora with pedicle of fat*

The fibrofatty Martius graft is introduced into the vagina via a tunnel along the inferior pubic ramus. It is sewn into place with five anchor sutures and the vagina repaired over it (Figures 6 and 7)

SPECIFIC SITES AND PROBLEMS

Complete destruction of the urethra

This occurs in 5% of affected women, especially when there is an obstruction low in the pelvis. The principle is to make a new urethra from the mucosa that remains. A U-shaped incision is made, with the bottom of the U being at the junction of the bladder or remnant of the urethra and the arms of the U reaching the position of the new meatus (Figure 8). The mucosa is then reflected from lateral to medial, with the resultant flaps being large enough to create a tube by suturing the two flaps over a Foley catheter (Figures 9 and 10). This is covered by the Martius graft and the vaginal mucosa is mobilised to cover the repair, or, if there is not sufficient tissue, labial skin flaps are used.

Urethral fistulas

These pose a particular problem in that, although the fistula may be closed successfully, residual stress incontinence may be as high as 50% because the continence mechanism is invariably partially

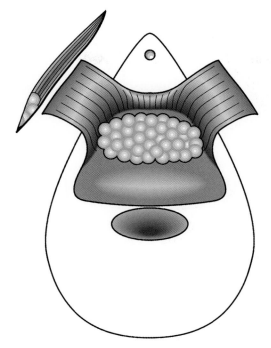

Figure 6 *Martius fibrofatty graft introduced into vagina under inferior pubic ramus and sewn over the repair*

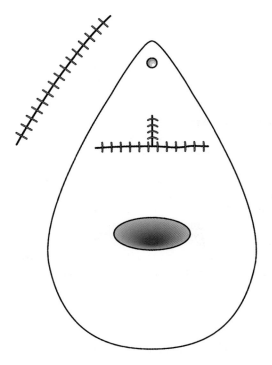

Figure 7 *Vagina and labia repaired*

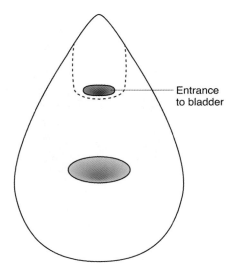

Figure 8 *Absent urethra with a U-shaped initial incision*

or completely destroyed, as observed personally at the Addis Ababa Fistula Hospital. If possible, dissection and closure should be in a vertical manner to maintain urethral length, and the urethra should be supported by the incorporation of extra sutures to elevate the bladder neck to the symphysis pubis.

Vesicocervical and vesicouterine fistulas

These can also be repaired via the vaginal route, the dissection being commenced in the same way as for a vaginal hysterectomy (Figure 11), exploring the space between the cervix and bladder until the fistula is identified and, after identifying the ureters (Figure 12), closure of the fistula, repair of the cervix and closure of the vaginal mucosa. Occasionally, the surgeon may need to opt for the abdominal route for repair if access is limited.

Closed/scarred vagina

Of the women presenting in Addis Ababa, 28% need some degree of vaginoplasty because of scarring,[5] but it appears that there may be a geographical variation between countries. The vagina needs to be opened first by either one, or more commonly two, Schuchardt incisions, one left and one right. The scar tissue is excised and the bladder is mobilised. However, after excision of the scar, it is often impossible to find any mucosa with which to cover the vagina. Labial flaps can be used by undermining the labia and bringing them into the vagina in order to keep it open. If there is a large rectal fistula with resultant scarring and tissue loss, then a flap of skin from the gluteal region can be rotated into the vagina to cover the posterior wall.

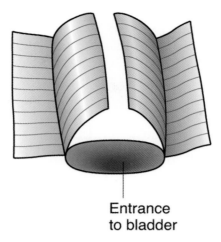

Entrance
to bladder

Figure 9 *Flaps formed from vaginal skin to create new urethra*

Devastating injuries with complete or near complete destruction of the bladder

Unfortunately for some women, their injuries are so severe as to completely destroy the bladder, when there can be no hope of a functional cure. The only option is for bladder augmentation if there is some bladder left, but this is not without complications of mucous plug formation, incomplete emptying, and the need for self-catheterisation, and of course it is necessary to have an adequately functioning urethra, which is rare in such extensive injuries. If the kidneys are suitable,

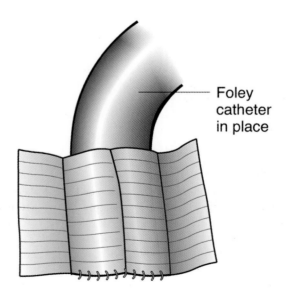

Foley
catheter
in place

Figure 10 *New urethra sewn over indwelling catheter*

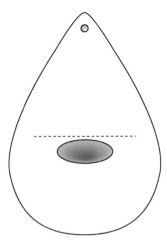

Figure 11 *Initial incision for cervicovaginal fistula repair*

then a Mainz II pouch can be an option if the woman's anal sphincter has adequate function. These women will then be continent per rectum, which some women find unacceptable. At the Addis Ababa Fistula Hospital an ileal conduit is more commonly formed. This restricts the woman so that she will not be able to return to her village owing to poor access to health care and no means of obtaining the necessary bags. These women have traditionally stayed at our hospital to work. They become excellent nursing aides, being compassionate to patients. They are also highly skilled. One such woman, Mamitu Gashe, although not having a conduit, has stayed at the hospital for other health reasons and has become so skilled that she can operate confidently by herself. She has

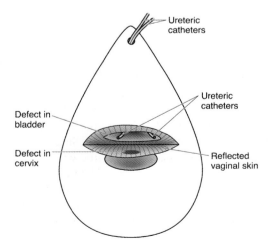

Figure 12 *Dissection: fistula and ureters identified; cervix and bladder are closed and vagina repaired*

cured nearly 2000 cases of VVF and is also cited on a gold medal for surgery from the Royal College of Surgeons of England!

Postoperative care

Meticulous postoperative care is needed to ensure adequate hydration and urine output, but more importantly to ensure continuous free drainage of the bladder so that no tension is placed on the repair site. A catheter is left on free drainage for 12–18 days depending on the site and size of the fistula. It is than clamped to test the repair with a full bladder and, if the woman is dry on clamping, the catheter is removed.

The vagina is packed after the operation and the packs are removed on the third day. However, the time is extended and the vagina may even be repacked if a large amount of vaginal scar tissue has been excised because this helps to keep it open during the healing phase.

INCONTINENCE AFTER REPAIR

With the above techniques, a closure rate of 92% can be expected.[29] Although most VVFs can be closed, a significant number of these women will remain with residual incontinence. The incidence has been variably reported as between 6.2% and 57%.[18,30] It is higher in two groups: women with urethral and bladder neck injuries, where the continence mechanism is partially or completely damaged;[31] and those with significant vaginal scarring and reduced bladder volume.[32] Various operations have been tried, but the most successful to date is a modification of an Aldridge sling. A sling is fashioned from rectus sheath and placed tension free under the mid-urethra. This is combined with retropubic dissection, mobilising the anterior urethra because it is often firmly scarred on to the posterior aspect of the symphysis pubis. To prevent the urethra from re-scarring on to the pubis and forming a 'drainpipe' urethra, a pedicle of omentum is interposed between the urethra and bone. This has a 67% success rate for total continence in urodynamically selected women at 14 months.[33] A novel way of preventing stress incontinence in those with bladder neck and urethral fistulas and those needing total urethral reconstruction is to make a sling of either ischiocavernosus muscle or fibrous tissue from the medial aspect of the inferior pubic ramus and place it under the urethra, again without tension. Early results in carefully selected women at the Addis Ababa Fistula Hospital seem promising.

THE CONTINUING PROBLEM

Prevention could be achieved with adequate obstetric care for all women, but, considering the status of women throughout most of the world and the lack of infrastructure and resources, this dream is a long way from being realised. It has been estimated that, if Nigeria was to eliminate fistulas, then 75 000 new obstetric units would have to be built.[34]

However, at the present time the work of caring for these women is touching only the surface. VVF was once a scourge in the West, but now, on going into the 21st century, this completely preventable condition is causing untold misery among the women of the developing world.

Surely, as obstetricians and gynaecologists, we should be the spearhead of this enormous task to rid the world of this tragic injury that blights the lives of millions of young women.

Let the words of the late revered gynaecologist, Professor Chasser Moir of Oxford, inspire us in this task: 'Nothing can equal the gratitude of the woman who, wearied by constant pain and desperate that her very presence is an offence to others finds suddenly that life has been given anew and that she has again become a citizen of the world'.[1]

References

1. Moir JC. *The Vesico-vaginal Fistula*. 2nd ed. London: Baillière Tindall; 1967.
2. Zacharin RF. *Obstetric Fistula*. New York: Springer-Verlag; 1988. p. 2,47,124.
3. Hilton P. Sims to SMIS – an historical perspective on vesico-vaginal fistula. *The Yearbook of the Royal College of Obstetricians and Gynaecologists, 1994.* London: RCOG Press; 1995. p. 7–16.
4. Mafouz BN. Urinary and recto-vaginal fistulae in women. *J Obstet Gynaecol Br Emp* 1929;37: 581–9.
5. Arrowsmith SD, Hamlin EC, Wall LL. Obstructed labor injury complex: obstetric fistula formation and the multifaceted morbidity of maternal birth trauma in the developing world. *Obstet Gynecol Surv* 1996:51:568–74.
6. Mahfouz N. Urinary fistula in women. *J Obstet Gynaecol Br Emp* 1957:64;23–34.
7. Warwick R, Williams PL. *Grays Anatomy*. Philadelphia, PA: Saunders; 1973. p. 1328–34, 1356–63.
8. McMinn RMH. *Lasts Anatomy*. Edinburgh: Churchill Livingstone; 1994. p. 381–4,392–400.
9. Hilton P. Urodynamic findings in patients with urogenital fistula. *Br J Urol* 1998;81;539–42.
10. Menefee SA, Elkins T. Urinary fistula. *Curr Opin Obstet Gynecol* 1996;8:380–3.
11. Bieler EU, Schnabel T. Pituitary and ovarian function in women with vesicovaginal fistulae after obstructed and prolonged labour. *S Afr Med J* 1976;50:257–66.
12. Wall LL. Obstetric fistula: a hope for a new beginning. *Int Urogynecol J* 1995;6;292–5.
13. Waaldijk K, Elkins TE. The obstetric fistula and peroneal nerve injury, an analysis of 947 consecutive patients. *Int Urogynecol J* 1994;5:183–7.
14. Reif ME. Bilateral common peroneal nerve palsy secondary to prolonged squatting in natural childbirth. *Birth* 1988;15:100–2.
15. Cockshott PW. Pubic changes associated with obstetric vesico vaginal fistulae. *Clin Radiol* 1973:224:241–7.
16. Kelly J. Vesico-vaginal and recto-vaginal fistulae. *J R Soc Med* 1992:85:257–8.
17. Liskin LS. Maternal morbidity in developing countries: a review and comment. *Int J Gynaecol Obstet* 1992;37:77–87.
18. Kelly J, Kwast BE. Epidemiological study of vesico-vaginal fistula in Ethiopia. *Int Urogynecol J* 1993:4;278–81.
19. Ampofo K, Out T, Uchelo G. Epidemiology of vesico-vaginal fistula in northern Nigeria. *West Afr J Med* 1990;9:98–102.
20. Federal Democratic Republic of Ethiopia Ministry of Health. *Health and health related indicators*. Addis Ababa: Planning and programming Department, Ministry of Health; 2001. p. 8.
21. Hilton P. Urogenital fistulae. In: MacLean AB, Cardozo C, editors. *Incontinence in Women*. London: RCOG Press; 2002. p. 163–80.
22. Waaldijk K. Fistula repairs in Nigeria and Niger. *Safe Mother* 1999;27:8.
23. Waaldijk K. *Step by Step Surgery of Vesicovaginal Fistula*. Edinburgh: Campion Press; 1994.
24. Margolis T, Mercer LJ. Vesicovaginal fistula. *Obstet Gynecol Surv* 1994;49:840–7.
25. Edwards JN. Principles of management of the vesicovaginal fistula. *S Afr Med J* 1982;62: 989–91.
26. Tomlinson AJ, Thorton JG. A randomised controlled trial of antibiotic prophylaxis for vesico-vaginal fistula repair. *Br J Obstet Gynaecol* 1998;105:397–9.
27. Zacharin RF. Grafting as a principle in the surgical management of vesicovaginal and rectovaginal fistulae. *Aus N Z J Obstet Gynaecol* 1980;20:10–17.

28. Rangnekar NP, Imdad Ali N, Kaul SA, Pathak HR. Role of the martius procedure in the management of urinary-vaginal fistulas. *J Am Coll Surg* 2000;191:259–63.

29. Muleta M. Obstetric fistula: a retrospective study of 1210 cases at the Addis Ababa Fistula Hospital. *J Obstet Gynaecol* 1997;17:68–70.

30. Murray C, Goh JT, Fynes M, Carey MP. Urinary and faecal incontinence following delayed primary repair of obstetric genital fistula. *BJOG* 2002;199:828–32.

31. Hilton P. Urodynamic findings in patients with urogenital fistulae. *Br J Urol* 1998;81:539–42.

32. Arrowsmith SD. Genitourinary reconstruction in obstetric fistulas. *J Urol* 1994;152:403–6.

33. Carey MP, Goh JT, Fynes MM, Murray CJ. Stress urinary incontinence after delayed primary closure of genitourinary fistula: a technique for surgical management. *Am J Obstet Gynecol* 2002;186:948–53.

34. Waaldijk K. *Evaluation Report XIV on VVF Projects in Northern Nigeria and Niger.* Katsina, Nigeria: Babber Ruga Fistula Hospital; 1998.

17

The rights of the pregnant woman in maternity care and the Human Rights Act 1998

Barbara Hewson

INTRODUCTION

The Human Rights Act 1998 came into force in October 2000. The Act introduced the European Convention on Human Rights into England and Wales. Separate arrangements were made for introducing the Convention into Scotland and Northern Ireland, but the focus of this chapter will be on the law of England and Wales, so I shall not comment further on these other jurisdictions.

The Act was intended to 'bring rights home', according to the Labour Government, but in the context of medicine, and maternity care in particular, the Act has not had much impact to date. There is a simple explanation for this. Patients in this country already possess a formidable array of legal rights under pre-existing law, and, as a result, the Act has not been a catalyst for dramatic change in the context of medical law. Nor has it made substantial inroads into the legal position of those who receive, and provide, maternity care. The *status quo* remains: despite various practical differences between pregnant women and other categories of patient, pregnant women continue to enjoy the same legal rights and expectations as patients in general, which most agree is no bad thing.

It is trite that, as only women become pregnant, those involved in maternity care are in the unusual position of caring for members of only one sex, at a critical stage of their lives. Pregnancy, labour and birth are not pathological, and indeed may be seen as a manifestation of health.[1] They are also watershed experiences in the life of a woman, her partner and her existing family. In a society with a declining birth rate, every pregnancy is important. Indeed, it is a matter of concern that women are increasingly postponing motherhood to a point when it becomes difficult, risky (in the sense of increased risk of fetal abnormality) or even impossible. These wider issues form the backdrop to this discussion.

Patients' rights in general derive from two main legal sources: common law (i.e. judge-made law) and statutes. It is fair to say that these rights in this country are well developed. However, individuals may not always be well informed about their rights, and therefore may find it difficult to exercise them effectively. The following is a basic overview of patients' rights. The Human Rights Act 1998, as will be shown, at best underpins or reinforces, but does not supersede, these rights.

CONSENT

Patients' rights at common law are well established and the right to self-determination is enshrined in a number of cases. The right to decide what is done to one's body is a fundamental legal right. A patient has the right to give, or to refuse, consent to medical advice, examination or treatment.

This includes the right to withdraw from a course of treatment. It also includes the right to refuse life-saving treatment. Patients are free to reject advice or treatment for reasons that are rational, irrational, or for no reason at all. The fact that a woman is pregnant makes no difference to her right to consent to, or to refuse treatment. Doctors are under no obligation to treat a woman who has exercised her right to refuse treatment.[2-8]

If a woman were subjected to a medical examination or treatment without her consent, this would be unlawful. This would constitute the tort of 'trespass', which could ground a civil action for damages. If the unwanted treatment caused very serious harm, it could also ground a criminal prosecution.

What about participation in clinical trials, or being seen or examined by medical students to facilitate their training and education? Patients' right to self-determination means that they have the right to decide whether or not they participate in clinical trials. If they do, but subsequently change their mind, they are free to withdraw.

INFORMATION

As the Department of Health points out, the provision of information is central to the consent process[9] Patients have the right to receive sufficient and comprehensible information, in order to make an informed choice about a proposed course of treatment, and to be informed of any significant risks.[4,10,11] Patients are entitled to be told, in language appropriate to them, what the proposed treatment is, its principal risks, benefits and alternatives, and the consequences of not receiving that treatment.

In addition, patients need to be given practical information, such as where the treatment is to take place, for how long they will be hospitalised, the likely after effects, etc.

The Department of Health states that the *presumption* must be that patients wish to be well informed about the risks and benefits of various options, and that when they make it clear (verbally or nonverbally) that they do not wish to be given this level of information, this should be documented.[12]

A doctor is also obliged to answer any questions that patients ask.[10] It is interesting to note, by way of an international comparison, that the New York State Department of Health tells patients to be assertive: 'you must speak up and ask questions'.[13] This of course presupposes that they are in a fit state to speak up and ask questions.

If a patient is misinformed, or if information that the patient has expressly or impliedly requested is withheld, the acceptance or refusal of treatment may be legally ineffective.[14]

DUTY OF CARE

Health professionals owe their patients a 'duty of care'. This means that they are expected to exercise reasonable care and skill in diagnosing, advising and treating their patients. Patients are entitled to receive a standard of care that a responsible body of medical opinion considers is appropriate for their medical condition.[15,16]

There may not always be consensus amongst responsible medical professionals about the type of care that should be provided in a particular case. A professional will not therefore be culpable, if he or she sides with one school of thought rather than another, provided that it reflects a responsible body of medical opinion.

If a professional breaches his or her duty of care to a patient, with the result that the patient is injured or suffers loss, the patient could seek compensation in an action for negligence.

INCAPACITY

The legal test for deciding whether persons have the capacity to make decisions about their treatment is, in summary:

- whether the person can understand and retain the information that is provided

- whether the person can weigh it up to make a choice.

Adults are presumed to have the capacity to make decisions about their care and treatment.[17]

Patients who are incapacitated either temporarily (e.g. as a result of an accident, shock, pain or drugs) or permanently (e.g. in a coma), so that they cannot communicate their wishes and cannot give effective consent, are nonetheless entitled to be treated in their 'best interests'.[2,3,6]

Contrary to what some people may believe, a relative or spouse does *not* have any legal right to consent to treatment on behalf of a patient.[2]

The only situation in which someone may legally consent to treatment on another's behalf is when a patient is under the age of 18 years, in which case their parent or other person with parental responsibility, or, ultimately, a family court judge exercising an inherent jurisdiction to protect child welfare, may consent on his or her behalf.[18,19]

As indicated above, when patients are incapacitated, the medical profession's duty is to provide them with whatever care and treatment is in their best interests. This does not mean just the provision of drugs and other therapies or procedures, it also includes attending to their basic needs, such as washing, providing food and hydration, etc.

AUTONOMY

UK law values personal autonomy highly. In *S* v. *McC* in 1972 Lord Reid said: 'There is no doubt that a person of full age and capacity cannot be ordered to undergo a blood test against his will.... The real reason is that English law goes to great lengths to protect a person of full age and capacity from interference with his personal liberty. We have too often seen freedom disappear in other countries not only by coups d'état but by gradual erosion: and often it is the first step that counts. So it would be unwise to make even minor concessions.'[20]

STATUS OF THE FETUS

A lot of ink has been spilt on the status of the fetus. Although this issue raises very interesting philosophical and moral questions, the law deals with it in a pragmatic way. The law is not metaphysical, and the quasi-theological idea of 'two persons in one' is not one that is acceptable to the law. UK law has always adopted the position that a fetus is not a person until it is born.[21,22] This has two consequences from a human rights perspective. First, it means that a fetus lacks the necessary legal standing to assert rights on its own behalf. Secondly, it means that a claim that (say) current abortion law is incompatible with a fetal 'right to life' would be very unlikely to succeed.

If a fetus were a 'person', it would be very difficult to justifying killing it simply because the woman did not want to carry or to give birth to a child (although, following the ruling in the Maltese 'conjoined twins' case,[23] a case for termination could be made out, based on the woman's right to bodily integrity and 'self-defence').

The UK reaffirmed its commitment to pregnant women's autonomy in the famous case of *St George's* v. *S* in 1998.[24] There, the Court of Appeal decided that, if a pregnant woman could be subjugated to save her own life or that of her fetus, that would annihilate the autonomy principle:

'How can a forced invasion of a competent adult's body against her will even for the most laudable of motives (the preservation of life) be ordered *without irremediably damaging the principle of self-determination?* When human life is at stake the pressure to provide an affirmative answer authorising unwanted medical intervention is very powerful. Nevertheless the autonomy of each individual requires continuing protection even, perhaps particularly, when the motive for interfering with it is readily understandable, and indeed to many would appear commendable: hence the importance of remembering Lord Reid's warning against making "even minor concessions"[25]. [emphasis added]

The Court went on to point out that, if this principle were breached, then logically any adult could be forced to undergo bodily invasion to save a child: 'If it has not already done so medical science will no doubt one day advance to the stage when a very minor procedure undergone by an adult would save the life of his or her child, or perhaps the life of a child of a complete stranger. The refusal would rightly be described as unreasonable, the benefit to another human life would be beyond value, and the motives of the doctors admirable. If, however, the adult were compelled to agree, or rendered helpless to resist, *the principle of autonomy would be extinguished*'.[26] [emphasis added]

The Law Commission of England and Wales, which is responsible for formulating proposals for law reform, also considered this issue in *Injuries to Unborn Children* (Report no. 60, 1974). A particular concern was to consider the type of legislation needed to ensure that babies born injured as a result of an accident while *in utero* could be compensated. Its recommendations led to Parliament passing the Congenital Disabilities (Civil Liability) Act 1976. The Law Commission decided that there were sound public policy reasons why a child should not be allowed to sue its mother for injuries sustained *in utero*, subject to one exception: where those injuries were sustained in a car accident where the mother was the driver, and hence insured. It also concluded that a child's right to sue a third party for prebirth injuries is parasitic upon the third party's duty to the mother.

Prenatally, the professional's duty of care is owed to the pregnant woman. If a baby is born injured as a result of prenatal negligence, it then acquires a right to sue, based on the breach of duty to its mother. Equally, if the injury is caused by a refusal by the woman to accept advice or treatment, the baby has no independent right to sue. This may seem harsh, but is generally thought to be the only pragmatic solution.[27,28]

In law, there is no duty to rescue.[29] If, therefore, a pregnant woman were to decide that she does not want medical treatment of some kind, the law does not mandate any forced benevolent act for the sake of her fetus (or her other children, assuming she has any).

There has been an isolated attempt by a public authority to detain a pregnant woman for a hospital birth, in 1988.[30] The London Borough of Bromley claimed that she had a hippy lifestyle and suffered from mental health problems. It tried to make her fetus a ward of court. It sought a court order for her arrest, to force her into hospital for the remainder of her pregnancy. Bromley's goal was to take the baby into care when it was born. The court hearing was conducted in the woman's absence. The judge refused to make the order sought. Bromley appealed to the Court of Appeal, which also refused to intervene.

The Court of Appeal explained why English law should uphold a woman's autonomy. First, English case law does not recognise fetuses as separate legal entities until they are born. Therefore, fetuses could not be made wards of court. Second, the question of whether pregnant women's civil liberties ought to be curtailed in this way is a matter for Parliament, and not for judges. Third, the judges thought that if fetuses could be made wards of court, this would create a most undesirable conflict in cases involving pregnant women. Ordinarily, in wardship cases, the welfare of the child is paramount. How could this 'welfare principle' be reconciled with a pregnant woman's autonomy?

SOME INTERNATIONAL COMPARISONS

The US Supreme Court, when considering the constitutionality of restrictions on access to abortion, has not accepted that a fetus is a 'person'.[31,32] Only one state supreme court in the USA has ruled that a fetus is a 'person' (*Whitner* v. *South Carolina* (1997)[33]). Whitner was a black drug addict who was successfully prosecuted for child abuse while pregnant and given a long jail sentence. The court's rationale was that child abuse laws cover acts that endanger a viable fetus. The majority accepted that its ruling could be used to punish pregnant women who drank or smoked, but seemed indifferent to such an outcome. The South Carolina Attorney-General's office intimated that doctors and women involved in post-viability abortions could now be tried for murder and sentenced to death.[34]

The US Supreme Court has ruled that a covert drug testing policy used by the Medical University of South Carolina hospital against pregnant women was illegal and unconstitutional (*Ferguson* v. *City of Charleston* (2001)[35]). The hospital operated the scheme in league with local police and prosecutors. The women targeted were mainly black. If a woman's urine tested positive for cocaine, the hospital would inform the police, who would come to arrest her. These women were not offered drug treatment programmes.

The Canadian Supreme Court, following the approach of the Law Commission of England and Wales, and of the English courts in *Re F (in utero)*, has held that the state has no power to detain a drug-abusing pregnant woman for the sake of her fetus (*Winnipeg Child & Family Services* v. *G* (1997)[36]).

In the Republic of Ireland, although article 40.3.3 of the Irish Constitution expressly guarantees the 'right to life of the unborn', the Supreme Court has said that this provision is concerned to prevent abortion only. Thus, it may not be invoked to prevent the deportation of a pregnant asylum seeker, notwithstanding evidence that her home state has a much higher infant mortality rate.[37]

THE NHS ACT 1977

Section 1 of the National Health Service Act 1977[38] provides:

(1)   It is the Secretary of State's duty to continue *the promotion* in England and Wales of a comprehensive health service designed to secure *improvement* –
  (a)   in the physical and mental health of the people of those countries, and
  (b)   in the prevention, diagnosis and treatment of illness, and for that purpose *to provide or secure the effective provision of services* in accordance with this Act.

(2)   The services so provided shall be free of charge except in so far as the making and recovery of charges is expressly provided for or by or under any enactment, whenever passed'. [emphasis added]

Pursuant to this statutory duty, the Secretary of State is obliged by section 3 to provide a range of facilities 'to such extent *as he considers necessary* to meet all *reasonable* requirements' [emphasis added], such as:

- hospital accommodation

- medical, dental, nursing and ambulance services

- such other facilities for the care of expectant and nursing mothers and young children as he considers are appropriate as part of the health service

- medical inspection of pupils in attendance at schools maintained by local authorities and the medical treatment of such pupils

- the giving of advice on contraception, the medical examination of persons seeking advice on contraception, the treatment of such persons and the supply of contraceptive substances and appliances.[38]

Section 1 does *not* impose a duty to provide a comprehensive health service, and such a service may never, for human, financial or other resource reasons, be achievable.[39] Section 3 gives a very significant degree of discretion to the Secretary of State, as to how he goes about discharging that duty (which, for practical purposes, is delegated to health authorities and trusts). The NHS Act 1977 has been amended to give patients a modest increase in rights: for example, section 28F permits regulations to be made that entitle patients to choose their GP, subject to the GP's consent and to the limit on patient numbers for that GP not being exceeded.

There is no mention of home births. Previously, the Midwives Act 1936[40] and then the National Health Service Act 1946[41] made express provision for a home birth service, to be provided by the local health authority. With the removal of that obligation, home birth services now represent only 2% of births.[42] According to the Expert Maternity Group, the demand for such a service remains unmet, with 22% of women surveyed by MORI saying that they would like a home birth.[43] Some NHS authorities provide a home birth service, but for many women the choice is simply not available, unless they can afford the services of an independent midwife.

Short of amending the existing 1977 Act to impose a statutory obligation on health authorities to provide such a service, there seems little prospect of this option becoming more widely available, unless purchasers and providers can be persuaded that home births are more economical.

DISCRIMINATION

Providers of medical services are subject to legislation, which prohibits discrimination on the grounds of sex, race or disability.[44–46] The Commission for Racial Equality used to have a code of practice specifically for the NHS; however, this does not appear to be still in print. The Disability Rights Commission recently issued a code of practice for service providers.

There has been relatively little litigation using this legislation concerning the provision of goods, facilities and services (compared with the enormous volume of litigation involving discrimination in the workplace). First, cases against service providers have to be brought in the county court, and litigants are at risk of an order for costs if they lose. This is in contrast to cases involving discrimination in the employment context, which go before employment tribunals, where usually no orders for costs are made against losing parties. Secondly, the NHS is legally required to provide care for all, free of charge; so the chances of overt (i.e. direct) discrimination are presumably much reduced.

HUMAN RIGHTS ACT 1998

Section 6 of the Act requires public authorities (which would include NHS trusts) to act compatibly with the European Convention on Human Rights. Section 7 gives a new right of action to people whose human rights have been infringed by a public authority to sue for damages.

The first point to stress is that the Convention does not contain any express right to health, or to health care of any description. Certain articles of the Convention may be particularly relevant in the context of healthcare provision:

- Article 2 requires that everyone's right to life shall be protected by law.

- Article 3 prohibits torture or inhuman or degrading treatment or punishment absolutely.

- Article 5 guarantees the right to liberty and security of person.

- Article 8 guarantees a right to respect for one's private and family life.

- Article 9 guarantees the right to freedom of thought, conscience and belief.

- Article 10 protects the freedom to give and to receive information.

- Article 14 provides: 'The enjoyment of the rights and freedoms set forth in this Convention shall be secured without discrimination on any ground such as sex, race, colour, language, religion, political or other opinion, national or social origin, association with a national minority, property, birth or other status.'

In a recent high-profile ruling concerning patient rights – the case of Ms B, the paralysed woman who wanted to be taken off a ventilator and allowed to die naturally[8] – the Act was not mentioned in the judgment, although it may have been discussed during legal argument. The case of *Pretty* v. *United Kingdom*, which went from the House of Lords to the European Court of Human Rights in Strasbourg, showed that the Act did not change UK law on euthanasia.[47] Article 2 of the Convention (which protects the right to life) has not so far been interpreted to include protection of fetal life.[48]

Article 3 prohibits torture and degrading treatment or punishment absolutely, but it requires a high threshold of maltreatment – the deliberate infliction of pain and suffering, which is most unlikely to arise in a therapeutic context. Placing a disabled person in detention without suitable sleeping or lavatory facilities has been held to constitute degrading treatment.[49]

Article 8 of the Convention is perhaps the most important in this context. It guarantees the right to respect for one's private and family life. This article encompasses the right to physical and moral integrity;[50] the right to refuse medical treatment;[51] and also the right to medical confidentiality.[52,53] Nevertheless, Article 8 may be subject to interference by the state on a number of specified grounds: 'There shall be no interference by a public authority with the exercise of this right except such as is in accordance with the law and is necessary in a democratic society in the interests of national security, public safety or the economic wellbeing of the country, for the prevention of disorder or crime, for the protection of health or morals, or for the protection of the rights and freedoms of others.'

Thus, it may be open to the state to justify a policy of universal vaccination on public health grounds.[54]

When child protection issues are raised in the context of a child about to be born, it should be noted that the European Court of Human Rights in Strasbourg has twice found that taking a newborn away from its mother in hospital, under an emergency care order, violated article 8 (*K & T* v. *Finland*[55] and *P, C & S* v. *United Kingdom*[56]). In the latter case, it stated: '…the removal of a baby from its mother at birth requires exceptional justification. It is a step which is traumatic for the mother and places her own physical and mental health under a strain, and it deprives the new-born baby of close contact with its birth mother and…of the advantages of breastfeeding'.[57]

Article 10, which guarantees the right to give and to receive information, may be pertinent in the field of maternity care, especially when taken together with article 14 (the right not to be discriminated against, in the enjoyment of one's convention rights). Therefore, state measures that involve giving pregnant women less information – and, consequently, less choice – than other categories of patient, may be vulnerable to a human rights challenge. At the time of writing, however, the Human Rights Act 1998 seems unlikely to effect major change to the position of individuals giving, or receiving, maternity care.

References

1. House of Commons Health Committee, *Second Report on Maternity Services*. London: HMSO; 1992. Vol. 1, para. 4.
2. *Re F (Mental Patient: Sterilisation)* [1990] AC 1, HL
3. *Airedale NHS Trust* v. *Bland* [1993] AC 789, HL
4. *Re T* [1993] Fam 95
5. *Re C (Adult: Refusal of Treatment)* [1994] 1 WLR 290
6. *Re MB (Medical Treatment)* [1997] 2 FLR 426
7. *St George's Healthcare NHS Trust* v. *S* [1999] Fam 26
8. *Re B (Adult: Refusal of Treatment)* [2002] 2 All ER 449
9. Department of Health. *Good Practice in Consent – Implementation Guide*. London: DoH; 2001. p. 17, para. 1.
10. *Sidaway* v. *Governor of Bethlem Royal Hospital* [1985] AC 871, HL
11. *Pearce* v. *UB NHS Trust* (1999) PIQR 53
12. Department of Health. *Good Practice in Consent – Implementation Guide*. London: DoH; 2001. p. 17 para. 2.
13. New York State Department of Health. *About Your Rights* [www.health.state.ny.us/nysdoh/hospital/english2.htm].
14. *Re T per* Lord Donaldson MR at 115B–C
15. *Bolam* v. *Friern HMC* [1957] 1 WLR 582
16. *Bolitho* v. *City of Hackney HA* [1996] 7 Med LR 1
17. *Re B (adult: refusal of treatment)* [2002] 2 All ER 449
18. *In re R (A Minor)* [1992] Fam 11
19. *In re W (A Minor)* [1993] Fam. 64
20. *S* v. *McC* [1972] AC 24 at 43
21. *Paton* v. *BPAS Trustees* [1979] QB 726
22. *Burton* v. *Islington HA* [1993] QB 204
23. *Re A (Conjoined Twins) (No. 1)* [2001] 2 WLR 480
24. *St George's* v. *S* [1999] Fam. 26
25. *St George's* v. *S* [1999] Fam. 46H–47A
26. *St George's* v. *S* [1999] Fam. 47B
27. Congenital Disabilities (Civil Liability) Act 1976. s. 1.
28. The Law Commission. *Report on Injuries to Unborn Children*. Report No. 60. Cm. 5709. 1974.
29. McIvor C. Expelling the myth of the parental duty to rescue. *Child Fam Law Q* 2000;12:229.
30. *Re F (in utero)* [1988] Fam 122
31. *Thornburgh* v. *ACOG* 476 US 747 (1986)
32. *Planned Parenthood* v. *Casey* 505 US 833 (1992)
33. *Whitner* v. *South Carolina* (1997) 492 SE 2d 777
34. Paltrow LM. Pregnant drug users, fetal persons, and the threat to *Roe v Wade*. *Albany Law Rev* 1999;63:999.
35. *Ferguson* v. *City of Charleston* 532 US 67 (2001)
36. *Winnipeg Child & Family Services* (1997) 3 BHRC 611

37.   *Baby O v. Minister for Justice, Equality and Law Reform* [2002] IESC 53 (6th June, 2002)
38.   National Health Service Act 1977. s. 3(1)(a), (c), (d); s. 5(1)(a), (b).
39.   *R v. North and East Devon HA ex p. Coughlan* [2000] 2 WLR 622
40.   Midwives Act 1936. s. 1(1).
41.   National Health Service Act 1946. s. 23(1).
42.   Midwives Information and Resource Service. *Place of Birth.* Informed Choice Leaflet for Professionals No. 10. Rev. ed. Cumbria: MIDIRS; 2003.
43.   Expert Maternity Group. *Changing Childbirth.* London: HMSO; 1993. Part 1, para. 2.6.1.
44.   Sex Discrimination Act 1975, part III
45.   Race Relations Act 1976, part III
46.   Disability Discrimination Act 1995, part III.
47.   *Pretty v. United Kingdom* (2002) 35 EHRR 1
48.   *Paton v. United Kingdom* (1980) 3 EHRR CD 408
49.   *Price v. United Kingdom* (2002) 34 EHRR 1285
50.   *X & Y v. Netherlands* (1986) 8 EHRR 235
51.   *Peters v. Netherlands* No. 21132/ 93, 77–A DR (1994)
52.   *MS v. Sweden* (1999) 28 EHRR 313
53.   *Z v. Finland* (1998) 25 EHRR 371
54.   *Acmanne v. Belgium* (1984) 40 DR 251
55.   *K & T v. Finland.* Judgment of the Grand Chamber, 12 July 2001
56.   *P, C & S v. United Kingdom.* Judgment of the Second Chamber, 16 July 2002
57.   *P, C & S v. United Kingdom.* Judgment of the Second Chamber, 16 July 2002. para. 131.

18

Urodynamics

Gordon Hosker

INTRODUCTION

Urodynamics is an umbrella term for measurements to describe and quantify the bladder and urethra's ability to store and expel urine. The report of the Second International Consultation on Incontinence[1] gives a comprehensive overview of the state of urodynamics up to 2001. Since then, the International Continence Society has reviewed and restated the standardisation of terminology of lower urinary tract dysfunction[2] and published a document describing good urodynamic practices.[3]

This chapter describes the following urodynamic investigations regularly used in assessing lower urinary tract function in women and examines their clinical usefulness in the light of these 'state of the art' reports and latest research:

- uroflowmetry

- filling cystometry

- pressure-flow studies

- urethral function tests.

UROFLOWMETRY

A woman's urinary flowrate is often assessed before other urodynamic investigations. She is asked to attend her appointment with a comfortably full bladder and is shown to a private room where she micturates on a commode/toilet fitted with a flow sensor. The equipment prints out a graph of flowrate as a function of time, together with some parameters derived from the graph.

Figure 1 shows normal voiding. Flowrate increases as the bladder empties and then decreases when the bladder is about half empty. Often the curve is bell-shaped and symmetrical as shown in this example. Parameters measured include the maximum flowrate (Q_{max}) and voided volume. For a woman voiding more than 150 ml, the normal maximum flowrate would be about 20 ml/s (and would rarely be below 12 ml/s).[4]

Figure 2 shows a typical trace from a woman with voiding difficulty; note the reduced maximum flowrate (8 ml/s) and protracted stream.

The flowmeter automatically calculates parameters from the graph of flowrate and time, such as: Q_{max} and average flowrate (Q_{ave}), voided volume, voiding time and flow time. However, it is important to look at the graph itself and perhaps recalculate some parameters because the software is currently incapable of distinguishing artefact from physiological data.

In Figure 3a, the woman has passed a loose stool during voiding and this has resulted in a sudden, large artefact. The software has measured the maximum flowrate as the height of this spike at 27 ml/s

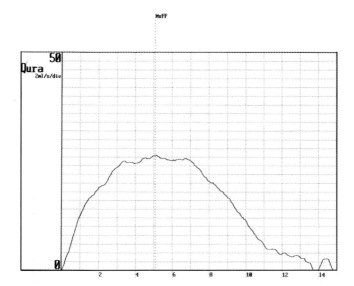

Figure 1 *Normal female urine flow (Q$_{max}$ 26 ml/s)*

but it is obvious that the 'real' maximum flowrate is much lower than this. For this reason, the International Continence Society has now defined Q$_{max}$ as that obtained after smoothing out such artefacts and rounding it to the nearest whole number.[3] Therefore, the correct maximum flowrate in this example is 7 ml/s (Figure 3b). Without such smoothing, it is recommended[3] that the computed maximum flowrate (27 ml/s) should be termed Q$_{max.raw}$.

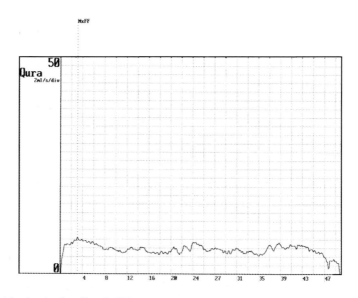

Figure 2 *Impaired female urine flow (Q$_{max}$ 8 ml/s)*

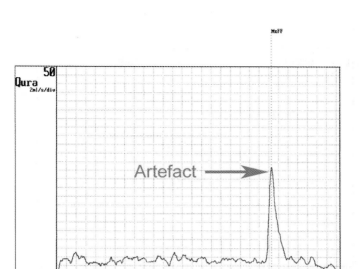

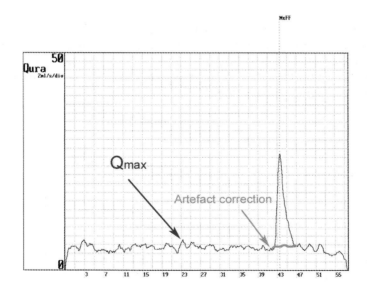

Figure 3 *(a) Flow curve with artefact giving incorrect Q_{max} of 27 ml/s ($Q_{max \cdot raw}$); (b) flow curve with artefact corrected giving true Q_{max} of 7 ml/s*

It is now recommended[3] that uroflowmetry should be documented in the format VOID: maximum flowrate/volume voided/post-void residual volume. Therefore, if the woman represented in Figure 2 had a post-void residual of 20 ml, then her flow measurement should be reported as VOID: 26/214/20.

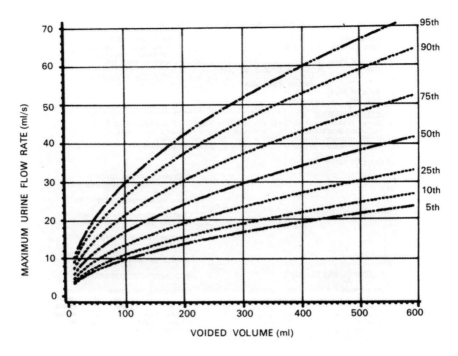

Figure 4 *The Liverpool nomogram for maximum flow rate in normal females (reproduced from: Haylen BT, Ashby D, Sutherst JR, Frazer MI, West CR. Maximum and average urine flow rates in normal male and female populations – the Liverpool nomograms.* Br J Urol *1989;64:30–8,[4] with permission from Blackwell Publishing)*

It has been a long-held view that flowrate is dependent on voided volume; the more urine passed, the greater the maximum flowrate (unless the bladder is overdistended, when flowrate tends to become slower). Nomograms have been generated in normal populations of women (such as the Liverpool nomograms shown in Figure 4) and illustrate the general dependency of flowrate on voided volume.[4] However, on an individual basis, this does not always hold true and, while some women show a strong volume dependence on maximum flowrate (Figure 5a), others' flowrates are independent of voided volume (Figure 5b).[5,6]

Urinary flowrate may not only depend on voided volume but also on the position a woman adopts during micturition. Hovering over a toilet seat (as many women do when away from their own toilet) can reduce flowrate considerably compared with the sitting position.[7] Although the measurement of free flowrate is one of the more physiological tests found in urodynamics, it can also be influenced by patient apprehension. There is evidence to suggest that higher flowrates are achieved on a second flowrate measurement,[8] when the woman has acclimatised to the machinery and surroundings. Therefore, if a poor flowrate is measured, it is prudent to ask whether the void was representative of that normally encountered and a second flowrate measurement may be necessary to confirm poor voiding.

The information gained from this simple, noninvasive test is not just limited to whether or not there is any voiding difficulty. There is some evidence to suggest that low pre-operative maximum flowrates predispose women to voiding difficulty after surgery for incontinence.[9,10]

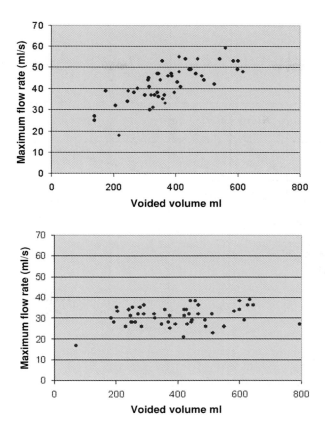

Figure 5 *(a) Normal female voiding – strong dependence of flow rate on voided volume; (b) normal female voiding – flow rate independent of voided volume*

FILLING CYSTOMETRY

One of the fundamental investigations within urodynamics is filling cystometry. This measures the bladder's ability to store urine.

Preliminaries: residual urine

Prior to filling cystometry it is common to assess the amount of any residual urine. It is currently thought that if a large residual volume is expected (e.g. the woman has neurological disease and does not self-catheterise) then filling cystometry should be carried out on top of any residual urine.[11] This also applies to a neurologically normal patient if there is evidence of hydronephrosis.[12] If the patient self-catheterises then the bladder should be emptied prior to filling cystometry.[12]

Preliminaries: testing for urinary tract infection

Prior to filling cystometry it is also prudent to check for urinary tract infection because this predisposes the patient to detrusor overactivity.[13] Infection is usually detected by microscopy and culture but, in a urodynamic setting, dipsticks sensitive to nitrites and leucocytes are a convenient, cheap and apparently accurate way of doing this[13] immediately prior to the investigation. If infection is detected by the dipstick then a specimen can be sent to the laboratory, the infection appropriately treated, and urodynamics carried out only if the symptoms persist when the urine is clear. Doubt was expressed in 2002 concerning the sensitivity and specificity of dipsticks in detecting infection,[14,15] so there needs to be more work to verify whether or not dipsticks should continue to be used in this way.

Preliminaries: setting up

Usually, a thin, fluid-filled pressure line is placed in the bladder (normally urethrally, but it can be done suprapubically), taped in place, and connected to a pressure transducer to measure bladder pressure (p_{ves}). Another catheter, placed alongside it, is used to fill the bladder (unless a double-lumen catheter is used).

Pressure changes within the bladder come from two sources: one is the intrinsic pressure generated by surface tension in the smooth muscle of the detrusor, the other is extrinsic pressure that arises from changes in abdominal pressure (such as when coughing, laughing, moving position etc.) impinging on the bladder. During urodynamic measurements, it is common practice to monitor these abdominal pressure changes (p_{abd}) and electronically subtract them from the pressures measured within the bladder (p_{ves}) to give pressures solely due to the activity of the detrusor muscle itself (p_{det}) (Figure 6).

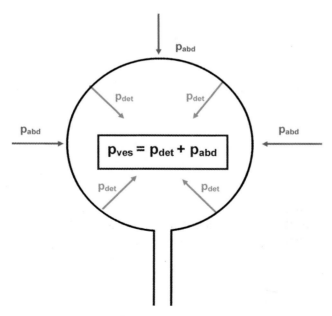

Figure 6 *Pressure in the bladder (p_{ves}) is a combination of the intrinsic pressure generated by the detrusor muscle (p_{det}) and the extrinsic abdominal pressure (p_{abd})*

Table 1 *Plausible pressures at the start of cystometry (with lower values of p_{ves} and p_{abd} being found in slim women in the supine position while higher values are associated with heavier women in the erect position); values outside these ranges are likely to indicate a technical problem, which should be rectified before cystometry commences (data abstracted from Schafer et al., 2002[3])*

	Minimum (cmH$_2$O)	Maximum (cmH$_2$O)
P$_{ves}$	5	50
P$_{abd}$	5	50
P$_{det}$	0	10

The abdominal pressure changes are usually measured by a fluid-filled pressure line placed in the rectum, which has a plastic flap or balloon at its tip to protect it from being blocked by faeces. However, it is equally valid to place a fluid-filled pressure line in the upper two-thirds of the vagina[16] or through an abdominal stoma.

After instrumentation, the pressure transducers should be levelled to the superior border of the symphysis pubis and the lines flushed through to exclude any air bubbles.[3] The intravesical and abdominal pressures should then be set to measure relative to atmospheric pressure and not relative to the initial resting pressures within the patient.[3] Before cystometry commences, the values of p$_{ves}$, p$_{abd}$ and p$_{det}$ should be plausible (Table 1) and the patient should cough to confirm that the resultant rise in abdominal pressure is recorded equally in the bladder and the rectum.

The complete technical details of ensuring accurate, plausible and interpretable recordings are published elsewhere.[3]

Alternative pressure sensors

Apart from external pressure transducers, it is possible to use catheter mounted pressure transducers, such as the so-called microtip or solid state pressure transducers, to measure intravesical and abdominal pressure.

These devices are relatively unaffected by artefacts caused by knocking or moving the pressure lines and this makes them ideal for ambulatory monitoring, but there has been some concern over their use for conventional urodynamics.

The pressure measured by these devices depends on the position of the sensor within the bladder and this is unknown. Theoretically, this could give rise to errors of up to 10 cmH$_2$O.[3] However, simultaneous measurements with these devices and external pressure transducers do not show great differences between the pressures[17] and concerns regarding their use in conventional urodynamics may be unfounded.

Normal filling cystometry

The bladder is filled with sterile water or physiological saline and the intravesical and abdominal pressure changes are monitored. For conventional urodynamics, a filling rate of between 50 and 100 ml/min is usually used. In women in whom there is neurological disease or marked detrusor overactivity, slower infusion rates of about 10 ml/min are more appropriate because this minimises the chance of provoking detrusor contractions that may result in complete micturition before voiding data can be collected.

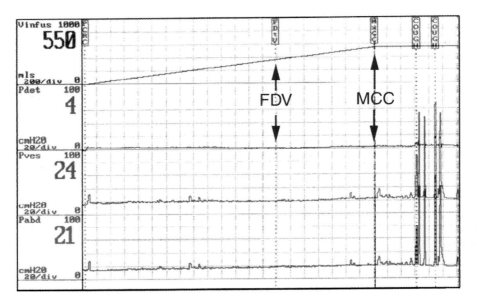

Figure 7 *Normal filling cystometrogram with the volume infused in the bladder (V_{infus}) displayed in the top trace; the pressure in the bladder (p_{ves}) and, the abdominal pressure (p_{abd}) are shown in the bottom two traces; the derived intrinsic pressure generated by the detrusor muscle ($p_{det} = p_{ves} - p_{abd}$) is the second trace from the top; the figures displayed on the left indicate the value of each parameter at maximum cystometric capacity; FDV = first desire to void; MCC = maximum cystometric capacity*

It is now recommended that filling rates, previously described as slow, medium or rapid,[18] should be defined simply as being physiological or nonphysiological and this is determined by dividing the patient's weight in kilograms by four.[2] If this figure is numerically less than the filling rate in millilitres per minute, then the filling rate is nonphysiological.[19]

Quality control should be carried out during the recording, with the patient coughing periodically (every minute or every 50 ml[3]) to ensure continued correct positioning of the pressure lines and to confirm that the system is still free of leaks and air bubbles.

In a normal cystometrogram (Figure 7) there is usually a small, gradual rise in detrusor pressure (approximately $1\,cmH_2O/100\,ml$) as the bladder fills. At some point during filling the woman will experience an awareness of the need to empty her bladder. This is termed the 'first desire to void'. Nevertheless, filling can be continued comfortably (with the same small gradual rise in detrusor pressure) until the woman can delay micturition no longer. This is the 'maximum cystometric capacity'. Values for these parameters vary from centre to centre but typical values are shown in Table 2. Other sensations can be recorded during cystometry; these are defined in the 'standardisation of terminology' document.[2]

Filling is often carried out in the supine position and, as this provides only a minimal challenge to the bladder in many instances, it is usual practice to ask the woman to move to an upright position and then carry out provocative manoeuvres such as heel bouncing, jogging, listening to running water, coughing, etc. In a normal bladder, there should be no fluctuations in detrusor pressure during any part of the filling cystometry, although there will be momentary pressure variations in intravesical and abdominal pressure when the patient moves (Figure 8).

Table 2 *Values of some urodynamic parameters in 72 women with normal urinary control; cystometry carried out with sterile water at body temperature at a rate of 100 ml/min (Hosker GL, Ward GH, unpublished data, 1982)*

	Mean	SD	Min	Max
Age (years)	41.4	10.1	25	75
Parity	2.3	1.6	0	7
Residual urine (ml)	11.0	13.0	0	6
FDV (ml)	304.0	116.0	60	640
MCC (ml)	543.0	94.0	360	800
Compliance (ml/cmH$_2$O)	124.0	150.0	31	800
MUCP (cmH$_2$O)	69.0	23.0	29	117

SD = standard deviation; FDV = first desire to void; MCC = maximum cystometric capacity; MUCP = maximum urethral closure pressure

Should the patient move position during the cystometry, it is important to reposition external transducers to the level of the symphysis pubis to record accurately the pressure relative to atmospheric pressure because pressure measured by a fluid-filled system is dependent on the vertical height of the transducer relative to the source of pressure (i.e. the higher the bladder or the rectum above the transducer, the greater the hydrostatic pressure on the measuring device).

Filling rate and temperature of the filling medium[20] may influence filling cystometry. It has also been thought that pH and osmolality[21,22] of the filling medium have an effect, but the results of work published in 2000[23] and 2002[24] suggest that this is not the case. However, high concentrations of sodium may influence sensations of bladder filling in patients with an overactive bladder and a cystometric capacity under 250 ml.[25] The range of filling media, temperatures and filling rates employed in the UK[26] are shown in Figure 9a–c.

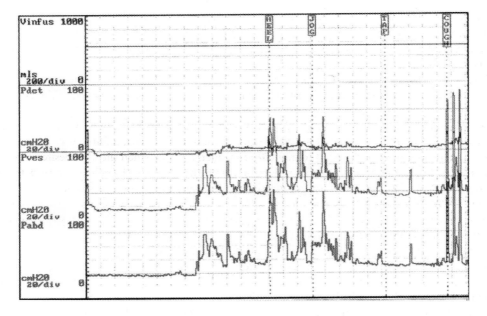

Figure 8 *Normal bladder behaviour during provocative manoeuvres of heel bouncing, jogging, listening to running water and coughing*

(a)

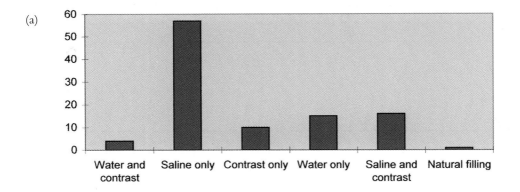

(b)

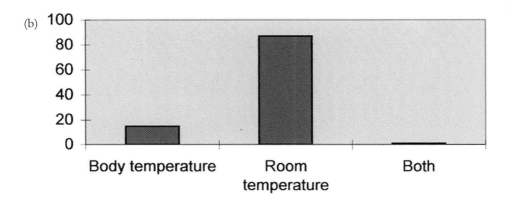

(c)

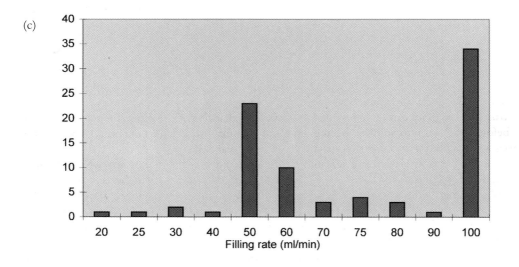

Figure 9 *(a) Infusion fluids used for cystometry in the UK; (b) temperature of infusion fluids used for cystometry in the UK; (c) filling rates used for cystometry in the UK; the vertical axis is the number of centres carrying out urodynamics*

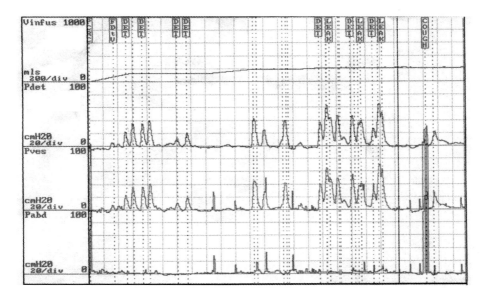

Figure 10 *Phasic detrusor overactivity during filling (with leakage episodes tagged at the top of the trace)*

Detrusor overactivity

A common finding in women undergoing urodynamic measurements is detrusor overactivity (this used to be termed detrusor instability). It is seen as involuntary detrusor contractions occurring during the storage phase of urodynamics (before 'permission to void' has been granted). A marked example is shown in Figure 10, where fluctuations are seen in both the p_{det} and in the p_{ves} recordings, but not p_{abd} during bladder filling. Another example is shown in Figure 11, when listening to running water has provoked uninhibited contractions.

However, not all activity seen in the p_{det} trace is detrusor overactivity. The fluctuations seen in the p_{det} recording in Figure 12 is not detrusor overactivity because they are seen in p_{abd} and not p_{ves}. They are simply rectal contractions.

Detrusor overactivity can be subdivided as phasic (i.e. characteristic pressure fluctuations at any stage before 'permission to void' has been granted) or terminal (i.e. a single involuntary contraction occurring at maximum cystometric capacity, resulting in leakage).[2]

Detrusor overactivity is of clinical significance if it is accompanied by symptoms such as urgency or leakage. The magnitude of the rise in p_{det} is irrelevant in determining whether any overactivity is clinically significant. Infection, inflammation, tumour, stone and neurogenic pathology can all be triggering factors for detrusor overactivity, and further investigation may be needed if overactivity is detected. However, many women have detrusor overactivity that appears to be idiopathic in nature. It can also be influenced by hormonal status.[27]

Detrusor overactivity can be detected (with a reasonable sensitivity and specificity of 80%) by simple cystometry.[28,29] This involves connecting a vertical tube to an intravesical catheter and observing whether the meniscus (the height of which is a measure of pressure) fluctuates. This is useful when conventional urodynamics is unavailable and in an elderly population.

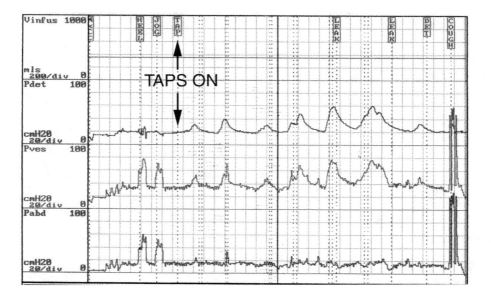

Figure 11 *Phasic detrusor activity after listening to running water*

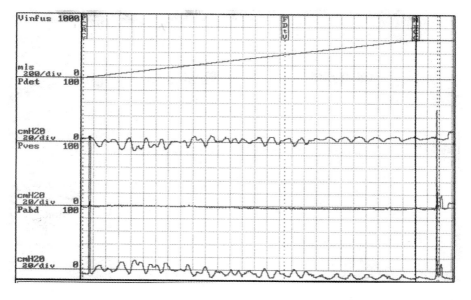

Figure 12 *Pressure fluctuations in the p_{det} trace due to rectal contractions rather than detrusor overactivity (note the absence of pressure fluctuations in the p_{ves} trace)*

Low-compliance bladders

The bladder can normally accommodate a reasonable amount of fluid without any major change in pressure while it does so. Some bladders become 'stiffer' as a result of structural changes such as those induced by radiotherapy. These are characterised by a large change in pressure as the bladder fills and often its capacity is reduced.

Compliance is defined as the change in volume measured relative to the change in pressure; in a low-compliance bladder this would be less than 30 ml/cmH$_2$O.

If there are indications of low compliance during filling cystometry, it is good practice to stop or reduce bladder filling temporarily and observe the detrusor pressure. If the detrusor pressure remains high then low compliance is the correct interpretation. If the detrusor pressure drops to normal levels then it simply means that the filling rate was too fast for that bladder to accommodate that amount of fluid.

High-compliance bladders

Some bladders can accept large volumes of fluid with little change in pressure. These 'floppy' bladders are generally neurogenic in origin and, although they can usually accommodate much more than one litre of fluid, it would probably be only of academic interest to fill these bladders with any more than this during cystometry.

Urodynamic stress incontinence

Another common finding during the storage phase of urodynamics is that of urodynamic stress incontinence (formerly termed genuine stress incontinence).[2] Leakage from the urethra is observed (or remotely detected) when the abdominal pressure is raised (usually by coughing) without any evidence of simultaneous detrusor activity (Figure 13).

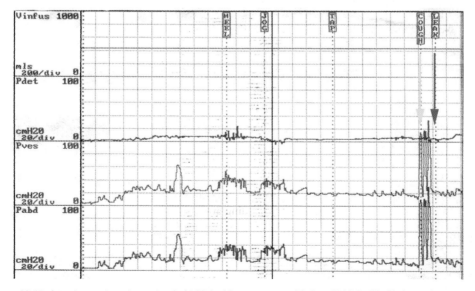

Figure 13 *Urodynamic stress incontinence (coughs highlighted by grey arrow and leakage highlighted by black arrow)*

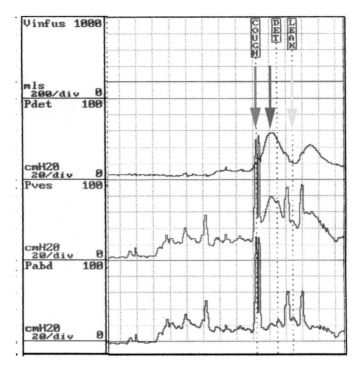

Figure 14 *Cough-induced detrusor overactivity (coughs highlighted by first black arrow, detrusor contraction highlighted by second black arrow and leakage highlighted by grey arrow)*

Coughing has also provoked leakage in the example shown in Figure 14. However, here the coughing has triggered some detrusor overactivity and it is this that has led to the leakage rather than an incompetent urethra.

PRESSURE-FLOW STUDIES

These are usually carried out at the end of filling cystometry. The filling catheter is removed from the bladder but the intravesical and abdominal pressure lines are left in place. The woman then sits on a flow meter and empties her bladder (preferably in private).

Figure 15 shows a normal pressure-flow study. The usual sequence of events is for the pelvic floor to relax, the bladder then to contract, and flow eventually occurs. The presence of a small diameter pressure line (or even a double-lumen catheter) should not impair flow to any great extent (provided it is no greater than 8 French gauge[1]) so the normal flowrates discussed in the free flowrate section are also applicable to this investigation. The detrusor pressure at the point of maximum flow ($p_{det.Qmax}$) for normal female voiding appears to be predominantly between 12 and 34 cmH$_2$O for a general cross-section of mainly parous women[30] and slightly higher 23–47 cmH$_2$O for young nulliparous women.[31]

There are some women who completely empty their bladders with a normal maximum flowrate but do not generate a detrusor contraction. They appear predominantly to relax the pelvic floor and urethra. This phenomenon seems to be a variation of normal and is more often encountered in women with urodynamic stress incontinence.[32]

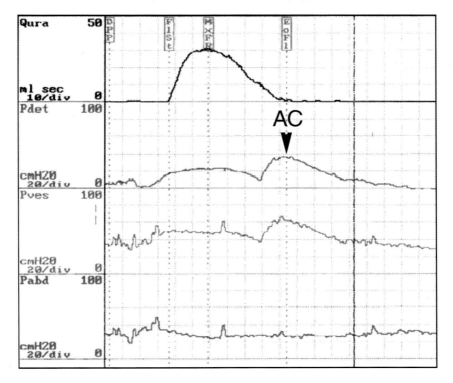

Figure 15 *Normal pressure-flow study with flow (top trace) preceded by a detrusor contraction (second from top trace); AC = after-contraction*

Occasionally, the detrusor pressure can rise at the end of the void and this is known as an after-contraction (Figure 15). This is sometimes an artefact caused by the pressure sensor hitting the wall of the bladder (and is more frequently seen with catheter mounted transducers). However, it can be a physiological event but its clinical significance is unknown.

Women can have obstructed voiding caused by a urethral stricture, kinking of the urethra by genitourinary prolapse, or even failure of the urethra to relax properly. Figure 16 shows a typical example with a long, poor, protracted stream being driven by an abnormally high detrusor pressure. Unlike male voiding, where there is a plethora of data on normal and abnormal voiding pressures and flow, the same does not exist for women. However, a composite diagram of the different schools of thought regarding parameters for female obstructed voiding appears in the report of the Second International Consultation on Incontinence.[1] Analysis of data presented in 1987, comparing voiding in women with normal diameter (≥ 8 mm) or reduced calibre (< 8 mm) urethras,[29] suggests a simple guideline: if the ratio of the maximum flowrate (in ml/s) to the detrusor pressure (in cmH_2O) at maximum flow is greater than one, then voiding is not obstructed. This cut off has a sensitivity of 89% and a specificity of 86%.

Women can also have poor flowrates because the detrusor is underactive and often this type of voiding is accompanied by abdominal straining. However, although it seems intuitively as if such women would be at most risk of developing voiding difficulty after incontinence surgery, there is no evidence that this is so.[9,33]

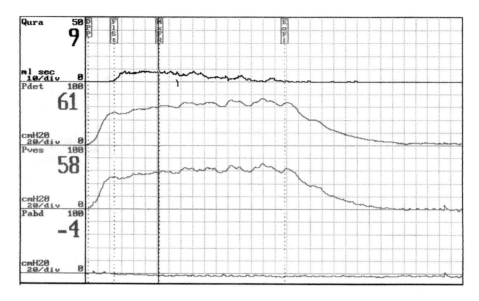

Figure 16 *Outflow obstruction in a woman; the figures displayed on the left indicate the value of each parameter at the point of maximum flow*

Indeed, pressure-flow studies have no predictive value for voiding difficulty after surgical intervention.[1] It appears that post-void residual assessment,[33] maximum flowrate,[9] and abdominal straining during voiding[10] fare better in this respect.

There has been a suggestion that detrusor pressure at the commencement of urine flow ($p_{det\ open}$) is predictive of success for colposuspension.[34] A report published in 2004 suggested that this is not the case, although elevation of this pressure (i.e. elevating the pressure needed to open the urethra and establish flow) is necessary for success.[35]

URETHRAL FUNCTION TESTS

Tests of the urethra's ability to contain urine within the bladder fall into two main categories: measurements of urethral pressure and measurements of leak point pressure.

Urethral pressure measurements

Several techniques to measure closure of the urethra have been used: the perfused side-hole catheter[36] (the 'Brown and Wickham' technique), liquid filled balloons,[37] air charged balloons,[38,39] and catheter mounted pressure transducers. Moving the device along the urethra from the bladder gives a urethral pressure profile (although, strictly speaking, devices which do not use air or fluid to interface with the transducer actually measure force and not pressure). The main parameters measured from such a profile are the maximum urethral closure pressure (MUCP), which is defined as the maximum pressure measured in the urethra relative to bladder pressure. The other is the functional profile length, or functional urethral length, which is defined as that length of the urethra that generates a pressure over and above bladder pressure. In a normal continent woman, MUCP and functional urethral length tend to be much greater (Figure 17) than in a woman with an incompetent urethra (Figure 18). However, there is a great deal of overlap between these, so the

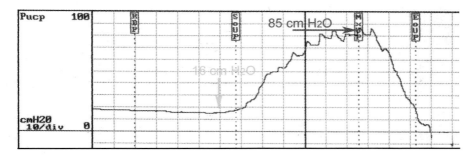

Figure 17 *Urethral pressure profile in a competent urethra with a maximum urethral closure pressure of 85–16 = 69 cmH₂O; the horizontal axis represents distance; "soUP" in the pressure at the bladder neck; the pressure to the left of "soUP" is bladder pressure; the pressure along the urethra is to the right of "soUP"*

measurement of urethral closure at rest cannot be used as a diagnostic test for an incompetent urethra.[40]

Over the last 25 years an MUCP of less than $20\,cmH_2O$ has been termed the 'low-pressure urethra' and has been particularly associated with intrinsic sphincter deficiency; an incompetent urethra in the absence of bladder neck hypermobility. Initial findings suggested that women treated with colposuspension were less likely to have a successful outcome if they had a low-pressure urethra,[41] but subsequent work has shown that women with a low-pressure urethra respond equally well to colposuspension or a sling procedure.[42] The success of tension-free vaginal tape appears to be unaffected by the presence of an MUCP of less than $20\,cmH_2O$ or by whether it is a secondary rather than a primary procedure.[43]

Apart from measuring urethral pressure at rest, it is possible to carry out a stress urethral pressure profile.[44] This involves recording increases in urethral pressure as a patient coughs or strains and measuring them relative to bladder pressure during the same manoeuvre. This test has not been proved to be clinically useful. However, a different technique of looking at the urethra under conditions of 'stress' emerged in 2002[45] and there may yet prove to be some value in it.

The whole subject of urethral pressure measurements was reviewed in 2002,[46] and it has been concluded that their clinical usefulness has yet to be demonstrated. They remain a research tool. Urethral pressure measurements are dependent on patient position, bladder volume, type and flexibility of the catheter, and orientation of the sensing device within the urethra. No standard has yet been established.

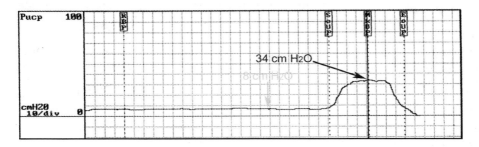

Figure 18 *Urethral pressure profile in an incompetent urethra with a maximum urethral closure pressure of 34–8 = 26 cmH₂O*

Originally, urethral pressure measurements were carried out in a retrograde fashion by putting a small funnel against the urethral meatus; fluid-filled tubing was attached to it and raised in height until the fluid started to flow along the urethra into the bladder.[47] The height of fluid required to do this is a measure of urethral pressure. Ethicon (Somerville, NJ) have taken this idea and produced a device that essentially does the same thing, the Gynecare MoniTorr[48]. It will be interesting to see if the measurement of urethral retro-resistance pressure proves to be a clinically useful tool in the assessment of urethral function.

Leak point pressures

Another way of assessing urethral closure is the measurement of Valsalva or cough leak point pressures.

For measurement of the Valsalva leak point pressure, abdominal pressure is gradually raised by the Valsalva manoeuvre until urinary leakage is detected at the meatus. The pressure required to do this (usually measured intravesically relative to atmospheric pressure) is the leak point pressure; the lower the leak point pressure, the less competent the urethra. It has been reported that a Valsalva leak point pressure of less than $60\,cmH_2O$ is equivalent to an MUCP of less than $20\,cmH_2O$ and that this is indicative of intrinsic sphincter deficiency.[49] This measurement is dependent on bladder volume,[50] size of urethral catheter,[51] patient position,[52] and what a woman interprets as a Valsalva manoeuvre.

In view of these difficulties and the nonphysiological nature of the Valsalva manoeuvre, coughing and gradually increasing its intensity until leakage occurs is another way of measuring leak point pressures.[53] This is technically more difficult to achieve and measure compared with Valsalva leak point pressures and has yet to demonstrate any conclusive clinical usefulness.

Apart from these two types of abdominal leak point pressures, it is also possible to measure detrusor leak point pressure. This is the value of the detrusor pressure, in the absence of any rise in abdominal pressure, when leakage occurs. It is of use in women with neurogenic lower urinary tract problems[1] because higher values are associated with greater risk of upper urinary tract damage.[54]

SUMMARY

Urodynamics is the only objective means of establishing the ability of the lower urinary tract to contain and expel urine. Although many of the tests still need refinement, urodynamics is essential for understanding the pathophysiology of lower urinary tract dysfunction and for measuring the functional changes induced by new therapeutic interventions

Urodynamic investigations show some variability[55] and may be worth repeating if initial testing fails to give a diagnosis. However, when conventional urodynamics has failed to give a diagnosis, or in selected primary cases, videourodynamics or ambulatory urodynamics may be appropriate.

Videourodynamics is a urodynamic investigation carried out with simultaneous imaging (usually radiography) of the lower urinary tract.[56] It can be carried out as a primary investigation (but the cost and significant exposure to X-rays probably limit its primary use to complicated continence problems). It is particularly useful in investigating women who have continuing urinary problems postoperatively.[57]

Ambulatory urodynamic monitoring is the use of a portable recorder to measure bladder pressures over a long period of time (usually four hours, but it can be up to 24 hours) while the patient is carrying out normal activities. A greater incidence of uninhibited detrusor contractions is seen during ambulatory urodynamics[58] so it is important to remember that only those associated with symptoms are likely to be of clinical significance.

In a clinical setting, it is not necessary for every woman with lower urinary tract dysfunction to undergo urodynamics. It is perfectly acceptable to treat urinary problems conservatively (with physiotherapy or pharmacological agents) after just taking a careful history and carrying out a clinical examination. However, history and examination should be supplemented by urodynamics (uroflowmetry, filling cystometry and pressure-flow studies) when surgical intervention is planned, in order to confirm the diagnosis and perhaps to aid procedure selection. It is also worth considering urodynamics when a patient has failed conservative therapy, even if further conservative therapy is being contemplated, to avoid wasting patients' time and healthcare resources by going down an inappropriate route because of an inaccurate diagnosis.

Urodynamics is a safe procedure with a small (2–3%) incidence of morbidity.[59,60] However, it is a skilled investigation and needs to be carried out by appropriately trained personnel, whether physician, nurse, clinical scientist, physiological measurement technician or other healthcare professional. The lack of appropriate training opportunities[61] has been a cause of concern for many years and has led to courses being set up nationally to address this problem. The process has now been further addressed by the Royal College of Obstetricians and Gynaecologists, with the Special Skills Committee setting up a training/accreditation module in June 2002.

References

1. Batista J, Bauer S, Griffiths D, Hilton P, Homma P, Kramer G, *et al*. Urodynamics. In: Abrams P, Cardozo L, Khoury S, Werin A, editors. *Incontinence*. Plymouth: Plymbridge Distributors; 2002. p. 317–72.

2. Abrams P, Cardozo L, Fall M, Griffiths D, Rosier P, Ulmsten U, *et al*. The standardisation of terminology of lower urinary tract function: report from the Standardisation Sub-committee of the International Continence Society. *Neurourol Urodyn* 2002;21:167–78.

3. Schafer W, Abrams P, Liao L, Mattiasson A, Pesce F, Spangberg A, *et al*. Good urodynamic practices: uroflowmetry, filling cystometry, and pressure-flow studies. *Neurourol Urodyn* 2002;21:261–74.

4. Haylen BT, Ashby D, Sutherst JR, Frazer MI, West CR. Maximum and average urine flow rates in normal male and female populations – the Liverpool nomograms. *Br J Urol* 1989;64:330–8.

5. Lavin J, Hosker G, Smith ARB. Voiding throughout the menstrual cycle in healthy females. *26th Annual Meeting of the International Continence Society, 27–30 August 1996, Athens, Greece*. p. 143–4. Abstract 179.

6. Timmerman A, van Mastrigt R. Volume dependence of maximum and average flowrate. *Neurourol Urodyn* 2002;21:340–1.

7. Moore KH, Richmond DH, Sutherst JR, Imrie AH, Hutton JL. Crouching over the toilet seat: prevalence among British gynaecological outpatients and its effect upon micturition. *Br J Obstet Gynaecol* 1991;98:569–72.

8. Hosker GL, Bryant AM, Wright G, Kilcoyne PM, Lord JC, Smith ARB. A comparison of normal saline and Urografin 150 for cystometry in women. *29th Annual Meeting of the International Continence Society, 23–26 August 1999, Denver, CO, USA*. p. 420–1. Abstract 345.

9. McLennan MT, Melick CF, Bent AE. Clinical and urodynamic predictors of delayed voiding after fascia lata suburethral sling. *Obstet Gynecol* 1998;92:608–12.

10. Bombier L, Freeman RM, Perkins EP, Williams MP, Shaw SR. Why do women have voiding dysfunction and *de novo* detrusor instability after colposuspension? *BJOG* 2002;109:402–12.

11. Garnett S, Abrams P. The role of urodynamics. In: MacLean AB, Cardozo L, editors. *Incontinence in Women*. London: RCOG Press; 2002. p. 61–75.

12. Abrams P. *Urodynamics*, 2nd ed. London: Springer-Verlag; 1997.

13. Nunns D, Smith AR, Hosker G. Reagent strip testing of urine for significant bacteriuria in a urodynamic clinic. *Br J Urol* 1995;76:87–9.

14. Buchsbaum G, Albushies D. Correlation between urine dipstick and urine culture in screening women with urinary incontinence for urinary tract infection. *32nd Annual Meeting of the International Continence Society, 28–30 August 2002, Heidelberg, Germany*. p. 260. Abstract 383.

15. Kenton K, Raza F, FitzGerald MP, Brubaker L. Accuracy of urine dipstick analysis in a urogynecologic population. *32nd Annual Meeting of the International Continence Society, 28–30 August 2002, Heidelberg, Germany*. p. 260–1. Abstract 384.

16. Wall LL, Hewitt JK, Helms MJ. Are vaginal and rectal pressures equivalent approximations of one another for the purpose of performing subtracted cystometry? *Obstet Gynecol* 1995;85:488–93.

17. Sullivan J, Lewis P, Howell S, Williams T, Shepherd A, Abrams P. The effect of pressure measurement technique in urodynamics. *Neurourol Urodyn* 2000;19:478–9.

18. Abrams P, Blaivas JG, Stanton S, Andersen JT. Standardisation of terminology of lower urinary tract function. *Neurourol Urodyn* 1988;7:403–26.

19. Klevmark B. Natural pressure:volume curves and conventional cystometry. *Scand J Urol Nephrol Suppl* 1999;201:1–4.

20. Sullivan J, Bulmer P, Lewis P, Howell S, Williams T, Shepherd A, *et al*. Small changes in filling medium temperature and filling rate affect urodynamic results. *Neurourol Urodyn* 2001;20:567–8.

21. Sethia KK, Smith JC. The effect of pH and lignocaine on detrusor instability. *Br J Urol* 1987;60:516.

22. Lavin JM, Hosker GL, Smith ARB. Does urinary pH influence micturition desire? *Neurourol Urodyn* 1997;16:396–7.

23. Swithinbank L, Rogers C, Ellis-Jones J, Abrams P. The effect of altering urinary pH on urinary symptoms in women. *Neurourol Urodyn* 2000;19:527–8.

24. Gluck T, Wagg A, Fry C, Malone-Lee J. The effects of biochemical changes to filling media during urodynamic testing in women with lower urinary tract symptoms. *Neurourol Urodyn* 2002;21:355.

25. Lee F, Susser J, Mundy A, Foxall P, Craggs M. Does urinary sodium affect bladder sensations in patients with an overactive bladder during urodynamics? *32nd Annual Meeting of the International Continence Society, 28–30 August 2002, Heidelberg, Germany*. p. 102–3. Abstract 181.

26. Hosker GL, Kilcoyne PM, Smith ARB. Urodynamic practice in the UK. *28th Annual Meeting of the International Continence Society, 14–17 September 1998, Jerusalem, Israel*. p. 66–7. Abstract 156.

27. Wall LL, Warrell DW. Detrusor instability associated with menstruation. Case report. *Br J Obstet Gynaecol* 1989;96:737–8.

28. Ouslander J, Leach G, Abelson S, Staskin D, Blaustein J, Raz S. Simple vs multichannel cystometry in the evaluation of bladder function in an incontinent, geriatric population. *J Urol* 1988;140:1482–6.

29. Sutherst JR, Brown MC. Comparison of single and multichannel cystometry in diagnosing bladder instability. *Br Med J (Clin Res Ed)* 1984;288:1720–2.

30. Hosker GL. The effect of reduced urethral calibre on voiding in women – impeded flow. *17th International Continence Society Meeting, 3–5 September 1987, Bristol, UK*. p. 74–5.

31. de Wachter S, Pauwels E, van Meel TD, Wyndaele J. Comparison of voiding dynamics in genuine stress incontinent women and normal healthy volunteers. *Neurourol Urodyn* 2002;21:432–3.

32. Karram MM, Partoll L, Bilotta V, Angel O. Factors affecting detrusor contraction strength during voiding in women. *Obstet Gynecol* 1997;90:723–6.

33. Kobak WH, Walters MD, Piedmonte MR. Determinants of voiding after three types of incontinence surgery: a multivariable analysis. *Obstet Gynecol* 2001;97:86–91.

34. Digesu GA, Khullar V, Cardozo L, Sethna F, Toozs-Hobson P, Bidmead J. Pre-operative pressure flow studies: do they predict the outcome of continence surgery? *Neurourol Urodyn* 2000;19:402–3.

35. Dolan LM, Smith ARB, Hosker GL. Opening detrusor pressure and the influence of age on success following colposuspension. *Neurourol Urodyn* 2004;23:10–15.

36. Brown M, Wickham JE. The urethral pressure profile. *Br J Urol* 1969;41:211–17.

37. Lose G. Simultaneous recording of pressure and cross-sectional area in the female urethra: a study of urethral closure function in healthy and stress incontinent women. *Neurourol Urodyn* 1992;11:55–89.

38. Davila GW, Pollak J, Neimark M. A comparison between air-charged and microtransducer catheters in the urodynamic evaluation of urethral function. *32nd Annual Meeting of the International Continence Society, 28–30 August 2002, Heidelberg, Germany*. p. 106–7. Abstract 186.

39. Pollak JT, Neimark M, Davila GW. A comparison between air-charged and microtransducer catheters in the urodynamic evaluation of urethral function. *Int Urogynecol J Pelvic Floor Dysfunct* 2002;13 Suppl 1:S9.

40. Hilton P, Stanton SL. Urethral pressure measurement by microtransducer: the results in symptom-free women and in those with genuine stress incontinence. *Br J Obstet Gynaecol* 1983;90:919.

41. Bowen LW, Sand PK, Ostergard DR, Franti CE. Unsuccessful Burch retropubic urethropexy: a case–controlled urodynamic study. *Am J Obstet Gynecol* 1989;160:452–8.

42. Sand PK, Winkler H, Blackhurst DW, Culligan PJ. A prospective randomized study comparing modified Burch retropubic urethropexy and suburethral sling for treatment of genuine stress incontinence with a low pressure urethra. *Am J Obstet Gynecol* 2000;182:30–4.

43. Rardin CR, Kohli N, Rosenblatt PL, Miklos JR, Moore R, Strohsnitter WC. Tension-free vaginal tape: outcomes among women with primary and recurrent stress urinary incontinence. *Obstet Gynecol*, 2002;100:893–7.

44. Bump RC, Copeland WE, Hurt WG, Fantl JMA. Dynamic urethral pressure/profilometry pressure transmission ratio determinations in stress-incontinent and stress-continent subjects. *Am J Obstet Gynecol* 1988;159:749–55.

45. Wolters M, Methfessel MD, Goepel C, Koelbl H. Computer-assisted virtual urethral pressure profile in the assessment of female genuine stress incontinence. *Obstet Gynecol* 2002;99:69–74.

46. Lose G, Griffiths D, Hosker G, Kulseng-Hanssen S, Perucchini D, Schafer W, *et al*. Standardisation of urethral pressure measurement: report from the Standardisation Sub-committee of the International Continence Society. *Neurourol Urodyn* 2002;21:258–60.

47. Bonney V. On diurnal incontinence of urine in women. *J Obstet Gynaecol Br Empire* 1923;30:358–65.

48. Slack M, Culligan P, Tracey M, Hunsicker, K, Patel B, Sumerary M. Relationship of urethral retro–resistance pressure to urodynamic measurements and incontinence severity. *Neurourol Urodyn* 2004;23:109–14.

49. McGuire EJ, Fitzpatrick CC, Wan J, Bloom D, Sanvordenker J, Ritchey M, *et al*. Clinical assessment of urethral sphincter function. *J Urol* 1993;150:1452–4.

50. Faerber GJ, Vashi AR. Variations in Valsalva leak point pressure with increasing vesical volume. *J Urol* 1998;159:1909–11.

51. Decter RM, Harpster L. Pitfalls in determination of leak point pressure. *J Urol* 1992;148:588–91.

52. Pajoncini P, Costantini E, Lombi R, Guercini F, Porena M. Does position modify the valsalva leak point pressure? *Neurourol Urodyn* 2002;21:342–3.

53. Peschers UM, Jundt K, Dimpfl T. Differences between cough and Valsalva leak-point pressure in stress incontinent women. *Neurourol Urodyn* 2000;19:677–81.

54. Combs AJ, Horowitz M. A new technique for assessing detrusor leak point pressure in patients with spina bifida. *J Urol* 1996;156:757–60.

55. MacLean AB, Cardozo L. Urodynamics and imaging for diagnosis (discussion). In: MacLean AB, Cardozo L, editors. *Incontinence in Women*. London: RCOG Press; 2002. p. 91–9.

56. McGuire EJ, Cespedes RD, Cross CA, O'Connell HE. Videourodynamic studies. *Urol Clin North Am* 1996;23:309–21.

57. Saxton HM. Urodynamics in the investigation of women with frequency, urgency, and incontinence and voiding difficulties. *Urol Radiol* 1991;13:48–57.

58. Heslington K, Hilton P. The incidence of detrusor instability by ambulatory monitoring and conventional cystometry pre and post colposuspension. *Neurourol Urodyn* 1995;14:416–17.

59. Steen W, Vejlsgaard R. Diagnostic catheterisation and bacteriuria in women with urinary incontinence. *Br J Urol* 1978;50:106–8.

60. Brostrom S, Jennum P, Lose G. Morbidity of urodynamic investigation in healthy women. *Int Urogynecol J Pelvic Floor Dysfunct* 2002;13 Suppl 1:S62.

61. Hosker GL, Kilcoyne PM, Lord JC, Smith AR. Urodynamic services, personnel and training in the United Kingdom. *Br J Urol* 1997;79:159–62.

19

First trimester ultrasound: a dating or a detailed scan?

Jon A Hyett

INTRODUCTION

The rapid development of ultrasound technology has led to substantial improvements in resolution so that it is now possible to examine fetal anatomy in detail by the end of the first trimester of pregnancy. Booking scans were initially introduced to allow accurate dating of pregnancy, but the improvements in resolution have shown that features such as increased nuchal translucency (NT) provide important information about fetal wellbeing. Early prenatal diagnosis is now more likely to be limited by our ability to determine whether an embryological process has been completed appropriately, or by our failure to recognise the features of primary pathology rather than those of secondary pathological change that we are used to seeing at more advanced gestations.

PREGNANCY DATING IN THE FIRST TRIMESTER

First trimester ultrasound was shown to be a reliable means of detecting fetal heart activity 30 years ago.[1] Further studies demonstrated that the crown–rump length could be accurately measured using this technique, and charts for determining gestational age with this measurement were constructed.[2] Indeed, the crown–rump length formula described by Robinson and Fleming[3] is still used in many ultrasound software programs that calculate gestational age.

The routine use of first trimester ultrasound has several potential benefits. Three percent of apparently normal pregnancies presenting for a first ultrasound examination at 12 weeks of gestation are not viable.[4] Diagnosis of miscarriage in an elective setting enables us to provide women with better medical and surgical care and improved psychological support. Dating pregnancy by menstrual history has been shown to be inaccurate in 11–42%.[5,6] This has implications for investigations such as biochemical screening for chromosomal abnormalities and for the timing of the second trimester anomaly scan. Inaccurate dating continues to cause problems up until delivery, with increased rates of induction of labour for postmaturity.[7] The accuracy of pregnancy dating is improved by offering a scan to measure fetal biometry at the first antenatal visit.[8] Dating is most precise when using crown–rump length measurements prior to 13 weeks of gestation and the biparietal diameter beyond this time.[9]

The performance of second trimester biochemical screening tests for chromosomal abnormalities is improved by ultrasound dating of pregnancy. Accurate dating reduces the variance of serum marker levels, improving the sensitivity and specificity of the test. For the triple test, the use of ultrasound improves detection for Down syndrome from 58% to 67% while maintaining a 5% false positive rate.[10] The inclusion of a routine ultrasound examination for dating purposes not only offers women a more efficient test, but is also cost-effective for healthcare providers.[11]

ULTRASOUND SCREENING IN THE FIRST TRIMESTER

Screening for chromosomal abnormality

Many centres in the UK now include a routine dating scan within the schedule of antenatal care. Although this has frequently been introduced for dating purposes, the potential for this investigation to become a cornerstone of antenatal screening is widely recognised. NT is increased in a large proportion of chromosomally abnormal fetuses at 11–14 weeks of gestation and has been shown to be the most powerful single marker for trisomy 21.[12] NT is best measured in a mid-sagittal section, which is also the best section for accurate assessment of crown–rump length. Algorithms for accurate risk assessment that take account of the fact that NT naturally increases with advancing gestation have been developed in a similar way to those used in serum screening programmes. The technique for NT measurement has been carefully described, a process of certified training introduced, and a system of continuous audit developed so that healthcare professionals involved in antenatal screening can have confidence in the reproducibility of risk assessment between individual sonographers in different centres. Data on the sensitivity and specificity of NT as a screening tool for chromosomal abnormalities has been reported in several large series of unselected women, showing a detection rate of 83.3% for a false positive rate of 5.7% (Table 1).[13–28]

Effective screening with NT relies on the availability of high-quality ultrasound machines, investment in staff training and the use of continuous audit to ensure that the quality of the ultrasound result is maintained.[29–31] The association between NT and trisomy 21 is, however, so well recognised, that many centres using other screening methods feel it would be inappropriate not to report or to offer karyotyping for a significant increase in NT. The implications of this policy also need to be examined. In one centre using an effective second trimester screening programme, only women with an NT ≥ 99th centile were counselled as being at high risk for pregnancy affected by

Table 1 *Screening studies reporting data for over 1000 women to describe the sensitivity and specificity of NT as a tool to screen for trisomy 21 at 10–14 weeks of gestation*

Reference	*n*	Screening cut off	FPR (%)	DR (%)
Szabo *et al.*, 1995[13]	3380	NT > 3.0 mm	1.6	28 of 31 (90)
Taipale *et al.*, 1997[14]	6939	NT > 3.0 mm	0.8	4 of 6 (67)
Hafner *et al*,. 1998[15]	4233	NT > 2.5 mm	1.7	3 of 7 (43)
Pajkrt *et al.*, 1998[16]	1473	NT > 3.0 mm	2.2	6 of 9 (67)
Theodoropoulos *et al.*, 1998[17]	3550	Risk > 1 in 300	4.9	10 of 11 (91)
Economides *et al.*, 1998[18]	2281	NT > 99th centile	0.4	6 of 8 (75)
Thilaganathan *et al.*, 1999[19]	11398	Risk > 1 in 200	4.7	16 of 21 (76)
Schwarzler *et al.*, 1999[20]	4523	Risk > 1 in 270	4.7	10 of 12 (83)
Krantz *et al.*, 2000[21]	5809	Risk > 1 in 250	5.0	26 of 33 (79)
Gasiorek-Wiens *et al.*, 2001[22]	21959	NT > 95th centile	9.6	174 of 210 (83)
Zoppi *et al.*, 2001[23]	12495	NT > 1.5 MoM	5.0	52 of 64 (81)
Brizot *et al.*, 2001[24]	2996	NT > 95th centile	5.8	7 of 10 (70)
Panbuarana *et al.*, 2001[25]	2353	NT > 2.5 mm	2.8	2 of 2 (100)
Wayda *et al.*, 2001[26]	7044	NT > 2.5 mm	4.5	17 of 17 (100)
Wapner, 2002[27]	8216	Risk > 1 in 270	11.9	50 of 61 (82.0)
Comas *et al.*, 2002[28]	8673	NT > 95th centile	5.0	43 of 43 (100)
Total	107322		5.7	454 of 545 (83)

FPR = false positive rate; DR = detection rate; MoM = multiples of the median

Table 2 *Studies examining the implementation of combined ultrasound (NT) and biochemical (pregnancy-associated plasma protein A and free beta-human chorionic gonadotropin) screening at 10–14 weeks of gestation*

Reference	n	False positive rate (%)	Detection rate for trisomy 21 (%)
Orlandi et al., 1997[34]	744	5.0	6 of 7 (86)
Biagiotti et al., 1998[35]	232	5.0	24 of 32 (75)
Benattar et al., 1999[36]	1656	5.0	5 of 5 (100)
De Biasio et al., 1999[37]	1467	3.3	11 of 13 (85)
de Graaf et al., 1999[38]	300	5.0	31 of 37 (84)
Spencer et al., 1999[39]	1156	5.0	187 of 210 (89)
Krantz et al., 2000[21]	5718	5.0	30 of 33 (91)
Spencer, 2001[40]	4088	5.0	6 of 7 (86)
Schuchter et al., 2002[41]	4939	5.0	12 of 14 (86)
Wapner et al., 2002[27]	8514	5.0	48 of 61 (79)
Total	28814	4.9	360 of 419 (86)

chromosomal abnormality. This group included 83% of pregnancies affected by trisomy 21, significantly reducing the prevalence of trisomy 21 in the population undergoing biochemical screening, with a six-fold reduction in the positive predictive value of this, second, test.[32] The problems related to sequential screening can be removed by combining risks from biochemical markers and ultrasound to give a single risk estimate for chromosomal abnormality. A prospective study (published in 2002) of 15000 women has shown that a test of this type, combining NT, beta-human chorionic gonadotrophin and PAPP-A at a single visit can detect 90% of trisomy pregnancies for a 5% false positive rate.[33] A further 11 studies reported in the literature support this view, showing that combined first trimester screening is an attractive (Table 2)[21,27,34–41] and cost-effective[42] option.

Although the first trimester combined test offers a comprehensive and effective form of screening for Down syndrome, there may be other markers that can also be taken into account, potentially improving detection rates or being used to reduce the false positive rate. Two ultrasound markers that have been put forward for this purpose are absence of the nasal bone and a Doppler sign, reversal of the A wave seen in the waveform of the ductus venosus. Down first described the features of children affected by trisomy 21 in 1866.[43] As well as including the feature we now describe in fetal life as NT he described these children as having small noses. Cicero et al.[44] examined the facial features of 701 fetuses prior to karyotyping in the first trimester. They showed that 73% of those affected by trisomy 21 had an absent nasal bone at this gestation, compared with only 0.5% of chromosomally normal fetuses. Using this marker in combination with NT could improve detection to 85%, at the same time reducing the false positive rate to 1%. Matias et al.[45] followed a similar (but separate) series of fetuses, assessing the ductus venosus waveform profile prior to karyotyping. The 'A wave' was reversed in 90.5% of chromosomally abnormal fetuses, but only in 3.1% of normal fetuses. This could also be used to improve the efficiency of first trimester screening prior to invasive testing.

Although both of these markers have been shown to perform well in a tertiary referral centre, some other publications are not so favourable. With less experience, it would be easy to report an 'absent' nasal bone because it had not been imaged successfully rather than being truly absent. Similarly, the skin edge of the nose may be mistaken as bony echogenicity in cases where the nose is in fact absent. Until the criteria for measurement of this marker are better established, and sonographers have been adequately trained in its measurement, it may be better not to rely on this finding for screening purposes. Demonstrating the ductus venosus waveform is also difficult, and this sign would therefore not appear to be useful as a routine screening tool. It has, however, been suggested that both these markers could be used after high-risk women are referred to a tertiary referral centre, prior to chorionic villus sampling being offered, and potentially enabling a reduction in the false positive rate associated with invasive testing.

An alternative approach to examining the use of markers in the first trimester is to look at the prevalence of those traditionally used at the time of the 20-week anomaly scan. A study of 5385 women in which three markers were examined – renal pyelectasis, intracardiac echogenic foci and choroid plexus cysts – found a prevalence of 0.9%, 0.6% and 2.2% respectively in chromosomally normal fetuses.[46] This was a similar prevalence to that seen in the same group at the time of the 20-week scan. Pyelectasis and intracardiac echogenic foci both appeared to be associated with chromosomal abnormality and would have improved detection for aneuploidy by 3% if these markers had been used in addition to the identification of increased NT (>99th centile) and major structural anomalies. Another study has suggested that the prevalence of isolated mild pyelectasis decreases with advancing gestation.[47] It may, therefore, be better to use this marker in the first trimester, assign a likelihood ratio for its presence, and therefore include the risk with that given by combined screening. Further work would need to be done so that a likelihood ratio and independence from other markers could be established. Certainly, the use of first trimester screening has such a strong effect on the prevalence of trisomic fetuses that it seems unlikely that markers will remain of any use at a later stage of pregnancy.[48]

Screening for structural anomalies

There are many case reports that demonstrate the ability of ultrasound to diagnose structural anomalies in the first trimester but few studies have examined the effectiveness of a routine first trimester anatomical survey. These studies suggest that, excluding nuchal abnormalities, between 25% and 45% of major anomalies may be detected by the end of the first trimester (Table 3).[49–53] Early diagnosis provides time to plan further follow-up and counselling about prognosis as well as allowing termination of pregnancy with fewer complications.

The earliest of these studies used a transvaginal approach for screening because many operators believe that the increased resolution this allows improves the definition of fetal anatomy.[54,55] Improvements in transabdominal probes mean, however, that fetal anatomy can normally be visualised adequately, and this approach has the advantage that the plane of ultrasound examination is easily altered so that appropriate fetal sections can be imaged. A sensible compromise may therefore be to complete as much of the examination as is possible using a transabdominal probe, switching to transvaginal assessment if these images are suboptimal.

Hernadi and Torocsik[49] evaluated prospectively a series of 3991 pregnancies to compare detection of fetal anomalies at 11–14 weeks of gestation with detection rates at 18 and 30 weeks of gestation. Systematic transvaginal ultrasound examination included evaluation of the anterior and posterior body contours, head, spine, stomach, kidneys, bladder and extremities; adequate views were obtained in 94% of the examinations. The prevalence of congenital anomalies in this essential low-risk population was 1.6%, including 21 pregnancies with isolated nuchal oedema or cystic hygromas (anomalies associated with high rates of chromosomal abnormality) diagnosed in the first trimester. When these 21 pregnancies are excluded, 14 (33%) of the remaining 43 fetal anomalies were detected at this stage. Although numbers become small, it appears that anomalies of some systems are easier to detect than those of others. The detection rate for central nervous system (CNS) anomalies was 42%, including the diagnosis of all cases of exencephaly and encephalocele but with poorer

Table 3 *Ultrasound detection of structural abnormalities in the late first trimester and mid second trimester of pregnancy; nuchal abnormalities (increased NT and cystic hygromas) are excluded*

Reference	Prevalence of structural anomalies %	Gestation of first scan (weeks)	Anomalies detected at first scan %	Detection of remaining anomalies at 20 weeks %	Overall detection %
Hernadi and Torocsik, 1997[49]	64/3991 (1.6)	11–14	14/43 (32.6)	9/29 (31.0)	23/43 (53.5)
D'Ottavio et al., 1997[50]	52/3490 (1.5)	13–15	17/52 (32.7)	25/35 (71.4)	42/52 (80.8)
Whitlow et al., 1999[51]	48/6443 (0.7)	11–14	22/48 (45.8)	19/26 (73.1)	41/48 (85.4)
Guariglia and Rosati, 2000[52]	40/3478 (1.2)	10–16	11/40 (27.5)	21/29 (72.4)	54/64 (84.4)
Carvalho et al., 2002[53]	66/2853 (2.3)	11–14	25/66 (37.9)	25/32 (78.1)	50/66 (75.8)
Total	270/20 255 (1.3)	–	89/249 (35.7)	99/151 (65.6)	210/273 (76.9)

detection of ventriculomegaly. Detection rates for renal/genitourinary and skeletal/limb anomalies were, however, only 13%. The poorer detection rate of some anomalies may be explained by difficulties in imaging a particular organ at such an early gestation, or the fact that the anomaly is not yet apparent at such an early stage of fetal development.

Two other series have examined prospectively the use of transvaginal ultrasound at 13–15 and 10–16 weeks of gestation.[50,51] They examined 3490 and 3478 pregnancies respectively. The detection rates for cystic hygromas and fetal hydrops (increased NT) were extremely high and these defects were frequently associated with chromosomal abnormalities. Detection rates for other structural anomalies were 33% and 28% and once again this was system dependent. CNS (45%) anomalies were often detected, but cardiac defects (17% detection) and anomalies of the face (25% detection) were frequently missed until the routine anomaly scan at 20 weeks of gestation.

Another prospective study found fetal anomalies in 92 of 6443 pregnancies (1.4%).[52] This included fetuses with increased NT, often associated with chromosomal abnormality. By excluding the data pertaining to chromosomally abnormal fetuses, it is possible to look at the detection rate of structural anomalies. Of the 48 cases with structural anomalies, 22 (45.8%) were successfully detected at 11–14 weeks of gestation. Once again, a first trimester scan appeared to be an effective means of detecting major CNS anomalies, such as anencephaly, although more subtle anomalies such as spina bifida were missed. Major abdominal wall defects were also successfully detected, but once again defects affecting the heart, the skeleton, limbs and the face were generally missed.

The fifth study, of 2853 women at 11–14 weeks of gestation, classified 130 (4.6%) fetuses with structural anomalies.[53] The apparently high prevalence was due to the inclusion of minor anomalies that would have little clinical significance postnatally, such as unilateral mild hydronephrosis. Some anomalies detected during the routine second trimester examination may not have been present at 12 weeks, an example being the two fetuses found to have ascites at this later stage. This, coupled with the fact that 910 women had no further ultrasound examination after the first trimester, makes direct comparison of first and second trimester findings more difficult. Sixty-six anomalies were classified as being major and 25 (37.8%) of these were successfully detected at 11–14 weeks. Once again, defects such as anencephaly were reliably detected while others such as skeletal and limb anomalies were frequently missed. It is interesting that the detection of cardiac defects was better in this series than in others (9 of 23 detected) and this may have been owing to a policy of detailed first trimester fetal echocardiography for all fetuses that had presented with increased NT.

The heterogeneous nature of these screening studies makes direct comparison difficult, but it appears that we should detect at least 35% of structural anomalies at this earlier stage of pregnancy, and that detection rates can be improved by developing strategies to focus on anomalies that have traditionally been missed. Further consideration of how this may be achieved is given below.

Detection of CNS anomalies

Anomalies such as anencephaly can be easily missed if the sonographer has not appreciated the fact that the ultrasound findings at this stage of pregnancy differ from those seen at 20 weeks of gestation. In one series, 8 of 31 (26%) cases were missed at the time of first trimester NT evaluation.[56] A review of the images suggested that this was because the sonographers had not recognised the signs of this major anomaly in the first trimester. The diagnosis can, however, be accurately made by demonstrating that there is acrania with no evidence of calcification of the calvarium in a transverse biparietal section. Inclusion of this view led to complete recognition of all cases in a follow-up audit. The diagnosis can be confirmed by examining a coronal section of the head, where the two cerebral lobes can be recognised 'floating' in the amniotic fluid. This has been called the 'Mickey Mouse' sign.[57]

Another cranial defect that may be diagnosed in the first trimester is an encephalocele. In 75% of cases the defect is occipital and the differential diagnosis from nuchal oedema may be made by demonstrating the bony skull defect. In one case report, the defect was noted first at 13 weeks as an empty cavity. This became a brain-filled defect at 14 weeks before resolving, until 19 weeks, when a persistent defect became obvious once again.[58] This suggests that these lesions may be dynamic in early pregnancy and cannot be ruled out by one examination alone. Indeed, another case had evidence of a bony defect at 11 weeks but no protruding sac until two weeks later.[59]

Holoprosencephaly describes a range of brain abnormalities resulting from incomplete cleavage of the forebrain. Alobar holoprosencephaly, characterised by a single monoventricular cavity and fusion of the thalami, may be recognised in the first trimester, but lobar holoprosencephaly may be more difficult to detect.[60] Holoprosencephaly is often associated with midline facial abnormalities as well as being associated with trisomy 13 and triploidy, both of which will be more prevalent in this first trimester population owing to the later effects of intrauterine lethality.[61]

CNS defects that remain difficult to detect in the first trimester include ventriculomegaly and spina bifida. The former is missed because it does not often develop before 14 weeks of gestation and the latter because it is not associated with the same signs as those that we have become accustomed to at the 20-week scan. In a first trimester screening clinic for chromosomal abnormalities, none of 29 cases of spina bifida was detected. This contrasted with the successful determination of spina bifida in three high-risk cases at 12–14 weeks of gestation.[62] This suggests that we are unlikely to detect this anomaly unless we specifically look for it, and underlines the fact that a sequential systemic examination is necessary to screen for fetal anomalies in the first trimester, just as is used at the time of the routine anomaly scan. The identification of these three cases was made primarily by the detection of the lumbosacral lesion and the demonstration of a lemon shaped head. Another group has since suggested that the shape of the head is more like an acorn than a lemon at this early gestation, and that closer examination of the cerebral peduncles shows that they run parallel to one another rather than being slightly splayed.[63] As the quality of ultrasound images continues to improve at these early gestations, brain anatomy has become easier to visualise, but it is important to review the process of embryological development to make full use of these images.

Detection of thoracic and cardiac anomalies

Cardiac anomalies are the most common cause of death due to congenital disease in infancy and childhood but are least likely to be detected during a routine 20-week anomaly scan.[64] Although specialist fetal echocardiography units achieve high levels of detection, screening a low-risk population using the four chamber view and outflow tracts has had varying success, often being dependent on operator training and experience.[65,66] A policy of referring 'high-risk' women for detailed echocardiographic assessment is also of limited benefit because only a small proportion (5%) of children born with major congenital heart disease fall into this group.[67]

Pathological studies investigating the underlying aetiology of increased NT have demonstrated an association between this first trimester sonographic finding and cardiac defects. The association is seen in both chromosomally abnormal and normal fetuses.[68,69] Retrospective analysis of a series of 30 000 pregnancies that were screened for chromosomal abnormality by measuring NT thickness at 10 + 4 to 13 + 6 weeks of gestation showed that the prevalence of major cardiac disease was halved in fetuses with an NT measurement below the 95th centile and significantly increased in fetuses with NT above the 95th centile. Indeed, referral of all fetuses with increased NT for detailed echocardiography would have allowed detection of 56% of the major cardiac defects.[70]

Several studies have now looked at this association prospectively, with variable results. The studies reported by Ghi *et al.*,[71] Mavrides *et al.*[72] and Michailidis *et al.*[73] were all conducted in London in units measuring NT in the same way, which allows relatively easy comparison. The detection rate for major cardiac disease ranged from 15% in one series to 36% in another. A fourth, Hungarian, study showed a detection rate of 51%.[74] These findings suggest that, although increased NT is not present in all cases of major congenital cardiac disease, it is a useful indicator of risk. The prevalence of cardiac disease for fetuses with NT above the 95th centile is consistently 5–7% in these studies, twice that seen in a diabetic population, reinforcing the fact that this group should be offered detailed fetal echocardiography.

Another thoracic anomaly that may be visualised at the time of the first trimester scan is a diaphragmatic hernia. The development of the diaphragm is normally complete by nine weeks of gestation. Herniation through a defect may occur at any stage beyond this, although it is more likely once the abdominal contents, which are involved in physiological herniation into the base of the cord, are returned, a process that may not be complete until 11 weeks. Although the traditional signs of a diaphragmatic hernia may, therefore, be seen at 11 weeks (demonstrating the stomach in the thorax) there may be some cases where this finding is not yet established.[75]

Nineteen cases of diaphragmatic hernia were reported in a series of 78 639 pregnancies that were scanned in the first trimester. The diagnosis was made at this stage in only one case, although it is likely that this was because anatomical assessment did not routinely include demonstration of a stomach bubble below the diaphragm rather than the fact that this sign rarely develops before the time of a later anomaly scan.[76] Seven cases (37%) had had increased NT in the first trimester and this group included five of the six neonatal deaths seen in the whole series, suggesting that increased NT may be an indicator of poor prognosis in these cases.[77]

Detection of abdominal anomalies

Herniation of the midgut into the base of the umbilical cord occurs from about eight weeks of gestation and return of the abdominal contents may not be complete until 11 weeks.[78] This feature of normal development complicates the diagnosis of exomphalos before 11 weeks of gestation, but beyond this point the diagnosis can be made by using the same criteria as those applied at the time of the traditional anomaly scan. This defect is commonly associated with trisomy 18, a chromosomal abnormality that has a high rate of intrauterine lethality. These fetuses are therefore more likely to be chromosomally abnormal when this finding is made at 11–14 weeks compared with 20 weeks of gestation.[79] Gastroschisis, a sporadic defect affecting approximately 1 in 5000 pregnancies, is also readily detected in the first trimester. In this instance the abdominal wall defect is lateral to the right side of a normally formed umbilicus, and free floating loops of bowel are seen in the amniotic pool.

The kidneys can be successfully visualised in 99% of cases by 12–13 weeks but renal agenesis may be overlooked at this gestation as the liquor volume is normal.[80] The detection of both infantile polycystic and multicystic dysplastic kidneys has been reported in the first trimester.[81,82] Detection is more likely in pregnancies known to be at risk of renal disease and may feature in the diagnosis of genetic conditions that affect multiple systems, such as Meckel–Gruber syndrome.[83] The fetal bladder can be visualised in about 50% of cases at ten weeks and in all cases by 13 weeks of gestation. The bladder is normally less than 7 mm in length at this gestation and an enlarged bladder is readily identified. Megacystis may resolve spontaneously, but karyotyping should be considered as this is also associated with chromosomal abnormalities. Extremely dilated bladders (>16 mm length) are found in fetuses with obstructive uropathy and such early diagnosis is associated with poor pregnancy outcome.[84]

Detection of skeletal and limb anomalies

Limb anomalies and skeletal defects were frequently missed in the low-risk populations screened by first trimester ultrasound (described above). This may, in part, be due to the fact that careful assessment of the limbs was not included in the sequential examination of the fetus, but may also be due to the difficulties with assessing fetal biometry at these early gestations. The upper limb in particular is relatively easy to examine at 11–14 weeks because the hands are virtually always placed in front of the face. The lower limbs can also be followed easily in transverse or longitudinal section, although it is important to remember that the natural position of the foot mimics mild talipes equinovarus. Joint position and movement can be demonstrated and will be abnormal in some severe neuromuscular abnormalities.[85] Reference ranges for long bone biometry in the first trimester of pregnancy have been published.[86] Although these seem to be helpful for the early diagnosis of some severe skeletal dysplasias, early biometric evaluation is unlikely to be helpful in less severe cases.[87] It is important to note, however, that many fetuses diagnosed with skeletal dysplasias in the first trimester of pregnancy have also been found to have increased NT.[88,89]

The placenta

The placenta is largely ignored during the 11–14-week scan but has an important place in the systematic evaluation of pregnancy. The hydatidiform mole has a similar, but subtler appearance in early pregnancy, being a complex, echogenic mass containing small cystic areas with a 'snowstorm' appearance.[90] This can be distinguished from localised areas of cystic change seen with a partial mole or with mesenchymal dysplasia.[91] Determining the position of the placenta may also be useful in predicting placenta praevia, although there will be a high false positive rate at this early gestation and 'at-risk' pregnancies should be reassessed in the third trimester.[92,93] The introduction of three-dimensional technology has led to the suggestion that calculation of placental volume may be a useful tool when screening for chromosomal abnormality; preliminary data suggest that placental volume is reduced in aneuploidy pregnancies.[94]

Multiple pregnancy

The early diagnosis of a twin pregnancy allows confident prediction of chorionicity by the demonstration of the 'λ' sign in dichorionic pregnancies and the 'T' sign in monochorionic pregnancies.[95] This is of importance because the risks of miscarriage, perinatal death, growth retardation and preterm delivery are all significantly increased in monochorionic pregnancies, which therefore require a higher degree of surveillance.[96] NT has been shown to be an effective screening test for chromosomal abnormalities in twin pregnancies, and many clinicians believe that it has a distinct advantage over biochemical screening in this respect.[97] Measurement of NT is an important part of sonographic assessment before continuing with multifetal pregnancy reduction, and in monochorionic twin pregnancies a disparity in NT measurements has been associated with an increased risk of the development of twin–twin transfusion syndrome in the second trimester.[98,99]

Conclusions

Improvements in image quality mean that the first trimester ultrasound scan is capable of offering us far more than a viability and dating service. Increased NT is now well recognised as being an important marker for chromosomal abnormality as well as for other conditions such as major cardiac disease and genetic syndromes. This has stimulated sonographers to examine the fetus more thoroughly in the first trimester, and a significant proportion of major anomalies can be detected at this stage. Data from studies that have looked at the effectiveness of first trimester ultrasound at detecting fetal abnormality do, however, show that a significant proportion of those missed will be detected at 20 weeks of gestation, so this later examination cannot be discarded. This situation will change as ultrasound technology continues to improve, as we become more disciplined with a sequential, systematic examination in the first trimester and as we gain more experience about the signs that various anomalies present at these early gestations. As we detect more anomalies in early pregnancy it may be sensible to consider the timing of the 20-week scan because greater flexibility may allow us to use ultrasound to screen for other potential obstetric complications.

References

1.   Robinson HP. Detection of fetal heart movement in first trimester of pregnancy using pulsed ultrasound. *BMJ* 1972;4:466–8.
2.   Robinson HP. Sonar measurement of fetal crown–rump length as means of assessing maturity in first trimester of pregnancy. *BMJ* 1973;4:28–31.
3.   Robinson HP, Fleming JE. A critical evaluation of sonar 'crown–rump length' measurements. *Br J Obstet Gynaecol* 1975;82:702–10.
4.   Pandya PP, Snijders RJ, Psara N, Hilbert L, Nicolaides KH. The prevalence of non-viable pregnancy at 10–13 weeks of gestation. *Ultrasound Obstet Gynecol* 1996;7:170–3.
5.   Barrett JM, Brinson J. Evaluation of obstetric ultrasonography at the first prenatal visit. *Am J Obstet Gynecol* 1991;165:1002–5.
6.   Peek MJ, Devonald KJ, Beilby R, Ellwood D. The value of routine early pregnancy ultrasound in the antenatal booking clinic. *Aust N Z J Obstet Gynaecol* 1994;34:140–3.
7.   Gardosi J, Vanner T, Francis A. Gestational age and induction of labour for prolonged pregnancy. *Br J Obstet Gynaecol* 1997;104:792–7.
8.   Crowther CA, Kornman L, O'Callaghan S, George K, Furness M, Wilson K. Is an ultrasound

assessment of gestational age at the first antenatal visit of value? A randomised clinical trial. *Br J Obstet Gynaecol* 1999;106:1273–9.

9. Taipale P, Hiilesmaa V. Predicting delivery date by ultrasound and last menstrual period in early gestation. *Obstet Gynecol* 2001;97:189–94.

10. Wald NJ, Cuckle HS, Densem JW, Kennard A, Smith D. Maternal serum screening for Down's syndrome: the effect of routine ultrasound scan determination of gestational age and adjustment for maternal weight. *Br J Obstet Gynaecol* 1992;99:144–9.

11. Benn PA, Rodis JF, Beazoglou T. Cost-effectiveness of estimating gestational age by ultrasonography in Down syndrome screening. *Obstet Gynecol* 1999;94:29–33.

12. Snijders RJM, Noble P, Sebire N, Souka A, Nicolaides KH. UK multicentre project on assessment of risk of trisomy 21 by maternal age and fetal nuchal translucency thickness at 10–14 weeks of gestation. Fetal Medicine Foundation First Trimester Screening Group. *Lancet* 1998;352:343–6.

13. Szabo J, Gellen J, Szemere G. First-trimester ultrasound screening for fetal aneuploidies in women over 35 and under 35 years of age. *Ultrasound Obstet Gynecol* 1995;5:161–3.

14. Taipale P, Hiilesmaa V, Salonen R, Ylostalo P. Increased nuchal translucency as a marker for fetal chromosomal defects. *N Engl J Med* 1997;337, 1654–8.

15. Hafner E, Schuchter K, Liebhart E, Philipp K. Results of routine fetal nuchal translucency measurement at weeks 10–13 in 4233 unselected pregnant women. *Prenat Diagn* 1998;18:29–34.

16. Pajkrt E, van Lith JM, Mol BW, Bleker OP, Bilardo CM. Screening for Down's syndrome by fetal nuchal translucency measurement in a general obstetric population. *Ultrasound Obstet Gynecol* 1998;12:163–9.

17. Theodoropoulos P, Lolis D, Papageorgiou C, Papaioannou S, Plachouras N, Makrydimas G. Evaluation of first-trimester screening by fetal nuchal translucency and maternal age. *Prenat Diagn* 1998;18:133–7.

18. Economides DL, Whitlow BJ, Kadir R, Lazanakis M, Verdin SM. First trimester sonographic detection of chromosomal abnormalities in an unselected population. *Br J Obstet Gynaecol* 1998;105:58–62.

19. Thilaganathan B, Sairam S, Michailidis G, Wathen NC. First trimester nuchal translucency: effective routine screening for Down's syndrome. *Br J Radiol* 1999;72:946–8.

20. Schwarzler P, Carvalho JS, Senat MV, Masroor T, Campbell S, Ville Y. Screening for fetal aneuploidies and fetal cardiac abnormalities by nuchal translucency thickness measurement at 10–14 weeks of gestation as part of routine antenatal care in an unselected population. *Br J Obstet Gynaecol* 1999;106:1029–34.

21. Krantz DA, Hallahan TW, Orlandi F, Buchanan P, Larsen JW, Macri JN. First trimester Down syndrome screening using dried blood biochemistry and nuchal translucency. *Obstet Gynecol* 2000;96:207–13.

22. Gasiorek-Wiens A, Tercanli S, Kozlowski P, Kossakiewicz A, Minderer S, Meyburg H, *et al.* Screening for trisomy 21 by fetal nuchal translucency and maternal age: a multicenter project in Germany, Austria and Switzerland. *Ultrasound Obstet Gynecol* 2001;18:646–8.

23. Zoppi MA, Ibba RM, Floris M, Monni G. Fetal nuchal translucency screening in 12495 pregnancies in Sardinia. *Ultrasound Obstet Gynecol* 2001;18:649–51.

24. Brizot ML, Carvalho MH, Liao AW, Reis NS, Armbruster-Moraes E, Zugaib M. First-trimester screening for chromosomal abnormalities by fetal nuchal translucency in a Brazilian population. *Ultrasound Obstet Gynecol* 2001;18:652–5.

25. Panbuarana P, Ajjimakorn S, Tungkajiwangoon P. First trimester Down syndrome screening by nuchal translucency in a Thai population. *Int J Gynaecol Obstet* 2001;75:311–12.

26. Wayda K, Kereszturi A, Orvos H, Horvath E, Pal A, Kovacs L, *et al*. Four years' experience of first-trimester nuchal translucency screening for fetal aneuploidies with increasing regional availability. *Acta Obstet Gynecol Scand* 2001;80:1104–9.

27. Wapner R, Thom E, Simpson JL, Pergament E, Silver R, Filkins K, *et al*. First trimester screening for trisomies 21 and 18. *N Engl J Med* 2003;349:1405–13.

28. Comas C, Torrents M, Munoz A, Antolin E, Figueras F, Echevarria M. Measurement of nuchal translucency as a single strategy in trisomy 21 screening: should we use any other marker? *Obstet Gynecol* 2002;100:648–54.

29. Monni G, Zoppi MA, Ibba RM, Floris M. Fetal nuchal translucency test for Down's syndrome. *Lancet* 1997;350:754–55.

30. Snjiders RJM, Thom EA, Zachary JM, Platt LD, Greene N, Jackson LG, *et al*. First trimester trisomy screening: nuchal translucency measurement training and quality assurance to correct and unify technique. *Ultrasound Obstet Gynecol* 2002;19:353–9.

31. Wojdemann KR, Christiansen M, Sundberg K, Larsen SO, Shalmi A, Tabor A. Quality assessment in prospective nuchal translucency screening for Down syndrome. *Ultrasound Obstet Gynecol* 2001;18:641–4.

32. Kadir RA, Economides DL. The effect of nuchal translucency measurement on second-trimester biochemical screening for Down's syndrome. *Ultrasound Obstet Gynecol* 1997;9:244–7.

33. Bindra R, Heath V, Liao A, Spencer K, Nicolaides KH. One-stop clinic for assessment of risk for trisomy 21 at 11–14 weeks: a prospective study of 15 030 pregnancies. *Ultrasound Obstet Gynecol* 2002;20:219–25.

34. Orlandi F, Damiani G, Hallahan TW, Krantz DA, Macri JN. First-trimester screening for fetal aneuploidy: biochemistry and nuchal translucency. *Ultrasound Obstet Gynecol* 1997;10:381–6.

35. Biagiotti R, Brizzi L, Periti E, d'Agata A, Vanzi E, Cariati E. First trimester screening for Down's syndrome using maternal serum PAPP-A and free beta-hCG in combination with fetal nuchal translucency thickness. *Br J Obstet Gynaecol* 1998;105:917–20.

36. Benattar C, Audibert F, Taieb J, Ville Y, Roberto A, Lindenbaum A, *et al*. Efficiency of ultrasound and biochemical markers for Down's syndrome risk screening. A prospective study. *Fetal Diagn Ther* 1999;14:112–17.

37. De Biasio, Siccardi M, Volpe G, Famularo L, Santi F, Canini S. First trimester screening for Down syndrome using nuchal translucency measurement with beta-hCG and PAPP-A between 10 and 13 weeks of pregnancy – the combination test. *Prenat Diagn* 1999;19:360–3.

38. de Graaf IM, Parkrt E, Bilardo CM, Leschot NJ, Cuckle HS, van Lith JM. Early pregnancy screening for fetal aneuploidy with serum markers and nuchal translucency. *Prenat Diagn* 1999;19:458–62.

39. Spencer K, Souter V, Tul N, Snijders R, Nicolaides KH. A screening program for trisomy 21 at 10–14 weeks using fetal nuchal translucency, maternal serum free beta-human chorionic gonadotropin and pregnancy-associated plasma protein-A. *Ultrasound Obstet Gynecol* 1999;13:231–7.

40. Spencer K. Age related detection and false positive rates when screening for Down's syndrome in the first trimester of pregnancy using fetal nuchal translucency and maternal serum free betahCG and PAPP-A. *BJOG* 2001;108:1043–6.

41. Schuchter K, Hafner E, Stangl G, Metzenbauer M, Hofinger D, Philipp K. The first trimester 'combined test' for the detection of Down syndrome pregnancies in 4939 unselected pregnancies. *Prenat Diagn* 2002;22:211–15.

42. Gilbert RE, Augood C, Gupta R, Ades AE, Logan S, Sculpher M, *et al*. Screening for Down's syndrome: effects, safety and cost effectiveness of first and second trimester strategies. *BMJ* 2001;323:1–6.

43. Down LJ. Observations on an ethnic classification of idiots. *Clin Lect Rep London Hosp* 1866;3:259–62.

44. Cicero S, Curico P, Papageorghiou A, Sonek J, Nicolaides K. Absence of nasal bone in fetuses with trisomy 21 at 11–14 weeks of gestation: an observational study. *Lancet* 2001;358:1665–7.

45. Matias A, Gomes C, Flack N, Montenegro N, Nicolaides KH. Screening for chromosomal abnormalities at 10–14 weeks: the role of ductus venosus blood flow. *Ultrasound Obstet Gynecol* 1998;12:380–4.

46. Whitlow BJ, Lazanakis ML, Kadir RA, Chatzipapas I, Economides DL. The significance of choroid plexus cysts, echogenic heart foci and renal pyelectasis in the first trimester. *Ultrasound Obstet Gynecol* 1998;12:385–90.

47. Guariglia L, Rosati P. Isolated mild fetal pyelectasis detected by transvaginal sonography in advanced maternal age. *Obstet Gynecol* 1998;92:833–6.

48. Thilaganathan B, Olawaiye A, Sairam S, Harrington K. Isolated fetal echogenic intracardiac foci or golf balls: is karyotyping for Down's syndrome indicated? *Br J Obstet Gynaecol* 1999;106:1294–7.

49. Hernadi L, Torocsik M. Screening for fetal anomalies in the 12th week of pregnancy by transvaginal sonography in an unselected population. *Prenat Diagn* 1997;17:753–9.

50. D'Ottavio G, Meir YJ, Rustico MA, Pecile V, Fischer-Tamaro L, Conoscenti G, *et al.* Screening for fetal anomalies by ultrasound at 14 and 21 weeks. *Ultrasound Obstet Gynecol* 1997;10:375–80.

51. Whitlow BJ, Chatzipapas IK, Lazanakis ML, Kadir RA, Economides DL. The value of sonography in early pregnancy for the detection of fetal abnormalities in an unselected population. *Br J Obstet Gynaecol* 1999;106:929–36.

52. Guariglia L, Rosati P. Transvaginal sonographic detection of embryonic-fetal abnormalities in early pregnancy. *Obstet Gynecol* 2000;96:328–32.

53. Carvalho MH, Brizot ML, Lopes LM, Chiba CH, Miyadahira S, Zugaib M. Detection of fetal structural abnormalities at the 11–14 week ultrasound scan. *Prenat Diagn* 2002;22:1–4.

54. Rottem S, Bronshtein M, Thaler I, Brandes JM. First trimester transvaginal sonographic diagnosis of fetal anomalies. *Lancet* 1989;i:444–5.

55. Timor-Tritsch IE. Transvaginal sonographic evaluation of fetal anatomy at 14 to 16 weeks. Why is this technique not attractive in the United States? *J Ultrasound Med* 2001;20:705–9.

56. Johnson SP, Sebire NJ, Snijders RJM, Tunkel S, Nicolaides KH. Ultrasound screening for anencephaly at 10–14 weeks of gestation. *Ultrasound Obstet Gynecol* 1997;9:14–16.

57. Chatzipapas IK, Whitlow BJ, Economides DL. The 'Mickey Mouse' sign and the diagnosis of anencephaly in early pregnancy. *Ultrasound Obstet Gynecol* 1999;13:196–9.

58. Bronshtein M, Zimmer EZ. Transvaginal sonographic follow-up on the formation of fetal cephalocele at 13–19 weeks' gestation. *Obstet Gynecol* 1991;78:528–30.

59. van Zalen-Spock M, van Vugt JMG, van der Harten HJ, van Geijn HP. Cephalocele and cystic hygroma: diagnosis and differentiation in the first trimester of pregnancy with transvaginal sonography. *Ultrasound Obstet Gynecol* 1992;2:289–92.

60. Blaas HG. Holoprosencephaly at 10 weeks 2 days (CRL 33 mm). *Ultrasound Obstet Gynecol* 2000;15:86–7.

61. Snijders RJ, Sebire NJ, Nayar R, Souka A, Nicolaides KH. Increased nuchal translucency in trisomy 13 fetuses at 10–14 weeks of gestation. *Am J Med Genet* 1999;86:205–7.

62. Sebire NJ, Noble PL, Thorpe-Beeston JG, Snijders RJM, Nicolaides KH. Presence of the lemon sign in fetuses with spina bifida at the 10–14 weeks scan. *Ultrasound Obstet Gynecol* 1997;10:403–5.

63. Buisson O, De Keersmaecker B, Senat MV, Bernard JP, Moscoso G, Ville Y. Sonographic diagnosis of spina bifida at 12 weeks: heading towards indirect signs. *Ultrasound Obstet Gynecol* 2002;19:290–2.

64. Office of Population Censuses and Surveys. *Mortality Statistics. Perinatal and Infant: Social and Biological Factors.* (Series DH3.) London: OPCS; 1997. p. 28.

65. Sharland GK, Allan LD. Screening for congenital heart disease prenatally: results of a 2? year study in South East Thames region. *Br J Obstet Gynaecol* 1992;99:220–5.

66. Bull C. Current and potential impact of fetal diagnosis on prevalence and spectrum of serious congenital heart disease at term in the UK. *Lancet* 1999;354:1242–7.

67. Maher JE, Colvin EV, Samdarshi TE, Owen J, Hauth JC. Fetal echocardiography in gravidas with historic risk factors for congenital heart disease. *Am J Perinatol* 1994;11:334–6.

68. Hyett JA, Moscoso G, Nicolaides KH. Abnormalities of the heart and great arteries in first trimester chromosomally abnormal fetuses. *Am J Med Genet* 1997;69:207–16.

69. Hyett JA, Perdu M, Sharland GK, Snijders RSM, Nicolaides KH. Increased nuchal translucency at 10–14 weeks of gestation as a marker for major cardiac defects. *Ultrasound Obstet Gynecol* 1997;10:242–6.

70. Hyett JA, Perdu M, Sharland GK, Snijders RSM, Nicolaides KH. Screening for congenital heart disease with fetal nuchal translucency at 10–14 weeks of gestation. *BMJ* 1999;318:81–5.

71. Ghi T, Huggon IC, Zosmer N, Nicolaides KH. Incidence of major structural cardiac defects associated with increased nuchal translucency but normal karyotype. *Ultrasound Obstet Gynecol* 2001;18:610–14.

72. Mavrides E, Cobian-Sanchez F, Tekay A, Moscoso G, Campbell S, Thilaganathan B, *et al.* Limitations of using first trimester nuchal translucency measurement in routine screening for major congenital heart defects. *Ultrasound Obstet Gynecol* 2001;17:106–10.

73. Michailidis GD, Economides DL. Nuchal translucency measurement and pregnancy outcome in karyotypically normal fetuses. *Ultrasound Obstet Gynecol* 2001;17:102–5.

74. Orvos H, Wayda K, Kozinszky Z, Katona M, Pal A, Szabo J. Increased nuchal translucency and congenital heart defects in euploid fetuses: the Szeged experience. *Eur J Obstet Gynecol* 2002;101:124–8.

75. Bronshstein M, Lewit N, Sujov P, Makhoul I, Blazer S. Prenatal diagnosis of congenital diaphragmatic hernia: timing of visceral herniation and outcome. *Prenat Diagn* 1995;15:695–8.

76. Blaas HG, Eik-Nes SH, Kiserud T, Hellevik LR. Early development of the abdominal wall, stomach and heart from 7 to 12 weeks of gestation: a longitudinal ultrasound study. *Ultrasound Obstet Gynecol* 1995;6:240–9.

77. Sebire NJ, Snijders RJM, Davenport M, Greenough A, Nicolaides KH. Fetal nuchal translucency thickness at 10–14 weeks of gestation and congenital diaphragmatic hernia. *Obstet Gynecol* 1997;90:943–6.

78. van Zalen-Sprock RM, Vugt JM, van Geijn HP. First-trimester sonography of physiological midgut herniation and early diagnosis of omphalocele. *Prenat Diagn* 1997;17:511–18.

79. Snijders RJM, Sebire NJ, Souka A, Santiago C, Nicolaides KH. Fetal exomphalos and chromosomal defects: relationship to maternal age and gestation. *Ultrasound Obstet Gynecol* 1995;6:250–5.

80. Rosati P, Guariglia L. Transvaginal sonographic assessment of the fetal urinary tract in early pregnancy. *Ultrasound Obstet Gynecol* 1996;7:95–100.

81. Bronshstein M, Bar-Hava I, Blumenfeld Z. Clues and pitfalls in the early prenatal diagnosis of 'late onset' infantile polycystic kidney. *Prenat Diagn* 1992;12:293–8.

82. Bronshstein M, Yoffe N, Brandes JM, Blumenfeld Z. First and early second-trimester diagnosis of fetal urinary tract anomalies using transvaginal sonography. *Prenat Diagn* 1990;10:653–66.

83. Sepulveda W, Sebire NJ, Souka A, Snijders RJ, Nicolaides KH. Diagnosis of the Meckel–Gruber syndrome at eleven to fourteen weeks' gestation. *Am J Obstet Gynecol* 1997;176:316–19.

84. Sebire NJ, Von Kaisenberg C, Rubio C, Snijders RJ, Nicolaides KH. Fetal Megacystis at 10–14 weeks of gestation. *Ultrasound Obstet Gynecol* 1996;8:387–90.

85. Hyett J, Noble P, Sebire NJ, Snijders R, Nicolaides KH. Lethal congenital arthrogryposis presents with increased nuchal translucency at 10–14 weeks of gestation. *Ultrasound Obstet Gynecol* 1997;9:310–13.

86. De Biasio P, Prefumo F, Lantieri PB, Venturini PL. Reference values for fetal limb biometry at 10–14 weeks of gestation. *Ultrasound Obstet Gynecol* 2002;19:588–91.

87. Gabrielli S, Falco P, Pilu G, Perolo A, Milano V, Bovicelli L. Can transvaginal fetal biometry be considered a useful tool for early detection of skeletal dysplasias in high-risk patients? *Ultrasound Obstet Gynecol* 1999;13:107–11.

88. Fisk NM, Vaughan J, Smidt M, Wigglesworth J. Transvaginal ultrasound recognition of nuchal edema in the first-trimester diagnosis of achondrogenesis. *J Clin Ultrasound* 1991;9:588–90.

89. Ben Ami M, Perlitz Y, Haddad S, Matilsky M. Increased nuchal translucency is associated with asphyxiating thoracic dysplasia. *Ultrasound Obstet Gynecol* 1997;10:297–8.

90. Benson CB, Genest DR, Bernstein MR, Soto-Wright V, Goldstein DP, Berkowitz RS. Sonographic appearance of first trimester complete hydatidiform moles. *Ultrasound Obstet Gynecol* 2000;16:188–91.

91. Jauniaux E, Nicolaides KH. Early ultrasound diagnosis and follow-up of molar pregnancies. *Ultrasound Obstet Gynecol* 1997;9:17–21.

92. Taipale P, Hilesmaa V, Ylostalo P. Diagnosis of placenta praevia by transvaginal sonographic screening at 12–16 weeks in a nonselected population. *Obstet Gynecol* 1997;89:364–7.

93. Rosati P, Guariglia L. Clinical significance of placenta previa detected at early routine transvaginal scan. *J Ultrasound Med* 2000;19:581–5.

94. Metzenbauer M, Hafner E, Schuchter K, Philipp K. First-trimester placental volume as a marker of chromosomal anomalies: preliminary results from an unselected population. *Ultrasound Obstet Gynecol* 2002;19:240–2.

95. Sepulveda W. Chorionicity determination in twin pregnancies: double trouble? *Ultrasound Obstet Gynecol* 1997;10:79–81.

96. Sebire NJ, Snijders RJ, Hughes K, Sepulveda W, Nicolaides KH. The hidden mortality of monochorionic twin pregnancies. *Br J Obstet Gynaecol* 1997;104:1203–7.

97. Sebire NJ, Snijders RJ, Hughes K, Sepulveda W, Nicolaides KH. Screening for trisomy 21 in twin pregnancies by maternal age and fetal nuchal translucency thickness at 10–14 weeks of gestation. *Br J Obstet Gynaecol* 1996;103:999–1003.

98. Monni G, Zoppi MA, Cau G, Lai R, Baldi M. Importance of nuchal translucency measurement in multifetal pregnancy reduction. *Ultrasound Obstet Gynecol* 1999;13:377–8.

99. Sebire NJ, D'Ercole C, Hughes K, Carvalho M, Nicolaides KH. Increased nuchal translucency thickness at 10–14 weeks of gestation as a predictor of severe twin-to-twin transfusion syndrome. *Ultrasound Obstet Gynecol* 1997;10:86–9.

20

Outpatient hysteroscopy

Tal Z Jacobson and Colin J Davis

DEFINITION

Hysteroscopy is the assessment of the cervical canal and uterine cavity by direct endoscopic visualisation. In the outpatient setting it is usually performed without anaesthetic or sedation. Outpatient hysteroscopy may be divided into diagnostic procedures and therapeutic procedures.

INTRODUCTION

Hysteroscopy is being applied increasingly in the outpatient or office setting. The development of new equipment has allowed both diagnosis and minor treatments to be carried out with no anaesthetic or under local anaesthetic. Patient selection, the correct equipment and instrumentation, and sufficient surgical experience and skills are essential to ensure the safety and success of an outpatient hysteroscopy clinic.

The advantages of outpatient hysteroscopy for the woman are the avoidance of a general anaesthetic, a more rapid assessment (especially if it is part of a one-stop assessment clinic), and less likelihood of cancellation. The environment may be less threatening than a conventional operating room and the woman has direct involvement in the procedure, with immediate feedback and faster recovery.[1,2]

For the medical staff there is the benefit of scheduling procedures in a dedicated clinic that provides excellent diagnostic efficacy and the possibility of treatment at the same time. Fewer staff are required than for the traditional theatre setup and there may be long-term cost savings.[3]

The procedure is accurate for the diagnosis of serious endometrial disease (i.e. cancer and hyperplasia) in women with abnormal uterine bleeding. Outpatient hysteroscopy is as accurate as traditional inpatient hysteroscopy.[4]

There are some disadvantages. The procedure may fail and a repeat operation under general anaesthetic may need to be scheduled. One study has reported a failure rate of 7.1% for diagnostic outpatient hysteroscopic vaginoscopy.[5] Another has shown a 12% failure rate for surgical procedures such as removal of an endometrial polyp or submucous fibroid.[6] Half of these women (6%) had their surgery completed at a second outpatient hysteroscopy and the other half (6%) needed admission for a day case procedure under general anaesthetic. Patient discomfort and pain levels are higher than with general anaesthesia, but generally the procedure is well tolerated. Operating times are limited to 15–20 minutes because of these factors. A large meta-analysis has demonstrated a failure rate for diagnostic procedures of 4.2% for outpatient hysteroscopy compared with 3.4% for inpatient procedures.[4] The dimensions of the outpatient instruments are reduced; this leads to an inevitable loss of resolution, but the quality of modern instruments is high enough to facilitate many operative procedures. Table 1 gives a summary of the advantages and disadvantages of outpatient hysteroscopy.

Table 1 *The potential advantages and disadvantages of outpatient hysteroscopy*

Advantages	Disadvantages
Avoids general anaesthetic	Procedure may fail
Faster recovery and return to work	Procedure may be painful
Outpatient procedure	Loss of resolution owing to smaller hysteroscopes
One-stop clinic	Some women may find it undignified or embarrassing
Less likely to be cancelled	Requires specific training and experience
Environment more patient friendly	Expensive initial equipment and dedicated facility costs
Immediate feedback to patient	
Fewer staff needed than conventional theatre setup	
Possible long-term cost savings	

TRAINING

The Royal College of Obstetricians and Gynaecologists (RCOG) has set guidelines for training in hysteroscopic surgery. Lecture based teaching and hands-on experience on simulators have been introduced through hysteroscopic and minimal access surgery courses. Subsequent experience should be gained through observation in practice and the careful supervision of a preceptor.

In June 2001 the British Society for Gynaecological Endoscopy introduced a formalised training and accreditation scheme for nurses leading to independent nurse practitioners in diagnostic outpatient hysteroscopy.[7] Further training in operative procedures is planned for the near future.

The RCOG has specified the stratification of levels of training that can be achieved based on the complexity of the surgical procedure[8] (Table 2). Not all of these procedures are appropriate for outpatient hysteroscopy and in practice the close interaction with the woman requires that a reasonable level of hysteroscopic skill and experience should be attained before attempting hysteroscopy in an outpatient setting.

CONSENT AND COUNSELLING

Appropriate counselling must be given and informed consent obtained from all women undergoing outpatient hysteroscopy. The informed consent must include the risks and benefits, and the alternatives to the proposed surgical procedure. Inherent in hysteroscopy is the small risk of

Table 2 *RCOG stratification of training level for hysteroscopic procedures (modified from RCOG 1994[8])*

Level	Procedure
1	Diagnostic hysteroscopy and targeted biopsy
	Simple polypectomy
	Intrauterine contraceptive device removal
2	Cannulation of proximal fallopian tube
	Removal of large polyps/pedunculated fibroids
	Minor Asherman syndrome
3	Resection of uterine septum
	Major Asherman syndrome
	Endometrial resection/ablation
	Resection of submucous fibroid
	Repeat endometrial resection or ablation

trauma to the cervix, infection, uterine perforation and bleeding. If electrosurgery is being used there is a slight risk of bowel injury should it be activated after a uterine perforation. If bleeding cannot be controlled there is a small risk of requiring hysterectomy. These risks and their potential consequences must be adequately explained to the woman prior to the operative procedure. Verbal consent is usually sufficient for these procedures but, if there is any doubt, written consent should be obtained.

INDICATIONS FOR OUTPATIENT HYSTEROSCOPY

Abnormal uterine bleeding such as menorrhagia, intermenstrual bleeding and postmenopausal bleeding are the most common reasons for hysteroscopy. Directed biopsy of suspicious lesions can be performed. The diagnosis and treatment of submucous fibroids and polyps is a frequent indication. This procedure can be considered in women with recurrent miscarriage or an abnormal hysterosalpingogram, ultrasound scan or saline instillation sonography. It is useful for visualising lost intrauterine contraceptive devices. The identification and treatment of uterine abnormalities or adhesions is a common indication.

PATIENT SELECTION

Appropriate patient selection is critical to the success of outpatient hysteroscopy. A detailed medical and gynaecological history should be taken.

Women with menstrual disorders or postmenopausal bleeding should have a transvaginal ultrasound scan to assess the endometrial thickness.[9] Saline instillation sonography involves scanning while introducing 10–20 ml of saline directly into the uterine cavity via a fine plastic tube. This technique is good at revealing intrauterine polyps and submucous fibroids. In our practice we do not generally proceed to hysteroscopy unless there is evidence of an ultrasound abnormality or persistent symptoms.[10] Some women will be unable to tolerate the hysteroscopy or find it too painful. If an operative procedure requires prolonged intrauterine surgery to remove pathology it is more appropriate to use a general anaesthetic.

Patient selection criteria for outpatient diagnostic hysteroscopy (adapted from: TJ Clark, personal communication) are:

- full patient counselling and consent

- negative pregnancy test if premenopausal.

Additional selection criteria for outpatient operative hysteroscopy (adapted from: TJ Clark, personal communication) are:

- woman tolerated diagnostic hysteroscopy well

- woman not actively bleeding

- malignancy not suspected

- focal pathology less than 4 cm diameter

- small pedunculated polyps/fibroids easier to remove than large sessile polyps/fibroids

- sidewall polyps/fibroids easier to remove than fundal lesions

- procedure feasible to complete within 20 minutes.

EQUIPMENT

Hysteroscopes

Modern hysteroscopes range in diameter from 2 mm to 4 mm. Most operators use a rigid rod lens system. A cold light source delivers illumination via a circumferential fibre optic light cable. Modern hysteroscopes provide a 60–90-degree outer field of view. This view is wider in gaseous than liquid media because of the lower refractive index. If the outer lens is centred along the axis of the telescope it is referred to as a zero degree hysteroscope. The distal outer lens may be offset to the axis of the telescope at various angles up to 30 degrees, providing a significantly expanded field of view when the lens is rotated. For operative procedures a 0–10-degree hysteroscope is preferable as this will keep the instruments in view. Customarily, the direction of the angle of view is always opposite the axis of the light cable connector. The hysteroscopic sheath sits over a matched hysteroscope. Simple diagnostic sheaths usually have one port for distension media. The continuous flow sheath has two separate channels fitted with stopcocks that serve independently to instil and remove distension media. The inner sheath carries the distension medium to the uterine cavity and a fitted outer sheath evacuates this medium by gravity or suction. A third channel allows the use of operative instruments.

Flexible hysteroscopes use a fibre optic cable bundle to transmit the image. They are expensive and cannot be autoclaved. They allow good visualisation and are suitable for diagnostic procedures or directed biopsy but cannot easily be used for operative procedures (Figure 1). They have been shown to cause slightly less pain but have a lower procedural success rate and longer operating time when compared with rigid hysteroscopes.[11]

The Versascope® (Gynecare, Edinburgh, UK) is a semirigid hysteroscope with an outer diameter of 1.8 mm. The optical system uses a set of 50 000 fused optical fibres. The observed image is the product of an array of individual optical fibres. A flexible disposable outer sheath gives the end of the hysteroscope a ten-degree tilt and provides an inflow channel and an outflow channel that also serves as an operative channel for 2 mm (7F) instruments.

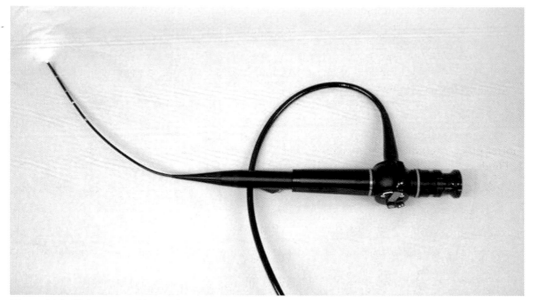

Figure 1 *Flexible hysteroscope (photo Andrew Kent)*

Video system

All hysteroscopic surgery should be undertaken using a video system rather than by direct visualisation through the hysteroscope. This allows a more comfortable and flexible operating position for the surgeon and a better training facility. The cameras themselves vary. Single CCD cameras are cheaper and smaller than three-chip cameras, but have inferior resolution and colour reproduction capabilities.

The ability to keep a record of the procedure by way of image capture or video recording is essential for the medical record and is an important part of clinical risk management. Modern systems allow stills and video of the procedure to be recorded on to CD or DVD, which can easily be reviewed and edited on a computer at a later date.

Light source

Xenon will provide the highest quality light for hysteroscopy. The light is transmitted via fibre optic cables to the hysteroscope. Although some of the heat generated by the light source is dissipated along the cable, it can still cause burns to the patient or the drapes and should be handled carefully.[12]

Distension media

A distension medium must be used to adequately distend the uterine cavity to provide a view of the endometrium and any pathology that is present. Gas or liquid can be used. The most commonly used gas is carbon dioxide. This requires a dedicated insufflator with an automatic pressure control. (A laparoscopic insufflator must not be used because the pressures would be too high.) It provides a good view of the cavity and is suitable for diagnostic procedures because of its spontaneous removal by ventilation, solubility in blood, ready availability, noncombustibility and convenience. Carbon dioxide has virtually the same index of refraction as air so it provides the best imaging. It is rarely appropriate for operative procedures because any bleeding rapidly obscures the view.

Liquid media allow continuous flushing of blood and debris and are more suitable for operative hysteroscopy. They are divided into electrolytic and nonelectrolytic solutions.

Glycine is a nonelectrolyte that provides a good view and is readily available. Unlike saline it can be used with monopolar instrumentation. The main disadvantage of glycine is that excess absorption of this fluid can lead to hyponatraemia. This is rare in outpatient hysteroscopy owing to the short operating times.

The development of bipolar instruments allows the use of normal saline as a distension medium and avoids the problem of hyponatraemia entirely, but simple fluid overload is still a risk. A comparison of saline with carbon dioxide as a distension medium has shown that saline leads to a shorter procedure time and to less lower abdominal pain, shoulder tip pain and nausea.[13]

Fluid media can be delivered in three ways:

- A gravity fall system involves raising the fluid bag to one metre above the patient, which gives a pressure of approximately 70 mmHg.

- A pressure cuff can be inflated around the bag.

- An automatic pressure infusion pump will allow presetting of the fluid flow rate and distension pressure.

For outpatient hysteroscopy, in view of the short operating times, the gravity fall or pressure bag system is usually sufficient.

Sterilisation

Nondisposable instruments must always be dismantled and cleaned of debris after use. They can then be adequately sterilised by soaking in 2% glutaraldehyde solution for at least 20 minutes. Fibre optic cables can simply be wiped with alcohol swabs between procedures, or disinfected together with the telescope. Hysteroscopic sheaths and resectoscope assemblies can be autoclaved. Ethylene oxide gas sterilisation is a cold system and does not damage sensitive equipment, but it is expensive and takes 72 hours, so an increased quantity of available hysteroscopes may be required.

Operative modalities

Miniaturised standard cold instruments such as scissors, graspers and biopsy forceps can be used with all outpatient hysteroscopes.

Monopolar electrosurgery uses the flow of electricity from the active electrode to the tissue to be treated and its return via the neutral electrode to the earth in the generator. This is employed with nonelectrolytic distension media and is the most common modality used for the traditional resectoscope with a general anaesthetic.

Bipolar electrosurgery passes current between two electrodes that are close together. A heated vapour pocket is formed and the tissue nearby or between the electrodes is desiccated. The patient is not part of the circuit. This procedure can be used with saline as a distension medium.

Laser surgery is a technique often used in ablative hysteroscopic procedures but it is less suitable for outpatient hysteroscopy.

STAFFING

All staff need to have a good understanding of the equipment. In addition to the surgeon there should be a nurse who can assist with instrumentation and control any equipment needed. Ideally, the nurse should be specially trained and experienced in outpatient hysteroscopy. Good communication with and cooperation from the patient is essential. It is preferable to have an additional member of staff to support and help the woman throughout the procedure.

ENVIRONMENT

There should be a well organised but relaxed environment in order to allow the woman to maintain her dignity and have some privacy during the operation. A recovery area is needed where she can sit afterwards. For high-risk women with significant medical conditions the procedure should be performed in a full operating theatre with an anaesthetist present to deal with any complications or to allow conversion to a general anaesthetic if appropriate.

RECORD KEEPING

The application of clinical governance has increased the need for full and contemporaneous records to be kept. The unique nature of endoscopic surgery allows stills and video images to be made. These should be considered as part of the surgical record and kept in the medical notes. The woman should be given the choice to view the procedure if she wishes. The ability to demonstrate the findings on a dedicated screen at the time of surgery is helpful in maintaining trust and cooperation.

ANALGESIA

Most women will require no anaesthesia, but a simple oral analgesic such as diclofenac can be given 30–60 minutes before the procedure.[14–16]

A local anaesthetic paracervical or intracervical block using Citanest® (Dentsply, Weybridge, Surrey) can be applied if the woman experiences discomfort during the procedure.

Some studies[17–19] have shown benefit with the use of a lignocaine spray or injection compared with placebo during diagnostic hysteroscopy but no difference in the success rate of the procedure. Other placebo controlled studies[20,21] have demonstrated no benefit with the use of local anaesthetic and good tolerance of the procedure without anaesthetic.

PROCEDURE

The procedure itself will not be described in detail because the use of anaesthetic, cervical preparation and cleansing, a tenaculum, a speculum etc. will vary, depending upon: the preferences of the surgeon, the hysteroscopic equipment being used, the planned procedure, and the woman's specific circumstances.[22]

In general the patient should be placed in the Lloyd-Davies position and a bimanual examination performed prior to the hysteroscopy to assess the direction of the cervical and uterine axis. The vaginoscopic technique advocates a hysteroscopically directed entry into the cervix without the use of a speculum. A systematic inspection of the uterine cavity and cervical canal should be performed[23] (Figure 2).

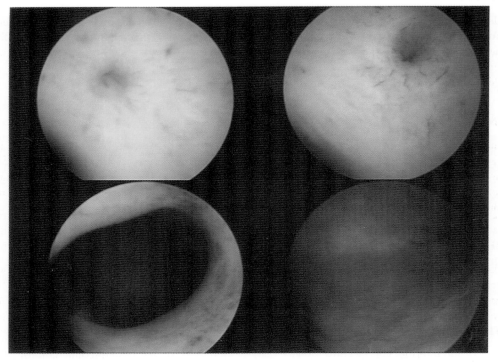

Figure 2 *Normal hysteroscopic views*

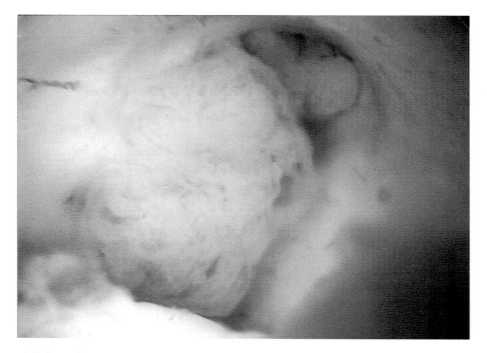

Figure 3 *Endometrial carcinoma*

Diagnostic hysteroscopy

The investigation of menstrual disorders is an ideal application for outpatient hysteroscopy. The combination of transvaginal ultrasound scanning and hysteroscopy leads to a high detection rate of intrauterine pathology and the opportunity to treat this at the same time if appropriate.[24–26]

Hysteroscopy is also useful for the elucidation of radiographic studies, such as hysterosalpingography, hysterosalpingo-contrast sonography or saline instillation sonography, which demonstrate the possibility of intrauterine pathology.[27,28] It can be used together with transvaginal ultrasound scanning and endometrial biopsy to assess postmenopausal bleeding or unscheduled bleeding on hormone replacement therapy.[29–31] It can also be considered in women with infertility or recurrent miscarriage and used in conjunction with fertiloscopy, which is an office or outpatient procedure used to assess the distal tubes and ovaries.[32]

Outpatient hysteroscopy is a reliable technique for the diagnosis of suspected endometrial carcinoma or hyperplasia (Figure 3). Focal lesions that may be missed inadvertently using a blind sampling technique such as a Pipelle biopsy alone can be identified hysteroscopically.[33] A biopsy sample should always be taken and sent for histological analysis at the time of hysteroscopy.[34,35]

The absolute and relative contraindications to hysteroscopy include cervical carcinoma, active pelvic inflammatory disease, pregnancy, active heavy bleeding and recent uterine perforation.

Therapeutic outpatient hysteroscopy

A lost intrauterine contraceptive device can be removed under hysteroscopic control after confirming its location by ultrasound (Figure 4).

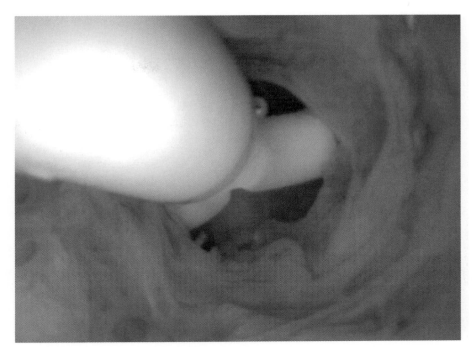

Figure 4 *Lost Mirena intrauterine contraceptive device*

For menorrhagia, second generation endometrial ablation techniques such as the use of thermal balloons, microwaves and cryosurgery can be performed as an outpatient procedure.[36] Hysteroscopy should be carried out just prior to the procedure to exclude previously unrecognised abnormalities.

The main intrauterine causes of abnormal uterine bleeding are endometrial polyps and submucous fibroids. Small polyps can be removed easily with graspers or by using bipolar diathermy to the polyp base (Figure 5).

Submucous fibroids that are associated with menorrhagia, dysmenorrhea, pelvic pain, infertility, recurrent miscarriage, premature labour or recurrent unscheduled bleeding while on hormone replacement therapy can be considered for hysteroscopic removal (Figure 6). For outpatient operative surgery, the number, location, size and distribution of the fibroids need to be considered.[37] In general they should be less that 3 cm in diameter. Submucous fibroids are classified into three grades according to their relative degree of intramural involvement. Grade 0 is essentially a pedunculated fibroid with the entire fibroid situated within the cavity. Grade 1 fibroids have more than 50% of the fibroid protruding into the cavity but part of it is intramural. Grade 2 fibroids have less than 50% of their bulk within the cavity and more than 50% is intramural. Grade 0 and small grade 1 fibroids are suitable for removal in the outpatient setting. Removal of grade 2 fibroids may be attempted by experienced surgeons but they sometimes require a two-stage procedure. This should also be considered for women with multiple submucous fibroids for whom fertility is an issue because adhesions may form between the scar sites of separate fibroids, leading to Asherman's syndrome.

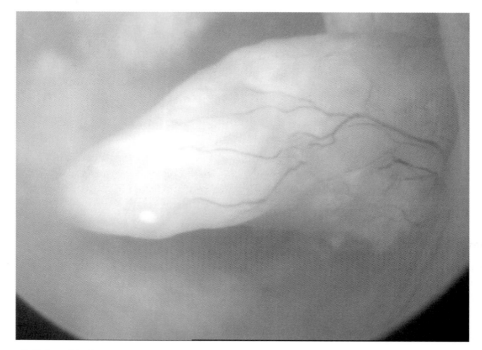

Figure 5 *Endometrial polyp*

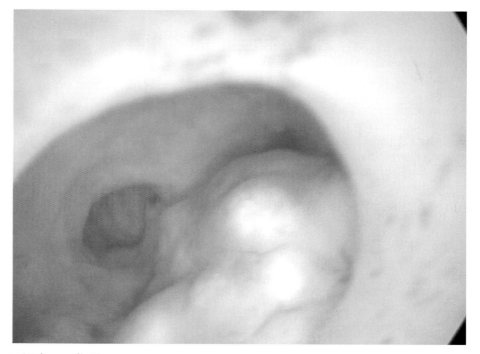

Figure 6 *Submucous fibroid*

Fallopian tube catheterisation can be performed hysteroscopically to investigate proximal tubal blockage or to insert intratubal devices for sterilisation, such as the Essure device. The synechiae of minor Asherman's syndrome can be treated as an outpatient but the majority of these women are likely to require a general anaesthetic. The excision of müllerian fusion defects such as uterine septae is possible in the outpatient setting but these procedures often require a simultaneous laparoscopy and are therefore more likely to be performed under general anaesthesia.

Downregulation

Gonadotrophin-releasing hormone analogue pretreatment prior to hysteroscopic surgery leads to improved visualisation, decreased operating time and less blood loss. It is particularly helpful for submucous fibroid resections in premenopausal women and, in selected patients, pretreatment may increase red cell mass and decrease the risks of the procedure.

COMPLICATIONS

Complications include cervical trauma, failure to enter more successfully the uterine cavity, producing a false passage, uterine perforation, bowel or bladder injury, infection, haemorrhage and fluid overload. These will be discussed individually below.

Perforation

The risk of uterine perforation can be reduced by accurate assessment of the cervico-uterine axes, gentle insertion of instruments, and introducing as well as advancing instruments only when good vision has been obtained. Operative procedures should be undertaken only when there is a clear view. The sudden loss of a clear view may be due to a loss of distension medium pressure secondary to perforation. The thickness of the uterine wall varies and is particularly thin near the tubal ostea. Great care should be taken at all stages of a procedure to avoid perforation, especially with an activated electrosurgical instrument. If perforation is suspected when using electrosurgery, a laparoscopy or laparotomy must be performed to assess the bowel and bladder.

Bowel injury

If uterine perforation does occur, injury to the bowel can ensue. In rare circumstances it is possible to produce a transmitted thermal injury to the bowel without complete perforation. A low threshold of suspicion should be maintained for women who have any symptoms of fever or pain after hysteroscopic surgery. Early investigations are required and laparoscopy or laparotomy should not be delayed if a bowel injury is suspected.

Haemorrhage

Bleeding may be a consequence of uterine perforation and this should therefore be considered as a cause of primary haemorrhage. If bleeding is from a fibroid or polyp base it can usually be controlled by electrosurgical coagulation and the use of oxytocics. Conversion to a general anaesthetic may be needed if control of the bleeding is difficult to obtain.

Infection

This complication is more likely to occur in the presence of previous pelvic inflammatory disease, in insulin dependent diabetics, and in women on high-dose steroids and others who are immunocompromised. These groups should be given prophylactic broad spectrum antibiotics.

Fluid overload

Uterine distension requires 60–75 mmHg of pressure. The aim of controlling fluid delivery for uterine distension is to maximise vision while minimising the amount of fluid intravasation (the absorption of fluid into the vascular system through uterine vessels). Intravasation is dependent upon the intrauterine pressure, the mean arterial pressure, the duration of surgery, and the vascularity and depth of myometrial penetration of the surgical procedure.

Excessive absorption of glycine can produce hypo-osmolar hyponatraemia leading to cerebral oedema. This is associated with nausea, vomiting, visual disturbance, headache and confusion. Convulsions, coma and death may follow. Treatment includes immediate termination of the surgical procedure, diuretic therapy, restriction of fluid intake, supplemental oxygen, and serial monitoring of electrolytes. In more severe cases, management should be in an intensive care setting with the help and expertise of intensive care specialists.

Normal saline is iso-osmolar. Excessive absorption of normal saline will not lead to the severe symptoms of hyponatraemia but fluid overload resulting in pulmonary oedema is a possibility. The best strategy for managing fluid overload is early detection and rapid initiation of treatment. Careful control of the infusion pressure, strict input and output monitoring, and limited operating time will decrease the risk of intravasation. In the outpatient setting the procedure should be stopped if the fluid deficit reaches 1000 ml. One advantage of performing hysteroscopy under local anaesthetic is that the earliest symptoms of encephalopathy (nausea, vomiting, weakness) will be more obvious to the surgeon and corrective measures can be taken more promptly than when the woman is under general anaesthesia.[38]

CONCLUSION

Outpatient hysteroscopy has evolved from the development of inpatient hysteroscopy and the introduction of many operative procedures, combined with technical developments that have allowed many of these procedures to be performed with the benefit of local anaesthetic. Good training, experience and equipment are essential to the implementation of outpatient hysteroscopy. The selection of suitable women and experienced appropriate support staff is critical in order to provide a good patient experience and a successful outcome of surgery.

Acknowledgements

We would like to thank Sian Jones, Pam Quinn, Helen Ludkin and Andrew Kent for providing additional information and images.

References

1. Kremer C, Duffy S, Moroney M. Patient satisfaction with outpatient hysteroscopy versus day case hysteroscopy: a randomised controlled trial. *BMJ* 2000;320:279–82.

2.   de Jong P, Doel F, Falconer A. Outpatient diagnostic hysteroscopy. *Br J Obstet Gynaecol* 1990;97:299–303.

3.   Ruach M, Hart R, Magos A. Outpatient hysteroscopy. *Contemp Rev Obstet Gynaecol* 1998;10:295–302.

4.   Clark TJ, Voit D, Gupta JK, Hyde C, Song F, Khan KS. Accuracy of hysteroscopy in the diagnosis of endometrial cancer and hyperplasia: a systematic quantitative review. *JAMA* 2002;288:1610–21.

5.   Paschopoulos M, Paraskevaidis E, Stefanidis K, Kofinas G, Lolis D. Vaginoscopic approach to outpatient hysteroscopy. *J Am Assoc Gynecol Laparosc* 1997;4:465–7.

6.   Farrugia M, McMillan L. Versapoint in the treatment of focal intra-uterine pathology in an outpatient clinic setting. *Gynecol Obstet* 2000;7:169–73.

7.   McGauren A. Doctoring the usual roles. *Health Serv J* 2002;(18 July):14–15.

8.   Royal College of Obstetricians and Gynaecologists. *Report of the RCOG Working Party on Training in Gynaecological Endoscopic Surgery*. London: RCOG Press; 1994.

9.   Royal College of Obstetricians and Gynaecologists. *The Management of Menorrhagia in Secondary Care*. Evidence-based Clinical Guideline No. 5 London: RCOG Press; 1998.

10. Vercellini P, Cortesi I, Oldani S, Moschetta M, De Giorgi O, Crosignani PG. The role of transvaginal ultrasonography and outpatient diagnostic hysteroscopy in the evaluation of patients with menorrhagia. *Hum Reprod* 1997;12:1768–71.

11. Unfried G, Wieser F, Albrecht A, Kaider A, Nagele F. Flexible versus rigid endoscopes for outpatient hysteroscopy. *Hum Reprod* 2001;16:168–71.

12. Mencaglia L, Hamou JE. *Manual of Hysteroscopy – Diagnosis and Surgery*. Tuttlingen: Endo-Press; 2002.

13. Nagele F, Bournas N, O'Connor H, Broadbent M, Richardson R, Magos A. Comparison of carbon dioxide and normal saline for uterine distension in outpatient hysteroscopy. *Fertil Steril* 1996;65:305–9.

14. De Iaco P, Marabini A, Stefanetti M, Del Vecchio C, Bovicelli L. Acceptability and pain of outpatient hysteroscopy. *J Am Assoc Gynecol Laparosc* 2000;7:71–5.

15. Tam W, Yuen PM. Use of diclofenac as an analgesic in outpatient hysteroscopy: a randomized, double-blind, placebo-controlled study. *Fertil Steril* 2001;76:1070–2.

16. Nagele F, Lockwood G, Magos AL. Randomised placebo controlled trial of mefenamic acid for premedication at outpatient hysteroscopy: a pilot study. *Br J Obstet Gynaecol* 1997;104:842–4.

17. Soriano D, Ajaj S, Chuong T, Deval B, Fauconnier A, Darai E. Lidocaine spray and outpatient hysteroscopy: randomized placebo-controlled trial. *Obstet Gynecol* 2000;96:661–4.

18. Davies A, Richardson RE, O'Connor H, Baskett TF, Nagele F, Magos AL. Lignocaine aerosol spray in outpatient hysteroscopy: a randomized double-blind placebo-controlled trial. *Fertil Steril* 1997;67:1019–23.

19. Esteve M, Schindler S, Machado S, Borges S, Santos C, Coutinho E. The efficacy of intracervical lidocaine in outpatient hysteroscopy. *Gynaecol Endosc* 2002;11:33–6.

20. Wong AY, Wong K, Tang LC. Stepwise pain score analysis of the effect of local lignocaine on outpatient hysteroscopy: a randomized, double-blind, placebo-controlled trial. *Fertil Steril* 2000;73:1234–7.

21. Lau WC, Tam WH, Lo WK, Yuen PM. A randomised double-blind placebo-controlled trial of transcervical intrauterine local anaesthesia in outpatient hysteroscopy. *BJOG* 2000;107:610–13.

22. Fraser IS. Personal techniques and results for outpatient diagnostic hysteroscopy. *Gynaecol Endosc* 1993;2:29–33.

23. Okeahialam MG, Jones SE, O'Donovan P. Early experience with the vaginoscopic approach to outpatient microhysteroscopy. *Gynaecol Endosc* 2001;10:57–9.

24. Okeahialam MG, Jones SE, O'Donovan PJ. Outcome of outpatient micro-hysteroscopy performed for abnormal bleeding while on hormone replacement therapy. *J Obstet Gynaecol* 2001;21:277–9.

25. Miskry T, Ruach M, Magos A. Hysteroscopy in women aged 30 years or less. *Gynaecol Endosc* 2000;9:315–17.

26. Tahir MM, Bigrigg MA, Browning JJ, Brookes ST, Smith PA. A randomised controlled trial comparing transvaginal ultrasound, outpatient hysteroscopy and endometrial biopsy with inpatient hysteroscopy and curettage. *Br J Obstet Gynaecol* 1999;106:1259–64.

27. Brown SE, Coddington CC, Schnorr J, Toner JP, Gibbons W, Oehninger S. Evaluation of outpatient hysteroscopy, saline infusion hysterosonography, and hysterosalpingography in infertile women: a prospective, randomized study. *Fertil Steril* 2000;74:1029–34.

28. World Health Organization Task Force on the Treatment of Infertility. Comparative trial of tubal insufflation, hysterosalpingography and laparoscopy with dye hydrotubation for assessment of tubal patency. *Fertil Steril* 1986;46:1101–7.

29. Nagele F, O'Connor H, Baskett TF, Davies A, Mohammed H, Magos AL. Hysteroscopy in women with abnormal uterine bleeding on hormone replacement therapy: a comparison with postmenopausal bleeding. *Fertil Steril* 1996;65:1145–50.

30. Gupta JK, Wilson S, Desai P, Hau C. How should we investigate women with postmenopausal bleeding? *Acta Obstet Gynecol Scand* 1996;75:475–9.

31. Alexopoulos ED, Simonis CD, Kidsley S, Fay TN. The value of outpatient hysteroscopy in the management of postmenopausal bleeding: a review of 862 cases. *Gynaecol Endosc* 2000;9:107–12.

32. Watrelot A, Dreyfus JM, Andine JP. Evaluation of the performance of fertiloscopy in 160 consecutive infertile patients with no obvious pathology. *Hum Reprod* 1999;14:707–11.

33. Agostini A, Shojai R, Cravello L, Rojat-Habib MC, Roger V, Bretelle F, *et al.* Endometrial biopsy during outpatient hysteroscopy: evaluation and comparison of two devices. *Eur J Obstet Gynecol Reprod Biol* 2001;97:220–2.

34. Lo KW, Yuen PM. The role of outpatient diagnostic hysteroscopy in identifying anatomic pathology and histopathology in the endometrial cavity. *J Am Assoc Gynecol Laparosc* 2000;7:381–5.

35. Bakour SH, Dwarakanath LS, Khan KS, Newton JR. The diagnostic accuracy of outpatient miniature hysteroscopy in predicting premalignant and malignant endometrial lesions. *Gynaecol Endosc* 1999;8:143–8.

36. Garry R for the Endometrial Ablation Group. Evidence and techniques in endometrial ablation: consensus. *Gynaecol Endosc* 2002;11:5–17.

37. Clark TJ, Mahajan D, Sunder P, Gupta JK. Hysteroscopic treatment of symptomatic submucous fibroids using a bipolar intrauterine system: a feasibility study. *Eur J Obstet Gynecol Reprod Biol* 2002;100:237–42.

38. Varol N, Maher P, Vancaillie T, Cooper M, Carter J, Kwok A, *et al.* A literature review and update on the prevention and management of fluid overload in endometrial resection and hysteroscopic surgery. *Gynaecol Endosc* 2002;11:19–26.

21

Forensic gynaecology

Ruhi Jawad and Jan Welch

Most gynaecologists will, at some point in their careers, be involved in the care of complainants of sexual assault. This chapter aims to provide an overview because good immediate management is essential in promoting recovery as well as in avoiding the loss of evidence, which is crucial to the investigation and prosecution of the crime. Currently only a small minority of allegations of rape result in a conviction; this is a major concern, especially as rapists can go on to commit further assaults.

INTRODUCTION

Sexual assault is defined as any form of nonconsenting sexual activity, and includes threats and attempts to commit sexual acts. Rape is a legal term and its definition varies between countries. In the UK it refers to nonconsensual penetration of the vagina or the anus by the penis; the earlier definition of rape has been broadened to include men as well as women. The word 'rape' derives from the Latin, *rapere:* 'to seize; to force; to have sexual intercourse'.

STATISTICS

In England and Wales, in the year ending March 2001, the police recorded 20 301 cases of indecent assault on women and 3530 on men, and 7929 rapes of women and 664 rapes of men.[1] These figures represent only a minority of such assaults, as the vast majority of those who have been sexually assaulted do not report to the police or consult a doctor.[2]

There is no 'traditional' terminology to use to refer to a person who has been sexually assaulted. Terms including 'victim', 'complainant', 'survivor' and 'patient', have been used. At the Haven (King's College Hospital, London) we use a broader term, 'client', which has the advantage of being neutral.

MANAGEMENT

The initial presentation after sexual assault is variable and the immediate management depends on where and when the client presents. A systematic approach helps to ensure both that the client receives optimal care and that the highest quality evidence is collected.

The client can present within hours or days after the assault, or sometimes after a much longer period, to the police, an accident and emergency department, a department of genitourinary medicine, a sexual health/family planning clinic, a general practitioner, a rape crisis centre, or a sexual assault centre. The client presenting to any one of the above venues should be triaged, escorted to a private area for the interview, and have the option of having a friend or relation present.

GENERAL MEASURES

The first priority is the management of serious physical injuries resulting from the assault. If the client's clothes need to be removed, care should be taken to preserve evidence and avoid contamination. It is important to take a mouth swab, and samples of urine and blood.

Reporting to the police

If the client requests police involvement, then the local police sexual offences investigating team should be contacted. At this point, neither further history nor examination should be performed. Hospital staff should avoid any interference with the forensic evidence provided that the client is clinically stable. She is then taken to a dedicated centre or examined in the accident and emergency department. The forensic medical examination is carried out by a specially trained forensic physician, who should if possible be female if a woman is to be examined.

Not reporting to the police

If the client does not want police involvement, then it is important for the doctor to take a comprehensive history, carry out an examination, and document the findings clearly and in detail. This information may be required as evidence later if the client subsequently decides to report to the police.

Consent

Specific informed consent must be obtained before any history is taken or examination is carried out. When discussing consent the client should be advised that the doctor cannot guarantee confidentiality of any material disclosed during the forensic examination, and therefore that she should not disclose information that is irrelevant but could be upsetting in court. She should also be advised that she can stop the examination at any time.

FORENSIC EXAMINATION

Forensic examination is a detailed procedure that should take place ideally within hours of the assault. The timing of the examination is based on the likelihood of recovering forensic evidence of assault, especially spermatozoa and biochemical evidence.[3-6]

In the absence of a suitably trained sexual offences examiner in the vicinity, a medical examination could be performed by a doctor with experience of the assessment of gynaecological normality and abnormality. If the assault took place less than seven days previously, this would mean that forensic DNA evidence that might otherwise have been found would be lost. If the sexual assault took place more than seven days previously, when DNA evidence would be most unlikely to be found, then the doctor can perform a medical evaluation of the client, making sure that all physical and genital findings are documented.

Appropriate trained personnel can be contacted via the local police, who will have a rota of doctors who work as forensic medical examiners or sexual offences examiners. In areas with sexual assault referral centres, appropriate services will be readily accessible.

It is reasonable to carry out a forensic medical examination within seven days of the assault. An examination can still be performed after this time to document any injuries.

Client support

A wide range of emotions and demeanours may be observed in those who have been sexually assaulted. Such individuals may be calm and show little emotion or they may be anxious and hysterical. The forensic examination team must demonstrate behaviour that is both empathetic and nonjudgemental to help the client during the examination. Someone should stay with the client throughout the examination to ensure a sense of safety. Formal psychological therapy is generally inappropriate at the initial assessment because most clients are acutely traumatised after the assault and may be exhausted.

History taking

The doctor should document carefully the details of the allegation as narrated, in an unrushed and sensitive manner. It is important that these notes are legible, reproducible and contemporaneous. They form part of the doctor's evidence and the basic reference from which a statement will be written if required.

The following details should be recorded, ideally on a standard proforma:

- date, day, time and venue of the examination
- persons present at the time of the examination
- written consent from the client or the appropriate adult (carer, parent, social worker, psychiatric nurse, etc.)
- history of the alleged assault
- narrated by police/client/others
- alleged assailant details (number, relationship, ethnicity, age)
- place of assault
- details of verbal threats, physical assault
- weapons or restraints used
- damage to clothing
- details of sexual assault
    - type of assault (vaginal, anal, oral intercourse)
    - relative positions during the sexual acts
    - condom used (ejaculation)
    - lubricant used
    - penetration of these orifices by other objects
    - other sexual acts (fingering, cunnilingus, rimming)
    - kissing, biting or licking parts of body
- bleeding from vagina or anus
- use of sanitary protection
- drug and alcohol used around time of the assault (date, time, quantity)
- whether the drugs were taken knowingly or unknowingly

- history post–assault
  - eaten, drank, brushed teeth
  - washed, wiped, bathed, showered, douched
  - changed clothes
  - changed sanitary protection
  - bowels opened
  - urine passed
  - self-harm

- general medical history

- occupation

- past medical, surgical, psychiatric history

- drug history (prescribed medications, allergies, over the counter medications, street drugs)

- obstetric and gynaecological history
  - present contraception
  - last menstrual period
  - number of children and mode of delivery
  - previous gynaecological surgery

- consensual/nonconsensual sexual intercourse two weeks prior to the alleged assault (partners, condom, lubricant use)

- sexual intercourse post-alleged assault (same details as above)

- presenting complaints.

Collection of clothing

The clothing worn by the client at the time of the alleged assault is collected for semen and other evidence, such as fibres, and for body fluids for toxicology and DNA testing. All sanitary protection used by the client during and after the assault should be sent for forensic analysis.

Examination

The genital examination can be difficult for someone who has been sexually assaulted, even when the client accepts the necessity of this procedure. The forensic examination is directed to a large extent by the history of the assault. Only disposable instruments taken from sealed packets should be used to retrieve forensic samples.[6] The examination should comprise:

- a general assessment and physical examination, with evaluation of any nongenital trauma

- measurement of height and weight

- a thorough anogenital examination using gross inspection and evaluation of the entire anogenital area, and colposcopy with video recording if appropriate (e.g. in cases of joint examinations with paediatricians, or where the findings may need another expert physician's opinion), and with consent

- collection of all physical evidence on the person and/or clothing of the client

- documentation on appropriate forms of the physical examination and all specimens and samples collected and submitted to the forensic science laboratory.

The forensic examination protocol will vary depending on the time since the sexual assault:

Assault within the last 3–5 days

- first aid

- forensic examination

- emergency contraception (levonorgestrel within 72 hours, intrauterine contraceptive device if within 120 hours of the earliest likely date of ovulation.)

- bacterial and/or anti-HIV prophylaxis

- follow-up.

Assault 7–14 days ago

- medical examination

- sexual health screen or prophylaxis

- counselling (GP, Victim Support, Survivors, social services).

Assault over 14 days ago

- sexual health screen

- counselling (GP, Victim Support, social services).

Forensic samples and swabs

Swabs are taken either for evidence or as control samples for comparison. Evidential swabs are from all areas of unwashed skin that have been in intimate contact with the alleged suspect and from the genital area and anus where appropriate. The control swabs should be taken from uncontaminated areas.

All samples should be packaged quickly and sealed to prevent contamination. The exhibits are labelled and sealed by the forensic doctor and each bears a unique identification code.

- combings and cuttings are taken from head and pubic hair to detect dried up body fluids, foreign hair and debris

- finger nail samples (could be debris from under the nails) or cuttings (provided that this is not detrimental to the client's appearance and self-esteem)

- mouth swab and saliva (taken from inside the mouth and around the teeth)

- body swabs should be slightly moistened (sterile water not saline): taken for blood, semen and saliva

- genital swabs
    - vulval swabs: Two swabs are taken from the external genitalia by rubbing the swabs over the labia and vestibule.

- low vaginal swabs: These are taken by separating the labia and passing a swab into the lower vagina under direct vision, avoiding contact with the external genitalia.
- foreign bodies: Any foreign body found in the vagina (e.g. tampon or condom) should be retrieved using a sterile disposable instrument and packaged as an exhibit (i.e. foreign body and instrument together).
- high vaginal swabs: After passing an appropriately sized speculum (Cuscos), two high vaginal swabs are taken from the fornices above the speculum. Vaginal swabs should be taken when only anal intercourse is alleged because semen can be found in and around the anus after vaginal intercourse. It is not likely to be found in the high vaginal swabs after only anal intercourse.[7]
- endocervical swabs: If the alleged assault has taken place more than 48 hours ago then two endocervical swabs should be taken as well as the high vaginal swabs because spermatozoa live longer in this area.[8]
- perianal swab: If anal penetration was attempted or achieved then swabs from the perianal area should be taken.
- internal anal and rectal swabs: A disposable proctoscope of the appropriate size, lubricated with water for injection, is inserted 1–2 cm into the anal canal. The obturator is removed and internal anal swabs are taken from beyond the edge of the proctoscope. The proctoscope is then withdrawn and a rectal swab is taken.

FOLLOW-UP

All clients should be offered a subsequent appointment to screen for sexually transmitted infections (STIs), and follow-up emergency contraception and any other medications and vaccinations given at the time of the forensic examination (bacterial prophylaxis, postexposure prophylaxis against HIV). Departments of genitourinary medicine can provide this care, as well as access to health advisers. These individuals can provide information and psychosocial support, usually immediately, as well as being able to arrange further psychological aftercare according to the client's needs and wishes.

SIGNIFICANCE OF INJURIES

General injuries

It is important to describe and record injuries accurately as their forensic significance may become apparent only much later. The doctor's contemporaneous notes may be scrutinised in court. Deficiencies in the notes may discredit both doctor and evidence, and thereby influence the outcome of the case.

Studies conducted since the mid-1980s have found that 31–82% of sexual assault victims sustain physical injuries, which are major in 5–10% and fatal in 0.1%.[9–11] Physical injuries most often involve the head, face, neck and extremities.[12] The risk of suffering physical injuries increases if the assailant was a stranger.[13]

The bodily injuries sustained in cases of sexual assault can range from minor abrasions to stab wounds. When describing the injuries it is essential to record the type of wound and its size, site and shape, and to use standard nomenclature when describing injuries, for example bruises (contusions), abrasions (scratches), lacerations (cuts, tears), incisions (slashes, stab wounds, penetrating wounds). A variety of injuries can coexist subsequent to trauma.

All injuries should be drawn accurately on body diagrams after measurement with a ruler or callipers; both the size of the injuries and their relation to fixed anatomical landmarks should be recorded. Tenderness, redness and swelling initially and transiently caused by trauma are not specific signs of injury. The ageing of injuries is one of the most contentious areas in forensic medicine.

Genital injuries

The pattern of genital injuries in female sexual assault victims has been much debated. Not all women who have been sexually assaulted have visible genital injuries; the reported frequency of such injury after rape (on naked eye examination, without using colposcopy or vaginal staining) has ranged from 16% to 61%.[14] Slaughter et al.[15] demonstrated positive colposcopic findings in 87% of female complainants of sexual assault, whereas gross visualisation identified positive genital findings in only 10–40% of cases.

Sexual offence examiners utilise the numbers on the face of a clock as a uniform method of designating the location of a structure or an injury. The 12 o'clock position is always superior (up), and the 6 o'clock always inferior (down). The external genitalia may be stretched, rubbed or be subject to blunt trauma at penile vaginal penetration. All types of injuries (bruises, tears, abrasions, redness and swelling) have been described at all sites on the external genitalia (i.e. posterior fourchette, labia majora, labia minora, hymen and fossa navicularis).

EMERGENCY CONTRACEPTION

Emergency contraception is an effective and safe method of preventing unwanted pregnancy after unplanned, unprotected intercourse.

Two methods of emergency contraception are currently recommended in guidance issued by the Faculty of Family Planning and Reproductive Health Care (FFPRHC).[16] Randomised controlled trials confirm the effectiveness of two 750 µg (0.75 mg) levonorgestrel tablets, taken 12 hours apart, within 72 hours of unprotected sexual intercourse.[17] To improve efficacy and compliance, clients should be encouraged to start the progesterone-only emergency contraception as soon as possible, but the second dose can be taken at a convenient time, as long as it is within 16 hours of the first dose.[16]

In situations where patient compliance is likely to be poor, progesterone-only emergency contraception may be given as a single dose of 1.5 mg levonorgestrel (FFPRHC guidance on emergency contraception, grade A recommendation, April 2003, update June 2003).[16]

An alternative method is insertion of a copper-containing intrauterine contraceptive device in the usual way within five days (120 hours) of the earliest likely date of ovulation in that menstrual cycle. Consideration should be given to the use of antibiotic prophylaxis against STIs to cover intrauterine device insertion after rape.

SEXUALLY TRANSMITTED INFECTIONS

The risk of STI after rape is high, from 4% to 56% in reported studies.[18] If untreated, the sequelae of gonorrhoea and chlamydia include pelvic inflammatory disease, ectopic pregnancy and infertility. The infections found reflect the local prevalence.

Diagnosis of STI

The diagnosis of an STI is usually unhelpful in court, except when the client is sexually inexperienced or at one of the extremes of age, as this finding can be used by the defence to denigrate her character. For this reason samples for STIs should generally not be taken at the time of forensic examination, but on a subsequent visit, by different staff. If there is any chance, however, that these investigations could be relevant, then there should be clear and detailed documentation ('chain of evidence'), which includes the identity of those taking and transporting the sample and carrying out laboratory tests. A protocol for such cases should also be agreed with laboratories so that appropriate procedures are followed for such samples, for example, ensuring that a senior member of staff oversees investigations and that additional tests, such as typing of gonorrhoea, are carried out if necessary.

STIs are commonly asymptomatic in women, and may be hard to diagnose. Even comprehensive sampling of genital and nongenital sites in optimal conditions will miss 12–15% of infections, which will be diagnosed only if further samples are taken at a follow-up visit. Repeated examinations – or even one in some cases – may, however, compound the trauma of the assault. An alternative is to offer antibiotic prophylaxis against gonorrhoea and chlamydia to those clients who seem unlikely to return for follow-up or who are reluctant to be examined. Suggested regimens are:

- ciprofloxacin 500 mg stat plus azithromycin 1 g stat

  or

- ciprofloxacin 500 mg stat plus doxycycline 100 mg twice daily for 7 days

  or (if pregnant or breastfeeding)

- amoxycillin 3 g plus probenicid 1 g stat plus erythromycin 500 mg twice daily for 14 days.

HIV infection

The acquisition of HIV infection from rape is rare in the UK. An individual risk assessment can be calculated as follows:

risk of acquisition of HIV from 1 episode of unprotected vaginal intercourse 1:1000

Risk of assailant having HIV infection

1 in 20 to 1 in 10 000 depending on population background and risk factors of assailant

$$1{:}1000 \times 1{:}20 - 1{:}1000 = 1{:}20\,000 - 1{:}10\,000\,000$$

The risk will, however, be greater if defloration, anal intercourse, trauma or multiple assailants were involved, or if the assailant is known to have HIV or risk factors for HIV such as a history of injecting drug use or coming from a high prevalence country.

Women are often concerned about their risk of acquiring HIV, so our practice in the Haven is to reassure that the risk is generally minute, but to carry out a risk assessment. If the risk is estimated to be significant, or the woman is extremely concerned about her risk and wishes to receive prophylaxis, then postexposure prophylaxis against HIV is offered. This is:

- Combivir® (zidovudine and lamivudine, GSK) one tablet twice daily with food

  and

- nelfinavir 1250 mg (five tablets) twice daily with food for 1 month.

It is our practice to supply a three-day starter pack, together with anti-emetics and antidiarrhoeals, followed by a review appointment. Sixty percent of our clients do not complete the month's course.

PSYCHOLOGICAL ASPECTS

The immediate and long-term psychological consequences of sexual assault vary from individual to individual.

Post-traumatic stress disorder

Post-traumatic stress disorder is 'an anxiety disorder in which exposure to an extreme mental or physical stress is followed, sometimes immediately, and sometimes not until 3 months or more after the stress, by persistent re-experiencing of the event, avoidance of stimuli associated with the trauma or numbing of general responsiveness, and manifestation of increased arousal'.[19]

Acute post-traumatic stress disorder usually lasts less than three months, while chronic post-traumatic stress disorder can last for three months or longer.

Female sexual abuse survivors, especially adolescents, are at increased risk for subsequent acting out behaviour, sexual promiscuity, physical and sexual abuse, anxiety, depression, chronic sleep disturbance, dissociate disorders, eating disorders, suicidal intentions and multiple associated psychiatric disorders.[20]

Rape trauma syndrome

Rape trauma syndrome refers to both the acute phase and the long-term reorganisation process that results from either a forcible or an attempted forcible rape. The syndrome consists of two phases: acute and reorganisation. Details are cited in the original work by Burgess and Holmstrom, 1974.[21]

There is major psychological and mental health morbidity associated with sexual assault; clients require sensitive care, therapy, information and follow-up. Psychological aftercare should be organised as a follow-up service according to the client's needs and wishes.

SPECIAL ISSUES

Child sexual abuse

Presentation

Presentation of child sexual abuse occurs in a number of ways, some of which clearly indicate the abuse, while, in some children, behavioural changes and psychosomatic or physical symptoms suggest the possibility of abuse. The health needs of the child are paramount in approaching any medical examination whatever the alleged circumstances leading to the need to gather forensic evidence.

The nature and timing of the physical examination of the sexually abused child or adolescent depends on the presenting complaint, the timing of the assault and the resources available in the community. The timing of the history and physical examination depends on the urgency for the collection of the forensic evidence. In most cases of child sexual abuse the last episode of abuse could have occurred weeks to months before the disclosure, and the physical examination can be delayed until a memorandum interview is taken.

In cases when children present with a history of sexual abuse or assault within 72 hours or with symptoms of suspicious genital discharge, bleeding or pain, a history and physical examination should be carried out as soon as possible to collect forensic evidence.

Paediatric forensic examinations

A forensic examination is required whenever a child has made a disclosure of sexual abuse or the referring agency or agencies strongly suspect that abuse has occurred. This consists of a full clinical history and examination, detailed documentation and photodocumentation, taking forensic samples, writing a report, case conferences and arranging any follow-up as required.

The forensic examination should be done as soon as possible after the sexual assault. Individual hospitals have protocols regarding acute and chronic sexual abuse. A colposcope is increasingly being used in forensic examination because this offers the advantages of light magnification, direct measurements, and photographic capabilities. Colposcopic photographs and video images can be used for teaching purposes with consent from the clients. Normal and abnormal genital anatomy can be reviewed by other experts and may be helpful in the courtroom.

Normal genital anatomy has been studied extensively, with cross-sectional and longitudinal studies providing the basis for comparisons with genital examination in sexually abused children.[22–26]

Adolescents

Adolescents are a vulnerable group who are at a high risk of sexual victimisation. Adolescent females are the most frequent victims of sexual assault.[27] Although nondisclosure or delayed disclosure also result in underestimation, both these factors put these clients at risk of unwanted pregnancy and STIs.

Young clients under the age of 16 years who are able fully to understand what is proposed, and its implications, are competent to consent to medical treatment regardless of age (Fraser Ruling, often termed 'Gillick competence'). If the young client is not Gillick competent, consent from the parent or carer with parental responsibility is necessary. Confidentiality is usually implicit when consent is given, although there are limits to confidentiality; for example, if sexual abuse or neglect has occurred because of parental neglect, then the child protection team should be notified. Young clients, under the age of 16 years, need an appropriate adult to be present at the time of the forensic examination, as the notes and results could have further implications in court.

The general physical examination should be carried out as discussed above. The breast examination is an important part of Tanner staging[28] in adolescent girls (and boys). The pelvic examination is carried out in the same way as that for an adult but, if the client has not previously been sexually active, or has not had a pelvic examination before, it is important to provide a careful explanation of the procedure. The hymen should be examined in detail and described using standard terms. The normal pubertal hymen may have a smooth curvilinear edge or extensive folds and notches. Perianal examination should also be conducted in detail.

With adolescent clients, genital injuries can be seen after both consensual and nonconsensual intercourse.[29] As with prepubertal clients, adolescents who have been sexually victimised often have normal genitalia.

Rape in pregnancy

Pregnancy has been postulated as being an especially vulnerable time for physical and sexual abuse. Abused women are more likely to begin their antenatal care in the third trimester than nonabused women.[30]

The pregnant client who has been subjected to sexual assault should receive the same medical forensic examination as the nonpregnant client, with special attention to her gravid status. If the client is known to be pregnant at the time of examination, medical consultation with an obstetric team should be available. If necessary the forensic examination should be carried out jointly by an obstetrician and a gynaecologist.

Rape of the older woman

Maltreatment of older women (aged over 60 years) is a problem that can be a combination of domestic violence and sexual assault. The prevalence tends to increase with age; the frail and the dependent are more at risk. Ramin et al.[31] reported a sexual assault frequency of 2% in women 50 years of age and older.

Patterns of sexual assault between postmenopausal and younger age female victims were reviewed by Hicks and Moon.[32] They found that older women had a lower frequency of oral and multiple sexual acts during assault, and that a much greater percentage (88%) of older women were assaulted by strangers; multiple assailants were involved for 21% of these clients.

Anal combined with vulval penetration was reported as the most common pattern of sexual acts during an assault.[31] Cartwright and Moore[33] found that elderly clients (aged 60–90 years) had a 52% incidence of genital trauma. Postmenopausal victims frequently do not report rape and may present with multiple injuries for medical treatment. Forensic medical examination and aftercare is dictated by the time of the assault, and by the presentation and needs and wishes of the client.

Drug-facilitated sexual assault

Since the mid-1990s there has been a dramatic increase in media reports on 'drug-facilitated sexual assault', which is a relatively new term. It is being used to define offences in which victims are subjected to nonconsensual sexual acts while they are incapacitated or semiconscious owing to the effect of alcohol.

Drug-facilitated sexual assault exists in a variety of formats. The drugs most commonly implicated are as follows.

- Rohypnol® (Roche) (the trade name for a drug called flunitrazepam) is commonly associated with drug rape.

- Gamma hydroxybutyrate (GHB) is a drug that can be home made and is not currently illegal to possess. It can be found in the club scene as a recreational drug. It is a colourless, odourless liquid, powder or capsule that is rapidly absorbed when taken orally. The half-life is 30 minutes,[34] and its effects can last from 45 minutes to 8 hours.[35]

- Ketamine is a commercially available anaesthetic for intravenous and intramuscular use. It is available on the street in powder, tablet and liquid form. It is smoked, sniffed or injected.

- Ethanol (alcohol) is a central nervous system depressant; the effects are dose related.

In a study published in 2001,[36] alcohol, either alone or in combination with other drugs, was by far the most common substance found, being present in urine collected from individuals who claimed to have been sexually assaulted and believed that drugs were involved. A study into drug-facilitated sexual assault was undertaken in the UK for the Home Office and reported in 2000 by Sturman.[37]

It is important that urine and blood are obtained from the client as soon as possible. The drugs will be detectable in urine for a longer period than in blood, but detection in blood will allow for the possibility of determining the dose given. This is followed by normal evidence gathering and forensic examination.

THE COURT PROCEDURE

The doctor may be called as a professional witness to give evidence and describe what was found at the time of the examination, after which he or she will be asked to give an opinion on what may have caused the findings or the lack of findings.

After the examination in chief, which in a criminal trial is conducted by the prosecution counsel, the doctor will be cross-examined by the defence counsel, who is allowed to ask leading questions. It is important when giving evidence to answer to the point, simply and briefly.

Before giving evidence in court it is important to study the case thoroughly and consider the differential diagnoses. The doctor is there to assist the court on the basis of his or her knowledge and experience. It is often helpful to the court, especially the jury, if the doctor giving evidence can explain genital anatomy and procedures by using diagrams and basic instruments used in the examination, for example, a Cuscos speculum and proctoscope.

THE FUTURE

Self-referrals

Most rape clients report directly to the police. Those who are unsure about police involvement often receive inappropriate care because they may have to wait for several hours in busy public areas in accident and emergency departments or genitourinary clinics, together with people who have acute medical problems. In addition they are often allowed to eat and drink or pass urine while they wait, thus destroying potential forensic evidence.

Self-referral clinics for those who have been sexually assaulted can bypass such problems. They can be set up in dedicated centres linked to local medical facilities, in which clients can be triaged and seen by the appropriate doctor or forensic nurse examiner. Clients can also be given choices about reporting to the police. The Havens are such centres; clients are given options that include direct liaison with the police, storage of forensic samples to support possible later reporting, or passing on anonymous intelligence and forensic samples to the police.

The Haven, Camberwell

The Haven is a specialist sexual assault referral centre based in the Department of Sexual Health of King's College Hospital, Southeast London, which opened in May 2000 as the pilot for London. It provides a comprehensive, client centred service to which clients can either present through the police or as self-referrals. A total of 1508 clients were seen at the Haven between May 2000 and July 2002, of whom 1188 (79%) were referred by the police and 320 (21%) self-referred. Sixty-six percent of police referrals are of white ethnicity compared with 52% self-referrals. Most clients were female (more than 95%); 16% were aged 12–15 years. Two further Havens are opening in 2004 to serve North London.

The Haven and other centres, such as St Mary's Centre in Manchester, are likely to be used as models for the future development of services in the UK because they have shown that the holistic approach offered at such centres provides not only comprehensive care for clients but also optimises evidence collection. Such models have been highly successful in the USA and Australia.

Sexual assault nurse examiner

The impetus to develop such a programme began in the USA. A forensic nurse examiner is a registered nurse who has been specially trained to provide comprehensive care to sexual assault survivors.

The role of nurse examiner involves providing comprehensive care for the client and working alongside medical colleagues. The forensic nurse examiner can conduct a complete medical forensic examination (following strict guidelines and protocols), advise and prescribe emergency contraception, advise on follow-up to screen for sexually transmitted diseases, and provide the rape client with information to assist her in anticipating what may happen next, and in making choices about reporting.

SUMMARY

The management of sexual assault may appear daunting, but when viewed in its component parts it is not difficult. Treatment should address physical injuries, pregnancy prophylaxis, sexually transmitted diseases and psychosocial sequelae.

Sensitive, supportive and well organised care after an assault can help to avoid medical problems and to initiate the process of recovery.

References

1. Home Office: Recorded crime statistics for England and Wales, 12 months to March 2001 [http://www.homeoffice.gov.uk].
2. Bowyer L, Dalton ME. Female victims of rape and their genital injuries. *Br J Obstet Gynaecol* 1997;104:617–20.
3. Allard JE. The collection of data from findings in cases of sexual assault and the significance of spermatozoa on vaginal, anal and oral swabs. *Sci Justice* 1997;37:99–108.
4. Graves HC, Sensabaugh GF, Blake ET. Postcoital detection of a male-specific semen protein. Application to the investigation of rape. *N Engl J Med* 1985;312:338–43.
5. Davies A, Wilson E. The persistence of seminal constituents in the human vagina. *Forensic Sci* 1974;3:45–55.
6. Rogers D, Newton M. Sexual assault examination. In: Stark MM, editors. *Forensic Science: a Physician's Guide to Clinical Forensic Medicine*. Clifton, NJ: Humana Press; 2000. p. 39–97.
7. Keating SM, Allard JE. What's in a name? Medical samples and scientific evidence in sexual assaults. *Med Sci Law* 1994;34:187–201.
8. Wilson EM. A comparison of the persistence of seminal constituents in the human vagina and cervix. *Police Surgeon* 1982;22:44–5.
9. Marchbanks PA, Lui KJ, Mercy JA. Risk of injury from resisting rape. *Am Epidemiol* 1990;132:540.
10. Rambow B, Adkinson C, Frost TH, Peterson GF. Female sexual assault: medical and legal implications. *Ann Emerg Med* 1992;21:727–31.
11. Tintinalli JE, Hoelzer M. Clinical findings and legal resolution in sexual assault. *Ann Emerg Med* 1985;14:447–53.
12. Satin AJ, Hemsell DL, Stone IC Jr, Theriot S, Wendel GD Jr. Sexual assault in pregnancy. *Obstet Gynecol* 1991;77:710–14.
13. Cartwright PS, Moore RA. The elderly victim of rape. *South Med J* 1989;82:988–9.
14. Bowyer L, Dalton ME. Female victims of rape and their genital injuries. *Br J Obstet Gynaecol*

1997;104:617–20.

15. Slaughter L, Brown CR, Crowley S, Peck R. Patterns of genital injury in female sexual assault victims. *Am J Obstet Gynecol* 1997;176:609–16.

16. Faculty of Family Planning and Reproductive Health Care Guidance. *J Fam Plann Reprod Health Care* 2003;29(2) [www.ffprhc.org.uk].

17. Randomised controlled trial of levonorgestrel versus the Yuzpe regimen of combined contraceptives for emergency contraception. Task Force on Postovulatory Methods of Fertility Regulation. *Lancet* 1998;352:428–33.

18. Lamba H, Murphy SM. Sexual assault and sexually transmitted infections: an updated review. *Int J STD AIDS* 2000;11:487–91.

19. Edgerton J. *American Psychiatric Glossary*, 7th ed. Washington, DC: American Psychiatric Press; 1994.

20. Jeffrey RT, Jeffrey LK. Psychologic aspects of sexual abuse in adolescence. *Curr Opin Obstet Gynecol* 1991;3:825–31.

21. Burgess AW, Holmstrom LI. Rape trauma syndrome. *Am J Psychiatry* 1997;133:413–17.

22. Emans SJ, Wood ER, Flagg NT, Freeman A. Genital findings in sexually abused, symptomatic and asymptomatic, girls. *Pediatrics* 1987;79:778–85.

23. Herman-Giddens ME, Forthingham TE. Prepubertal female genitals: examination for evidence of sexual abuse. *Pediatrics* 1987;80:203–8.

24. Pokorny SF, Kozintz CA. Configuration and other anatomic details of the pubertal hymen. *Adolesc Pediatr Gynecol* 1988;1:97–103.

25. McCann J, Voris J, Simon M, Wells R. Comparison of genital examination techniques in prepubertal girls. *Pediatrics* 1990;85:182–7.

26. Jenny C, Kuhns ML, Arakawa F. Hymens in newborn female infants. *Pediatrics* 1987;80:399–400.

27. Adams JA, Girardin B, Faugno D. Signs of genital trauma in adolescent rape victims examined acutely. *J Pediatr Adolesc Gynecol* 2000;13:88.

28. Tanner JM, Whitehouse RH. Clinical longitudinal standards for height, weight, height velocity, weight velocity, and stages of puberty. *Arch Dis Child* 1976;51:170–9.

29. Kempthorne JV. Sexual abuse and sexual assault of adolescents. In: Olshanker JS, Jackson CM, Smock WS, editors. *Forensic Emergency Medicine*. Philadelphia, PA: Lippincott Williams & Wilkins; 2001. p. 119–51.

30. McFarlane J, Parker B, Soeken K, Bullock L. Assessing for abuse during pregnancy. Severity and frequency of injuries and associated entry into prenatal care. *JAMA*, 1992;267:3176–8.

31. Ramin SM, Satin AJ, Stone IC Jr, Wendel GD Jr. Sexual assault in postmenopausal women. *Obstet Gynecol* 1992;80:860–4.

32. Hicks D, Moon D. Sexual assault of the older woman. In: Office of Criminal Justice Planning. *California Medical Protocol for Examination of Sexual Assault Victims: In Formulation Guide 1987* [www.csaia.org/SART.htm].

33. Cartwright PS, Moore RA. The elderly victim of rape. *South Med J* 1989;82:988–9.

34. Ferrera SD, Zotti S, Tedeshi L, Frison G, Castagna F, Gallimberti L, *et al.* Pharmacokinetics of gamma-hydroxybutyric acid in alcohol dependent patients after single and repeated oral doses. *Br J Clin Pharmacol* 1992;34:231–5.

35. Luby S, Jones J, Zalewski A. GHB use in South Carolina. *Am J Public Health* 1992;82:128.

36. Hindmarch I, Sohly E, Salamone S. Forensic urinalysis of drug use in cases of alleged assault. *J Clin Forens Med* 2001;8:197–205.

37. Sturman P. *Drug Assisted Sexual Assault: a Study for the Home Office Under the Police Research Award Scheme*. London: Home Office; 2000.

22

Selective and nonselective fetal reduction

Sailesh Kumar

INTRODUCTION

One of the difficult issues with which fetal medicine specialists are faced is the issue of termination of pregnancy in multiple gestation. This problem is further clouded when the pregnancy itself is the result of assisted reproductive techniques (ART) in a woman who was previously infertile, raising ethical issues that are not easily resolved. In high-order multiple pregnancies (triplets or greater) there is a clear benefit in terms of perinatal outcome when multifetal pregnancy reduction (MFPR) is carried out. However, when fetal reduction is performed for twins, the advantages are far from obvious.

Fetal reduction can be either selective or nonselective. In selective fetal reduction one of the fetuses may be discordant for an anomaly that may be lethal or its continued presence may jeopardise the survival of its co-twins. Nonselective fetal reduction is usually performed in high-order multiple pregnancies earlier in gestation to reduce the likelihood of high-order births with all their attendant complications. The choice of which fetus to terminate is therefore not dependent on any selection criteria but is often random.

Fetal reduction therefore has the dual objective of preventing the birth of a baby who may have a significant abnormality as well as obviating the significant risk of preterm delivery, which is frequently associated with multiple pregnancy. The decision to terminate any pregnancy is difficult but is arguably more contentious in a multiple pregnancy setting.

INCIDENCE AND EPIDEMIOLOGY OF MULTIPLE PREGNANCY

In the developed world, multiple pregnancy rates have increased significantly, with twin births doubling and triplets increasing three-fold.[1] ART are responsible for a significant increase in multiple births. In the UK almost half the babies born after *in vitro* fertilization (IVF) now come from a multiple pregnancy.[2] In Sweden[3] two-thirds of the increase in multiple births is the result of IVF or ovulation induction and indeed this trend is seen worldwide.

There is some evidence to suggest that spontaneous dizygotic twinning rates have slightly increased.[4] In contrast, monozygotic twinning rates have remained fairly constant over the last few decades[5] and across different racial groups.[6] However, the overall increase in the frequency of multiple births over the last three decades has largely been due to an increase in dizygotic twinning, which appears to be due primarily to gonadotrophin use for ovulation induction and ART.[7]

There has also been an increase in monozygotic twinning as a result of ART, with ovulation induction resulting in a three-fold greater incidence of monozygotic twins compared with after spontaneous conception, and a 2–3-fold increase after conventional IVF.[8] Intracytoplasmic sperm injection appears to produce the highest incidence of monozygotic twins, with some authors reporting rates up to 13-fold higher than spontaneous monozygotic twinning rates.[9]

COMPLICATIONS AND CONSEQUENCES OF MULTIPLE PREGNANCY

Maternal morbidity is associated with the mode of delivery. The National Sentinel Caesarean Section Audit Report published in the UK in 2001[10] stated that 59% of twin pregnancies were delivered by caesarean section, with 51% performed before 37 weeks of gestation. Multiple pregnancy caesarean sections contributed 14% to the overall section rate. Preterm caesarean sections (14% in twins and 36% in triplets) are also much more likely with multiple pregnancies.

Severe maternal obstetric haemorrhage is 2–3-fold more common with multiple pregnancy.[11] Surprisingly, assisted conception twins have a significantly higher rate of haemorrhage when compared with spontaneously conceived twins (10.6% versus 4%).[12] Multiple pregnancy is also associated with increased rates of maternal anaemia and the need for haematinic supplementation.

The incidence of pre-eclampsia is increased with twins[13] and triplets.[14] This risk is further increased if ART are responsible for the multiple pregnancy. This increased risk appears to be independent of the higher incidence of multiple pregnancies.[15] However, the incidence of pre-eclampsia and ART could be mediated by an increased incidence of the background rates of acquired thrombophilia or autoimmune disorders in the ART group.[16]

In addition to increased maternal risks, the perinatal risks are also enhanced. Preterm delivery and intrauterine growth restriction are the predominant determinants of neonatal morbidity and mortality in multiple pregnancies. In the UK in 1999, 41% of all live multiple births were before 30 weeks of gestation.[6] For triplets, in the UK, the perinatal morbidity was 56.2/1000 live births. This is two-fold greater than the perinatal morbidity for twins (33.1/1000) and eight-fold greater than that of singletons (7.4/1000).[6]

Bergh et al.[3] demonstrated that preterm births occurred in 30% of all IVF pregnancies compared with 6% in the general population. Low birthweight occurred in 27% of IVF pregnancies versus 5% in the general population. The overall perinatal mortality after IVF was two-fold greater compared with the general population. These authors ascribed these adverse outcomes to a higher incidence of multiple pregnancies rather than the technique itself. However, it is interesting that there also appears to be increased perinatal morbidity and mortality after ART, which is independent of multiple pregnancies because this increased risk is also apparent when singleton pregnancies are considered alone.

Neonatal problems such as respiratory distress syndrome, necrotising enterocolitis and intraventricular haemorrhage appear to be similar in triplets, twins and singletons when adjusted for both weight and gestation.[17] The incidence of congenital anomalies after IVF is somewhat ambiguous. Some authors[16] suggest that there is an increased risk after ART; however, this association disappeared after correction for maternal age. Bergh et al.[3] concluded that the majority of congenital anomalies occurring after IVF were primarily related to the increased incidence of multiple pregnancy rather than to the technique itself.

Multiple pregnancies in general, when compared with singletons, have an increased risk of neurological sequelae. Patterson et al.[18] reported a 47-fold increase in cerebral palsy in triplet pregnancies and an eight-fold increase in twins compared with singletons. Pharoah and Cooke[19] reported that the prevalence of cerebral palsy in registered births in the UK was 2.3/1000 in singletons, 12.6/1000 in twins and 44.8/1000 in triplets. In monochorionic pregnancies the risk of perinatal mortality and cerebral palsy is considerably greater if there is intrauterine death of the co-twin.[20]

The psychological costs of multiple pregnancies should not be underestimated. Thorpe *et al.*[21] demonstrated that a significantly higher proportion of mothers of twin pregnancies had depression compared with mothers of singletons of the same age. Mothers of twins where one infant had died were three times more likely to suffer depression than mothers of singletons. For triplets, almost all the families had sought psychological help and 36% of the mothers studied had severe enough depression to require antipsychotic therapy. A substantial minority expressed regrets about having triplets.[22]

The economic costs of multiple pregnancies lie particularly in the long-term costs of caring for a preterm infant. Hospital costs have increased substantially, not just in terms of numbers of babies but also through the greater incidence of prematurity, low birthweight and neurological handicap. In the UK, although the majority of IVF treatment cycles are privately funded, the cost of multiple pregnancies comes out of the NHS budget.

GESTATION AT FETAL REDUCTION

Unless there is discordance between the fetuses for an anomaly that may result in a significant risk of handicap, most fetal terminations are performed before 24 weeks of gestation under clause C of the Abortion Act. The majority of these are performed between 11 and 14 weeks of gestation. There are several reasons for choosing this gestation interval. Technically, it is more difficult to perform transabdominal procedures before 10 weeks because of the small fetal size and the accessibility involved in reaching the fetuses when the uterus is still essentially a pelvic organ. In addition, before this time the spontaneous loss of a fetus may occur, which would obviate the need to perform an MFPR. Transabdominal MFPR is usually performed between 11 and 14 weeks, primarily because of a lower miscarriage rate (5.4% versus 12%) and has almost entirely replaced the transvaginal technique.[23] This gestation has a number of advantages. Waiting until after this period will reduce the risk of spontaneous reduction of the surviving fetuses. Secondly, a limited anomaly scan can be performed, which would allow the detection of gross structural anomalies and features of aneuploidy, as well as sexing of the fetuses in order to guide fetal selection for reduction.[24] Although fetal sexing may raise a number of ethical issues, it is important in families at risk of X-linked disorders. Thirdly, screening for aneuploidy using nuchal translucency (NT) can also be performed prior to MFPR, again to help to guide selection if there is discordance of the NT measurement. There appears to be no significant change in pregnancy outcome if invasive prenatal diagnosis by chorionic villus sampling is performed prior to fetal reduction.[25] If there are no structural anomalies and the NT risks of aneuploidy are concordant and low, the fetus furthest away from the cervix is normally selected for reduction. There is some evidence that the incidence of aneuploidy in multifetal pregnancies is less than would be expected.[26] Therefore, with a low risk on NT screening, concerns for the risk of aneuploidy in the remaining fetuses after MFPR is not a major issue.

METHODS OF FETAL REDUCTION

This depends on the gestation and chorionicity of the pregnancy. Early in pregnancy the usual method of selective termination involves intracardiac injection of potassium chloride, usually by the transabdominal route, although some authors have also used the transvaginal route. This is the method of choice in dichorionic pregnancies regardless of the gestation because the demise of one fetus does not usually result in any significant co-twin sequelae. In monochorionic pregnancies the situation is different because selective termination of one fetus without consideration of possible vascular communications with the other fetus could result in the other fetus either succumbing at the time of the termination of its co-twin or suffering serious neurological consequences due to profound hypotension. Cord occlusion is the method of choice in monochorionic pregnancies that require selective termination later in pregnancy (after 16 weeks); although intensified laser may also be used, depending on the gestation.

There has been a steady improvement in the miscarriage rate and perinatal outcome owing to a combination of improved high-resolution ultrasound as well as the learning curve of the physicians performing the technique.[23]

RESULTS OF MULTIFETAL PREGNANCY REDUCTION

MFPR has been used over the last 10 years to reduce high-order multiple pregnancies in the late first trimester, usually down to twins, with the perinatal outcome of reduced twins approaching, but not quite ever reaching, that of spontaneous twins. This has therefore led to the reduction of higher order multiple pregnancies to a finishing number of two to be standard practice because many groups believe that the perinatal mortality and morbidity of twin pregnancies are acceptable.

In the most recent analysis from the International Registry, in 3513 women undergoing MFPR before 24 weeks of gestation at 11 centres, the overall pregnancy loss rate was 9.6%, with 3.7% preterm deliveries between 25 and 28 weeks of gestation,[23] both of which appear to be substantially better than the published outcomes for unreduced multiple pregnancies.[27-29] There was a strong correlation between the starting number of fetuses and the finishing number after MFPR, and the likelihood of poor pregnancy outcome (losses and prematurity). For fetal starting numbers of between four and six, the loss rate was between 12% and 22%, with a severe prematurity rate of 4–11%. The equivalent loss and prematurity rates for triplets were 6% and 3% respectively, and for twins they were 6% and 1.3%. With respect to finishing number, there was a sequential decrease in the risk of pregnancy loss and prematurity from a finishing number of three (20% loss, 6.5% severe prematurity), two (9% and 4%) and one (9% and 1.6%) respectively.

TRIPLETS TO TWINS

It is clear that there are improved perinatal and obstetric outcomes after reduction from high-order multiple pregnancies. However, until 2003 the evidence regarding whether triplets reduced to twins fare better than unreduced triplets was somewhat controversial.

In the International Registry the pregnancy loss rate from reducing triplets to twins was 4.6%.[23] However, the main problem with these data is that there was no control unreduced triplet group for comparison. Wimalasundera et al.[30] therefore undertook a meta-analysis of all studies of more than 20 women published on the MEDLINE computerised medical literature database between 1984 and 2001 in which triplets were reduced to twins. These were compared with a meta-analysis of outcome measures for unreduced triplets published during the same period. The outcome measures investigated were the pregnancy loss rate before 24 weeks of gestation, delivery between 24 and 28 weeks, delivery before 32 weeks, perinatal mortality rate, and take-home baby rate. Overall there were 11 studies of MFPR in which any of the above outcome measures could be derived from a total of 2230 cases, which were compared with 12 studies of unreduced triplets representing 604 cases. The pregnancy loss rate before 24 weeks for triplets reduced to twins was 5.6% compared with 11.5% for expectantly managed triplets (relative risk [RR] 0.45 [0.3–0.6]; $P < 0.0001$). The extreme preterm delivery rate before 28 weeks was also lower for the reduced group (2.9% versus 8.4%; RR 0.35 [0.2–0.6]; $P = 0.0001$), as was the rate of preterm delivery before 32 weeks (10.1% versus 20.3%; RR 0.5 [0.37–0.66]; $P < 0.0001$). Perinatal mortality was lower for surviving twins in the MFPR group (26.6/1000 live births) compared with unreduced triplets (92.2/1000; RR 0.3 [0.2–0.5]; $P < 0.0001$) and the take-home baby rate was greater for the reduced twin group (93%) than the unreduced triplet group (78.6%; RR 0.3 [0.2–0.7]; $P = 0.002$). Based on the above evidence it would appear that the reduction of triplets to twins significantly improves the perinatal outcome compared with unreduced triplets.

However, a number of studies have indicated that MFPR has a significant psychological impact on the parents. Bergh et al.[3] suggested that the parents' recall of the events surrounding the MFPR were of 'chaos and emotional disturbance' and in one of 13 cases the mother 'regretted the decision'. Berkowitz et al.[31] performed a retrospective telephone survey of parents' emotional reactions and attitudes to MFPR. More than 65% of the respondents recalled acute emotional pain, stress and fear, with 18% reporting feelings of guilt and anger.

There are also the ethical issues of terminating the lives of presumably healthy fetuses in order to increase the potential for the others in a multifetal pregnancy. Infertile women who conceive after ART are often nulliparous and invariably anxious to have children, therefore the ethical dilemma of a decision to undergo MFPR is considerable. If all life is sacred to the individual couple then they should be counselled to continue the triplet pregnancy. If, however, their primary concern is to reduce the complications of a triplet pregnancy, they should be guided towards MFPR.

Although MFPR improves perinatal outcome, it is far from an optimal solution to the problems associated with multifetal pregnancies. Prevention of multiple pregnancies has to be a primary objective of those performing ART. Notwithstanding this, when multifetal pregnancies result, it is now the standard of care to offer MFPR in all trichorionic triplet pregnancies as well as in higher order multiple pregnancies.

CONCLUSIONS

The introduction of various methods of assisted reproduction over the last 15 years has enabled many couples to have children. However, it has also increased the risk of multiple pregnancies with all their attendant problems. Although selective termination of pregnancy may be an acceptable option for couples where there is discordance for aneuploidy or a severe malformation among the fetuses, nonselective termination in order to reduce maternal and perinatal complications is a more contentious issue. Nevertheless, it must remain an option because it is an acceptable way of decreasing maternal and fetal morbidity and mortality. The final decision should be made by the couple after comprehensive counselling by medical staff who are familiar with the issues (both medical and ethical) involved.

References

1. Wood R. Trends in multiple births, 1938–1995. *Popul Trends* 1997;(87):29–35.
2. Human Fertilisation and Embryology Authority. *2000 Annual Report and Accounts.* London: Stationery Office; 2000.
3. Bergh T, Ericson A, Hillensjo T, Nygren KG, Wennerholm UB. Deliveries and children born after *in-vitro* fertilisation in Sweden 1982–95: a retrospective cohort study. *Lancet* 1999;354:1579–85.
4. Bortolus R, Parazzini F, Chatenoud L, Benzi G, Bianchi MM, Marini A. The epidemiology of multiple births. *Hum Reprod Update* 1999;5:179–87.
5. Botting BJ, Davies IM, Macfarlane AJ. Recent trends in the incidence of multiple births and associated mortality. *Arch Dis Child* 1987;62:941–50.

6.   Office of National Statistics. Series DH3 No. 33. London: HMSO;1999.

7.   Dawood MY. *In vitro* fertilization, gamete intrafallopian transfer, and superovulation with intrauterine insemination: efficacy and potential health hazards on babies delivered. *Am J Obstet Gynecol* 1996;174:1208–17.

8.   Schachter M, Raziel A, Friedler S, Strassburger D, Bern O, Ron-El R. Monozygotic twinning after assisted reproductive techniques: a phenomenon independent of micromanipulation. *Hum Reprod* 2001;16:1264–9.

9.   Tarlatzis BC, Qublan HS, Sanopoulou T, Zepiridis L, Grimbizis G, Bontis J. Increase in the monozygotic twinning rate after intracytoplasmic sperm injection and blastocyst stage embryo transfer. *Fertil Steril* 2002;77:196–8.

10.   Thomas J, Paranjothy S. *The National Sentinal Caesarean Section Audit Report*. London: RCOG Press; 2001.

11.   Waterstone M, Bewley S, Wolfe C. Incidence and predictors of severe obstetric morbidity: case–control study. *BMJ* 2001;322:1089–93.

12.   Daniel Y, Ochshorn Y, Fait G, Geva E, Bar-Am A, Lessing JB. Analysis of 104 twin pregnancies conceived with assisted reproductive technologies and 193 spontaneously conceived twin pregnancies. *Fertil Steril* 2000;74:683–9.

13.   Sibai BM, Hauth J, Caritis S, Lindheimer MD, MacPherson C, Klebanoff M, *et al.* Hypertensive disorders in twin versus singleton gestations. National Institute of Child Health and Human Development Network of Maternal-Fetal Medicine Units. *Am J Obstet Gynecol* 2000;182:938–42.

14.   Mastrobattista JM, Skupski DW, Monga M, Blanco JD, August P. The rate of severe preeclampsia is increased in triplet as compared to twin gestations. *Am J Perinatol* 1997;14:263–5.

15.   Lynch A, McDuffie R Jr, Murphy J, Faber K, Orleans M. Preeclampsia in multiple gestation: the role of assisted reproductive technologies. *Obstet Gynecol* 2002;99:445–51.

16.   Lambalk CB, van Hooff M. Natural versus induced twinning and pregnancy outcome: a Dutch nationwide survey of primiparous dizygotic twin deliveries. *Fertil Steril* 2001;75:731–6.

17.   Wolf EJ, Vintzileos AM, Rosenkrantz TS, Rodis JF, Lettieri L, Mallozzi A. A comparison of pre-discharge survival and morbidity in singleton and twin very low birth weight infants. *Obstet Gynecol* 1992;80:436–9.

18.   Patterson B, Nelson KB, Watson L, Stanley F. Twins, triplets, and cerebral palsy in births in Western Australia in the 1980s. *BMJ* 1993;307:1239–43.

19.   Pharoah PO, Cooke T. Cerebral palsy and multiple births. *Arch Dis Child Fetal Neonatal Ed* 1996;75:F174–7.

20.   Pharoah PO. Cerebral palsy in the surviving twin associated with infant death of the co-twin. *Arch Dis Child Fetal Neonatal Ed* 2001;84:F111–16.

21.   Thorpe K, Golding J, MacGillivray I, Greenwood R. Comparison of prevalence of depression in mothers of twins and mothers of singletons. *BMJ* 1991;302:875–8.

22.   Garel M, Salobir C, Blondel B. Psychological consequences of having triplets: a 4-year follow-up study. *Fertil Steril* 1997;67:1162–5.

23.   Evans MI, Berkowitz RL, Wapner RJ, Carpenter RJ, Goldberg JD, Ayoub MA, *et al.* Improvement in outcomes of multifetal pregnancy reduction with increased experience. *Am J Obstet Gynecol* 2001;184:97–103.

24.   Lipitz S, Shulman A, Achiron R, Zalel Y, Seidman DS. A comparative study of multifetal pregnancy reduction from triplets to twins in the first versus early second trimesters after detailed fetal screening. *Ultrasound Obstet Gynecol* 2001;18:35–8.

25.   Brambati B, Tului L. First trimester fetal reduction: its role in the management of twin and

higher order multiple pregnancies. *Hum Reprod Update* 1995;1:397–408.

26. Cuckle H. Down's syndrome screening in twins. *J Med Screen* 1998;5:3–4.

27. Yaron Y, Bryant-Greenwood PK, Dave N, Moldenhauer JS, Kramer RL, Johnson MP, *et al.* Multifetal pregnancy reductions of triplets to twins: comparison with nonreduced triplets and twins. *Am J Obstet Gynecol* 1999;180:1268–71.

28. Sebire NJ, D'Ercole C, Sepulveda W, Hughes K, Nicolaides KH. Effects of embryo reduction from trichorionic triplets to twins. *Br J Obstet Gynaecol* 1997;104:1201–3.

29. Ziadeh SM. Perinatal outcome in 41 sets of triplets in Jordan. *Birth* 2000;27:185–8.

30. Wimalasundera RC, Trew G, Fisk NM. Reducing the incidence of twins and triplets. *Best Pract Res Clin Obstet Gynaecol* 2003;17:309–29.

31. Berkowitz RL, Lynch L, Stone J, Alvarez M. The current status of multifetal pregnancy reduction. *Am J Obstet Gynecol* 1996;174:1265–72.

23

New approaches to endometrial carcinoma

Frank Lawton

INTRODUCTION

The traditional approach to the management of women with endometrial carcinoma has been to use surgery and radiotherapy, usually both modalities and in various combinations; overall this leads to about a 75% five-year survival rate. Compared with survival for cervical and ovarian cancer this is impressive but our apparent success should be viewed with caution to prevent therapeutic complacency.

Stage for stage survival rates are similar to those seen with cervical and epithelial ovarian cancer (Table 1), our apparent success arising from the fact that about three-quarters of women with endometrial cancer present with stage I disease, not because of medical intervention or screening but by referral because of symptoms, usually postmenopausal bleeding. However, presented another way, a 75% five-year survival means that one in four women with endometrial cancer will be dead within five years of diagnosis. It should be emphasised that these are data related to pure adenocarcinoma of the endometrium; those related to clear cell or serous papillary uterine tumours are much inferior (Table 2). This is not a 'benign' cancer.

While undoubtedly women with endometrial cancer, because of their age and the intercurrent morbidity associated with the cancer – obesity, diabetes, hypertension – have been regarded as of a degree of surgical/anaesthetic risk too great to consider surgery more aggressive than hysterectomy and bilateral salpingo-oophorectomy alone, it has been claimed that extended surgery – lymphadenectomy, omentectomy – may not only be of diagnostic significance, as per FIGO staging criteria, but may also be of therapeutic value. The Medical Research Council's ASTEC study (i.e. A Study in the Treatment of Endometrial Cancer) should provide further data to determine if this is indeed true.

Table 1 Gynaecological cancer: stage at presentation and five-year survival

Stage	Endometrium		Cervix		Ovary (epithelial)	
	Presentation (%)	5-year survival (%)	Presentation (%)	5-year survival (%)	Presentation (%)	5-year survival (%)
I	75	75	38	77	24	67
II	11	58	32	57	16	42
III	11	30	26	29	42	27
IV	3	10	4	9	18	10

Table 2 Endometrial cancer: five-year survival by histology

Histology	5-year survival (%)
Adenocarcinoma	75
Serous papillary	50
Adenosquamous	47
Clear cell	35

HISTORICAL REVIEW: COMBINED SURGERY AND RADIOTHERAPY

Over 100 years ago Thomas Cullen proposed that the choice of treatment for women with endometrial cancer was abdominal hysterectomy and bilateral salpingo-oophorectomy.[1] Even with the introduction of radium and its use in cervical carcinoma, surgery remained of prime importance. During the 1920s, however, influential researchers suggested, with little clinical data to support their theories, that a combination of surgery and radiotherapy was the best method to treat corpus cancer.[2] Nevertheless, during the 1940s Javert and Douglas began to question the efficacy of radiotherapy and recommended exploratory laparotomy including lymph node sampling as first-line treatment, reserving postoperative radiotherapy for those women found to be node positive.[3] However, over the same time period, other workers noted that women treated with preoperative irradiation had fewer vaginal recurrences than those treated by surgery alone. In 1975, in an excellent review article of 23 publications and over 6000 patients, Jones showed that the five-year survival rate for women treated by surgery alone was almost the same as those who were treated by radiation plus surgery (75% versus 78%).[4] It appeared that survival for women with well or moderately differentiated tumours was similar regardless of the extent of postoperative radiotherapy (vaginal brachytherapy with or without teletherapy) and even for those with poorly differentiated tumours the five-year survival rate for those who received additional pelvic radiotherapy, although better, was not statistically significantly so.[5]

In 1977 Joslin et al.[6] reported on a study that divided patients into two groups: those with disease confined to the endometrium only and those with myometrial invasion (broadly speaking, those with disease confined to the endometrium would have a 0% chance of nodal disease). The former group were treated with intravaginal radiation while the latter received both intravaginal and external therapy.[6] The results were impressive, with only three cases of vaginal recurrence in 256 women and an increased survival for those with myometrial invasion.

The realisation that myometrial penetration was seen to be a risk factor had encouraged Stallworthy's team some years before Joslin's report to undertake extended surgical staging, including pelvic lymph node sampling prior to radiotherapy.[7] They reported that, in women with clinical stage I disease, 6% with well differentiated tumours and over 25% of those with grade 3 disease had pelvic node metastases. The significance of this was that, since most women would be treated surgically by total abdominal hysterectomy and bilateral salpingo-oophorectomy (TAHBSO) only, either a high proportion would have undetected metastatic disease or, if they all also received radiotherapy (pre- or post-surgery), many would be receiving unnecessary adjuvant treatment.

Some years later the Gynecologic Oncology Group (GOG) in the USA produced a number of articles from a much larger study of over 600 women.[8,9] Results were similar, with 25% with either deep myometrial penetration or positive peritoneal cytology, 27% with capillary-like space invasion, and 18% with poorly differentiated tumours having positive pelvic nodes. It is interesting to note at this point that Boronow et al.[8] reported that the majority of women in the study were at low risk for nodal metastases and did not support the idea of more extended surgery for all women with endometrial cancer.

However, in 1988, FIGO announced new staging criteria, which included tumour grade, depth of myometrial penetration, endocervical glandular or stromal involvement, and nodal disease (Table 3). At the time there were reservations about determining nodal status and some clinicians believed that lymphadenectomy was merely a method by which gynaecological oncologists would prevent general gynaecologists from operating on women with endometrial cancer! Some 20 years later the establishment of gynaecological cancer centres provoked similar suspicions!

LYMPHADENECTOMY

That nodal status has to be known to fulfil FIGO staging requirements is obvious. In addition, of course, such data would allow a more rational approach to the use of postoperative radiotherapy. Women in whom nodal status is known are less likely to receive postoperative radiotherapy than those who undergo TAHBSO only.[10] There are also data to suggest that lymphadenectomy may be of therapeutic benefit. In a large retrospective study from the USA all patients underwent hysterectomy and bilateral salpingo-oophorectomy with peritoneal cytology and, in addition, 212 women had multiple site pelvic node sampling, defined as nodes taken from at least four different sites, 205 had 'limited sampling' (nodes taken from fewer than four sites), and 208 had no node sampling at all. The reasons for the degree, or absence, of lymphadenectomy were many: woman's general health, obesity, surgeon's skill or knowledge of the possibility of nodal disease, institutional practices etc., and the results of the study must be viewed in that context. Overall survival for those women who underwent multiple node sampling was significantly better than those who had hysterectomy only and this trend persisted when patients were categorised into high- and low-risk groups based on tumour grade, myometrial penetration and extrauterine disease, and was also seen in those women who received neither pre- nor postoperative radiotherapy. Recurrence rates were higher in the non-node sample group but neither the pattern of recurrence (pelvic, distant or both) nor the interval thereto was affected by lymphadenectomy.[11] However, this possible therapeutic effect has not been shown in other studies.[12,13]

Table 3 FIGO staging of endometrial cancer[a]

I	IA	Tumour limited to the endometrium
	IB	Invasion into <50% myometrium
	IC	Invasion into >50% myometrium
II	IIA	Endocervical glandular involvement only
	IIB	Cervical stromal involvement
III	IIIA	Tumour invades serosa and/or adnexa and/or positive peritoneal cytology
	IIIB	Metastases to pelvic and/or para-aortic lymph nodes
IV	IVA	Invasion of bladder and/or bowel mucosa
	IVB	Distant metastases including intra-abdominal and/or inguinal lymph nodes

[a]In addition, stages IA–IVA are further subdivided by degree of tumour grade (G1, 2, 3 = well, moderately or poorly differentiated)

PATIENT SELECTION FOR EXTENDED SURGERY

The majority of women with endometrial cancer will be node negative and lymphadenectomy may add to the morbidity of surgery, so attempts have been made to determine if women can be selected for more radical surgery based on the measurement of tumour markers or results of imaging studies. Serum CA125 levels are normal in over 90% of women with disease confined to the uterus and elevated in up to 90% of those with extrauterine disease.[14,15] The accuracy of ultrasound, computed tomography and magnetic resonance imaging in determining the depth of myometrial invasion has been compared. Of the three modalities, magnetic resonance imaging is superior with an 89% accuracy, 90% sensitivity and 88% specificity.[16]

Visual assessment of the depth of myometrial invasion has been reported as 90% accurate, a similar figure to that obtained by frozen section analysis.[17,18] Tumour size also correlates well with the incidence of nodal disease, with Schink et al.[19] reporting rates of 6%, 21% and 40% with a tumour size of less or more than 2 cm or occupying the whole uterine cavity. To date, the requirements of FIGO staging notwithstanding, there is no consensus on the extent of surgical endeavour in women with early endometrial cancer. An interesting study used a clinical algorithm to determine in 190 hypothetical patients whether extended surgical staging, TAHBSO plus radiotherapy as indicated by histological findings, or extended staging for only those patients with myometrial invasion determined by frozen section, was the most cost-effective strategy.[20] The most cost-effective was extended surgical staging for all patients because this reduced the expense of both postoperative radiotherapy and intraoperative frozen section analysis.

The morbidity of lymphadenectomy, particularly in obese, older women with coexisting disease typical of those with endometrial cancer has been used by some surgeons to argue against extended surgery. However, most series have shown no increase in morbidity or mortality from this approach.[21,22]

An interesting report from Naumann et al.[10] addressing the question of the beliefs of gynaecological oncologists concerning the therapeutic role of lymphadenectomy compared with their actual clinical practice is illuminating. In this study, although 65% of members of the predominantly US based Society of Gynecologic Oncologists who responded to the questionnaire believed that lymphadenectomy was of therapeutic benefit, only 45% of them actually carried out the surgical procedure (complete pelvic lymph node dissection) routinely. The fact should be emphasised that these practitioners, regardless of their belief, or otherwise, in the merits of the procedure, have no evidence from randomised controlled trials on which to support their contention.

Surgical staging has shown conclusively that the risk of nodal metastases, and hence the need for pelvic teletherapy, depends upon depth of myometrial penetration and tumour grade, which, in turn, are associated with the risk of adnexal or extrapelvic disease. However, reliance on these factors to direct radiotherapy to the pelvic sidewall without knowledge of nodal status is flawed. This question was addressed in the management, at King's College Hospital, of 40 consecutive patients with clinical stage I disease, all of whom underwent hysterectomy and surgical staging. Fifty-three percent of women with greater than 50% myometrial penetration were node negative, as were 45% of those who would be included in the GOG 'high-risk group'.[23] These women would have in all probability been scheduled for postoperative pelvic teletherapy, but it seems illogical to treat the pelvic sidewall and add to the morbidity of treatment in node negative women.

POSTOPERATIVE RADIOTHERAPY

Many institutions have reported on their results with women who, without surgical staging, were treated with postoperative radiotherapy – vault or teletherapy only or both in combination – and there can be no doubt that the results are excellent. In the study of Eltabbakh *et al.*[24] women with grade 1 or 2 lesions, with less than 50% myoinvasion after TAHBSO alone, received postoperative vaginal vault radiotherapy only, which led to an almost 100% five-year disease-free survival.[24] These results are impressive but whether or not this group requires any post-surgical therapy is questionable. In addition, women in a higher risk category – poorly differentiated tumours or greater than 50% myoinvasion – treated with a similar protocol, had only a 74% relapse-free five-year survival.[25] Received wisdom suggests that brachytherapy is a necessary adjunct to TAHBSO alone for women with grade 3 lesions and/or greater than 50% myoinvasion, and possibly for those with cervical involvement.

What then is the situation regarding postoperative radiotherapy for women who have had comprehensive surgical staging? Proponents of such surgical staging quote reports that quantify the morbidity that results from external beam radiotherapy after surgical staging compared with a selective use of brachytherapy only in node negative patients. The GOG reported a 37% complication rate for women treated with external radiotherapy after surgical staging compared with just 4% for those treated with vaginal brachytherapy only.[26] Five-year survival rates of between 86% and 100% have been achieved for women with stage IB disease and above by using only brachytherapy after surgical staging.[27–29] Randomised controlled trials investigating the role of postoperative radiotherapy in endometrial cancer are notable by their rarity; there are only two (plus one abstract) in the literature. The first was published over 20 years ago and undoubtedly has had a major influence on overall management.[5] In this study, carried out over a six-year period from 1968, 540 women with clinical stage I disease underwent TAHBSO without surgical staging followed by intravaginal radium delivering 6000 rad (60 Gy) to the vaginal vault. They were then randomised to receive either no further treatment (the control group) or a further 4000 rad (40 Gy) by teletherapy to the rest of the pelvis (the treatment group). During the follow-up period of 3–10 years there was a significant reduction in vaginal and pelvic recurrences in the treatment group (1.9% versus 6.9%; *P* < 0.01), but the distant metastasis rate in the treatment group was 9.9% compared with 5.5% in the controls. The results meant that five-year survival rates were almost identical (91% for controls compared with 89%). When the results of the GOG study are examined, the reason for the disappointing results is obvious. Within a group of women with apparent stage I disease there is a substantial proportion with extrapelvic disease, sites that would be untreated by pelvic radiotherapy. Aalders *et al.*[5] proposed that overall survival would be improved for high-risk patients (i.e. those with poorly differentiated tumours with. 50% myoinvasion, and incidentally for those with lymphovascular space involvement) by postoperative and pelvic radiotherapy. However, they also recommended that postoperative vaginal radiotherapy should be offered to all other patients to reduce vault recurrence. This report defined the use of post-surgical radiotherapy for almost two decades and remains immensely influential. Most gynaecologists would expect their radiation oncology colleagues to recommend vault irradiation and would probably have discussed this with the woman before referral. The second trial was published 20 years later.[30] In this so-called PORTEC (Post-operative Radiation Therapy I Endometrial Carcinoma) study 715 women were treated by TAHBSO alone (i.e. no surgical staging) and were then randomised to no further treatment or to receive 46 Gy pelvic radiotherapy. The rate of locoregional recurrence was 14% in the surgery only arm compared with 4% in the surgery plus radiotherapy arm, but, once again, five-year actuarial survival rates were almost identical (85% and 81% respectively). Almost three-quarters of the recurrences were at the vaginal vault and the majority of non-irradiated patients (79%) were salvageable by radiotherapy. Most complications were mild but the complication rate was 25% in the irradiated arm versus 6% in the surgery only group. The authors considered that radiotherapy produced such a marginal benefit for women with grade 2, superficially invasive tumours or for those aged 60 years or less, that it need not be given, particularly as the salvage at relapse (79%) was so good. For some women, however, those aged over 60 with grade 1–2 tumours with greater than 50% myoinvasion, and those with grade 3 disease, had an 18% locoregional failure rate and the authors thought that adjuvant radiotherapy should be offered, even though there may be no survival benefit, there being such a small recurrence rate in the irradiated arm.

It should be noted that both of these randomised studies reached similar conclusions regarding which women are at high enough risk of relapse to justify adjuvant radiotherapy based on tumour grade and depth of myometrial invasion, although Aalders et al.[5] and the PORTEC group were at odds in recommending vault radiotherapy for all. It would seem reasonable to believe that women with medium-risk disease are all but cured by surgery alone or have a high chance of salvage by radiotherapy at relapse.

It has been estimated that 67% of locoregional recurrences in non-irradiated patients can be cured by utilising 70 Gy radiotherapy.[31] It would be expected that toxicity at a dose of 70 Gy would be higher than that with adjuvant therapy (around 40 Gy) but, with perhaps only a quarter of the women requiring radiotherapy in the first place, overall toxicity and cost would be reduced considerably.

LAPAROSCOPIC SURGERY

Minimal access surgery has been demonstrated to yield as good a lymph node harvest as open laparotomy and there is no doubt that laparoscopically assisted vaginal hysterectomy is superior in terms of morbidity and inpatient stay.[32,33] The conversion rate to open laparotomy is less than 5% and is usually due to patient obesity preventing laparoscopic surgery. It has been proposed that laparoscopic surgery should be the operation of choice for women with endometrial cancer; however, reports of port site recurrences have appeared in the literature.[34–36] Kadar[34] suggested that such recurrences were merely a function of advanced disease at the time of surgery because both of his patients had microscopic stage III disease, but Faught and Fung Kee Fung's patient had stage IC disease.[36] It has been proposed that the increased time taken for laparoscopic surgery compared with open laparotomy and the pressure created by the pneumoperitoneum may increase the incidence of port site metastases.

CHEMOTHERAPY AND HORMONAL THERAPY

At the time of death due to endometrial cancer many patients will have locoregional recurrence but tumour will be found in sites outside of traditional pelvic radiotherapy fields and these are usually the cause of death. It should be noted that about 10% of women with apparent stage I disease have omental metastases and around 14% will have positive peritoneal cytology.[37–39] If survival is to be improved in these women then these extrapelvic tumour sites must be treated.

The role of postoperative or adjuvant chemotherapy in women with poor prognosis disease has not been defined. It is apparent that, although the pelvis may be affected at the time of relapse, there is often disease in the upper abdomen or thorax and, in addition, extra-abdominal disease at diagnosis is a characteristic of nonendometrioid cancers. Clearly, therefore, there is a need for postoperative systemic therapy in a number of patients. Active regimens include combinations of cyclophosphamide, doxorubicin and platinum (CAP) but high response rates of reasonable duration are rarely reported. A typical response rate would be around 25% with a median overall survival of only seven months.[39]

The majority of studies, however, have been in relapsed disease but there are few reports that contain large patient numbers. Other drugs shown to be active in relapsed patients include paclitaxel and ifosfamide, with response rates of up to 40% as single agents and higher in combination. There have been a number of reports of the use of cytotoxic and hormonal therapy in combination. Most regimens use megestrol or medroxyprogesterone acetate in combination with CAP, but patient numbers are usually small (less than 50), with responses varying from 33% to 60%. This may be superior to chemotherapy alone but there are no data available from randomised phase III trials. Hormonal treatment of endometrial cancer is dependent on receptor status. Biologically aggressive tumours tend to be receptor negative and therefore resistant to hormonal therapy and, even in receptor positive disease, response to hormonal manipulation is usually of a finite duration. Tamoxifen can induce synthesis of progesterone receptors in tumours with low levels thereof but once again the duration of this effect is limited. In a nude mouse model the growth of transplanted endometrial cancers can be stopped with a combination of tamoxifen and progestogens but only for about four to five months before 'resistance' occurs, mimicking the situation seen clinically.[40]

FAMILIAL ENDOMETRIAL CANCER

Familial clustering of endometrial cancers have been reported and by far the majority are seen in association with colon cancer in families with hereditary nonpolyposis colon cancer syndrome. This is an autosomal dominant condition caused by germline mutations in DNA mismatch repair genes and is characterised by the development of colon cancer at a much younger age than that in the general population. In such families, as well as colon cancer, cases of endometrial, ovarian, renal and biliary tract cancer may be seen and it has been estimated that the lifetime risk of developing endometrial cancer may be over 40%.[41] Recommendations regarding endometrial surveillance in such families have not been established but some authors have suggested that prophylactic TAHBSO should be considered.[42]

Somatic mutations/amplification in mismatch repair genes have also been reported. K-*ras* oncogene mutations have been demonstrated in both endometrial hyperplasia and carcinoma, and such mutation may be an early event in the genesis of endometrial cancer.[43] p53 mutations occur commonly in early stage serous papillary cancers but not in endometrioid tumours, suggesting variable genetic pathways for these different endometrial cancers.[44] As with all potential gene therapies, clinical or therapeutic use of these gene abnormalities is some years away.

THE (NEAR) FUTURE

The results of a number of randomised clinical trials will probably define the role of lymphadenectomy and postoperative radiotherapy in endometrial cancer in the next few years, and the 25% of women with true high-risk disease who are most likely to benefit from adjuvant radiotherapy will be identified by extended surgical staging. Overall, the surgical workload is likely to grow in line with the increase in women's life expectancy and perhaps secondary to the more frequent use of tamoxifen in women with breast cancer, their unaffected relatives and other high-risk groups. The use of laparoscopic surgery is also likely to increase. However, an overall improvement in survival will not be apparent or at least will not be demonstrable because such randomised studies currently recruiting or planned will not be large enough to reveal small differences in outcome. An overall survival of more than 70% will make it difficult, or even unethical, to recruit large numbers of women. Improvements in outcome will be small and confined to specific patient subgroups. Most patients will continue to be diagnosed with FIGO I disease and will be cured by surgery alone or salvaged by radiotherapy at relapse. It is likely that more use will be made of chemotherapy and at an earlier point in treatment.

Statistical considerations apart, the results of some of the above will benefit individual women in terms of quality, and quantity, of life. These are worthy endpoints.

References

1.   Cullen TH. *Cancer of the Uterus*. Philadelphia: Saunders; 1900.

2.   Arneson A. Clinical results and histologic changes following the radiation treatment of cancer of the corpus uteri. *Am J Roentgenol* 1936;36:461–6.

3.   Javert CT, Douglas R. Treatment of endometrial carcinoma. *Am J Roentgenol* 1956;75:508–14.

4.   Jones HW. Treatment of adenocarcinoma of the endometrium. *Obstet Gynecol Surv* 1975;30:147–69.

5.   Aalders JG, Abeler V, Kolstad P, Onsrud M. Postoperative external irradiation and prognostic parameters in stage I endometrial carcinoma: clinical and histopathologic study of 540 patients. *Obstet Gynecol* 1980;56:419–26.

6.   Joslin CA, Vaishampayan GV, Mallik A. The treatment of early cancer of the corpus uteri. *Br J Radiol* 1977;50:38–45.

7.   Lewis BV, Stallworthy JA, Cowdell R. Adenocarcinoma of the body of the uterus. *J Obstet Gynaecol Br Cwlth* 1970;77:343–8.

8.   Boronow RC, Morrow CP, Creasman WT, Di Saia PJ, Silverberg SG, Miller A, *et al*. Surgical staging in endometrial cancer: clinical-pathologic findings of a prospective study. *Obstet Gynecol* 1984;63:825–32.

9.   Creasman WT, Morrow CP, Bundy BN, Homesley HD, Graham JE, Heller PB. Surgical pathologic spread patterns of endometrial cancer. A Gynecologic Oncology Group study. *Cancer* 1987;60:2035–41.

10. Naumann RW, Higgins RV, Hall JB. The use of adjuvant radiation therapy by members of the Society of Gynaecologic Oncologists. *Gynecol Oncol* 1999;75:4–9.

11. Kilgore LC, Partridge EE, Alvarez RD, Austin JM, Shingleton HM, Noojin F, *et al*. Adenocarcinoma of the endometrium: survival comparisons with and without pelvic node sampling. *Gynecol Oncol* 1995;56:29–33.

12. Belinson JL, Lee KR, Badger GJ, Pretorius RG, Jarrell MA. Clinical stage I adenocarcinoma of the endometrium – analysis of recurrences and the potential benefit of staging lymphadenectomy. *Gynecol Oncol* 1992;44:17–23.

13. Trimble EL, Kosary C, Park RC. Lymph node sampling and survival in endometrial cancer. *Gynecol Oncol* 1998;71:340–3.

14. Niloff JM, Klug TL, Schaetzl E, Zurawski VP Jr, Knapp RC, Bast RC Jr, *et al*. Elevation of serum CA125 in carcinomas of the fallopian tube, endometrium and endocervix. *Am J Obstet Gynecol* 1984;148:1057–8.

15. Sood AK, Buller RE, Burger RA, Dawson JD, Sorosky JI, Berman M. Value of preoperative Ca 125 level in the management of uterine cancer and prediction of clinical outcome. *Obstet Gynecol* 1997;90:441–7.

16. Kim SH, Kim HD, Song YS, Kang SB, Lee HP. Detection of deep myometrial invasion in endometrial carcinoma: comparison of transvaginal ultrasound, CT, and MRI. *J Comput Assist Tomogr* 1995;19:766–72.

17. Larson DM, Connor GP, Broste SK, Krawisz BR, Johnson KK. Prognostic significance of gross myometrial invasion with endometrial cancer. *Obstet Gynecol* 1996;88:394–8.

18. Shim JU, Rose PG, Reale FR, Soto H, Tak WK, Hunter RE. Accuracy of frozen-section diagnosis at surgery in clinical stage I and II endometrial carcinoma. *Am J Obstet Gynecol* 1992;166:1335–8.

19. Schink JC, Lurain JR, Wallemark CB, Chmiel JS. Tumour size in endometrial cancer: a prognostic factor for lymph node metastases. *Obstet Gynecol* 1987;70:216–19.

20. Barnes MN, Roland PY, Straughn M, Kilgore LC, Alvarez RD, Partridge EE. A comparison of treatment strategies for endometrial adenocarcinoma: analysis of financial impact. *Gynecol Oncol* 1999;74:443–7.

21. Larson DM, Johnson K, Olson KA. Pelvic and para-aortic lymphadenectomy for surgical staging of endometrial cancer: morbidity and mortality. *Obstet Gynecol* 1992;79:998–1001.

22. Homesley HD, Kadar N, Barrett RJ, Lentz SS. Selective pelvic and periaortic lymphadenectomy does not increase morbidity in surgical staging of endometrial carcinoma. *Am J Obstet Gynecol* 1992;167:1225–30.

23. Lawton FG. The management of endometrial cancer. *Br J Obstet Gynaecol* 1997;104:127–34.

24. Eltabbakh GH, Piver MS, Hempling RE, Shin KH. Excellent long-term survival and absence of vaginal recurrences in 332 patients with low-risk stage I endometrial adenocarcinoma treated with hysterectomy and vaginal brachytherapy without formal staging lymph node sampling: report of a prospective trial. *Int J Radiat Oncol Biol Phys* 1997;38:373–80.

25. Weiss E, Hirnle P, Arnold-Bofinger H, Hess CF, Bamberg M. Adjuvant vaginal high-dose-rate afterloading alone in endometrial carcinoma: patterns of relapse and side effects following low-dose therapy. *Gynecol Oncol* 1998;71:72–6.

26. Morrow GP, Bundy BN, Kurman RJ, Creasman WT, Heller P, Homesley HD, et al. Relationship between surgical-pathological risk factors and outcome in clinical stage I and II carcinoma of the endometrium. *Gynecol Oncol* 1991;40:55–65.

27. Orr JW Jr, Holiman JL, Orr PF. Stage I corpus cancer: is teletherapy necessary? *Am J Obstet Gynecol* 1997;176:777–89.

28. Ng TY, Perrin LC, Nicklin JL, Cheuk R, Crandon AJ. Local recurrence in high-risk node-negative stage I endometrial carcinoma treated with postoperative vaginal vault brachytherapy. *Gynecol Oncol* 2000;79:490–4.

29. Fanning J. Long term survival of intermediate risk endometrial cancer (stage IG3, IC, II) treated with full lymphadenectomy and brachytherapy without teletherapy. *Gynecol Oncol* 2001;82:371–4.

30. Creutzberg CL, van Putten WL, Koper PC, Lybeert ML, Jobsen JJ, Warlam-Rodenhuis CC, et al. Surgery and postoperative radiotherapy versus surgery alone for patients with stage-1 endometrial carcinoma: multicentre randomised trial. PORTEC Study Group: Post-operative Radiation Therapy in Endometrial Carcinoma. *Lancet* 2000;355:1404–11.

31. Ackerman I, Malone S, Thomas G, Franssen E, Balogh J, Dembo A. Endometrial carcinoma – relative effectiveness of adjuvant irradiation vs therapy reserved for relapse. *Gynecol Oncol* 1996;60:177–83.

32. Childers JM, Brzechffa PR, Hatch KD, Surwit EA. Laparoscopically assisted surgical staging (LASS) of endometrial cancer. *Gynecol Oncol* 1993;51:33–8.

33. Fram KK. Laparoscopically assisted vaginal hysterectomy versus abdominal hysterectomy in stage I endometrial cancer. *Int J Gynecol Cancer* 2002;12:57–61.

34. Kadar N. Port-site recurrences following laparoscopic operations for gynaecological malignancies. *Br J Obstet Gynaecol* 1997;104:1308–13.

35. Wang PH, Yen MS, Yuan CC, Chao KC, Ng HT, Lee WL, et al. Port-site metastases after laparoscopic-assisted vaginal hysterectomy for endometrial cancer: possible mechanisms and prevention. *Gynecol Oncol* 1997;66:151–5.

36. Faught W, Fung Kee Fung M. Port-site recurrences following laparoscopically managed early stage endometrial cancer. *Int J Gynecol Cancer* 1999;9:256–8.

37. Chen SS, Spiegel G. Stage I endometrial carcinoma. Role of omental biopsy and omentectomy. *J Reprod Med* 1991;36:627–9.

38. Nieto JJ, Gornall R, Toms E, Clarkson S, Hogston P, Woolas RP. Influence of omental biopsy on adjuvant treatment in clinical Stage I endometrial carcinoma. *BJOG* 2002;109:576–8.

39. Price FV, Chambers SK, Carcangiu KE, Kohorn EI, Schwartz PE, Chambers JT, *et al.* Intravenous cisplatin, doxorubicin and cyclophosphamide in the treatment of uterine papillary serous carcinoma (UPSC). *Gynecol Oncol* 1993;51:383–9.

40. Mortel R, Zaino RJ, Satyaswaroop PG. Designing a schedule of progestin administration in the control of endometrial carcinoma growth in the nude mouse model. *Am J Obstet Gynecol* 1990;162:928–6.

41. Dunlop MG, Farrington SM, Carothers AD, Wyllie AH, Sharp L, Burn J, *et al.* Cancer risk associated with germline DNA mismatch repair gene mutations. *Hum Mol Genet* 1997;6:105–10.

42. Burke W, Peterson G, Lynch P, Botkin J, Daly M, Garber J, *et al.* Recommendations for follow-up care of individuals with an inherited predisposition to cancer. I: Hereditary nonpolyposis colon cancer. Cancer Genetics Studies Consortium. *JAMA* 1997;227:915–19.

43. Enomoto T, Inoue M, Perantoni AO, Buzzard GS, Miki H, Tanizawa O, *et al.* K-*ras* activation in premalignant and malignant epithelial lesions of the human uterus. *Cancer Res* 1991;51:5308–14.

44. Lax SF, Kendall B, Tashiro H, Slebos RJ, Hedrick L. The frequency of p53, K-*ras* mutations, and microsatellite instability differs in uterine endometrioid and serous carcinoma: evidence of distinct molecular genetic pathways. *Cancer* 2000;88:814–24.

24

Ovarian cysts in pregnancy

Christopher Lee and Davor Jurkovic

INTRODUCTION

The reported prevalence of ovarian cysts has risen significantly since the 1970s.[1,2] A likely cause of this trend is the increasing use of ultrasound examination in pregnancy. In addition to the traditional anomaly scan at 20 weeks of gestation, many women are now also being offered ultrasound scans in the first trimester. The indications for this vary and include pregnancy dating, suspected early pregnancy failure, and first trimester screening for chromosomal abnormalities. The routine visualisation of the adnexae is a standard part of ultrasound examination in obstetrics and gynaecology. This practice has introduced an informal 'screening process' whereby a large number of asymptomatic pregnant women are screened for adnexal pathology.

The presence of an ovarian cyst is traditionally considered to be an indication for operative intervention owing to fear of ovarian cancer and acute complications of ovarian cysts such as torsion, rupture and obstruction of labour. However, these risks are difficult to quantify and it is possible that many asymptomatic women with cysts are being overtreated. This is of particular concern in pregnancy, when the risks of operative complications are increased. In this chapter we will summarise current data on epidemiology, pathology and clinical significance of ovarian cysts in pregnancy, and discuss various management strategies that could be used during pregnancy.

EPIDEMIOLOGY

The prevalence of ovarian cysts in pregnancy depends on the sensitivity of the screening test, diagnostic criteria to define an ovarian cyst, and the timing of examination in pregnancy. Two studies described the prevalence of ovarian cysts in pregnancy before the use of ultrasound, when diagnosis was based on the clinical examination of women with symptoms suggestive of an adnexal mass.[1,3] They showed a prevalence of ovarian tumours of approximately 1:1000.

With the introduction of routine second trimester obstetric ultrasound examination the reported prevalence of ovarian cysts increased. Hogston and Lilford[4] reviewed the results of 26 110 routine ultrasound scans and they found 137 adnexal cysts, giving a prevalence of 1:190. Only 45% of these cysts could also be detected on clinical examination.[4] A later study by Hill *et al.*[5] included 7996 women, 55% of whom were examined before 20 weeks of gestation. A total of 335 adnexal cysts were found. The prevalence of cysts was 1:24 (4%), which is ten times higher than in the findings of Hogston and Lilford.[4] A screening study in our department was conducted at the time of the 11–14-week nuchal translucency scan. A total of 728 cysts were found in 2925 women, a prevalence of 24.9%.[2]

The increased prevalence in the latter studies may be partly due to improved resolution of modern ultrasound machines. However, it is more likely that the increase is due to the more liberal use of ultrasound in early pregnancy. During the first it is much easier to visualise the ovaries than later in gestation. Furthermore, the prevalence of ovarian cysts is much higher earlier in pregnancy.

A cross-sectional study by Hill *et al.*[5] showed that the prevalence of ovarian cysts is four times higher at 13–15 weeks of gestation compared with 34–39 weeks. Our longitudinal study showed that 85% of cysts detected during the first trimester resolve spontaneously during pregnancy.[2] The resolution rate was observed even for large complex cysts. These results indicate that the vast majority of ovarian cysts are functional in nature and that their reported prevalence is likely to increase in the future with the widespread use of transvaginal scanning in early pregnancy when there is suspected early pregnancy failure.

PATHOLOGICAL CHARACTERISTICS

Functional cysts

The vast majority of adnexal cystic masses detected in early pregnancy are functional, such as corpus luteum or follicular cysts. The corpus luteum is formed from postovulatory follicles and synthesises progesterone, providing hormonal support for the pregnancy in the first trimester. It normally resolves by the 16th week of gestation. Serum progesterone levels increase during the first two weeks after conception and then decrease slightly and level off until a luteoplacental shift occurs.[6] By 8.5 weeks of gestation the placenta and corpus luteum are contributing equal amounts of progesterone.[7]

Kobayashi *et al.*[8] carried out a study designed to follow changes in the size of functional cysts observed on ultrasonography during early pregnancy.[8] They looked retrospectively at the results of 6357 first trimester ultrasound reports and identified 250 women with adnexal masses. They classified a functional cyst as being smooth, round and thin walled, without evidence of internal echoes or nodularity on ultrasonography. They found that maximum functional cyst size is reached at about seven weeks of gestation, with gradual diminution thereafter. They further observed that there is wide variation in the way functional cysts behave, and they cannot be defined in terms of a maximum cyst diameter, or in terms of persistence beyond a certain gestation, as has previously been described.

Corpus luteum cysts, however, are not uncommonly observed to contain areas of mixed internal echoes representing haemorrhage. This may have a fine 'web-like' appearance, form a 'jelly-like' area across the cyst, or have a ground-glass appearance like an endometrioma, depending on how organised the blood in the cyst cavity has become. Cysts demonstrating these ultrasound features would not fulfil the diagnostic criteria proposed by Kobayashi *et al.*[8]

It appears therefore that the most important feature in confirming a diagnosis of functional cyst is the transient nature of these structures. Thus the diagnosis is normally confirmed on noting spontaneous resolution at a follow-up scan 4–6 weeks after the initial scan.

Dermoid cysts

Dermoid cysts or mature cystic teratomas are the most common complex ovarian masses encountered in pregnancy, making up 24–40% of all pregnancy related ovarian tumours.[9] They are characterised on ultrasound examination as cystic masses containing multiple areas of hyperechogenicity arising from hair, bone and calcified areas within the cyst. Acoustic shadows may also be cast behind these structures due to high impedance to ultrasound wave transmission.

Common ovarian cysts in young women can usually be characterised accurately by ultrasound examination. Jermy *et al.*[10] have shown that the positive predictive value of transvaginal ultrasound for the diagnosis of dermoid cysts and endometriomas is 97.1% and 96.7% respectively. Using colour flow Doppler imaging, few dermoid cysts appear to have detectable flow,[11–13] however the functional ovarian tissue adjacent to the cyst capsule may display variable degrees of vascularity. Although Whitecar et al.[14] stated that, in their department, pre-operative ultrasound was not helpful in differentiating tumours of low malignant potential from benign neoplasms, a benign dermoid cyst, which is the most common complex ovarian cyst detected during pregnancy, reportedly demonstrates pathognomonic features with an accuracy of 97–100% on ultrasound.[14]

Complications associated with dermoid cysts are uncommon, but may include torsion and rupture. During pregnancy, the rate of such complications is thought to be increased because of the increasing size of the uterus. In addition, dermoid cysts may complicate labour by presenting a mechanical obstruction to the birth canal. Caspi et al.[15] followed 49 women with ultrasonically diagnosed ovarian dermoid cysts smaller than 6 cm for assessment of possible complications during pregnancy and labour in 68 pregnancies. They performed serial ultrasound scans before and during pregnancy, and after delivery, in order to detect changes in the size of the dermoid cyst. None of the women included in the study suffered any of the classic complications attributable to dermoid cysts in pregnancy, such as torsion, rupture and dystocia. They concluded that ovarian dermoid cysts smaller than 6 cm in diameter can be conservatively followed during pregnancy and labour. Their study also showed no evidence of growth of any dermoid cysts throughout pregnancy.[15]

In our own study, 18 dermoid cysts were managed expectantly with no adverse outcomes. They constituted 6.1% of the total cysts included in the study and 40% of persistent cysts. These results indicate that expectant management is appropriate for the majority of dermoids detected in pregnancy. However, an operative intervention may be considered for large dermoids greater than 10 cm in diameter, as the risk of complications may be higher.

Endometrioma

Ovarian endometriomas represent an advanced stage of endometriosis. Although many reports describe them as having typical ultrasound features, they are a common source of a false positive diagnosis of malignancy. They are typically seen on ultrasound examination as well circumscribed thick walled cysts that contain homogeneous low-level internal echoes. This so-called 'ground glass' appearance is due to altered blood. The fluid is often hypoechoic so in some cases it may be necessary to increase the gain setting to detect the low-level echogenicity.[16] The wall may contain hyperechoic foci and sometimes the internal wall is covered with 'sludge'.[17] Additional information may be obtained by the application of gentle pressure with the tip of the transvaginal probe, which may reveal tenderness and reduced mobility of the pelvic viscera. Internal septations have been described in 10–30% of all endometriotic cysts seen.[18–20] If the lesion is bilateral, both ovaries may be adherent in the midline, a feature sometimes referred to as 'kissing ovaries'.

Although they may be asymptomatic, the majority of endometriomas have characteristic features and a clinical history to support the diagnosis.

Pregnancy complicated by endometriomas has been reported as being rare because of their association with infertility.[21] However, in our study, endometriomas were found to be the second most common persistent benign ovarian cyst diagnosed in pregnancy, constituting 3% of the total number of cysts included in the study and 20% of persistent cysts. There are variable reports on the behaviour of endometriosis in pregnancy. Some women show marked progression of endometriosis or a significant increase in the size of endometriomas during pregnancy.[22,23] In animal models such as rats and mice, pregnancy has been shown to confer a beneficial effect on endometriosis.[24] It has also been observed that pregnancy provides subjective and objective improvements in many women with extensive pelvic endometriosis and this has become the basis for some forms of medical treatment.

Benign epithelial ovarian tumours

Epithelial tumours are derived from the coelomic epithelium overlying the embryonic gonadal ridge, from which develop müllerian and wolffian structures, whereas mucinous cystadenomas develop along endocervical pathways and serous cystadenomas develop along tubal pathways. These benign cysts are most common in women over the age of 40 years, although they tend to occur at a slightly younger age than their malignant counterparts[25] and make up 1.5% of ovarian cysts diagnosed during pregnancy and 10% of ovarian cysts persisting throughout pregnancy.

Serous cystadenomas are the most common benign epithelial tumours across all age ranges and about 10% are bilateral. They are usually unilocular and papillary processes are often seen projecting from the internal capsule into the cyst cavity. The epithelium on the inner surface is cuboidal or columnar and may be ciliated. The cyst fluid is usually thin and serous.[25] Mucinous cystadenomas constitute 15–25% of all ovarian tumours. However, they are far less common in women of reproductive age. Typically, they are large, unilateral and multilocular with a smooth internal capsule. The cyst fluid is generally thick and gelatinous[26].

Tubal pathology

Although not strictly ovarian cysts, a section on tubal pathology encompassing fimbrial cysts and dilated fallopian tubes is included because disorders of the fallopian tube contribute a significant proportion of cystic adnexal masses diagnosed during pregnancy, and can pose similar management dilemmas. Indeed they are a common source of false positive diagnoses of ovarian cysts.

Fimbrial cysts are usually seen on ultrasound examination as thin walled anechoic, unilocular adnexal masses. They have a smooth internal capsule and minimal blood flow revealed by colour flow Doppler interrogation. Importantly, from a diagnostic viewpoint, they can be identified separately from the ovary on ultrasound examination. This observation may be facilitated by gentle pressure applied with the tip of the ultrasound probe while visualising both ovary and cyst.

Hydrosalpinx is caused by fluid accumulation within the fallopian tube due to occlusion of the distal fimbrial portion of the tube. The most common aetiology of tubal occlusion is previous salpingitis, which may have been clinical or subclinical. Prevalence varies with geographical location and population studied. In our screening study, tubal pathology was the cause of 1.2% of adnexal masses detected in pregnancy and 12.1% of persistent adnexal masses requiring surgical intervention.

Ultrasound examination reveals a tubular anechoic structure with thickened mucosal folds (incomplete septations) and nodular projections into the lumen. They may be thin or thick walled and these have been described as different pathological entities.[16,27] The appearance of internal echoes in the distended lumen with the absence of blood flow suggests pyosalpinx. However, acute pelvic infection in pregnancy is rare.

Malignant ovarian tumours

Although rare, ovarian cancer is the second most common gynaecological cancer diagnosed during pregnancy, after cervical carcinoma.[28] The incidence of ovarian cancer associated with pregnancy is estimated as 1/12 000 to 1/25 000 births.[29] Earlier reports suggested that 2–5% of ovarian cysts in pregnancy are malignant but that the prognosis is relatively good.[30–33] It is unclear whether the prognosis is good because of earlier diagnosis by antenatal ultrasound screening, or because ovarian malignancy in pregnancy is of lower grade than in nonpregnant women, or a combination of both.[34] The distribution of ovarian tumour subtypes in pregnancy is different from that seen in the general population. This is not surprising because pregnant women comprise a relatively young segment of the population. It seems that, in general, the incidence of ovarian cancer in pregnancy parallels that in women of childbearing age.[29,35] Consequently, one would expect a greater proportion of germ cell tumours than in the general population, and this indeed proves to be the case. Copeland and Landon[36] reviewed the literature on ovarian cancer occurring during pregnancy and found that 45% are germ cell tumours (dysgerminomas in particular) and only 37.5% are epithelial. This contrasts with figures for the general population, in whom epithelial tumours constitute approximately 90% of all ovarian cancers.[25]

Borderline tumours (or tumours of low malignant potential) have been shown to constitute 33–50% of ovarian cancers in pregnancy.

Ovarian cancers diagnosed during pregnancy seem to be associated with a better maternal prognosis because they are more likely to be of lower stage at diagnosis. However, stage for stage the prognosis appears to be the same as for nonpregnant women.[35,37]

CLINICAL SIGNIFICANCE

The main concerns associated with ovarian cysts detected during pregnancy centre around the following clinical issues:

- accurate discrimination between benign and malignant pathology in persistent or morphologically 'suspicious' ovarian cysts
- prompt diagnosis and treatment of adnexal torsion
- the rare complication of labour dystocia secondary to mechanical obstruction of the birth canal by an ovarian cyst located low in the pelvis.

Differential diagnosis of adnexal masses

Ultrasound diagnosis

The ability of ultrasound examination to discriminate between benign and malignant ovarian tumours varies between different reports. The main factor that determines the success of ultrasound diagnosis appears to be the experience of the operator.[38] Since the early 1990s, a number of scoring systems and multiparameter diagnostic tests have been proposed in an attempt to standardise the assessment of ovarian tumours and reduce the dependence of ultrasound diagnosis on the quality of the operator.[39–41] Although the initial reports were encouraging, the prospective assessment of the proposed models showed much lower diagnostic accuracy than expected.[42] It has also been shown that the models are less accurate than an experienced ultrasound operator in detection of ovarian malignancy.[43] It is important to stress that none of the diagnostic models was developed for use in pregnancy, which affects morphological characteristics of cysts and significantly increases the vascularity of pelvic tumours.

It has been shown, however, that subjective assessment can be used to exclude ovarian malignancy in the vast majority of women with simple unilocular cysts, dermoids, endometriomas and tubal pathology, which account for the majority of persistent cysts in pregnancy.[43] For a persistent cyst with uncertain morphology, referral for expert examination should be considered.

Magnetic resonance imaging

Magnetic resonance imaging (MRI) gives no radiation exposure and is a useful adjunct in the evaluation of adnexal masses. It provides clear anatomical delineation of masses because of its multiplanar imaging capability and excellent spatial resolution. There is no impediment by bowel gas or bone as with ultrasound. It may be beneficial as an adjunct to ultrasound in selected patients in whom diagnostic need sufficiently warrants such an intervention.[44] Shetty and Lamki[44] advocate the use of MRI in all cases in which ultrasound demonstrates a solid suspicious mass or is unable adequately to define the site of origin of a mass. However, no randomised controlled trial comparing ultrasound with MRI for the diagnosis of pelvic abnormalities has been published and it is likely that the accuracy of MRI will also be largely dependent on the experience of the operator in interpreting images. Clearly, requirements for such intervention will vary depending on the ability and experience of the ultrasound operator.

Biochemical indices

The measurement of serum CA125 has been widely used as a second-line investigation of persistent ovarian cysts detected on ultrasound. This is because elevated CA125 levels are observed in more than 80% of women with ovarian cancer. It has been noted, however, that serum CA125 levels are altered in pregnancy.[45] Aslam *et al.*[46] measured serum CA125 in 188 women with uncomplicated pregnancies between 11 and 14 weeks of gestation at the routine nuchal translucency screening visit. All women included in the study had morphologically normal ovaries observed on ultrasound examination. The study showed that 20% of pregnant women with morphologically normal ovaries exceed a serum CA125 level of 35 iu/ml, which corresponds to the 99th centile in the nonpregnant population. The authors therefore concluded that the CA125 level is physiologically increased at 11–14 weeks of gestation and cut off values, which are used to assess the nature of ovarian cysts in nonpregnant women, cannot be applied to pregnant women at this gestation. A new cut off level for maternal CA125 at 11–14 weeks of gestation of 112 iu/ml was proposed in order to achieve a discriminatory power similar to that in nonpregnant women because this value corresponded to the 99th centile in the study.

Adnexal torsion

Adnexal torsion is one of the few causes of the acute abdomen that is more common in pregnancy than in the nonpregnant state.[47] The potential danger of adnexal torsion is the permanent destruction of the organs involved by prolonged ischaemic insult. Presentation is typically with unilateral lower quadrant pain, often acute in onset. Nausea, vomiting, fever and leucocytosis are all common features, although their specificity is low, particularly in pregnancy. Ultrasound examination is usually helpful, considered in conjunction with the clinical picture. Typical B mode findings include visualisation of a tender adnexal mass. Ovarian stromal volume is normally increased because of interstitial oedema secondary to impaired venous return. Colour flow Doppler interrogation may reveal the absence of ovarian blood flow if torsion is complete.[47]

Traditional management of adnexal torsion without pregnancy has been moulded by the belief that untwisting of the adnexa and conservation of the involved ovary would be likely to precipitate acute thrombotic events such as pulmonary embolism. This has meant that the accepted treatment has been salpingo-oophorectomy. Zweizig *et al.*[48] retrospectively reviewed 94 cases of ovarian torsion between 1989 and 1991, 65% of which were treated by untwisting of potentially viable adnexa and ovarian cystectomy (termed conservative management), and 35% of which were treated by the more traditional approach of salpingo–oophorectomy. They reported no thromboembolic complications or increase in postoperative morbidity, although they did comment that their sample size was too small to demonstrate a lack of increased morbidity from pulmonary embolus when adnexa are untwisted in appropriate patients. A literature review failed to find any cases of thromboembolic morbidity associated with the practice of untwisting of the adnexa as treatment for adnexal torsion.[47] In a recent series of 54 women with black-bluish ovaries all underwent detorsion with sparing of the affected ovary; 93% were documented on follow-up scan to have normal ovarian volume with follicular development. The authors concluded that ovarian torsion should be treated by untwisting regardless of colour and that cystectomy should be performed instead of oophorectomy.[49]

Dystocia

Labour dystocia is a rare complication associated with ovarian cysts in pregnancy. The main risk factors appear to be large cyst size (typically over 10 cm diameter) and cysts located low in the pelvis. Obstetricians are alerted to the requirement for intervention by failure of engagement of the fetal head in the pelvis in late gestation.

When intervention is deemed necessary, the decision on the nature of the intervention is based on the morphological characteristics of the cyst. If the cyst is simple, anechoic with no solid component and no increased vascularity demonstrable on colour flow Doppler examination, ultrasound guided fine needle aspiration is the treatment of choice for prevention/treatment of labour dystocia (see below). However, if the cyst displays complex morphology on ultrasound examination, prevention/treatment of labour dystocia is achieved through delivery by caesarean section. Ovarian cystectomy may be performed during the procedure.

MANAGEMENT OF OVARIAN CYSTS IN PREGNANCY

There are several key questions that need to be addressed when considering how best to manage adnexal masses detected during pregnancy:

- Is intervention warranted or is expectant management possible?

- What type of intervention is most appropriate?

- When should intervention take place?

Reedy et al.[50] compared fetal outcome variables between laparoscopy and laparotomy performed during pregnancy with use of the Swedish Health Registries from 1973 to 1993. When they compared infants born after maternal laparoscopy or laparotomy during pregnancy with all infants born, they found a significant increase in low-birthweight infants, delivery before 37 weeks, and an increase in growth restricted infants.

Platek et al.[51] carried out a retrospective study evaluating pathological features and outcomes of pregnancies complicated by a persistent adnexal mass that was managed conservatively or with surgical intervention. Only women with adnexal masses ≥6 cm were included in the study, irrespective of morphological characteristics or symptomatology. Those with cysts that resolved during pregnancy prior to delivery were not included. Women with a cyst diagnosed incidentally at delivery were also not included (i.e. at caesarean section). Of the 43 372 records examined, persistent ovarian cysts meeting the above criteria were identified in 31 women (0.07%), of whom 19 (61%) had an operative intervention at a mean gestational age of 18.6 weeks (range 15–22 weeks). Of those operated on during pregnancy, all underwent laparotomy (74% by low transverse incision, 26% by midline incision). Histology revealed that, of these 19, nine were functional cysts, six were dermoid cysts, two were paratubal cysts, one was an endometrioma and one a hyperreactio lutealis. There were adverse outcomes in two of the 19 women operated on (11%). One had a spontaneous miscarriage at 17 weeks of gestation within 24 hours of the operation to remove a paratubal cyst. The other had spontaneous rupture of the membranes at 20 weeks of gestation at the time of extubation from anaesthesia after bilateral ovarian cystectomy for endometriomas. She did, however, go on to have a normal delivery of a healthy baby at term. Twelve of the 31 (39%) had nonsurgical management of the adnexal masses, including fine needle aspiration of simple ovarian cysts (five) and spontaneous resolution postpartum after expectant management (two). Two women suspected to have dermoid cysts were operated on postpartum, at which time this diagnosis was confirmed.

The management decision was made at the discretion of the obstetrician after consultation with the woman. There is no indication of whether this was based on symptoms and/or ultrasound morphology. However, of those who underwent surgical management, 14 of 19 (74%) of the masses were complex in appearance at the initial ultrasound diagnosis, whereas 5 of the 19 (26%) had simple ultrasound appearances. There were no instances of ovarian torsion or emergency surgical intervention in this series. Platek et al.[51] subsequently proposed a strategy for the management of ovarian cysts in pregnancy.

Using this management strategy, any complex mass ≥6 cm persisting beyond 16 weeks of gestation should be treated by surgical intervention in pregnancy (laparotomy or laparoscopy). Using the figures from their study, 14 of 31 persistent cysts ≥6 cm in diameter were complex in appearance. This means one would expect a surgical intervention rate of at least 45.2% with this model. This prediction does not take into account simple cysts or dermoid cysts that require emergency intervention because of symptoms.

In 2001 we carried out a prospective screening study at King's College Hospital, looking at women with uncomplicated normal pregnancies attending clinic for ultrasound assessment of nuchal thickness for screening for Down syndrome at 11–14 weeks.[2] Ovarian cysts were detected in 24.9% of the women scanned. Simple cysts less than 5 cm in diameter were detected in 13.7%. Complex cysts or simple cysts greater than 5 cm in diameter were detected in 11.2%.

Asymptomatic women were managed expectantly with follow-up scans regardless of the size of the cyst, unless ultrasound features were strongly suggestive of ovarian cancer or the cyst showed rapid growth. Intervention was generally reserved for symptomatic women. Of 328 cysts of complex morphology or simple and ≥5 cm in diameter, 90% were managed expectantly and 10% were subject to surgical intervention; 84.7% resolved spontaneously. Surgery was carried out during pregnancy in only 2 (0.6%) women and at caesarean section in 4 (1.2%); 27 women (8.2%) were managed by postpartum surgery, while 11 (3.4%) with ovarian cysts were managed expectantly postpartum.

There were no cases of ovarian cancer among the 2925 women scanned. The conclusions of this study were that expectant management is suitable for most women found to have an ovarian cyst in pregnancy, and surgery should be performed only if clinically indicated or if the cyst shows rapid growth on a follow-up scan 4–6 weeks after the initial scan. Using this approach, surgical intervention during pregnancy is reserved for women in whom symptoms necessitate intervention. The predicted surgical intervention rate during pregnancy is 0.6% when using data from this study, which is significantly less compared with the management strategy proposed by Platek.[51]

SURGICAL MANAGEMENT

The traditional detection of ovarian cysts in pregnancy was by symptoms and clinical examination followed by operation. Prior to the advent of diagnostic ultrasound and acceptance of laparoscopy, symptomatic women with a clinically detectable adnexal mass were diagnosed and treated at laparotomy. Treatment would have been by oophorectomy or ovarian cystectomy.

Ultrasound guided fine needle aspiration

Ultrasound guided cyst aspiration offers a less invasive alternative to the traditional techniques employed for the surgical management of ovarian cysts in pregnancy. It is particularly useful for symptomatic cysts that are shown on ultrasound to be simple benign appearing cysts. As mentioned above, the use of high-resolution ultrasound to distinguish benign from malignant disease is remarkably effective.[43] There are several features that make this an attractive management option. The procedure can be performed in an outpatient setting with no requirement for general anaesthesia; the reported procedure-related complication rate is extremely low,[52] and symptom relief is prompt in the majority of women.

The main limitation of the procedure is that a high proportion of women managed in this way will require further intervention at a later date. Caspi *et al.*[52] reported a recurrence rate of 40% in their series of ten women. Two required laparotomy during pregnancy; two had laparotomy in the postpartum period. Guariglia *et al.*[53] reported a 33.3% recurrence rate after one aspiration and 11.1% after two aspirations.

Ultrasound guided cyst aspiration may therefore be thought of as a minimally invasive safe and effective means of symptom control in selected women, with the added benefit of deferring definitive treatment, when required, until the postpartum period.

Laparoscopy versus laparotomy

There are several studies that have shown significant rates of adverse outcomes associated with surgery for removal of adnexal masses during pregnancy. In Japan, Usui *et al.*[54] reviewed 69 women diagnosed with adnexal masses that required surgery during pregnancy. Sixty-eight had laparotomy for treatment, one had ultrasound guided fine needle aspiration. Twelve percent of these women had preterm deliveries and 3.3% experienced spontaneous abortion. There were three perinatal deaths, two of which were due to major anomalies.

Whitecar *et al.*[14] reviewed 130 cases of women undergoing surgical intervention during pregnancy. Of these, 86 underwent exploratory laparotomy before delivery, and 43 extirpation of the mass at the time of caesarean section. One women underwent ultrasound guided cyst aspiration. There were adverse pregnancy outcomes, defined as perinatal death or preterm delivery, in 14 of 56 (25%) women who underwent laparotomy and for whom fetal records were available.

In the nonpregnant population it has been well documented that laparoscopic surgery has the potential to reduce both postoperative morbidity and recovery time and unnecessary bed occupancy compared with open abdominal surgery. These features in turn may reduce the danger of thromboembolism.

In the past, concerns expressed regarding the use of laparoscopic surgery during pregnancy have included potential direct trauma to the uterus or fetus, compromise of uteroplacental perfusion due to increased intra-abdominal pressure associated with carbon dioxide insufflation, and carbon monoxide poisoning as a result of exposure to smoke generated by thermal energy in the form of laser surgery or bipolar diathermy.[55]

Moore and Smith[56] reported on 14 women with adnexal masses diagnosed during the second trimester of pregnancy and managed laparoscopically. The average gestational age was 16 weeks, with an average operating time of 84 minutes and a hospital stay of two days. There were no postoperative complications or episodes of preterm labour associated with the surgery. The authors concluded that laparoscopic surgery during pregnancy can be performed for significant adnexal masses.

A possible impact of laparoscopic surgery on fetal or neonatal outcome was evaluated by analysis of the Swedish Health Registry from 1973 to 1993.[50] The authors compared the fetal outcome of 2233 laparoscopies and 2491 laparotomies performed in women with a singleton pregnancy at between 4 and 20 weeks of gestation. There were no significant differences in birthweight, gestational duration, intrauterine growth restriction, infant death or fetal malformation.

However, there was a significant increase in low-birthweight infants($<2500\,g$), delivery before 37 weeks of gestation, and the number of growth restricted neonates when comparing infants born after laparoscopy or laparotomy with all infants born.

When to intervene

In most women, surgery can be safely postponed until after delivery. The intervention should be delayed until the second trimester in all asymptomatic women. In all cases of asymptomatic first trimester cysts the scan should be repeated 4–6 weeks after the initial diagnosis to avoid operating on functional cysts that would otherwise resolve spontaneously.

Whitecar et al.[14] found that there were significantly fewer adverse pregnancy outcomes (defined as perinatal death or preterm delivery) in those women who underwent laparotomy before 23 weeks of gestation compared with after 23 weeks of gestation. Lavie et al.,[57] however, reported that, when surgical intervention is indicated, diagnostic and therapeutic laparoscopy should be considered as an elective first-line modality as far as the 16th week of gestation. Beyond this gestational age these authors are of the opinion that the size of the gravid uterus is a technical obstacle forcing the use of laparotomy as the primary surgical procedure.

The second trimester is considered the safest time to perform laparoscopic surgery for several reasons:[58]

- The miscarriage rate attributable to surgery is 5.6% in the second trimester compared with 12% in the first trimester.

- The rate of preterm labour in the second trimester is low.

- The uterus is still small enough not to obliterate the operative field compared with the third trimester.

- The theoretical risk of teratogenesis in the second trimester is low.

Laparoscopic technique in pregnancy

The woman can be placed in the dorsal lithotomy position in the first half of pregnancy. Later in pregnancy, slight left lateral tilting of the operating table is desirable in order to alleviate impaired venous return. No instrument should be applied to the cervix or inserted into the uterine cavity. Owing to the enlarged gravid uterus, care should be taken with trocar insertion. The primary trocar should be inserted after determining the height of the uterine fundus. The trocar may be inserted by an open technique or alternatively at the supraumbilical, subxiphoid midline or left upper quadrant (Palmer's point). Depending on the height of the uterus, the second trocars are inserted higher than those in nonpregnant women and they should be inserted under direct vision.

Maintaining the intra-abdominal pressure to less than 12 mmHg and minimising the length of operative time will decrease the possible risk of maternal hypercapnia and fetal acidosis.[58] Prophylactic tocolysis is not usually needed, but it can be administered if the woman experiences uterine irritability or contraction. Some authors have administered glucocorticoids to women in the late second trimester or in the third trimester of pregnancy to enhance lung maturity.

Laparotomy

An open procedure may be unavoidable in women with large complex cysts deemed unlikely to be amenable to laparoscopic removal, and in late pregnancy when the gravid uterus occupies a large proportion of the abdominal cavity, precluding the safe insertion of the trocars.

Tocolysis is usually administered prior to commencement of the procedure. A midline incision may be necessary to afford sufficient access in cases warranting laparotomy; the alternative is a paramedian incision above the cyst itself.

CONCLUSION

The prevalence of ovarian cysts detected during pregnancy is increasing and will continue to do so as first trimester scanning becomes available to a wider sector of the pregnant population and the sensitivity of ultrasound to detect ovarian cysts continues to improve.

All women with cysts other than simple unilocular cysts less than 5 cm in diameter should be offered a rescan 4–6 weeks later. The majority of cysts detected are asymptomatic and expectant management is appropriate. Intervention should be limited to women in whom the risk of complications may be high, as with large or fast growing cysts, cysts located low in the pelvis, and cysts with a large solid component. Intervention may also be indicated for treatment of symptoms.

In cases where there is a high index of suspicion for malignancy, women should be referred to centres where there is expertise in the ultrasound assessment of ovarian tumours in order to reduce the false positive rate of ultrasound diagnosis.

When an intervention is needed for a presumed benign cyst, laparoscopy between 12 and 16 weeks of gestation is the optimal surgical approach. Later in pregnancy a laparotomy should be used. When there is a strong suspicion of cancer, these women should be referred to a regional cancer centre.

References

1. Beischer NA, Buttery BW, Fortune DW, Macafee CA. Growth and malignancy of ovarian tumours in pregnancy. *Aus N Z J Obstet Gynaecol* 1971;11:208–20.
2. Salim R, Woelfer B, Aslam N, Elson J, Jurkovic D. The value of routine ultrasound screening for adnexal masses at the 11–14 weeks early anomaly scan. Abstracts of the 11th World Congress on Ultrasound in Obstetrics and Gynecology, 23–28 October 2001, Melbourne, Australia. *Ultrasound Obstet Gynecol* 2001;18 Suppl 1:9. Abstract CEG-15.
3. White KC. Ovarian tumours in pregnancy. A private hospital ten-year survey. *Am J Obstet Gynecol* 1973;116:544–50.
4. Hogston P, Lilford RJ. Ultrasound study of ovarian cysts in pregnancy: prevalence and significance. *Br J Obstet Gynaecol* 1986;93:625–8.
5. Hill LM, Connors-Beatty DJ, Nowak A, Tush B. The role of ultrasonography in the detection

and management of adnexal masses during the second and third trimesters of pregnancy. *Am J Obstet Gynecol* 1998;179:703–7.

6.   Johansson EDB. Plasma levels of progesterone in pregnancy measured by a rapid competitive protein binding technique. *Acta Endocrinol (Copenh)* 1969;61:607–17.

7.   Perkins KY, Johnson JL, Kay HH. Simple ovarian cysts: clinical features on a first-trimester ultrasound scan. *J Reprod Med* 1997;42:440–4.

8.   Kobayashi H, Yoshida A, Kobayashi M, Yamada T. Changes in size of the functional cyst on ultrasonography during early pregnancy. *Am J Perinatol* 1997;14:1–4.

9.   Templeman CL, Fallat ME, Lam AM, Perlman SE, Hertweck SP, O'Connor DM. Managing mature cystic teratomas of the ovary. *Obstet Gynecol Surv* 2000;55:738–45.

10.   Jermy K, Luise C, Bourne T. The characterisation of common ovarian cysts in premenopausal women. *Ultrasound Obstet Gynecol* 2001;17:140–4.

11.   Tekay A, Joupilla P. Validity of pulsatility and resistance indices in classification of adnexal tumors with transvaginal color Doppler ultrasound. *Ultrasound Obstet Gynecol* 1992;2:338–44.

12.   Zanetta G, Vergani P, Lissoni A. Color Doppler ultrasound in the preoperative assessment of adnexal masses. *Acta Obstet Gynecol Scand* 1994;73:637–41.

13.   Chou C, Chang CH, Yao BL, Kuo HC. Color Doppler ultrasonography and serum CA 125 in the differentiation of benign and malignant ovarian tumors. *J Clin Ultrasound* 1994;22:491–6.

14.   Whitecar MP, Turner S, Higby MK. Adnexal masses in pregnancy: a review of 130 cases undergoing surgical management. *Am J Obstet Gynecol* 1999;181:19–24.

15.   Caspi B, Levi R, Appelman Z, Rabinerson D, Goldman G, Hagay Z. Conservative management of ovarian cystic teratoma during pregnancy and labor. *Am J Obstet Gynecol* 2000;182:503–5.

16.   Tailor A, Hacket E, Bourne TH. Ultrasonography of the ovary. In: Anderson JC, editor. *Gynaecological Imaging*. London: Churchill Livingstone; 1999. p. 332–3.

17.   Timmerman D, Deprest J, Bourne T. *Ultrasound and Endoscopic Surgery in Obstetrics and Gynaecology. A Combined Approach to Diagnosis and Treatment*. London: Springer-Verlag; 2003. p. 189–203.

18.   Athey PA, Diment DD. The spectrum of sonographic findings in endometriomas. *J Ultrasound Med* 1989;8:487–91.

19.   Kupfer MC, Schwimer SR, Lebovic J. Transvaginal sonographic appearance of endometriomata: spectrum of findings. *J Ultrasound Med* 1992;11:129–33.

20.   Volpi E, De Grandis T, Zuccaro G, La Vista A, Sismondi P. Role of transvaginal sonography in the detection of endometriomata. *J Clin Ultrasound* 1995;23:163–7.

21.   Gregora M, Higgs P. Endometriomas in pregnancy. *Aust N Z J Obstet Gynaecol* 1998;38:106–9.

22.   Johnson TR Jr, Woodruff JD. Surgical emergencies of the uterine adnexae during pregnancy. *Int J Gynaecol Obstet* 1986;24:331–5.

23.   Vercellini P, Ferrari A, Vendola N, Carinelli SG. Growth and rupture of an ovarian endometrioma in pregnancy. *Int J Gynaecol Obstet* 1992;37:203–5.

24.   Cummings AM, Metcalf JL. Effects of surgically induced endometriosis on pregnancy and effect of pregnancy and lactation on endometriosis in mice. *Proc Soc Exp Biol Med* 1996;212:332–7.

25.   Girling JC, Soutter WP. Benign tumours of the ovary. In: Shaw RW, Soutter WP, Stanton SL, editors. *Gynaecology*. 2nd ed. Edinburgh: Churchill Livingstone; 1997. p. 615–25.

26.   Herrmann UJ. Sonographic patterns of ovarian tumours. *Clin Obstet Gynecol* 1993;36:375–83.

27.   Brosens IA, Gordon AG. *Tubal Infertility*. Philadelphia, PA: Lippincott; 1989. p. 26–9.

28. Jolles CJ. Gynecologic cancer associated with pregnancy. *Semin Oncol* 1989;16:417–24.

29. Antonelli N, Dotters DJ, Katz VL, Kuller JA. Cancer in pregnancy: a review of the literature, Part 1. *Obstet Gynecol Surv* 1996;51:125–34.

30. Jubbe ED. Primary ovarian carcinoma in pregnancy. *Am J Obstet Gynecol* 1963;85:345.

31. Creasman WT, Rutledge F, Smith JP. Carcinoma of the ovary associated with pregnancy. *Obstet Gynecol* 1971;38:111–16.

32. Chung A, Birnbaum SJ. Ovarian cancer associated with pregnancy. *Obstet Gynecol* 1977;41:211.

33. Lutz MH, Underwood PB, Rozier JC, Putney FW. Genital malignancy in pregnancy. *Am J Obstet Gynecol* 1977;129:536–42.

34. Thornton JG, Wells M. Ovarian cysts in pregnancy: does ultrasound make traditional management inappropriate? *Obstet Gynecol* 1987;69:717–20.

35. Boulay R, Podczaski E. Ovarian cancer complicating pregnancy. *Obstet Gynecol Clin North Am* 1998;25:385–99.

36. Copeland LJ, Landon MB. Malignant disease in pregnancy. In: Gabbe SG, Niebyl JR, Simpson JL, editors. *Obstetrics: Normal and Problem Pregnancies.* 3rd ed. New York: Churchill Livingston; 1996. p. 1155–81.

37. Otton G, Higgins S, Phillips K, Quinn M. A case of early-stage epithelial ovarian cancer in pregnancy. *Int J Gynecol Cancer* 2001;11:413–17.

38. Timmerman D, Schwarzler P, Collins WP, Claerhout F, Coenen M, Amant F, *et al.* Subjective assessment of adnexal masses with the use of ultrasonography: an analysis of interobserver variability and experience. *Ultrasound Obstet Gynecol* 1999;13:11–16.

39. Sassone M, Timor-Tritsch IE, Artner A, Westhoff C, Warren WB. Transvaginal sonographic characterization of ovarian disease: evaluation of a new scoring system to predict ovarian malignancy. *Obstet Gynecol* 1991;78:70–6.

40. Jacobs I, Oram D, Fairbanks J, Turner J, Frost C, Grudzinskas JG. A risk of malignancy index incorporating CA125, ultrasound and menopausal status for the accurate preoperative diagnosis of ovarian cancer. *Br J Obstet Gynaecol* 1990;97:922–9.

41. Tailor A, Jurkovic D, Bourne TH, Collins WP, Campbell S. Sonographic prediction of malignancy in adnexal masses using multivariate logistic regression analysis. *Ultrasound Obstet Gynecol* 1997;10:41–7.

42. Aslam N, Tailor A, Lawton F, Carr J, Savvas M, Jurkovic D. Prospective evaluation of three different models for the pre-operative diagnosis of ovarian cancer. *BJOG* 2000;107:1347–53.

43. Valentin L, Hagen B, Tingulstad S, Eik-Nes S. Comparison of 'pattern recognition' and logistic regression models for discrimination between benign and malignant pelvic masses: a prospective cross validation. *Ultrasound Obstet Gynecol* 2001;18:357–65.

44. Shetty MK, Lamki N. Imaging of pelvic masses during pregnancy. *J Womens Imaging* 2001;3:63–8.

45. Kobayashi F, Sagawa N, Nakamura K, Nonogaki M, Ban C, Fujii S, *et al.* Mechanism and clinical significance of elevated CA125 levels in the sera of pregnant women. *Am J Obstet Gynecol* 1989;160:563–6.

46. Aslam N, Ong C, Woelfer B, Nicolaides K, Jurkovic D. Serum CA125 at 11–14 weeks gestation in women with morphologically normal ovaries. *BJOG* 2000;107:689–90.

47. Sharp HT. The acute abdomen during pregnancy. *Clin Obstet Gynecol* 2002;45:405–13.

48. Zweizig S, Perron J, Grubb D, Mishell D. Conservative management of adnexal torsion. *Am J Obstet Gynecol* 1993;168:1791–5.

49. Cohen SB, Oelsner G, Seidman DS, Admon D, Mashiach S, Goldenberg M. Laparoscopic detorsion allows sparing of the twisted ischaemic adnexa. *J Am Assoc Gynecol Laparosc* 1999;6:139–43.

50. Reedy MB, Kallen B, Kuehl TJ. Laparoscopy during pregnancy: a study of five fetal outcome parameters with use of the Swedish Health Registry. *Am J Obstet Gynecol* 1997;177:673–9.

51. Platek DN, Henderson CE, Goldberg GL. The management of a persistent adnexal mass in pregnancy. *Am J Obstet Gynecol* 1995;173:1236–40.

52. Caspi B, Ben-Arie A, Appelman Z, Or Y, Hagay Z. Aspiration of simple pelvic cysts during pregnancy. *Gynecol Obstet Invest* 2000;49:102–5.

53. Guariglia L, Conte M, Are P, Rosati P. Ultrasound-guided fine needle aspiration of ovarian cysts during pregnancy. *Eur J Obstet Gynecol Reprod Biol* 1999;82:5–9.

54. Usui R, Minakami H, Kosuge S, Iwasaki R, Ohwada M, Sato I. A retrospective survey of clinical, pathologic, and prognostic features of adnexal masses operated on during pregnancy. *J Obstet Gynaecol Res* 2000;26:89–93.

55. Seidman D. S, Nezhat C, Nezhat F, Nezhat C, Yuval Y, Oelsner G, *et al*. Is laparoscopic surgery safe during pregnancy? Abstracts of the American Pediatric Society and the Society for Pediatric Research, 6–10 May 1996, Washington, DC. *Pediatr Res* 1996;39 Suppl 2):112. Abstract 657.

56. Moore RD, Smith WG. Laparoscopic management of adnexal masses in pregnant women. *J Reprod Med* 1999;44:97–100.

57. Lavie O, Neuman M, Beller U. The management of a persistent adnexal mass in pregnancy. *Am J Obstet Gynecol* 1996;175:750.

58. Al-Fozan H, Tulandi T. Safety and risks of laparoscopic surgery in pregnancy. *Curr Opin Obstet Gynecol*;14:375–9.

25

Subtotal abdominal hysterectomy

Isaac Manyonda

INTRODUCTION

Abdominal hysterectomy is the most common major gynaecological operation in both the UK[1] and the USA.[2] It ranks second only to caesarean section as the most frequently performed major gynaecological operation in the USA, where an estimated 633 000 are carried out annually.[3] It rates highest in satisfaction scores compared with other modalities of treatment for dysfunctional uterine bleeding.[4] However, since hysterectomy disrupts the anatomical relationships and local nerve supply, it has seemed teleologically sound to suppose that pelvic organ function could be adversely affected. Because subtotal hysterectomy minimises anatomical disruption, it may ameliorate the potential adverse effects of total hysterectomy.

In a series of publications in 1983–1985, Kilkku *et al.*[5–7] extolled the virtues of subtotal hysterectomy with respect to urinary and sexual function. They interviewed 105 women before total abdominal hysterectomy with bilateral salpingo-oophorectomy, and again at six weeks, six months and one year postoperatively. They also interviewed 107 women who underwent subtotal hysterectomy with bilateral salpingo-oophorectomy. Their conclusion was that subtotal hysterectomy conferred significant advantages over total hysterectomy with respect to bladder and sexual function. The impact of the reports was so profound that, in Finland, where the research was undertaken, 53% of abdominal hysterectomies carried out between 1981 and 1986 were subtotal. However, subsequent studies by Virtanen *et al.*,[8] from the same institute, did not concur with Kilkku *et al.*'s findings and, by 1991, the rate of subtotal hysterectomy had dropped to 13%.[9] On closer scrutiny, the two studies were not comparable because Kilkku *et al.* compared total and subtotal hysterectomy, while the study conducted by Virtanen *et al.* was a longitudinal assessment of total hysterectomy only.

The debate on total versus subtotal hysterectomy was thrown wide open, with gynaecologists having no evidence base to advise their patients, and the popular press jumping on the bandwagon of this uncertainty. The fundamental issues were whether subtotal hysterectomy conferred any benefits over total hysterectomy with regard to bladder, bowel and sexual functions, as well as in recovery and complication rates. The concern that cancer could develop in the cervical stump was no longer considered a justification for the routine use of total abdominal hysterectomy. Screening had been shown to reduce the incidence of invasive cancer,[10] and the risk of cervical cancer after subtotal abdominal hysterectomy was estimated at less than 0.1%.[11] However, injury to the urinary tract, which occurs in 0.5–3.0% of patients,[12] is the most frequent cause of litigation after total abdominal hysterectomy.[13] Subtotal hysterectomy requires less mobilisation of the bladder and minimises the risk of injury to the ureters. Research had also suggested that the subtotal procedure was associated with lower rates of wound infection and haematoma,[14] and avoided symptomatic vault granulation.[15] The suggestion that subtotal hysterectomy could be more beneficial with regard to sexual function captured the public's imagination and drew the popular press into the foray, with gynaecologists being frequently pilloried for performing total hysterectomy instead of the subtotal procedure. It was only in 2002 that definitive data became available that should resolve the long-standing controversy of total versus subtotal hysterectomy.[16]

HISTORICAL PERSPECTIVES

Charles Clay performed the first recorded hysterectomy (subtotal) in 1843, but the woman died in the immediate postoperative period. He tried again the next year, and this time the woman lived for 15 days. The cause of her subsequent demise is disputed, but the widely accepted explanation is that careless porters dropped her on the floor while the nurses were changing the bedlinen.[17] Early hysterectomies were all subtotal, the first total hysterectomy being attributed to EH Richardson in 1929.[18] From then on there was a gradual increase in the frequency of performing total hysterectomy, but it was not until the 1940s, which heralded antibiotics, blood transfusion, modern anaesthesia and improved surgical techniques, that total hysterectomy became the mainstay procedure. With the recognition that cancer occasionally developed in the cervical stump, subtotal hysterectomy became such an anathema that authors apologised for including a description of the operation in manuals of operative gynaecology, condemning it to the repertoire of the inexperienced surgeon.[19] The results of a postal survey published in 1998 confirmed this view and showed that subtotal hysterectomy is an unpopular operation in the UK.[20] This is also confirmed in national statistics,[21] where subtotal hysterectomy accounts for less than 5% of the total number of hysterectomies performed.

The reports from Kilkku et al.[5-7] referred to above, the changing perspective of the risk of cancer in the cervical stump, the risk of bladder and ureteric injury, and the prevailing litigious climate in medical practice, as well as patient demand and media interest, have forced British gynaecologists to re-examine their attitude to subtotal hysterectomy.

WHY HYSTERECTOMY MAY AFFECT PELVIC ORGAN FUNCTION

Anatomical considerations

Hysterectomy alters the relative anatomical spatial relationships among the pelvic organs, and disrupts their innervation. The pelvic plexus, which is of paramount importance in the coordinated contractions of the smooth muscle of the bladder and bowel, is formed by the junction of the pelvic parasympathetic and sympathetic nerves. This plexus is intimately related to the bladder, cervix and vagina, and the nerve supply of the pelvic organs is derived from it.[22] During the operation of total hysterectomy, the pelvic plexus may be at risk in four areas. First, the main branches of the plexus passing beneath the uterine arteries may be damaged during the division of the cardinal ligaments.[23] Secondly, the major part of the vesical innervation, which enters the bladder base before spreading throughout the detrusor muscle, may be damaged during blunt dissection of the bladder from the uterus and cervix. Thirdly, the extensive dissection of the paravaginal tissue may disrupt the pelvic neurons passing from the lateral aspect of the vagina.[24] Finally, the removal of the cervix will result in the loss of a large segment of the plexus, which is intimately related to it. The remaining portion of the plexus may be inadequate to deal with afferent impulses from the rectum and the bladder, leading possibly to bladder and rectal dysfunction.[25] It is therefore conceivable that damage to this autonomic innervation during pelvic surgery may result in functional disorders of the pelvic viscera, and it has been suggested that constipation after hysterectomy may be caused by autonomic denervation of the hindgut.[26] Similarly, sympathetic damage produces loss of proximal urethral pressure and parasympathetic damage could cause detrusor areflexia.[27] Disturbance of the innervation of the cervix and the upper vagina after total hysterectomy could also interfere with lubrication and orgasm. The so-alled internal orgasm is essentially a cervical orgasm, caused by stimulation of nerve endings in the uterovaginal plexus, which intimately surround the cervix and attach to the upper vagina. Much of the sensory and autonomic information from the pelvic organs, including the uterus, is channelled through the uterovaginal plexus, so it is understandable that the loss of a major portion of the uterovaginal plexus by excision of the cervix could have an adverse effect on sexual arousal and orgasm in women who previously experienced an internal orgasm. Women who achieve orgasm through clitoral stimulation may not be affected. In those who had experienced both types of orgasm or in whom sexual response is blended, a decrease in sexual response after hysterectomy may be noted.[25] Vaginal shortening and vaginal dryness due to a reduction in cervical mucous[28] may also contribute to sexual problems.

It should, however, be borne in mind that hysterectomy may include the removal of structures that are a source of symptoms, including endometriomas, myomas, pelvic adhesions and adenomyosis, which may be more significant than the anatomical distortions and interruptions of the nerve supply referred to above.

Psychological considerations

Few operations raise more passions than hysterectomy. Depending on a variety of factors such as cultural beliefs and education, women's views on the role of the uterus may well influence how they will react to hysterectomy. Historically, the uterus has been regarded as the regulator and controller of important physiological functions, a sexual organ, a source of energy and vitality, and a maintainer of youth and attractiveness.[29] It is little wonder, therefore, that the removal of such an organ may be expected to alter women's perception of self, especially with regard to femininity, attractiveness, sexual desire and ability to respond sexually.[30] This in turn affects quality of life and psychological parameters, which are important considerations because the vast majority of hysterectomies are performed to improve quality of life rather than to cure life threatening disease.

INFLUENCE OF HYSTERECTOMY ON SEXUAL FUNCTION

The issue of whether hysterectomy affects sexual function is complex because both physical and psychological factors have varying and unquantifiable influences on human sexuality. Psychological studies suggest that post-hysterectomy sexual function is influenced by a wide range of patient characteristics. For example, poor knowledge of reproductive anatomy, negative prehysterectomy expectations of sexual recovery after surgery, pre-operative psychiatric morbidity, and unsatisfactory pre-operative sexual relations are all associated with poor outcome.[31,32] Prehysterectomy factors that are associated with positive postsurgery sexuality include frequency of coitus, frequency of desire, and orgasmic response.[33] In other words, those women who retained an overall desire for sexual activity, and were presumably hampered by negative physical symptoms, may be expected to experience an improvement in their sexual function after hysterectomy.

Interest in the influence of anatomical changes was brought into sharp focus by the series of studies from Scandinavia by Kilkku et al.[5–7] in the early to mid-1980s. They compared coital frequency, dyspareunia, libido and frequency of orgasm before surgery and at six weeks, six months, one year and three years postsurgery in 105 women who underwent total hysterectomy and 107 who had the subtotal procedure. Both groups showed an equal but slight reduction in coital frequency, dyspareunia decreased in both groups, but statistically more in the subtotal abdominal hysterectomy group; the frequency of orgasm was significantly reduced in the total abdominal hysterectomy group but not in the subtotal group. Such findings lent credence to Masters and Johnson's[34] observation that 'many women will certainly describe cervical sexual pressure as a trigger mechanism for coital responsivity'. Such women may be handicapped sexually when such a trigger mechanism is removed surgically. However, subsequent studies from the institute where Kilkku carried out her work suggested that the negative effect of total hysterectomy on sexual function was not so great as originally perceived,[8] thus triggering debate and controversy that may have been resolved only recently.[16]

BLADDER FUNCTION AFTER HYSTERECTOMY

In a retrospective questionnaire, Milson et al.[35] found a significant increase in urinary incontinence in women who had previously undergone hysterectomy compared with those who had not (20.8% versus 16.4%). However, retrospective data comparing hysterectomised with nonhysterectomised women is unreliable because a degree of vesicourethral dysfunction may be present prior to surgery.[7,36,37] Parys et al.[24] therefore carried out a prospective study with both subjective and objective assessments of urinary function and found subjective symptoms in 58.3% of women prior to hysterectomy, although urodynamic dysfunction was found in only 38.9%. Postoperatively, they found an increase in urinary symptoms (75%), new urodynamic abnormalities (an additional 30%), and pelvic neuropathy, as evidenced by sacral nerve reflex latencies. In contrast, Langer et al.[38] evaluated 16 asymptomatic premenopausal women and performed cystometry and uroflowmetry pre-operatively, and again at four weeks and four months post-hysterectomy, and found no difference in symptoms or urodynamic results. Although some have found no more urinary symptoms after hysterectomy than after dilatation and curettage,[39] others compared urinary symptoms after transcervical resection of the endometrium and similarly found no difference.[40] Another study even reported a statistically significant decrease in stress incontinence, frequency and nocturia 12 months after total abdominal hysterectomy.[8] It has been hypothesised that decreased urinary stress incontinence after hysterectomy may be due to elevation of the bladder neck by fixation of the vaginal vault to the uterosacral ligaments.[39] Apparent urodynamic or neurological changes post-hysterectomy may not necessarily cause symptoms. Prior et al.[41] found an increase in vesical sensitivity after hysterectomy, irrespective of whether the vaginal or abdominal approach was used; this persisted for at least six months but was not always associated with urinary symptoms. Although there are few data on the effect of vaginal as opposed to abdominal hysterectomy, it has been reported that urgency more often follows a vaginal procedure.[42]

Does the less disruptive subtotal hysterectomy confer any advantages over total hysterectomy with regard to urinary function? In the same group of women in whom they compared sexual function after total or subtotal hysterectomy, Kilkku et al.[5–7] found statistically significant differences in urinary symptoms between the two operations. In the total hysterectomy group, 28.6% of the women reported pre-operative incomplete bladder emptying, which fell to 22.1% post-surgery. In contrast, 35.5% of the subtotal hysterectomy group reported incomplete bladder emptying prior to surgery, and by one year this figure had fallen to only 10.3%. Similar trends were found for urinary incontinence and frequency. The authors therefore concluded that subtotal hysterectomy was more advantageous.[7] However, once again subsequent studies by Virtanen et al.[8] from the same institute did not concur with Kilkku's findings, although in reality the two studies are not comparable because Kilkku compared total and subtotal hysterectomy while the study conducted by Virtanen was a longitudinal assessment of total hysterectomy only.

Other workers have also studied the effects of total versus subtotal hysterectomy on bladder function. Kujansuu et al.[43] evaluated urethral closure function pre-operatively and postoperatively in 31 nonrandomised patients who underwent subtotal ($n = 13$) and total ($n = 18$) hysterectomy. They found no operation-induced changes in urethral relaxation and functional length, closure pressure or resistance to stress associated with either operation. Lalos and Bjerle[44] performed a randomised comparison of 22 women, equally divided between total and subtotal hysterectomy. They found no differences in either urodynamic evaluation or subjective symptoms such as frequency and incontinence. The numbers in these studies were so small that the findings were not statistically significant. The poor quality of these previous studies is best illustrated by the fact that, in 2000, a systematic review[45] of studies comparing the effects of subtotal abdominal hysterectomy and total abdominal hysterectomy on urinary function identified only three studies[7,44,46] of sufficiently high methodological quality to be included in the analysis. Two were observational studies that showed an increased risk of incontinence among women who had undergone total abdominal hysterectomy.[7,46] The third[44] was a small randomised controlled trial showing no advantages of one operation over the other.

IMPACT OF HYSTERECTOMY ON BOWEL FUNCTION

Women often date the onset of bowel symptoms to previous gynaecological surgery. However, bowel dysfunction is common among women with gynaecological symptoms,[47–50] even in the absence of surgery. Most studies on the effect of hysterectomy on bowel function[26,51–53] have been retrospective, with small numbers of women and a lack of adequate controls, while some have not even defined the type or route of the hysterectomy. The following examples illustrate the quality of studies in the literature.

Taylor et al.[51] conducted a case–control study through detailed questionnaires in which post-hysterectomy women and controls were compared, and showed that women with previous hysterectomy were more likely to report infrequent defaecation and firmer stool consistency. However, they excluded women who had undergone extensive bowel operations and those with irritable bowel syndrome in the matched controls, while the same exclusions were not applied to the hysterectomy group. Conversely, Prior et al.[54] observed that, after hysterectomy, constipation was more likely to disappear than to develop. They also found no change in whole gut transit times in 26 women before and six months after hysterectomy.

A retrospective study of 593 women who underwent hysterectomy (abdominal, vaginal, radical or subtotal) against a control group of 100 women who had laparoscopic cholecystectomy found a significantly increased rate of bowel dysfunction in the hysterectomy group (3% versus 9%).[55] No significant difference in incidence of bowel symptoms was noted for the various types of hysterectomy. It was also observed that, in women with changes in bowel function, alterations in bladder function were observed more frequently ($P < 0.001$) than in the group with no deterioration of bowel function after hysterectomy. Interesting though these findings were, this was nevertheless a retrospective study that depended on the recall of symptoms going back over a five-year period, and the validity of a comparison between hysterectomy and cholecystectomy patients is highly questionable.

Goffeng et al.[56] conducted a longitudinal study, pre-operatively and at 3 and 11–18 months after hysterectomy. Detailed interviews enquiring about bowel function were performed, together with rectal manometry measurements and the whole gut transit time. Anorectal physiology was normal after hysterectomy and no adverse bowel symptoms were noted except for a significant improvement in abdominal pain. There was no difference between total hysterectomy and subtotal hysterectomy. A prospective study designed to determine the incidence of symptoms suggestive of irritable bowel syndrome arising after hysterectomy concluded that hysterectomy had little if any effect on the *de novo* development of this condition.[54]

QUALITY OF LIFE AND PSYCHOLOGICAL SEQUELAE OF HYSTERECTOMY

In contemporary clinical research, it is now widely recognised that it is not sufficient simply to measure the outcome of a clinical intervention in terms of morbidity and mortality. Quality of life is an important outcome variable,[57,58] and its measurement prospectively and concurrently complements morbidity and mortality measures. Psychiatric symptoms can arise as a result of physical illness, or may influence the manifestation and/or outcome of the treatment of that illness, so it is also highly informative to use the tools now available to study the psychological sequelae of clinical interventions. Indeed it has been argued that the functional impact of a clinical intervention should be the definitive arbiter of treatment success, and measurement of quality of life has been recommended for outcome assessment of treatments for menorrhagia.[59]

Research results published in 1997[60] and 2001[61] present compelling evidence that hysterectomy improves quality of life. Crosignani et al.[60] reported improvement in quality of life when using SF-36 in women after vaginal hysterectomy compared with endometrial resection, and Sculpher et al.[62] compared abdominal hysterectomy with transcervical resection of the endometrium and also found an improvement in quality of life. Similarly, others have reported symptom relief after hysterectomy, associated with marked improvement in quality of life.[63] It is reasonable to suppose that women feel better because they no longer suffer the symptoms that meant they had to have a hysterectomy in the first place. Kjerulff et al.[64] reported that at 12 and 24 months after hysterectomy symptoms were resolved completely or mostly in 95.8% and 96% of women respectively, while 85.3% and 81.6% respectively reported an improvement in health.

Hysterectomy has traditionally been considered to be associated with adverse psychiatric sequelae.[30,65,66] However, the earlier studies often lacked conceptual clarity and had methodological flaws, many being retrospective analyses with inadequate measures of outcome. Over about the last five years, more robust instruments have been employed to study psychological outcome after clinical interventions. Thus, studies published since the mid-1970s on the psychological sequelae of hysterectomy, using the General Health Questionnaire or equivalent tools, have arrived at entirely different conclusions.[67–72] In general, research has indicated that women with pre-operative depression are at increased risk for depression after surgery.[67,71–74] This is consistent with the Maryland study, the largest prospective study to date (on 1299 women), which reported a substantial decrease in depression and anxiety levels after hysterectomy.[57]

Thus the consensus from most research evidence suggests that hysterectomy improves quality of life and psychological measures. Thakar et al. (personal communication, 2002) have compared quality of life measures and psychological sequelae in women undergoing total versus subtotal hysterectomy and concluded that both procedures improve quality of life and reduce psychiatric symptoms, with no advantage for one operation over the other. Since, in general, hysterectomy and other treatments for menstrual disturbance are administered to improve quality of life rather than to cure life threatening conditions, quality of life measurements should be an integral part of any evaluation of treatment modalities, and should be studied concurrently with clinical measures.

COMPLICATIONS AND RECOVERY RATES

With total abdominal hysterectomy, much of the operative time, cost and morbidity is associated with the removal of the cervix.[75] There can be no argument that, compared with total, vaginal or laparoscopic hysterectomy, subtotal abdominal hysterectomy is a safer operation, whatever the skill of the surgeon. There is less or no mobilisation of the bladder, and minimal, if any, risk to the ureters. It is well to remember that, in the UK as well as the USA, injury to the urinary tract, estimated at between 0.5% and 3%,[12] is the biggest cause of litigation after hysterectomy.[13] If surgical outcome in terms of cure rates and patient satisfaction is similar between subtotal and the other types of hysterectomy, there may be a strong argument for adopting the safer procedure. Additional advantages of subtotal hysterectomy are that haematomas and wound infections are reported to be less common.[14] The higher incidence of the latter associated with total abdominal hysterectomy is often attributed to contamination of the abdominal cavity by vaginal flora during the procedure. Vault granulations do not complicate subtotal hysterectomy, but they occur in 21% of women after total hysterectomy, even if polygalactide sutures are used, and they almost always cause symptoms.[15]

There are, however, potential disadvantages with subtotal hysterectomy. Although the risk of cervical cancer after subtotal abdominal hysterectomy is small, estimated at less than 0.1%,[11] it cannot be ignored altogether. The incidence of cyclical bleeding after subtotal hysterectomy has been variably reported, and many women would be disappointed to find that they continue to menstruate after having undergone major surgery to eradicate menses. Even small amounts of residual endometrial tissue can result in abnormal bleeding and complicate the use of hormone replacement therapy. Finally, there is uncertainty on the issue of vaginal vault versus cervical stump prolapse after abdominal hysterectomy. Although, theoretically, subtotal hysterectomy could decrease the incidence of post-hysterectomy prolapse of the vaginal vault by preserving the connective tissue support of the upper vagina, earlier studies reported cervical prolapse after subtotal hysterectomy, and careful long-term follow-up studies are required to resolve this issue.

TOTAL VERSUS SUBTOTAL ABDOMINAL HYSTERECTOMY: THE RESOLUTION OF A LONG-STANDING CONTROVERSY

Thakar et al.,[16] in what was described in an accompanying editorial[76] as the largest and most comprehensive randomised trial to date comparing the effects of total and subtotal hysterectomy, tested the hypothesis that subtotal confers advantages over total hysterectomy. They conducted a prospective, randomised, double blind multicentre trial in which 279 women undergoing hysterectomy for benign disease were randomly allocated to total ($n = 146$) or subtotal ($n = 133$) hysterectomy. The main outcome measures were bladder, bowel and sexual functions, postoperative recovery/complication rates, and quality of life and psychological measures.

These authors found no significant differences between the two groups pre- and postoperatively for the important parameters of urinary, bowel and sexual functions. After surgery, fewer women in both groups had urinary frequency, nocturia, interrupted stream or incomplete emptying. On urodynamic assessment, the first desire to void, strong desire to void, and maximum capacity, were significantly increased over time. Women with fibroids had high urinary frequency pre-operatively and a greater postoperative reduction in this symptom. Neither operation had an adverse impact on sexual function, and deep dyspareunia was significantly reduced in both groups postoperatively. Women in the total hysterectomy group stayed longer in hospital and had a higher incidence of pyrexia and antibiotic use. In the subtotal hysterectomy group, 7% developed cyclical bleeding and two women had cervical prolapse.[16]

Thakar et al.[16] concluded that neither total nor subtotal hysterectomy adversely affects pelvic organ function. Indeed, both may significantly improve aspects of bladder and sexual function. Subtotal hysterectomy appears to have early advantages with respect to recovery and complications, but is also associated with longer term cyclical bleeding and possibly cervical prolapse. They also found that hysterectomy, whether total or subtotal, improves quality of life and reduces psychiatric symptoms.

WHY TOTAL OR SUBTOTAL HYSTERECTOMY DOES NOT ADVERSELY AFFECT PELVIC ORGAN FUNCTION

It is biologically plausible that the disruption of local innervation and anatomical relationships caused by hysterectomy could lead to pelvic organ dysfunction, yet the consistently high satisfaction rates reported in association with simple hysterectomy,[4,73,77–79] and the findings in the study reported in 2002 by Thakar et al.,[16] suggest that major postoperative morbidity in terms of pelvic organ dysfunction is not a common occurrence after total or subtotal hysterectomy. Work carried out by Butler-Manuel et al.[80] provides a rational and plausible anatomical explanation concerning why simple hysterectomy may not adversely affect bladder, bowel and sexual functions. They showed that the nerve content of the uterosacral ligaments and cardinal ligaments differs along their length, with a significantly greater nerve content in the middle to lateral thirds towards their origin at the pelvic side wall compared with the medial third towards the insertion of these ligaments into the uterine body and cervix. During simple hysterectomy, the ligaments, and therefore the nerves within them, are divided close to the uterus and the cervix. Thus, only the nerves innervating the uterus and cervix are interrupted, while those innervating the surrounding structures, including the bladder and rectum, remain intact. In contrast, radical hysterectomy, in which the ligaments are divided more laterally, has been associated with greater disturbance of pelvic organ function.[81] This is also consistent with the observation that laparoscopic uterine nerve ablation for endometriosis and dysmenorrhoea[82,83] does not adversely affect bladder function. Finally, as nerve damage during simple hysterectomy does not adversely affect urinary or bowel function, subtotal hysterectomy would not be expected to confer any advantages with respect to pelvic organ function.

CONCLUDING REMARKS

Although alternatives to hysterectomy for benign gynaecological disease are now widely available, including the Mirena intrauterine system (Schering Health Care Ltd, Burgess Hill, West Sussex, UK), endometrial ablation, uterine artery embolisation for fibroids, and pharmacological approaches, hysterectomy is the only definitive cure for abnormal uterine bleeding, improving quality of life and rating highest in satisfaction scores compared with the other modalities of treatment for dysfunctional uterine bleeding. The vast majority of hysterectomies are performed via the abdominal route. Over the last decade or more, the issue of whether subtotal hysterectomy confers benefits over the total procedure has been hotly debated. The largest and most comprehensive trial to date comparing the effects of total and subtotal hysterectomy found no differences between the two operations with respect to bladder, bowel or sexual function up to one year after surgery. Thus, although these data suggest that subtotal confers no benefits over total hysterectomy, longer term follow-up is required, especially with regard to post-hysterectomy vaginal vault prolapse. It would also be important to establish whether the improvement in aspects of urinary function after both types of operation will be maintained in the long term.

Hysterectomy has been a mainstay of gynaecological therapy for over 100 years, and is likely to be so for the foreseeable future, simply because it is highly efficacious. The total versus subtotal hysterectomy debate has largely been resolved. Other questions that should be addressed include: the issue of the widely and wildly varying hysterectomy rates; whether vaginal hysterectomy is advantageous over abdominal hysterectomy and, if so, how more gynaecologists can be encouraged to adopt this approach; the true place of the conservative surgical approaches to the management of menorrhagia; and the optimal approaches to the management of uterine fibroids, since the latter are currently the most common indication for hysterectomy. In terms of counselling women who require hysterectomy for a benign indication, they can now be reassured that neither total nor subtotal abdominal hysterectomy adversely affects pelvic organ function. Subtotal abdominal hysterectomy is easier to perform than total abdominal hysterectomy, and has less risk of ureteric damage, but it requires that women have regular cervical smears and may result in cyclical bleeding in a small proportion of women. The key to optimal counselling may lie in providing women with as much information as possible, and inviting them to participate in the decision making about the type of hysterectomy they should undergo. Such empowerment may well improve satisfaction rates after surgery.[84]

References

1. Department of Health. *Hospital Episode Statistics 1998–1999*. London: DoH; 2000.
2. Lepine LA, Hillis SD, Marchbanks PA, Koonin LM, Morrow B, Kieke BA, *et al.* Hysterectomy surveillance – United States, 1980–1993. *MMWR CDC Surveill Summ* 1997;46:1–15.
3. Hall MJ, Owings MF. *2000 National Hospital Discharge Survey. Advance Data from Vital and Health Statistics, No. 329.* (Department of Health and Human Services publication no. (PHS) 2002-1250.) Hyattsville, MD: National Center for Health Statistics, 2002.
4. Dwyer N, Hutton J, Stirrat GM. Randomised controlled trial comparing endometrial resection with abdominal hysterectomy for surgical treatment of menorrhagia. *Br J Obstet Gynaecol* 1993;100:237–43.
5. Kilkku P, Gronoos M, Hirovnen T, Rauramo L. Supravaginal uterine amputations vs. hysterectomy. Effects on libido and orgasm. *Acta Obstet Gynecol Scand* 1983;62:147–52.
6. Kilkku P. Supravaginal uterine amputation vs. hysterectomy. Effects on coital frequency and dyspareunia. *Acta Obstet Gynecol Scand* 1983;62:141–5.
7. Kilkku P. Supravaginal uterine amputation versus hysterectomy with reference to subjective bladder symptoms and incontinence. *Acta Obstet Gynecol Scand* 1985;64:375–9.
8. Virtanen HS, Makinen JI, Tenho T, Kiiholma P, Pitkanen Y, Hirvonen T. Effects of abdominal hysterectomy on urinary and sexual symptoms. *Br J Urol* 1993;72:868–72.
9. Virtanen HS, Makinen JI, Kiilholma PJ. Conserving the cervix at hysterectomy. *Br J Obstet Gynaecol* 1995;102:587.
10. Herbert A. Cervical screening in England and Wales: its effect has been underestimated. *Cytopathology* 2000;11:471–9.
11. Kilkku P, Gronoos M. Peroperative electrocoagulation of the endocervical mucosa and later carcinoma of the cervical stump. *Acta Obstet Gynecol Scand* 1982;61:265–7.
12. Hendry W. Urinary tract injuries during gynaecological surgery. In: Studd J, editor. *Progress in Obstetrics and Gynaecology*, Vol. 5. Edinburgh: Churchill Livingstone; 1985. p. 362.
13. Whitelaw JM. Hysterectomy: a medical–legal perspective, 1975 to 1985. *Am J Obstet Gynecol* 1990;162:1451–8.
14. Nathorst-Boos J, Fuchs T, von Schoultz B. Consumers' attitude to hysterectomy. The experience of 678 women. *Acta Obstet Gynecol Scand* 1992;71:230–4.
15. Manyonda IT, Welch CR, McWhinney NA, Ross LD. The influence of suture material on vaginal vault granulations following abdominal hysterectomy. *Br J Obstet Gynaecol* 1990;97:608–12.
16. Thakar R, Ayers S, Clarkson P, Stanton S, Manyonda I. Outcomes after total versus subtotal abdominal hysterectomy. *N Engl J Med* 2002;347:1318–25.
17. Sutton C. Hysterectomy: a historical perspective. *Baillieres Clin Obstet Gynaecol* 1997;11:1–22.

18. Richardson EH. A simplified technique for abdominal panhysterectomy. *Surg Gynecol Obstet* 1929;48:248–51.

19. Howkins J, Stalworthy J. *Bonney's Gynaecological Surgery*. London: Baillière Tindall; 1974. p. 282.

20. Thakar R, Manyonda I, Robinson G, Clarkson P, Stanton S. Total versus subtotal hysterectomy: a survey of current views and practice amongst British gynaecologists. *J Obstet Gynaecol* 1998;18:267–9.

21. Department of Health. *Hospital Episodes Statistics 1994-1995*. London: DoH; 1996.

22. Warwick R, Williams PL, editors. *Gray's Anatomy*, 31st edn. Edinburgh: Longmans; 1980. p. 1203–4.

23. Smith PH, Ballantyne B. The neuroanatomical basis of denervation of the urinary bladder following major pelvic surgery. *Br J Surg* 1968;55:929–33.

24. Parys BT, Haylen BT, Hutton JL, Parsons KF. The effect of simple hysterectomy on vesicourethral function. *Br J Urol* 1989;64:594–9.

25. Hasson HM. Cervical removal at hysterectomy for benign disease. Risks and benefits. *J Reprod Med* 1993;38:781–90.

26. Smith AN, Varma JS, Binnie NR, Papachrysostomou M. Disordered colorectal motility in intractable constipation following hysterectomy. *Br J Surg* 1990;77:1361–5.

27. Benson JT. Neurophysiology of the female pelvic floor. *Curr Opin Obstet Gynecol* 1994;6:320–3.

28. Jewett JF. Vaginal length and incidence of dyspareunia following total abdominal hysterectomy. *Am J Obstet Gynecol* 1952;63:400–7.

29. Sloan D. The emotional and psychosexual aspects of hysterectomy. *Am J Obstet Gynecol* 1978;131:598–605.

30. Polivy J. Psychological reactions to hysterectomy: a critical review. *Am J Obstet Gynecol* 1974;118:417–26.

31. Dennerstein L, Wood C, Burrows GD. Sexual responses following hysterectomy and oophorectomy. *Obstet Gynecol* 1977;49:92–6.

32. Helström L, Sörbom D, Bäckström T. Influence of partner relationship on sexuality after subtotal hysterectomy. *Acta Obstet Gynecol Scand* 1995;74:142–6.

33. Helström L, Lundberg PO, Sörbom D, Bäckström T. Sexuality after hysterectomy: factor analysis of women's sexual lives before and after subtotal hysterectomy. *Obstet Gynecol* 1993;81:357–62.

34. Masters WH, Johnson V. *Human Sexual Response*. Boston, MA: Little, Brown; 1966. p. 117.

35. Milsom I, Ekelund P, Molander U, Arvidsson L, Areskoug B. The influence of age, parity, oral contraception, hysterectomy and menopause on the prevalence of urinary incontinence in women. *J Urol* 1993;149:1459–62.

36. Yarnell JW, Voyle GJ, Richards CJ, Stephenson TP. The prevalence and severity of urinary incontinence in women. *J Epidemiol Community Health* 1981;35:71–4.

37. Jecquier AM. Urinary symptoms and total hysterectomy. *Br J Urol* 1976;48:437–41.

38. Langer R, Neuman M, Ron-el R, Golan A, Bukovsky I, Caspi E. The effect of total abdominal hysterectomy on bladder function in asymptomatic women. *Obstet Gynecol* 1989;74:205–7.

39. Griffith-Jones MD, Jarvis GJ, McNamara HM. Adverse urinary symptoms after total abdominal hysterectomy – fact or fiction? *Br J Urol* 1991;67:295–7.

40. Bhattacharya S, Mollison J, Pinion S, Parkin DE, Abramovich DR, Terry P, et al. A comparison of bladder and ovarian function two years following hysterectomy or endometrial ablation. *Br J Obstet Gynaecol* 1996;103:898–903.

41. Prior A, Stanley K, Smith AR, Read NW. Effect of hysterectomy on anorectal and urethrovesical physiology. *Gut* 1992;33:264–7.

42. Vervest HA, Kiewiet du Jong M, Vervest TM, Barents JW, Hospels AA. Micturition symptoms and urinary incontinence after non-radical hysterectomy. *Acta Obstet Gynecol Scand* 1988;67:141–6.

43. Kujansuu E, Teisala K, Punnonen R. Urethral closure function after total and subtotal hysterectomy measured by urethrocystometry. *Gynecol Obstet Invest* 1989;27:105–6.

44. Lalos O, Bjerle P. Bladder wall mechanics and micturition before and after subtotal and total hysterectomy. *Eur J Obstet Gynecol Reprod Biol* 1986;21:143–50.

45. Brown JS, Sawaya G, Thom DH, Grady D. Hysterectomy and urinary incontinence: a systematic review. *Lancet* 2000;356:535–9.

46. Iosif CS, Bekassy Z, Rydhstrom H. Prevalence of urinary incontinence in middle-aged women. *Int J Gynaecol Obstet* 1988;26:255–9.

47. Preston DM, Lennard-Jones JE. Severe chronic constipation of young women: idiopathic slow transit constipation. *Gut* 1986;27:41–8.

48. Prior A, Whorwell PJ. Gynaecological consultation in patients with the irritable bowel syndrome. *Gut* 1989;30:996–8.

49. Longstreth GF, Preskill DB, Youkeles L. Irritable bowel syndrome in women having diagnostic laparoscopy or hysterectomy: relation to gynecologic features and outcome. *Dig Dis Sci* 1990;35:1285–90.

50. Hogston P. Irritable bowel syndrome as a cause of chronic pain in women attending a gynaecology clinic. *BMJ* 1987;294:934–5.

51. Taylor T, Smith AN, Fulton PM. Effect of hysterectomy on bowel function. *BMJ* 1989;299:300–1.

52. Roe AM, Bartolo DC, Mortensen NJ. Slow transit constipation. Comparison between patients with or without previous hysterectomy. *Dig Dis Sci* 1988;33:1159–63.

53. Karasick S, Spettell CM. The role of parity and hysterectomy on the development of pelvic floor abnormalities revealed by defecography. *AJR Am J Roentgenol* 1997;169:1555–8.

54. Prior A, Stanley K, Smith AR, Read NW. Relation between hysterectomy and the irritable bowel syndrome: a prospective study. *Gut* 1992;33:814–17.

55. van Dam JH, Gosselink MJ, Drogendijk AC, Hop WC, Schouten WR. Changes in bowel function after hysterectomy. *Dis Colon Rectum* 1997;40:1342–7.

56. Goffeng AR, Andersch B, Antov S, Berndtsson I, Oresland T, Hulten L. Does simple hysterectomy alter bowel function? *Ann Chir Gynaecol* 1997;86:298–303.

57. Spilker B. *Quality of Life Assessment in Clinical Trials.* New York: Raven Press; 1990.

58. Padilla GV, Grant MM, Ferrell B. Nursing research into quality of life. *Qual Life Res* 1992;1:341–8.

59. Coulter A, Peto V, Jenkinson C. Quality of life and patient satisfaction following treatment for menorrhagia. *Fam Pract* 1994;11:399–401.

60. Crosignani PG, Vercellini P, Apolone G, De Giorgio O, Cortesi I, Meschia M. Endometrial resection versus vaginal hysterectomy for menorrhagia: long term clinical and quality-of-life outcomes. *Am J Obstet Gynecol* 1997;177:95–101.

61. Rannestad T, Eikeland OJ, Helland H, Qvarnström U. The quality of life in women suffering from gynecological disorders is improved by means of hysterectomy. Absolute and relative differences between pre- and postoperative measures. *Acta Obstet Gynecol Scand* 2001;80:46–51.

62. Sculpher MJ, Dwyer N, Byford S, Stirrat GM. Randomised trial comparing hysterectomy and transcervical resection: effect on health related quality of life and costs two years after surgery. *Br J Obstet Gynaecol* 1996;103:142–9.

63.   Carlson KJ, Millar BA, Fowler FJ Jr. The Maine Women's Health Study: I. Outcomes of hysterectomy. *Obstet Gynecol* 1994;83:556–65.

64.   Kjerulff KH, Rhodes JC, Langenberg PW, Harvey LA. Patient satisfaction with results of hysterectomy. *Am J Obstet Gynecol* 2000;183:1440–7.

65.   Barker MG. Psychiatric illness after hysterectomy. *BMJ* 1968;2:91–5.

66.   Richards DH. Depression after hysterectomy. *Lancet* 1973;ii:430–3.

67.   Martin RL, Roberts WV, Clayton PJ. Psychiatric status after hysterectomy. *JAMA* 1980;244;350–3.

68.   Alexander AD, Naji AA, Pinion SB, Mollison J, Kitchener HC, Parkin DE, *et al.* Randomised trial comparing hysterectomy with endometrial ablation for dysfunctional uterine bleeding: psychiatric and psychosocial outcome. *BMJ* 1996;312:280–4.

69.   Gath D, Cooper P, Day A. Hysterectomy and psychiatric disorder: I. Levels of psychiatric morbidity before and after hysterectomy. *Br J Psychiatry* 1982;140:335–42.

70.   Gath D, Rose N, Bond A, Day A, Garrod A, Hodges S. Hysterectomy and psychiatric disorder: are the levels of psychiatric morbidity falling? *Psychol Med* 1995;25:277–83.

71.   Ryan MM, Dennerstein L, Pepperell R. Psychological aspects of hysterectomy. A prospective study. *Br J Psychiatry* 1989;154:516–22.

72.   Moore JT, Tooley DH. Depression following hysterectomy. *Psychosomatics* 1976;17:86–9.

73.   Kjerulff KH, Langenberg PW, Rhodes JC, Harvey LA, Guzinski GM, Stolley PD. Effectiveness of hysterectomy. *Obstet Gynecol* 2000;95:319–26.

74.   Gath D, Cooper P, Bond A, Edmonds G. Hysterectomy and psychiatric disorder: II. Demographic psychiatric and physical factors in relation to psychiatric outcome. *Br J Psychiatry* 1982;140:343–50.

75.   Munro MG, Deprest J. Laparoscopic hysterectomy: does it work? A bicontinental review of the literature and clinical commentary. *Clin Obstet Gynecol* 1995;38:401–25.

76.   Schaffer JI, Word A. Hysterectomy – still a useful operation. *N Engl J Med* 2002;347:1360–2.

77.   Gannon MJ, Holt EM, Fairbank J, Fitzgerald M, Milne MA, Crystal AM, *et al.* A randomised trial comparing endometrial resection and abdominal hysterectomy for the treatment of menorrhagia. *BMJ* 1991;303:1362–4.

78.   Pinion SB, Parkin DE, Abramovich DR, Naji A, Alexander DA, Russell IT, *et al.* Randomised trial of hysterectomy, endometrial laser ablation and transcervical endometrial resection for dysfunctional uterine bleeding. *BMJ* 1994;309:979–83.

79.   Weber AM, Walters MD, Schover LR, Church JM, Piedmonte MR. Functional outcomes and satisfaction after abdominal hysterectomy. *Am J Obstet Gynecol* 1999;181:530–5.

80.   Butler-Manuel SA, Buttery LD, A'Hern RP, Polak JM, Barton DP. Pelvic nerve plexus trauma at radical hysterectomy and simple hysterectomy: the nerve content of the uterine supporting ligaments. *Cancer* 2000;89:834–41.

81.   Butler-Manuel SA, Summerville K, Ford AM, Blake P, Riley AJ, Sultan AH, *et al.* Self assessment of morbidity following radical hysterectomy for cervical cancer. *J Obstet Gynaecol* 1999;19:180–3.

82.   Sutton CJ, Ewen SP, Whitelaw N, Haines P. Prospective, randomised, double-blind, controlled trial of laser laparoscopy in the treatment of pelvic pain associated with minimal, mild and moderate endometriosis. *Fertil Steril* 1994;62:696–700.

83.   Sutton CJ, Pooley AS, Ewen SP, Haines P. Follow-up report on a randomised controlled trial of laser laparoscopy in the treatment of pelvic pain associated with minimal to moderate endometriosis. *Fertil Steril* 1997;68:1070–4.

84.   Drife JO. Conserving the cervix at hysterectomy. *Br J Obstet Gynaecol* 1994:101:563–4.

26

HRT and breast disease: the surgeon's perspective

Jo Marsden and Nigel Sacks

INTRODUCTION

Breast cancer is the most common female malignancy in the UK, with an overall lifetime risk of one in ten and approximately 42 000 new cases diagnosed annually. Reproductive factors are implicated in both sporadic and familial breast cancer, so concern exists regarding the impact that hormone replacement therapy (HRT) may have on the incidence and prognosis of breast cancer, this in turn having a significant negative impact on long-term continuance with HRT. Clinical studies have shown that long-term use of HRT is associated with a small increase in breast cancer incidence (i.e. developing breast cancer) but that overall breast cancer mortality, the most important endpoint, may not be adversely affected at all. Considerably less is known of the epidemiology and role of HRT in benign breast disorders and pre-invasive, *in situ* breast cancer, which constitute a considerable part of the practice of breast surgeons.

BREAST ANATOMY AND PHYSIOLOGY

The prepubertal breast consists of only a few ducts embedded in fat. During puberty these develop into an extensive branching system, leading to the terminal ductal-lobular unit (TDLU), the epithelium of which has the highest mitotic rate in the breast. Four types of lobule development are recognised, progressing from poorly differentiated 'primitive' type I lobules that have high proliferation rates and oestrogen receptor (ER) expression and predominate in nulliparous women, to type III and IV lobules that differentiate as a result of pregnancy and lactation respectively and have a reduced proliferation rate and ER content. Most breast cancers arise in the TDLU and are classified according to their origin (i.e. invasive ductal or lobular carcinoma) or whether the basement membrane is breached or not (i.e. invasive or *in situ* disease). Type I lobules are thought to be the site of origin of most ductal and lobular carcinoma *in situ* (DCIS, LCIS) and invasive lobular carcinoma.[1]

Oestrogen is essential for initiating breast development at puberty, stimulating the growing duct, TDLU and connective tissue elements. With the commencement of ovulatory menstrual cycles and exposure to both serum oestrogen and progesterone, breast epithelium exhibits maximal mitosis in the luteal phase of the menstrual cycle, followed by apoptosis, which may occur in response to falling levels of these hormones.[2] During pregnancy, progesterone is necessary for lobular differentiation. Other hormones required for optimal development of the breast include insulin, growth hormone and corticosteroids. Prolactin also exerts a mitotic effect but serum levels are elevated only towards the end of the last trimester of pregnancy and during lactation. From the age of about 35 years, the breast begins to undergo involutional change and, by the age of the menopause, only a few ducts remain, fat having replaced the regressed epithelial and connective tissue. Breast involution is attributed to hormone withdrawal because it commences at an age when serum follicle stimulating hormone level begins to rise, although serum oestradiol usually remains stable until the onset of the menopausal transition.

Since both oestrogen and progesterone have such an obvious and important role in normal breast development, it could be assumed that reproductive factors and, therefore HRT, would be equally relevant in the development of benign breast disorders, *in situ* disease and breast carcinoma, but available epidemiological data do not support this.

THE EPIDEMIOLOGY OF BENIGN BREAST DISORDERS

The term 'benign breast disorders' encompasses a diverse range of different conditions and has been subject to a variety of classification systems using both clinical and histological criteria. This has resulted in difficulty in the interpretation of epidemiological studies and therefore with obtaining a clear understanding of their biological behaviour and the potential impact of exogenous oestrogen and progestogens. Currently, two classifications are commonly used. The first, Aberrations in Normal Development and Involution (ANDI), is based on the concept (but disputed by and not popular with breast pathologists) that most benign breast conditions develop from variations in the normal physiological processes in the breast, changes ranging from normal to slight abnormality (aberration) to disease (Table 1).[3] Reproductive factors are important in the normal development and involution of breast tissue, so it is surprising that, with the exception of altered prolactin metabolism, only weak associations of endocrine factors with ANDI have been reported.[4]

The second classification, which is more widely used and recognised, categorises benign breast conditions according to histological type, with specific reference to proliferative activity and the presence of atypia and the associated risk of subsequent breast cancer development. Women with nonproliferative benign lesions do not have an increased risk of breast cancer, whereas risk is approximately doubled in those with proliferative lesions and elevated five-fold in women with atypical ductal or lobular hyperplasia (Table 2).[5] Epidemiological studies based on this histological classification have shown a consistent relationship only with obesity; other endocrine related factors are reported to have weak or no positive association with benign proliferative lesions.[6]

Table 1 *ANDI classification of benign breast disease*

Physiological stage	Normal	Aberration	Disease
Early reproductive (15–25 years)	Lobular development Stromal development Nipple eversion	Fibroadenoma Adolescent hypertrophy Nipple inversion	Giant fibroadenoma Gigantomastia Subareolar abscess/mammary duct fistula
Mature reproductive (25–40 years)	Cyclical changes of menstruation	Cyclical mastalgia/nodularity	
Involution (35–55 years)	Lobular involution Duct involution	Cysts, sclerosing lesions Duct ectasia/nipple retraction	
	Epithelial turnover	Simple hyperplasia	Atypical hyperplasia

HRT AND BENIGN BREAST DISORDERS

HRT appears to reverse the changes of breast involution and therefore, with its use, benign conditions such as fibroadenomas, cysts and mastalgia may persist in the menopause.[7,8] There are no data showing whether this effect of HRT is determined according to the regimen prescribed, but studies published in 1999 evaluating the impact of HRT on mammographic breast density and epithelial proliferation suggest that this may be relevant. The placebo controlled Postmenopausal Estrogen/Progestin Interventions (PEPI) trial demonstrated that oestrogen alone (i.e. conjugated equine [CEE] oestrogen 0.625 mg) did not increase the proportion of women developing increased mammographic breast density, whereas a significant increase was found with both cyclical and continuous combined HRT (19.4%, 95% confidence interval [CI] 9.9–28.9; and 23.5%, 95% CI 11.9–35.1 in women prescribed CEE 0.625 mg plus cyclical medroxyprogesterone acetate [MPA] 10 mg/day for 12 days/cycle or continuous MPA 2.5 mg).[9] Biopsies of tissue from areas of abnormal mammographic breast density in women using HRT have also shown a significant increase in the number and size of proliferating breast epithelial cells compared with women who are not exposed to HRT, but only in those taking combined therapy.[10]

Although HRT does appear to influence the incidence of benign breast disorders, some studies have reported that the risk of subsequent breast cancer in women with atypical hyperplasia is reduced in postmenopausal compared with premenopausal women, suggesting that exposure to HRT will increase the risk of malignant change.[11] In the few studies where accurate histological classification of benign breast disorders has been performed, HRT has not been shown to increase subsequent breast cancer risk in women with biopsy proven atypia, but further supportive evidence is necessary given the small number of incident breast cancer cases upon which these risk estimates are based (Table 2).[12,13]

THE EPIDEMIOLOGY OF PRE-INVASIVE, IN SITU BREAST CANCER AND HRT

The two distinct forms of *in situ* breast disease, DCIS and LCIS, are characterised by malignant epithelial cells that have not breached the basement membrane of the TDLU and therefore lack the potential for regional nodal or distant metastases. DCIS is not a discrete pathological entity (subtypes that have differing malignant potential have been identified), whereas LCIS is usually of

Table 2 *Histological classification of benign breast disease and breast cancer risk with oestrogen replacement therapy[5,12] (reproduced from: Marsden J. Hormone replacement therapy and breast cancer. In: Barter J, Hampton N, editors.* The Year in Gynaecology 2001. *Oxford: Clinical Publishing; 2001. p. 180,[75] with permission from the publisher)*

	Without ERT		With ERT	
	No. cases	RR (95% CI)	No. cases	RR (95% CI)
Proliferative disease with atypical cell changes (atypical ductal or lobular hyperplasia)	5	2.53 (1.00–6.30)	7	2.87 (1.30–6.30)
Proliferative disease without atypia (multiple cysts, duct papillomata, sclerosing adenosis)	21	1.13 (0.69–1.90)	29	1.37 (0.88–2.10)
All nonproliferative benign disease (duct ectasia, solitary cysts, fibroadenoma)	26	1.27 (0.81–2.00)	36	1.52 (1.00–2.30)

ERT = oestrogen replacement therapy; RR = relative risk; CI = confidence interval low nuclear and histological grade. DCIS is a major risk factor for breast cancer, with 90% of recurrences (both *in situ* and invasive) occurring in the ipsilateral breast within five years of diagnosis.[14,15] Management is therefore aimed at achieving local control within the breast.

Mastectomy is appropriate for widespread change in the breast but, for localised disease, depending on the grade and extent of the lesion, and hence malignant potential, the optimal treatment after local surgical excision remains uncertain. The effectiveness of adjuvant radiotherapy and tamoxifen is being addressed in large randomised trials.[16–19] LCIS, in contrast, is now considered to be a risk marker for developing invasive breast cancer in the future because subsequent risk applies equally to both breasts, with more than 50% of cancers being diagnosed after 15 years.[15] The standard management of LCIS in the UK is mammographic surveillance, but some women may opt for what should really be regarded as prophylactic mastectomy.

Characteristically, DCIS is now associated with impalpable microcalcification that is usually detected by mammography; therefore it has increased in incidence since the introduction of mammographic screening programmes. The incidence of DCIS is approximately 20% of all mammographically detected cancers.[20] LCIS has no specific mammographic features, rarely presents as symptomatic disease, and is therefore usually an incidental finding after a breast biopsy performed for another indication and, as such, the incidence is low, ranging from 0.5% to 3.6%.[14]

The low incidence rate of *in situ* disease renders it difficult to establish its epidemiology and, in particular, whether there are aetiological factors common to both *in situ* and invasive breast cancer. Current evidence suggests that some reproductive risk factors for *in situ* disease are shared with invasive disease, such as late age at first full-term pregnancy but other associations remain to be clarified, including the role of HRT.[21] Preliminary results from large randomised tamoxifen breast chemoprevention trials (i.e. the National Surgical Adjuvant Breast and Bowel Programme tamoxifen chemoprevention trial [NSABP-P1] and the International Breast Cancer Intervention Study [IBIS-I]) provide indirect evidence that HRT may be important in the development of *in situ* disease because statistically significant reductions in DCIS have been found in high-risk women exposed to tamoxifen, of the order of 50% ($P < 0.002$) and 69% (odds ratio 0.31, 95% CI 0.12–0.82) respectively.[22,23] Although available observational studies have reported HRT to increase the risk of developing *in situ* disease, surveillance bias cannot be excluded, given that women who use HRT are more likely to attend for mammographic breast screening.[21,24–30] The results of the placebo controlled Women's Health Initiative (WHI) study published in 2003 failed to demonstrate any increase in the risk of *in situ* disease in women allocated to receive continuous combined HRT (i.e. CEE 0.625 mg and MPA 2.5 mg) after a mean follow-up of 5.6 years (hazard ratio 1.18, 95% CI 0.77–1.72).[31] Although early detection bias can be discounted, the lack of an effect may simply reflect that this large randomised trial was underpowered to detect a small change in incidence of *in situ* disease, which constitutes approximately one-fifth of all screen detected cancers.[20] The WHI study findings as they stand should not be interpreted as evidence that the use of HRT in women after a diagnosis of DCIS or LCIS is without risk, particularly in the ER positive (ER+ve) subtypes.

BREAST CANCER

Evidence for the hormone dependency of breast cancer

Epidemiological studies have demonstrated a clear and consistent relationship between reproductive function and breast cancer risk because disease incidence increases after puberty and falls by an estimated 2.7% (95% CI 2.1–3.2) per year after the onset of the menopause.[32] The reduced risk observed with early age at first birth and high parity probably reflects enhanced differentiation of the epithelium in the terminal ducts and lobules of the breast, rendering cells less susceptible to malignant transformation. In postmenopausal women, whose ovaries no longer function, serum oestrogen is produced by aromatisation of androgens to oestrogen in peripheral adipose tissue and this is assumed to account for the association of postmenopausal obesity with increased breast cancer risk. Support for this hypothesis and the importance of serum oestrogen, even at low circulating levels, in the promotion of transformed breast cancer cells is provided by review of studies demonstrating positive correlations between risk and elevations in serum oestrogen and androgens,[33] the Multiple Outcomes of Raloxifene Evaluation (MORE) study, which found raloxifene to confer maximal reduction in the incidence of ER+ve breast cancer in women with the highest circulating levels of serum oestradiol[34] and, most recently, in 2002, preliminary data from the Arimidex, Tamoxifen, Alone or in Combination (ATAC) adjuvant breast cancer trial, in which disease-free survival was significantly improved in women randomised to receive this aromatase inhibitor that results in oestrogen levels so low as to be undetectable by established assay techniques.[22]

In premenopausal women, breast cancer prognosis appears in some studies to be improved if surgery is performed during the mid to late luteal rather than the follicular phase of the menstrual cycle.[35] This has been interpreted as support for a protective effect of progesterone, particularly as higher circulating levels (i.e. >4 ng/ml) at the time of initial breast surgery have been associated with improved survival.[36] However, in postmenopausal women, clinical evidence regarding the effect of progestogens on the breast is largely drawn from studies of combined HRT, which have shown an adverse effect on breast cancer incidence.

HRT AND BREAST CANCER INCIDENCE: EVIDENCE FROM CLINICAL STUDIES

Observational studies

Reliable estimation of any associated risk of postmenopausal breast cancer with exposure to either unopposed or combined HRT has been limited owing to a lack of sufficiently powered placebo controlled randomised trials. Advice to women has therefore depended on risk estimates drawn from observational studies, the reanalysis of which provide evidence that HRT confers a similar degree of risk as that of delaying the menopause (i.e. 2.3% per year of exposure) and that risk is increased significantly with long-term use, although the associated relative and absolute risk is small.[32] Expressed as absolute risk, the use of HRT from the age of 50 years has been estimated to account for two extra cancers per 1000 women who use it continuously for five years, and six additional cancers with ten years' exposure. Less than 5% of the women had been exposed to combined HRT but, despite the small patient numbers, the risk appeared to be greater than that observed with oestrogen alone (relative risk with more than 5 years' exposure 1.53, standard error 0.23). Subsequent individual observational studies have also reported an increased risk with combination therapy over unopposed oestrogen.[37–44] Until the publication of the Million Women Study, the number of breast cancer events in these studies has been too small for reliable subgroup analysis to determine whether risk is influenced by the class of progestogen and pattern of progestogen administration.[44]

The Million Women Study[44] provided detailed information about exposure to a diverse range of HRT regimens and breast cancer risk from approximately 25% of women in the UK aged between 50 and 64 years who attended the National Health Service Breast Screening Programme (NHSBSP) between 1996 and 2001. During the average follow-up for cancer incidence of 2.6

years, 9364 incident breast cancers were diagnosed (at a mean of 1.2 years from recruitment). The relative risk of breast cancer for current HRT users (mean duration 5.8 years) was 1.66 (95% CI 1.58–1.75); the risk increased with lengthening total duration of use, but past use had no significant effect.[45] Estimates varied by the HRT type (i.e. unopposed oestrogen relative risk 1.30, 95% CI 1.21–1.40; combined HRT relative risk 2.00, 95% CI 1.88–2.12; tibolone relative risk 1.45, 95% CI 1.25–1.68) but were unaffected by the specific oestrogen or progestogen prescribed, the pattern of progestogen administration, or the route of administration (vaginal preparations were not evaluated). In contrast to other observational data and randomised trials (the latter are discussed in the next section), breast cancer risk was reported to be elevated with less than one year's exposure. It is important, however, to appreciate that the data on HRT use in this study are cross-sectional and not prospective. If HRT use continued after recruitment (particularly in those who had only just commenced HRT), the duration of HRT use presented is likely to underestimate total exposure. Adding an average of 1.2 years (i.e. the mean time to cancer diagnosis from recruitment) to each of the duration categories for current HRT users shifts the pattern of risk to one that is more consistent with other data. The Million Women Study, although large, is observational, and the results should be interpreted in the context of continuing randomised trials. If differences exist between women attending the NHSBSP and those who do not, and between attendees who agreed or declined to participate in the study, this could bias the reported results.

Randomised studies

Continuing or completed placebo controlled trials of HRT in healthy women in which breast cancer is a primary endpoint are summarised in Table 3.[31,46–53] Most conclusions about HRT and breast cancer incidence have been drawn from the two largest randomised trials, the Heart and Estrogen/Progestin Replacement Study (HERS)[50] and the WHI study,[31] both of which examined the effect of continuous combined HRT (i.e. CEE 0.625 mg and MPA 2.5 mg). Owing to an excess of adverse breast cancer events, the combined HRT arm of the WHI study was closed prematurely in July 2002. The Medical Research Council discontinued in 2002 the Women's International Study of Long-Duration Oestrogen use after Menopause (WISDOM)[51,52] in the UK because this used the same HRT regimen as WHI and HERS, the reason being that continuation would not add further to clinical practice. Unfortunately, the sample sizes of two randomised trials that have allocated different combined HRT preparations are too small for definitive conclusions to be drawn.[49,53]

As yet there is no randomised evidence to support an increase in breast cancer risk with exposure to unopposed oestrogen, although the only completed trial (i.e. Women's Estrogen for Stroke Trial, WEST) was of a short duration (i.e. mean 33 months +/−17 months standard deviation).[46] The unopposed oestrogen arm (i.e. CEE 0.625 mg daily) of the WHI study is continuing after an interim analysis at 5.2 years because no evidence has emerged to date of an excess of breast cancer events.[48]

The main finding of the continuous combined arm of the WHI study was that, with a mean follow-up of 5.6 years (estimated mean duration of use 3.1 years), the hazard ratio for invasive and *in situ* breast cancer combined was 1.24 (95% CI 1.02–1.50), with risk beginning to increase three years after randomisation.[31] Risk appeared to be restricted to women with a history of HRT exposure prior to study entry, supporting a duration effect and predictions from previous observational studies.[32] In absolute terms, the event rate per 1000 women using combined HRT is one extra *in situ* cancer and four extra invasive cancers with five years of use. For invasive cancers, this equates with an excess risk of 1 in 250.

The risk of breast cancer falls after the cessation of HRT (by five years, risk is no greater than that in women who have never been exposed to HRT) and implies that HRT promotes the

Table 3 *HRT and breast cancer incidence: continuing or completed placebo controlled randomised trials with breast cancer as a primary endpoint*

HRT	HRT regimen (all oral preparations)	*n*	Follow-up (years)	No. events		RR (95% CI)
				HRT	Placebo	
Oestrogen						
Viscoli et al., 2001 (WEST)[46]	E$_2$ 2 mg	664	2.8	5	5	1.00 (0.30–3.50)
ESPRIT-UK team, 2002[47]	E$_2$ 2 mg	1017	2	4	4	0.98 (0.25–3.91)
WHI Study[48]	CEE 0.625 mg	10739	>5.2	–	–	Interim analysis – no excess risk
Cyclical combined HRT						
Nachtigall et al., 1992[49]	CEE 2.5 mg + MPA 10 mg	168	10	0	4	*P* = 0.12
Continuous combined HRT						
Hulley et al., 1998 (HERS)[50]	CEE 0.625 mg + MPA 2.5 mg	2763	4.1	34	25	1.38 (0.82–2.31)
Cheblowski et al., 2003 (WHI)[31]	CEE 0.625 mg + MPA 2.5 mg	16608	5.6	199	150	1.24 (1.01–1.54)
WISDOM[51,52]	CEE 0.625 mg + MPA 2.5 mg	5700	–	–	–	–
Høibraaten et al., 2000 (EVTET)[53]	E$_2$ 2 mg + NEA 1 mg	140	2	–	–	

RR = relative risk; CI = confidence interval; WEST = Women's Estrogen for Stroke Trial; E$_2$ = oestradiol; ESPRIT = oEStrogen in the Prevention of ReInfarction Trial; CEE = conjugated equine oestrogen; MPA = medroxyprogesterone acetate; HERS = Heart and Estrogen/Progestin Replacement Study; WHI = Women's Health Initiative Study; WISDOM = Women's International Study of Long Duration Oestrogen after Menopause; EVTET = Estrogen in Venous ThromboEmbolism Trial; NEA = norethisterone acetate

growth of cells that have already undergone malignant transformation.[32,44] Although it could be anticipated that tumours developing in women using HRT at presentation are more likely to be clinically advanced and have a worse prognosis, observational data have shown the converse.[32,54] HRT associated cancers would also be expected to be ER+ve given that the benefit of endocrine breast cancer treatment and chemoprevention therapy is restricted to hormone sensitive disease, and observational evidence does support this.[55–58] The randomised WHI study, however, reported that tumours developing in women allocated to HRT were larger, although the mean size difference was small (i.e. 2 mm, *P* = 0.04) and more likely to be node positive (proportion of positive nodes with HRT [*n* = 25] 25.9%, 95% CI 19.5–30; placebo [*n* = 21] 15.8%, 95% CI 10–23.1).[31] This trend is of borderline significance (*P* = 0.08) and the wide, overlapping confidence intervals raise uncertainty about whether additional breast cancer events would weaken or strengthen this association. No difference was reported between treatment groups with respect to tumour grade, histological type, and hormone receptor positivity, but the WHI study is almost certainly underpowered to detect such differences. Most postmenopausal tumours are ER+ve and invasive lobular cancers constitute only about 10% of all invasive disease. Thus, approximately 1000 breast cancer events would be needed to detect a 5% difference compared with placebo, but there were only 349 invasive cancers in the latest WHI report.

Eight deaths were reported in the WHI study, four in each of the HRT and placebo groups. Based on the phenotypes of tumours diagnosed in women allocated to HRT and to placebo in the WHI study, calculation of prognosis with the validated and widely used Nottingham Prognostic Index does not place HRT associated cancers in a worse prognostic group compared with placebo, and the difference is small in estimated ten-year survival based on mean tumour size, a mean tumour grade of 2, and weighting according to the proportion of node positive disease (i.e. 62.5% for HRT versus 61% for placebo).[59] If the increased risk of node positivity as reported by WHI is accurate, then the likely impact on long-term survival is likely to be small.

The Million Women Study reported an increased breast cancer mortality in current HRT users (relative risk 1.22, 95% CI 1.00–1.48) but this was of borderline statistical significance ($P = 0.05$).[44] Although this contrasts with previous observational studies, it does not necessarily imply that HRT associated cancers are more advanced; it may simply reflect that more cancers were diagnosed in women with a history of HRT exposure. In the absence of details about the phenotype, stage and treatment of the incident cancers these data are difficult to interpret.

The unavailability of other randomised trials evaluating different combined regimens makes it is difficult to know with any certainty whether it is correct to extrapolate the risk estimates from the WHI study to all types of combination therapy. The results of the Million Women Study, however, suggest that risk is increased irrespective of progestogen type and route of administration.[44] If the assumption that increased mammographic density is an accurate surrogate of breast cancer risk in postmenopausal women is correct, data from the placebo controlled PEPI trial supports the finding that risk is increased equally with both cyclical and continuous progestogen administration. Unopposed oestrogen (i.e. CEE 0.625 mg) had no significant effect.[9]

HRT AND MAMMOGRAPHIC BREAST CANCER SCREENING

Delayed mammographic detection has been cited as an explanation for the more adverse prognostic features of HRT associated breast cancers in the WHI study. However, although there was a statistically significant increase in the number of abnormal mammograms in women allocated to HRT compared with those allocated to placebo ($P < 0.01$) from the first year of follow-up, the proportional increase in the various categories of mammographic abnormality in HRT users compared with the placebo group was similar; therefore, HRT may not result in the misclassification of only abnormal mammographic appearances, potentially increasing mammographic inaccuracy. The absence of details about screening sensitivity, specificity and quality assurance within the WHI study (women were screened at over 3000 centres), combined with the fact that no established national or regional screening programmes perform annual two-view mammography (the screening method used in WHI), makes it difficult to extrapolate the results to the performance of other screening programmes and draw any definite conclusions about the impact that HRT may have on the potential breast cancer mortality reduction from the NHSBSP. About half (53%) of the 33% of women attending the NHSBSP currently use combined HRT.[45] In view of the PEPI trial results, the likely proportion expected to develop any density increase would be approximately 5%.[9] Invasive breast cancer detection rates in the NHSBSP have exceeded predicted targets since 1994, so combined HRT use in women attending for screening would not appear to have a significant adverse effect on performance.[20]

FAMILIAL BREAST CANCER

Approximately 10% of women diagnosed with breast cancer have a family history of the disease; half of them have an identifiable genetic mutation. Women from families with an inherited genetic predisposition are characterised by young age of onset (i.e. less than 40 years at diagnosis), clustering of cases affecting first degree relatives, and an increased incidence of bilateral disease. Most currently identifiable mutations affect the *BRCA1* and *BRCA2* tumour suppressor genes, which have an associated lifetime breast cancer risk of up to 80%. Tumours developing in *BRCA1* mutation carriers are slightly more likely to have a hormone resistant phenotype in that they are more often high grade and both ER and progesterone receptor (PR) negative. Current data suggest that, although *BRCA2* tumours are usually high grade, the expression of ER does not appear to differ significantly from sporadic cancers.[60]

Studies evaluating the effect of HRT on the risk of subsequent breast cancer in women with an affected first degree relative have not shown risk to be any greater than that conferred by HRT in women without a family history (Table 4) but, in the absence of more detailed information, conclusions about the effect of HRT in women with a likely inherited genetic predisposition cannot be made.[32,39,44,58,61,62] Despite the biological characteristics of *BRCA1* associated tumours suggesting that reproductive factors are unlikely to influence their incidence, prophylactic tamoxifen and oophorectomy have been shown to reduce the risk of invasive breast cancer in mutation carriers, although the numbers of women treated in these studies are small.[63-65] It is interesting and important that the use of add-back HRT for the amelioration of oestrogen deficiency symptoms after oophorectomy in *BRCA1* mutation carriers has not been shown to reduce the benefit of ovarian ablation.[65]

THE USE OF HRT IN BREAST CANCER SURVIVORS

In view of the known hormone dependency of most breast cancers, HRT is contraindicated in breast cancer survivors. However, many of these women experience oestrogen deficiency symptoms as an adverse effect of their treatment and discussion of symptom management is becoming commonplace in breast cancer follow-up clinics.[66] Unfortunately, many of the prescription medicines and complementary therapies that are recommended as 'safe' alternatives to HRT have not been evaluated in placebo controlled trials and, for those that have, the studies are of short duration and of insufficient power to determine whether there is any potential antagonism with respect to symptom or cancer control with concomitantly administered breast cancer therapy. This particularly applies to many of the most frequently used complementary therapies for the menopause, many of which have oestrogenic activity (e.g. phyto-oestrogens, Agnus Castus, ginseng, hops, Dong quai) and should be subject to rigorous controlled evaluation in trials in this patient population.[67,68]

Several observational studies have now been published in which the outcome has been reported of breast cancer survivors who have elected to use HRT after their diagnosis and treatment. None has shown HRT to impair disease-free or overall survival, the majority being reviewed in 2001 in a meta-analysis in which the annual risk of recurrence was not reported to be increased with the use of HRT for a median duration of 30 months (relative risk 0.82, 95% CI 0.58–0.93).[69] Unfortunately, there are no data on histological subtype or hormone receptor status of recurrent tumours diagnosed in women who have elected to use HRT after their cancer diagnosis. No reduction in disease-free, cause-specific or overall mortality has been reported in women using HRT whose primary tumour was ER+ve or who were concomitantly taking tamoxifen, but the

Table 4 *HRT and breast cancer risk in women with a family history of breast cancer affecting a first degree relative*

	Breast cancer risk RR (95% CI)[a]	Duration of HRT use
Collaborative Group re-analysis, 1997[32]	1.06 (SE 0.199)	>5
Sellers *et al.*, 1997[61]	1.35 (0.72–2.53)	>5
Magnusson *et al.*, 1999[39]	1.98 (1.02–3.81)	>5
Olssen *et al.*, 2001[62]	1.86 (1.27–2.56)	>4[b]
Ursin *et al.*, 2002[58]	0.99 (0.84–1.17)	>5

[a] Ever versus never used; [b] Standardised incidence rate; RR = relative risk; SE = standard error

number of breast cancer events in these subsequent studies are far too small for reliable estimation of risk.[70] Indirect evidence supporting a lack of antagonism between tamoxifen and oestrogen replacement therapy was found in the Italian chemoprevention trial in which women taking both agents had a decreased incidence of breast cancer (cumulative frequency of breast cancer 0.92%, 95% CI 0.17–1.66 versus 2.58%, 95% CI 1.30–3.85) in women using oestrogen replacement therapy alone, although the numbers were small.[71] Retrospective data on surveillance mammography in breast cancer survivors who are prescribed HRT suggest that it does not appear to impede screening for contralateral primaries or ipsilateral recurrence.[72] Although this may also reflect small patient numbers and a lack of appropriate controlled groups for comparison, concurrent use of tamoxifen may explain this finding. Breast cancer mortality has been reported in only one study, which failed to show any reduction in survival (relative risk 0.34, 95% CI 0.13–0.91). However, with a total number of fatal breast cancer events of five, this evidence is no more than anecdotal.[73]

Based on the WHI study, the estimated hazard ratio with two years' HRT exposure is 0.72 (95% CI 0.47–1.10), and adjustment for the period between baseline and cancer diagnosis in the Million Women Study results in an emerging increase in risk after 2.2 years of combined HRT use. If risk for incidence can be applied to the potential for recurrence, this also suggests that short-term HRT exposure may not significantly increase the risk of progressive breast cancer.

The continuing *ad hoc* prescription of HRT to symptomatic women with breast cancer will not add to our knowledge of its impact in this group of women; to answer this uncertainty, large randomised trials are necessary. Since the successful implementation of a pilot randomised study in the UK, larger-scale trials, in which disease-free survival and overall survival are the primary endpoints, are now being conducted in the UK and Scandinavia in symptomatic women with early stage breast cancer.[74]

SUMMARY

Although randomised controlled trials support estimations from observational studies of breast cancer risk with long-term exposure to combined HRT, there are still many questions about this relationship that remain unanswered by current data, in particular, whether HRT has any effect on breast cancer mortality and recurrence. Despite the number of studies that have been conducted, it is still not possible to identify which women may be placed at this increased risk if they take HRT. Understanding the role of HRT in the aetiology and outcome of breast cancer is rendered more difficult by the fact that the natural history of breast cancer development is poorly understood. No clear association has been shown between HRT use and the incidence or progression of either benign breast disorders or pre-invasive *in situ* breast cancer; however, current evidence is limited owing to bias or insufficient sample size. There is an obvious need to continue with clinical trials but, until more reliable data become available, ensuring adequate informed consent of women prior to initiation of HRT must allow for this clinical uncertainty.

References

1. Hughes LE, Mansel RE, Webster DJT. Breast anatomy and physiology. In: Hughes LE, Mansel RE, Webster DJT, editors. *Benign Disorders and Diseases of the Breast*. 2nd ed. Edinburgh: Saunders; 2000. p. 7–20.

2. Anderson TJ, Ferguson DJ, Raab GM. Cell turnover in the 'resting' human breast: influence of parity, contraceptive pill, age and laterality. *Br J Cancer* 1982;46:376–82.

3.   Hughes LE, Mansel RE, Webster DJ. Aberrations of normal development and involution (ANDI): a new perspective on pathogenesis and nomenclature of benign breast disorders. *Lancet* 1987;ii:1316–19.

4.   Parlati E, Liberale I, Travaglini A, Morelli P, Menini E, Dell'Acqua S. Endocrine aspects of benign breast disease. *Cancer Detect Prev* 1992;16:25–6.

5.   Dupont WD, Page DL. Risk factors for breast cancer in women with proliferative breast disease. *N Engl J Med* 1985;312:146–51.

6.   Goehring C, Morabia A. Epidemiology of benign breast disease, with special attention to histologic types. *Epidemiol Rev* 1997;19:310–27.

7.   Marsh MS, Whitcroft S, Whitehead MI. Paradoxical effects of hormone replacement therapy on breast tenderness in postmenopausal women. *Maturitas* 1994;19:97–102.

8.   Brenner RJ, Bein ME, Sarti DA, Vinstein AL. Spontaneous regression of interval benign cysts of the breast. *Radiology* 1994;193:365–8.

9.   Greendale GA, Reboussin BA, Sie A, Singh R, Olson LK, Gatewood O, et al. Effects of estrogen and estrogen-progestin on mammographic parenchymal density. Postmenopausal Estrogen/Progestin Interventions (PEPI) Investigators. *Ann Intern Med* 1999;130:262–9.

10. Hofseth LJ, Raafat AM, Osuch JR, Pathak DR, Slomski CA, Haslam SZ. Hormone replacement therapy with estrogen or estrogen plus medroxyprogesterone acetate is associated with increased epithelial proliferation in the normal postmenopausal breast. *J Clin Endocrinol Metab* 1999;84:4559–65.

11. Schnitt SJ. Benign breast disease and breast cancer risk: potential role for antiestrogens. *Clin Cancer Res* 2001;7(12 Suppl):4419s–22s.

12. Dupont WD, Page DL, Parl FF, Plummer WD Jr, Schuyler PA, Kasami M, et al. Estrogen replacement therapy in women with a history of proliferative breast disease. *Cancer* 1999;85:1277–83.

13. Byrne C, Connolly JL, Colditz GA, Schnitt SJ. Biopsy confirmed benign breast disease, postmenopausal use of exogenous female hormones, and breast carcinoma risk. *Cancer* 2000;89:2046–52.

14. Silverstein MJ. Ductal carcinoma *in situ* of the breast. *BMJ* 1998;317:734–9.

15. Frykberg ER. Lobular carcinoma *in situ* of the breast. *Breast J* 1999;5:296–302.

16. Fisher B, Dignam J, Wolmark N, Mamounas E, Costantino J, Poller W, et al. Lumpectomy and radiation therapy for the treatment of intraductal breast cancer: findings from National Surgical Adjuvant Breast and Bowel Project B-17. *J Clin Oncol* 1998;16:441–52.

17. Julien JP, Bijker N, Fentiman IS, Peterse JL, Delledonne V, Rouanet P, et al. Radiotherapy in breast-conserving treatment for ductal carcinoma *in situ*: first results of the EORTC randomised phase III trial 10853. EORTC Breast Cancer Cooperative Group and EORTC Radiotherapy Group. *Lancet* 2000;355:528–33.

18. Fisher B, Dignam J, Wolmark M, Wickerham DL, Fisher ER, Mamounas E, et al. Tamoxifen in treatment of intraductal breast cancer: National Surgical Adjuvant Breast and Bowel Project B-24 randomised controlled trial. *Lancet* 1999;353:1993–2000.

19. Houghton J, George WD, Cuzick J, Duggan C, Fentiman IS, Spittle M, et al. Radiotherapy and tamoxifen in women with completely excised ductal carcinoma *in situ* of the breast in the UK, Australia, and New Zealand: randomised controlled trial. *Lancet* 2003;362:95–102.

20. Blanks RG, Moss SM, Patnick J. Results from the UK NHS breast screening programme 1994–1999. *J Med Screen* 2000;7:195–8.

21. Claus EB, Stowe M, Carter D. Breast carcinoma *in situ*: risk factors and screening patterns. *J Natl Cancer Inst* 2001;93:1811–17.

22. Baum M, Budzer AU, Cuzick J, Forbes J, Houghton JH, Klijn JG, et al. Anastrozole alone or in combination with tamoxifen versus tamoxifen alone for adjuvant treatment of

postmenopausal women with early breast cancer: first results of the ATAC randomised trial. *Lancet* 2002;359:2131–9.

23. Cuzick J, Forbes J, Edwards R, Baum M, Cawthorn S, Coates A, *et al*. First results from the International Breast Cancer Intervention Study (IBIS-I): a randomised prevention trial. *Lancet* 2002;360:817–24.

24. Brinton LA, Hoover R, Fraumeni JF Jr. Menopausal oestrogens and breast cancer risk: an expanded case–control study. *Br J Cancer* 1986;54:825–32.

25. Schairer C, Byrne C, Keyl PM, Brinton LA, Sturgeon SR, Hoover RN. Menopausal estrogen and estrogen-progestin replacement therapy and risk of breast cancer (United States). *Cancer Causes Control* 1994;5:491–500.

26. Stanford JL, Weiss NS, Voight LF, Daling JR, Habel LA, Rossing MA. Combined estrogen and progestin hormone replacement therapy in relation to risk of breast cancer in middle-aged women. *JAMA* 1995;274:137–42.

27. Longnecker MP, Bernstein L, Paganini-Hill A, Enger SM, Ross RK. Risk factors for *in situ* breast cancer. *Cancer Epidemiol Biomarkers Prev* 1996;5:961–5.

28. Henrich JB, Kornguth PJ, Viscoli CM, Horwitz RI. Postmenopausal estrogen use and invasive versus *in situ* breast cancer risk. *J Clin Epidemiol* 1998;51:1277–83.

29. Trentham-Dietz A, Newcomb PA, Storer BE, Remington PL. Risk factors for carcinoma *in situ* of the breast. *Cancer Epidemiol Biomarkers Prev* 2000;9:697–703.

30. Seeley T. Do women taking hormone replacement therapy have a higher uptake of screening mammograms? *Maturitas* 1994;19:93–6.

31. Chlebowski RT, Hendrix SL, Langer RD, Stefanick ML, Gass M, Lane D, *et al*. Influence of estrogen plus progestin on breast cancer and mammography in healthy postmenopausal women: the Women's Health Initiative Randomized Trial. *JAMA* 2003;289:3243–53.

32. Collaborative Group on Hormonal Factors for Breast Cancer. Breast cancer and hormone replacement therapy: collaborative reanalysis from 51 individual epidemiological studies of 52,705 women with breast cancer and 108,411 women without breast cancer. *Lancet* 1997;350:1047–59.

33. Endogenous Hormones and Breast Cancer Collaborative Group. Endogenous sex hormones and breast cancer in postmenopausal women: reanalysis of nine prospective studies. *J Natl Cancer Inst* 2002;94:606–16.

34. Cummings SR, Duong T, Kenyon E, Cauley JA, Whitehead M, Krueger KA, *et al*. Serum estradiol level and risk of breast cancer during treatment with raloxifene. *JAMA* 2002;287:216–20.

35. Badwe RA, Gregory WM, Chaudary MA, Richards MA, Bentley AE, Rubens RD, *et al*. Timing of surgery during the menstrual cycle and survival of premenopausal women with operable breast cancer. *Lancet* 1991;337:1261–4.

36. Mohr ME, Wang DY, Gregory WM, Richards MA, Fentiman IS. Serum progesterone and prognosis in operable breast cancer. *Br J Cancer* 1996;73:1552–5.

37. Colditz GA, Rosner B, for the Nurses' Health Study Research Group. Use of estrogen plus progestin is associated with greater increase in breast cancer risk than estrogen alone. *Am J Epidemiol* 1998;147 Suppl:64S.

38. Persson E, Weiderpass R, Bergkvist L, Bergstrom R, Schairer C. Risks of breast and endometrial cancer after estrogen and estrogen-progestin replacement therapy. *Cancer Causes Control* 1999;10:253–60.

39. Magnusson C, Baron JA, Correia N, Bergström R, Adami HO, Persson I. Breast-cancer risk following long-term oestrogen and oestrogen-progestin replacement therapy. *Int J Cancer* 1999;81:339–44.

40. Schairer C, Lubin J, Troisi R, Sturgeon S, Brinton L, Hoover R. Menopausal estrogen and estrogen–progestin replacement therapy and breast cancer risk. *JAMA* 2000;283:485–91.

41. Ross RK, Paganini-Hill A, Wan PC, Pike MC. Effect of hormone replacement therapy and breast cancer risk: estrogen versus estrogen plus progestin. *J Natl Cancer Inst* 2000;92:328–32.

42. Moorman PG, Kuwabara H, Millikan RC, Newman B. Menopausal hormones and breast cancer in a biracial population. *Am J Public Health* 2000;90:966–71.

43. Newcomb PA, Titus-Ernstoff L, Egan KM, Trentham-Dietz A, Baron JA, Storer BE, et al. Postmenopausal estrogen and progestin use in relation to breast cancer risk. *Cancer Epidemiol Biomarkers Prev* 2002;11:593–600.

44. Million Women Study Collaborators. Breast cancer and hormone-replacement therapy in the Million Women Study. *Lancet* 2003;362:419–27.

45. Beral V, Million Women Study Collaborators. Patterns of use of hormone replacement therapy in one million women in Britain, 1996–2000. *BJOG* 2002;109:1319–30.

46. Viscoli CM, Brass LM, Kernan WN, Sarrel PM, Suissa S, Horwitz RI. A clinical trial of estrogen-replacement therapy after ischemic stroke. *N Engl J Med* 2001;345:1243–9.

47. Cherry N, Gilmour K, Hannaford P, Heagerty A, Khan MA, Kitchener H, et al. Oestrogen therapy for prevention of reinfarction in postmenopausal women: a randomised placebo controlled trial. *Lancet* 2002;360:2001–8.

48. Women's Health Initiative [www.whi.org].

49. Nachtigall MJ, Smilen SW, Nachtigall RD, Nachtigall RH, Nachtigall LE. Incidence of breast cancer in a 22-year study of women receiving estrogen-progestin replacement therapy. *Obstet Gynecol* 1992;80:827–30.

50. Hulley S, Grady D, Bush T, Furberg C, Herrington D, Riggs B, et al. Randomized trial of estrogen plus progestin for secondary prevention of coronary heart disease in postmenopausal women. Heart and Estrogen/progestin Replacement Study (HERS) Research Group. *JAMA* 1998;280:605–13.

51. Vickers M. The MRC long-term randomised controlled trial of hormone replacement therapy: background, design and objectives. *J Br Menopause Soc* 1996;2:9–13.

52. MRC Media Release. MRC stops study of long-term use of HRT (reference MRC/51/02) [www.mrc.ac.uk].

53. Høibraaten E, Qvigstad E, Arnesen H, Larsen S, Wickstrom E, Sandset PM. Increased risk of recurrent venous thromboembolism during hormone replacement therapy – results of the randomized, double-blind, placebo-controlled estrogen in venous thromboembolism trial (EVTET). *Thromb Haemost* 2000; 84:961–7.

54. Nanda K, Bastian LA, Schulz K. Hormone replacement therapy and the risk of death from breast cancer: a systematic review. *Am J Obstet Gynecol* 2002;186:325–34.

55. Buzdar AU, Come SE, Brodie A, Ellis M, Goss PE, Ingle JN, et al. Proceedings of the First International Conference on Recent Advances and Future Directions in Endocrine Therapy for Breast Cancer: summary consensus statement. *Clin Cancer Res* 2002;7(12 Suppl):4335s–7s.

56. Li CI, Weiss NS, Stanford JL, Daling JR. Hormone replacement therapy in relation to risk of lobular and ductal breast carcinoma in middle-aged women. *Cancer* 2000;88:2570–7.

57. Chen CL, Weiss NS, Newcomb P, Barlow W, White E. Hormone replacement therapy in relation to breast cancer. *JAMA* 2002;287:734–41.

58. Ursin G, Tseng CC, Paganini-Hill A, Enger S, Wan PC, Formenti S, et al. Does menopausal hormone replacement therapy interact with known factors to increase risk of breast cancer? *J Clin Oncol* 2002;20:699–706.

59. Kollias J, Murphy CA, Elston CW, Ellis IO, Robertson JF, Blamey RW. The prognosis of small primary breast cancers. *Eur J Cancer* 1999;35:908–12.

60. Lakhani SR, van de Vijer MJ, Jacquemier J, Anderson TJ, Osin PP, McGuffog L, et al. The pathology of familial breast cancer: predictive value of immunohistochemical markers, estrogen receptor, progesterone receptor, HER-2 and p53 in patients with mutations in BRCA1 and BRCA2. J Clin Oncol 2002;20:2310–18.

61. Sellers TA, Mink PJ, Cerhan JR, Zheng W, Anderson KE, Kushi LH, et al. The role of hormone replacement therapy in the risk for breast cancer and total mortality in women with a family history of breast cancer. Ann Intern Med 1997;127:973–80.

62. Olsson H, Bladstrom A, Ingvar C, Moller TR. A population-based cohort study of HRT use and breast cancer in southern Sweden. Br J Cancer 2001;85:674–7.

63. Narod SA, Brunet JS, Ghardirian P, Robson M, Heimdal K, Neuhausen SL, et al. Tamoxifen and risk of contralateral breast cancer in BRCA1 and BRCA2 mutation carriers: a case–control study. Hereditary Breast Cancer Clinical Study Group. Lancet 2000;356:1876–81.

64. King MC, Wieand S, Hale K, Lee M, Walsh T, Owens K, et al. Tamoxifen and breast cancer incidence among women with inherited mutations in BRCA1 and BRCA2: National Surgical Adjuvant Breast and Bowel Project (NSABP-P1) Breast Cancer Prevention Trial. JAMA 2001;286:2251–6.

65. Rebbeck TR, Levin AM, Eisen A, Snyder C, Watson P, Cannon-Albright L, et al. Breast cancer risk after bilateral prophylactic oophorectomy in BRCA1 mutation carriers. J Natl Cancer Inst 1999;91:1475–9.

66. Carpenter JS, Andrykowski MA, Cordova M, Cunningham L, Studts J, McGrath P, et al. Hot flashes in postmenopausal women treated for breast carcinoma: prevalence, severity, correlates, management, and relation to quality of life. Cancer 1998;82:1682–91.

67. Liu J, Burdette JE, Xu H, Gu C, van Breemen RB, Bhat KP, et al. Evaluation of estrogenic activity of plant extracts for the potential treatment of menopausal symptoms. J Agric Food Chem 2001;49:2472–9.

68. Amato P, Christophe S, Mellon PL. Estrogenic activity of herbs commonly used as remedies for menopausal symptoms. Menopause 2002;9:145–50.

69. Col NF, Hirota LK, Orr RK, Erban JK, Wong JB, Lau J. Hormone replacement therapy after breast cancer: a systematic review and quantitative assessment of risk. J Clin Oncol 2001;19:2357–63.

70. Dew JE, Wren BG, Eden JA. Tamoxifen, hormone receptors and hormone replacement therapy in women previously treated for breast cancer: a cohort study. Climacteric 2002;5:151–5.

71. Veronesi U, Maisonneuve P, Sacchini V, Rotmensz N, Boyle P, Italian Tamoxifen Study Group. Tamoxifen for breast cancer among hysterectomised women. Lancet 2002;359:1122–4.

72. Reddy M, Miller P, Furicchia N, Frazier R, Song T, Decker DA, Consequences of estrogen replacement therapy (ERT) on breast density in breast cancer survivors treated with ERT and breast conservation. 2001;abstract 202 [http://www.sabcs.org/abstractOnline.html].

73. O'Meara ES, Rossing MA, Daling JR, Elmore JG, Barlow WE, Weiss NS. Hormone replacement therapy after a diagnosis of breast cancer in relation to recurrence and mortality. J Natl Cancer Inst 2001;93:754–62.

74. Marsden J, Whitehead MI, A'Hern R, Baum M, Sacks N. Are randomised trials of hormone replacement therapy in symptomatic breast cancer patients feasible? Fertil Steril 2000;73:292–9.

27

Bacterial vaginosis, late miscarriage and preterm birth

M Ruth Mason and Ronald F Lamont

INTRODUCTION

With technological advances and the improvement in operator skills in obstetric ultrasound, preterm birth (delivery before 37 completed weeks of gestation) caused by spontaneous preterm labour (SPTL, as opposed to induced preterm birth) has replaced congenital malformations as the major cause of perinatal and neonatal death and handicap in the developed world. Worldwide, approximately 13 million preterm births occur annually, ranging from an incidence of 5.6% in Oceania to 11% in the USA.[1] Despite the use of tocolytics to delay or prevent preterm birth,[2] the use of antepartum glucocorticoids to reduce the incidence and severity of idiopathic respiratory distress syndrome,[3] and the improvements in neonatal intensive care unit (NICU) facilities, the mortality and morbidity from preterm birth has remained relatively constant over the last 20 years. Following delivery at 24 weeks of gestation, 80% of babies die and it is not until 30 weeks of gestation that neonatal mortality drops to 10%. Although most preterm births occur after 35 weeks of gestation, virtually all of the associated mortality and morbidity occurs in the babies born before that time.[4] The EPICure study[5] examined the outcome of more than 1100 babies born at between 22 and 26 weeks of gestation in the UK and Ireland over a nine-month period in 1995. Approximately 65% of these babies died in the delivery suite or in the NICU. Of those who could be followed up to 30 months of age, approximately half were found to be suffering from some form of disability and in half of these the disability was severe. Only 13% of all the preterm infants delivered before 26 weeks were alive and intact at follow-up to 30 months of age.

COST OF PRETERM BIRTH

In the USA, the provision of neonatal intensive care is estimated to be US$10,000 per baby per week. If a baby is disabled and requires life-long residential care, it is estimated that this will cost US$450,000. The total cost of neonatal intensive care in the USA annually is thought to be US$5 billion.[6] Bearing in mind the population of the USA is approximately five times that of the UK, that the incidence of preterm birth is approximately double that of the UK and that a higher proportion of gross domestic product is invested in health in the USA than in the UK, it is likely that the cost of provision of NICU unit facilities in the UK annually is approximately £340 million. Using information available from the National Perinatal Epidemiology Unit in Oxford, an attempt can be made to identify as objectively as possible the economic and other consequences of preterm birth. The respective costs of neonatal intensive care and long-term health care during the first eight years of life are quadruple and double for babies with a birthweight less than 1000 g compared with those of birthweight more than 1500 g.[7] The cost to the health service for childhood hospital admissions is 20 times higher in infants born before 28 weeks of gestation compared with those born after 37 weeks.[7] Other economic implications are more difficult to cost and these include additional educational assistance owing to a higher rate of school failure and increased risk of school year repetition for babies born preterm. It is also difficult to quantify the reduction in family income or the intangible cost associated with the emotional and physical effects on the parents, the isolation of the mother, the restriction of social contact, and the increased risk of marital break-up.

NORMAL AND ABNORMAL GENITAL TRACT FLORA

Normally the vagina is dominated by *Lactobacillus* spp., which, by producing lactic acid renders the vagina acid (pH < 4.5), at which low pH the growth of other organisms is suppressed. With increasing gestational age, the total number of organisms in the vagina, both aerobes and anaerobes, increases, although aerobic organisms dominate. As a result, by term, the vagina is colonised by organisms of low virulence that pose no significant threat to the baby at the time of birth. At low vaginal pH, lactobacilli readily produce hydrogen peroxide, which is toxic to bacteria. When the pH of the vagina increases as a result of bleeding, sexual intercourse or vaginal douching, lactobacilli are less able to produce hydrogen peroxide. As a result, the normal lactobacillus-dominated flora is replaced by a 1000-fold overgrowth of anaerobic organisms and other organisms such as *Gardnerella vaginalis*, *Mycoplasma hominis* and *Mobiluncus* spp. By producing keto acids such as succinate, the chemotactic response of polymorphonuclear leucocytes and their killing ability is reduced. As a result, there is a synergistic increase in the number of potentially pathogenic organisms despite no cellular inflammatory response. There is no inflammation present, so there is no vaginitis and the condition is known as bacterial vaginosis.

PREVALENCE OF BACTERIAL VAGINOSIS

The reported prevalence of bacterial vaginosis varies widely from 5% to 51% depending on the population.[8] In a general gynaecology clinic in Harrow, Middlesex, UK, the incidence was 11%[9] and in an antenatal clinic in the same hospital the incidence was 15%.[10] In women attending for routine smear tests in general practice, the incidence of bacterial vaginosis was 9%.[11] A higher incidence of 28% was found in women undergoing termination of pregnancy[12] or *in vitro* fertilisation (24.6%).[13] In the USA, a high incidence of bacterial vaginosis was reported in an inner-city population of pregnant women (32.5%),[14] but the highest incidence has been reported in rural Uganda where over 50% of women had bacterial vaginosis, 80% of whom were asymptomatic.[15] Bacterial vaginosis has emerged as a co-factor for sexually transmitted infections and, more importantly, the acquisition of HIV in women. If ways of reducing the prevalence of bacterial vaginosis can be found, this may be a means of reducing the incidence of sexually transmitted HIV infection.[15]

DIAGNOSIS OF BACTERIAL VAGINOSIS

Bacterial vaginosis may be diagnosed clinically by the finding of a white homogeneous adherent vaginal discharge, which may have an offensive fishy smell due to increased levels of polyamines and trimethylamines. Diagnosis may, however, be more difficult because up to 50% of women with bacterial vaginosis may be asymptomatic. In others, bacterial vaginosis remits and relapses spontaneously. Current antibiotic treatments restore the normal lactobacillus-dominated flora in the short term, but approximately 30% of these women relapse within one month.[16] Historically, the diagnosis of bacterial vaginosis has been made from composite clinical criteria using the Amsell classification.[17] Three out of four clinical criteria must be present: a homogeneous white or grey adherent vaginal discharge; vaginal pH > 4.5; clue cells on wet preparations; and a characteristic amine or fishy smell on addition of a 10% solution of the alkali potassium hydroxide.

This technique is clumsy, has low reproducibility and is unpleasant. It has now been superseded by Gram stain examination of vaginal secretions. Gram stain diagnosis of bacterial vaginosis is both specific and sensitive and can be achieved by using a low vaginal swab.[18] This can be self-administered and obtained by the woman herself.

Using Gram staining of an air dried smear of vaginal secretions, vaginal flora can be classified as grade I: normal (predominantly lactobacillus morphotypes); grade II: intermediate (reduced lactobacillus morphotypes mixed with other bacterial morphotypes); or grade III: bacterial vaginosis (a few or no lactobacillus morphotypes with greatly increased numbers of *G. vaginalis* and other morphotypes). Gram staining can also be quantified according to Nugent's criteria, a reliable and reproducible method of diagnosis.[19] By examining the detailed microbiology of different Gram stain grades of genital flora during pregnancy a different distribution of bacterial species can be observed. Some organisms, such as *Lactobacillus* spp. decrease linearly from 91% in grade I to 66% in grade II and 38% in grade III. Others such as alpha-haemolytic streptococcus or *Corynebacterium* spp. show a linear increase in colonisation from grades I to III (9% to 36% to 56% and 36% to 56% to 84% respectively). Some organisms such as coagulase negative *Staphylococcus* spp. were isolated from a similar number of women with grade I (58%), grade II (78%) and grade III (74%) smears. Other organisms, such as *G. vaginalis*, *Mycoplasma hominis* and many anaerobes, were rarely isolated in grade I and grade II and were fully manifest only with high isolation rates in grade III Gram stain specimens. In this way, it is possible using a cheap and simple test such as Gram staining of vaginal secretions to predict the likelihood of the presence of particular organisms in pregnancy.[20] *G. vaginalis* is present in the vagina of 50–60% of healthy women without bacterial vaginosis and this isolation from cultures of vaginal swabs is not diagnostic of bacterial vaginosis. A more comprehensive review of the incidence, epidemiology, aetiology, and natural history, diagnosis, obstetric and gynaecological complications of bacterial vaginosis was reviewed in 2002.[21]

EVIDENCE IMPLICATING INFECTION AS A CAUSE OF, AND BIOCHEMICAL MECHANISMS OF, SPTL AND PRETERM BIRTH

Infection as a cause

The aetiology of preterm birth is multifactorial but there is strong evidence to implicate infection as a possible cause and this has been reviewed elsewhere.[22] Whereas 25 years ago 40% of preterm births were thought to be idiopathic, we now know that, with careful examination of the mother, the fetus and the placenta, at least one cause of preterm birth will be identified in 96% of cases and two or more causes in 56%. In up to 40% of these mothers, infection can be identified as an aetiological factor.[23]

Biochemical mechanisms of spontaneous preterm labour and preterm birth

Labour is a dual process involving a decrease in cervical resistance leading to progressive effacement and dilatation of the cervix accompanied by an increase in uterine contractility, resulting in longer, stronger more frequent and more synchronous uterine contractions. Prostaglandins are intimately involved in both of these processes and are synthesised from their obligate precursor, arachidonic acid. Arachidonic acid is released by the action of phospholipase enzymes on glycerophospholipids in the cell membrane and some organisms are known to produce phospholipase A_2.[24] Bacteria also produce other enzymes such as proteases, mucinases, collagenases and elastases, which permit them to resist local secretory immunoglobulin A, penetrate the cervical mucous plug, and disrupt the extraplacental membranes. By producing endotoxins, microorganisms also induce macrophages to produce pro-inflammatory cytokines such as interleukin (IL)-1, IL-6, IL-8, which are found in significantly increased concentrations in the amniotic fluid of women with infection who are in SPTL compared with those without infection.[25] Babies born before term as a result of SPTL with an infectious aetiology in whom there can be found funisitis (inflammation of the umbilical cord), or increased concentrations of white cells or pro-inflammatory cytokines, are statistically significantly more likely to develop periventricular leucomalacia,[26] bronchopulmonary dysplasia[27] or cerebral palsy by the age of three years.[28]

BACTERIAL VAGINOSIS AND THE PREDICTION OF LATE MISCARRIAGE, SPTL AND PRETERM BIRTH

First-trimester miscarriage has a different aetiology from second-trimester miscarriage, and early preterm birth can be considered on a continuum with late second-trimester miscarriage.

Although there is undeniable evidence to associate bacterial vaginosis and other forms of abnormal genital tract flora with SPTL and preterm birth, by the time a woman is admitted in SPTL there may be irreversible changes in the uterine cervix that render attempts to inhibit the process unsuccessful, so there is logic in using abnormal genital tract flora diagnosed by Gram stain of vaginal secretions as a means of predicting SPTL and preterm birth.

Eight cohort studies from Europe, the USA and the Far East[10,29–35] and three case–control studies from the USA, Sweden and Australia[36–38] used different methods but nevertheless found an association with bacterial vaginosis or bacterial vaginosis-related organisms and an adverse outcome of pregnancy.

In a UK study, bacterial vaginosis detected before 16 weeks of gestation was associated with a five-fold increased risk of mid-trimester pregnancy loss[10] and its association was confirmed by a study in Denver USA that reported a more than three-fold increased association between bacterial vaginosis and second trimester loss.[14] Another study reported an association between previous second trimester miscarriage and bacterial vaginosis, but not between recurrent first trimester loss and bacterial vaginosis.[39] In a prospective cohort study of 1216 pregnant women reported in 2002, bacterial vaginosis was not strongly predictive of early miscarriage but was predictive of miscarriage between 13 and 15 weeks of gestation.[40] Many of these studies from different countries, which have confirmed the association between bacterial vaginosis and SPTL and preterm birth, have used different diagnostic techniques at varying gestational ages of screening. Most of the studies have shown a statistically significant association between abnormal genital tract flora and adverse pregnancy outcome. More importantly, the degree of risk of SPTL and preterm birth was found to be greater the earlier in pregnancy at which the abnormal genital tract flora was detected. Detection at around 26 weeks of gestation was associated with a 1.4–1.9-fold increased risk of preterm birth.[29,30,33,41] In contrast, abnormal genital tract colonisation detected in the second trimester was associated with a 2–6.9-fold increased risk of adverse outcome.[10,31,34,35] In a longitudinal study of women in Indonesia,[34] the risk was almost double in those diagnosed with bacterial vaginosis in early pregnancy (21%) compared with women who developed the condition later in pregnancy (11%). Using a multiple regression analysis, bacterial vaginosis diagnosed before

16 weeks of gestation was found to be associated with a five-fold increased risk of preterm birth or late miscarriage, independently of recognised risk factors such as previous preterm birth, black race or smoking.[10] As a result, antibiotics given prophylactically to reduce the incidence of preterm birth in women with bacterial vaginosis should be used early in pregnancy.

Bacterial vaginosis is also associated with an increased risk of preterm, prelabour rupture of the membranes, chorioamnionitis, amniotic fluid colonisation, low-birthweight infants and postpartum endometritis.[42,43]

PROPHYLACTIC ANTIBIOTICS FOR WOMEN WITH ABNORMAL GENITAL TRACT FLORA IN EARLY PREGNANCY

A number of studies have examined the use of antibiotics for the prevention of preterm birth in women identified as being at risk of preterm birth as a result of abnormal genital tract flora in early pregnancy. Unfortunately, the studies used different doses of different antibiotics administered by different routes and regimens in women with varying risk and, not surprisingly, showed different outcomes. With respect to the route of administration, there is logic in using intravaginal antibiotics because the 1000-fold increase in genital tract flora associated with bacterial vaginosis may require a heavy local loading dose of antibiotics to the vagina. If, however, the abnormal genital tract flora has existed from early pregnancy, then locally administered vaginal antibiotics may not eradicate those organisms that have already gained access to the decidua by ascending colonisation. Under these circumstances there would be merit in considering systemic antibiotics. The antibiotics used should be active against bacterial vaginosis or bacterial vaginosis associated organisms. The degree of abnormality of the genital tract flora is also potentially important. In a subgroup analysis of a tricentre, randomised, double blind, placebo controlled trial,[44] women with grade III flora on Gram staining of vaginal smears were found to respond better to clindamycin vaginal cream than those with either grade II flora or grades II and III combined, resulting in a greater reduction in the incidence of SPTL and preterm birth.[45]

The gestational age at the time of treatment is also important. Treatment administered at 24 weeks of gestation has not been shown to be of any benefit.[46] In the largest study ever conducted using antibiotics in pregnancy to prevent preterm birth in women with bacterial vaginosis, no benefit was found when using a 2 g stat dose of metronidazole given orally.[47] However, the study was criticised for a number of reasons.[48] Only a small proportion of eligible women were entered into the study, and women with symptomatic bacterial vaginosis were excluded. Some eight weeks could evolve between the diagnosis of bacterial vaginosis and the administration of antibiotics, by which time the grade of Gram stain had changed in 25% of the women. Although the study was purported to be on low-risk unselected women, nearly 85% were either black or Hispanic. Finally, 50% of the women were treated after 20 weeks of gestation and none before 16 weeks of gestation, emphasising the fact that late treatment is unlikely to be of benefit. Three studies of the use of clindamycin vaginal cream have been published.[35,44,49] In one,[35] 100% of the women were treated after 20 weeks of gestation and in another[49] 60% were treated after 20 weeks. In contrast, in a randomised, double blind, placebo controlled trial of clindamycin vaginal cream, 100% of the women were treated before 20 weeks of gestation and 60% before 16 weeks, resulting in a 60% reduction in the incidence of preterm birth from 10% in the placebo group to 4% in the treated group.[44] In the same study, women who initially had abnormal genital tract flora but who reverted to normal flora, and who were therefore not recruited to the study, were followed up and found to have an adverse outcome that was comparable with women with abnormal flora who had been given placebo.[45] The rate of adverse outcome was similar in women with untreated abnormal genital tract flora and those with abnormal flora who reverted to normal; thus it is likely that the inflammatory process resulting from ascending colonisation of the upper genital tract occurred early, before the genital tract flora reverted to normal. This further emphasises the importance of the early administration of antibiotics.

CONCLUSION

Infection is an important cause of SPTL and preterm birth. Abnormal genital tract flora in early pregnancy is a useful predictor of subsequent pregnancy loss either in the form of late miscarriage or preterm birth. The earlier in pregnancy at which this abnormal colonisation is detected, the greater is the risk of a subsequent adverse outcome. It has been reported that, of women in whom bacterial vaginosis was detected at the start of pregnancy (16–20 weeks at the time of screening) and who progressed beyond 32 weeks of gestation, 50% still had bacterial vaginosis. Among those in whom bacterial vaginosis was not present at 16 weeks of gestation, only 2% subsequently developed this condition.[50] Although antibiotics have the potential to prevent SPTL, late miscarriage and preterm birth, if they are to be successful it is likely that they will have to be administered early in pregnancy. The antibiotics should be active against the organisms associated with bacterial vaginosis and are most likely to be successful if used in women with the greatest degree of abnormal genital tract flora. We do not as yet have a means of identifying women with a genetic predisposition to produce pro-inflammatory cytokines in response to abnormal genital tract flora. Until we do, antibiotics have to be administered early before abnormal colonisation proceeds to infection and then to inflammation with the production of pro-inflammatory cytokines, which cause tissue damage leading to periventricular leucomalacia, bronchopulmonary dysplasia and cerebral palsy.

References

1. Villar J, Ezcurra E, Gurtner de la Fuente V, Campodonico L. Pre-term delivery syndrome: the unmet need. In: Kierse MJNC, editor. New perspectives for the effective treatment of pre-term labour – an international consensus. *Res Clin Forums* 1994;16:9–38.
2. Greenfield PJ, Lamont RF. The contemporary use of tocolytics. *Curr Obstet Gynaecol* 2000;10:218–24.
3. Crowley P, Chalmers I, Kierse MJ. The effects of corticosteroid administration before preterm delivery: an overview of the evidence from controlled trials. *Br J Obstet Gynaecol* 1990;97:11–25.
4. Magowan BA, Bain M, Juszczak E, McInneny K. Neonatal mortality amongst Scottish preterm singleton births (1985–1994). *Br J Obstet Gynaecol* 1998;105:1005–10.
5. Wood NS, Marlow N, Costeloe K, Gibson AT, Wilkinson AR. Neurologic and developmental disability after extremely preterm birth. EPICure Study Group. *N Engl J Med* 2000;343:378–84.
6. Kierse MJ. New perspectives for the effective treatment of preterm labor. *Am J Obstet Gynecol* 1995;173:618–28.
7. Petrou S. Economic consequences of preterm birth and low birthweight. *BJOG* 2003;110 Suppl 20:17–23.
8. Hay PE. Bacterial vaginosis and pregnancy. In: MacLean A, Regan L, Carrington D, editors. *Infection and Pregnancy*. London: RCOG Press; 2001. p. 158–71.

9.   Hay PE, Taylor-Robinson D, Lamont RF. Diagnosis of bacterial vaginosis in a gynaecology clinic. *Br J Obstet Gynaecol* 1992;99:63–6.

10.   Hay PE, Lamont RF, Taylor-Robinson D, Morgan DJ, Ison C, Pearson J. Abnormal bacterial colonisation of the genital tract as a marker for subsequent preterm delivery and late miscarriage. *BMJ* 1994;308:295–8.

11.   Lamont RF, Morgan DJ, Wilson SD, Taylor-Robinson D. Prevalence of bacterial vaginosis in women attending one of three general practices for routine cervical cytology. *Int J STD AIDS* 2000;11:495–8.

12.   Blackwell AL, Emery SJ, Thomas PD, Wareham K. Universal prophylaxis for *Chlamydia trachomatis* and anaerobic vaginosis in women attending for suction termination of pregnancy: an audit of short-term health gains. *Int J STD AIDS* 1999;10:508–13.

13.   Ralph SG, Rutherford AJ, Wilson JD. Influence of bacterial vaginosis on conception and miscarriage in the first trimester: cohort study. *BMJ* 1999;319:220–3.

14.   McGregor JA, French JL, Parker R, Draper D, Paterson E, Jones W, *et al.* Prevention of premature birth by screening and treatment of common genital tract infections: results of a prospective controlled evaluation. *Am J Obstet Gynecol* 1995;173:157–67.

15.   Mayaud P. Tackling bacterial vaginosis and HIV in developing countries. *Lancet* 1997;350:530–1.

16.   Larsson PG. Treatment of bacterial vaginosis. *Int J STD AIDS* 1992;3:239–47.

17.   Amsel R, Totten PA, Spiegal CA, Chen KC, Eschenback D, Holmes KK. Nonspecific vaginitis. Diagnostic criteria and microbial and epidemiologic associations. *Am J Med* 1983;74:14–22.

18.   Morgan DJ, Aboud CJ, McCaffrey IM, Bhide SA, Lamont RF, Taylor-Robinson D. Comparison of Gram-stained smears prepared from blind vaginal swabs with those obtained at speculum examination for the assessment of vaginal flora. *Br J Obstet Gynaecol* 1996;103:1105–8.

19.   Nugent RP, Krohn MA, Hillier SL. Reliability of diagnosing bacterial vaginosis is improved by a standardized method of gram stain interpretation. *J Clin Microbiol* 1991;29;297–301.

20.   Rosenstein IJ, Morgan DJ, Sheeham M, Lamont RF, Taylor-Robinson D. Bacterial vaginosis in pregnancy: distribution of bacterial species in different gram-stain categories of the vaginal flora. *J Med Microbiol* 1996;45:120–6.

21.   Boyle D, Adinkra P, Lamont RF. Bacterial vaginosis. *Prog Obstet Gynaecol* 2002;14:185–210.

22.   Lamont RF. Infection in preterm labour. In: MacLean A, Regan L, Carrington D, editors. *Infection and Pregnancy*. London: RCOG Press; 2001. p. 305–17.

23.   Lettieri L, Vintzileos AM, Rodis JF, Albini SM, Salafia CM. Does 'idiopathic' preterm labour resulting in preterm birth exist? *Am J Obstet Gynecol* 1993;168:1480–5.

24.   Bejar R, Carbelo V, Davis C, Gluck L. Premature labour II. Bacterial sources of phospholipase. *Obstet Gynecol* 1981;57:479–81.

25.   Romero R, Gomez R, Mazor M, Ghezzi F, Yoon BH. The preterm labor syndrome. In: Elder MG, Lamont RF, Romero R, editors. *Preterm Labour*. New York: Churchill Livingstone; 1997. p. 29–49

26.   Yoon BH, Romero R, Yang SH, Jun JK, Kim IO, Choi JH, *et al.* Interleukin-6 concentrations in umbilical cord plasma are elevated in neonates with white matter lesions associated with periventricular leukomalacia. *Am J Obstet Gynecol* 1996;174;1433–40.

27.   Yoon BH, Jun JK, Romero R, Park KH, Gomez R, Choi JH, *et al.* Amniotic fluid inflammatory cytokines (interleukin-6, interleukin-1 beta, and tumor necrosis factor-alpha), neonatal brain white matter lesions, and cerebral palsy. *Am J Obstet Gynecol* 1997;177:19–26.

28. Yoon BH, Romero R, Park JS, Kim CJ, Kim SH, Choi JH, *et al*. Fetal exposure to an intra-amniotic inflammation and the development of cerebral palsy at the age of three years. *Am J Obstet Gynecol* 2000;182:675–81.

29. Hillier SL, Nugent RP, Eschenbach DA, Krohn MA, Gibbs RS, Martin DH, *et al*. Association between bacterial vaginosis and preterm delivery of a low-birth-weight infant. The Vaginal Infections and Prematurity Study Group. *N Engl J Med* 1995;333:1737–42.

30. Meis PJ, Goldenberg RL, Mercer B, Moawad A, Das A, McNellis D, *et al*. The Preterm Prediction Study: significance of vaginal infections. National Institute of Child Health and Human Development Maternal-Fetal Medicine Units Network. *Am J Obstet Gynecol* 1995;173:1231–5.

31. Kurki T, Sivonen A, Renkonen OV, Savia E, Ylikorkala O. Bacterial vaginosis in early pregnancy and pregnancy outcome. *Obstet Gynecol* 1992;80:173–7.

32. Gratacos E, Figueras F, Barranco M, Vila J, Cararach V, Alonson PL, *et al*. Spontaneous recovery of bacterial vaginosis during pregnancy is not associated with an improved perinatal outcome. *Acta Obstet Gynecol Scand* 1998;77:37–40.

33. Gravett MG, Nelson HP, DeRouen T, Critchlew C, Eschenbach DA, Holmes KK. Independent association of bacterial vaginosis and *Chlamydia trachomatis* infection with adverse pregnancy outcome. *JAMA* 1986;256:1899–903.

34. Riduan JM, Hillier SL, Utomo B, Wiknjosastro G, Linnan M, Kandan N. Bacterial vaginosis and prematurity in Indonesia: association in early and late pregnancy. *Am J Obstet Gynecol* 1993;169:175–8.

35. McGregor JA, French JI, Jones W, Milligan K, McKinney PJ, Patterson E, *et al*. Bacterial vaginosis is associated with prematurity and vaginal fluid mucinase and sialidase: results of a controlled trial of topical clindamycin cream. *Am J Obstet Gynecol* 1994;170:1048–60.

36. Wennerholm UB, Holm B, Mattsby-Baltzer I, Nielsen T, Platz-Christensen J, Sundell G, *et al*. Fetal fibronectin, endotoxin, bacterial vaginosis and cervical length as predictors of preterm birth and neonatal morbidity in twin pregnancies. *Br J Obstet Gynaecol* 1997;104:1398–404.

37. Holst E, Goffeng AR, Andersch B. Bacterial vaginosis and vaginal microorganisms in idiopathic premature labor and association with pregnancy outcome. *J Clin Microbiol* 1994;32:176–86.

38. Eschenbach DA, Gravett MG, Chen KC, Hoyme UB, Holmes KK. Bacterial vaginosis during pregnancy. An association with prematurity and postpartum complications. *Scand J Urol Nephrol Suppl* 1984;86:213–22.

39. McDonald HM, O'Loughlin JA, Jolley P, Vigneswaran R, McDonald PJ. Prenatal microbiological risk factors associated with preterm birth. *Br J Obstet Gynaecol* 1992;99:190–6.

40. Llahi-Camp JM, Rai R, Ion C, Regan L, Taylor-Robinson D. Association of bacterial vaginosis with a history of second trimester miscarriage. *Hum Reprod* 1996;11:1575–8.

41. Oakeshott, P, Hay P, Hay S, Steinke F, Rink E, Kerry S. Association between bacterial vaginosis or chlamydial infection and miscarriage before 16 weeks' gestation: prospective community based cohort study. *BMJ* 2002;325:1334–6.

42. Silver HM, Sperling RS, St Calir PJ, Gibbs RS. Evidence relating bacterial vaginosis to intraamniotic infection. *Am J Obstet Gynecol* 1989;161:808–12.

43. Martius J, Eschenbach DA. The role of bacterial vaginosis as a cause of amniotic fluid infection, chorioamnionitis and prematurity – a review. *Arch Gynecol Obstet* 1990;247;1–13.

44. Lamont RF, Duncan SL, Mandal D, Bassett P. Intravaginal clindamycin to reduce preterm birth in women with abnormal genital tract flora. *Obstet Gynecol* 2003;101:516–22.

45. Rosenstein IJ, Morgan DJ, Lamont RF, Sheehan M, Dore CJ, Hay P, *et al*. Effect of intravaginal clindamycin cream on pregnancy outcome and on abnormal vaginal microbial flora of pregnant women. *Infect Dis Obstet Gynecol* 2000;8:158–65.

46. McDonald HM, O'Loughlin JA, Vigneswaran R, Jolley PT, Harvey JA, McDonald PJ. Impact of metronidazole therapy on preterm birth in women with bacterial vaginosis flora (*Gardnerella vaginalis*): a randomised, placebo controlled trial. *Br J Obstet Gynaecol* 1997;104:1391–7.

47. Carey JC, Klebanoff MA, Hauth JC, Hillier SL, Thom TA, Ernest JM, *et al*. Metronidazole to prevent preterm delivery in pregnant women with asymptomatic bacterial vaginosis. National Institute of Child Health and Human Development Network of Maternal-Fetal Medicine. *N Engl J Med* 2000;342:534–40.

48. Lamont RF. Antibiotics for the prevention of preterm birth. *N Engl J Med* 2000;342:581–3.

49. Joesoef MR, Hillier SL, Wiknjosastro G, Sumampouw H, Linnan M, Norojono W, *et al*. Intravaginal clindamycin treatment for bacterial vaginosis: effects on preterm delivery and low birth weight. *Am J Obstet Gynecol* 1995;173:1527–31.

50. Hay PE, Morgan DJ, Ison CA, Bhide SA, Romney M, McKenzie P, *et al*. A longitudinal study of bacterial vaginosis during pregnancy. *Br J Obstet Gynaecol* 1994;101:1048–53.

28

The re-emergence of the vaginal approach to hysterectomy

Karl S Oláh

Based on the RCOG/Wyeth Historical Lecture given at the Royal College of Obstetricians and Gynaecologists,
29 November 2002.

INTRODUCTION

The surgical technique of vaginal hysterectomy in the absence of significant prolapse is considered by many gynaecologists to be the operation that separates the gynaecologist from the surgeon. The vaginal approach to hysterectomy is a gynaecological procedure *par excellence*, and as such has enjoyed popularity of varying degrees through the years. This chapter documents the development of the operation, and the resurgence of interest in the technique.

THE HISTORY OF VAGINAL HYSTERECTOMY

Early history

All of the early operations were done for prolapse or inversion of the uterus. The idea of removing the uterus through the vagina originated with Soranus in AD 120, who was a distinguished obstetrician in Rome and Ephesus during the reign of the Emperor Hadrian.[1] The first authenticated description of removal of the uterus through the vagina was given by Berengarius of Bologna, in 1507.[1] In many of the women operated on before 1800 the diagnosis was uncertain. In most instances the operation was performed for simple or complicated inversion of the uterus, often with the inverted portion being ligated and the ischaemic portion then being allowed to slough.[1,2] Instances of partial or complete removal of the uterus carried out by a midwife were reported by Hildanus (1646),[1] Bernhard (1802)[3] and Wrisberg (1785).[4] In the case reported by Bernhard the inverted uterus was removed by the midwife with a razor. The profuse haemorrhage was controlled by the introduction of fragments of ice into the vagina and the woman recovered.

The authenticated history of intentional complete removal of the uterus dates back to 1813. In 1810, Wrisberg[4] discussed his 1787 paper on the propriety and feasibility of vaginal hysterectomy in a prize essay read before the Vienna Royal Academy of Medicine. On 13 April 1812, Paletta[5] unwittingly undertook a vaginal hysterectomy. The extent of the disease is unknown, but a tumour occupied the lower segment of the uterus. Using obstetric forceps and his hand, the uterus was brought down to the vaginal outlet. The upper part of the vagina was incised with a pair of curved scissors. After separating the lower segment of the uterus a hard body could be felt at the base of the tumour. This hard body proved to be the fundus of the uterus, which remained in connection with the tumour. The woman died at the end of the third day. Paletta did not intend to remove the entire uterus with the tumour, and the extent of the operation became evident only after its completion, upon careful examination of the specimen.

The first deliberate and well planned vaginal hysterectomy for carcinoma was performed in 1813 by CJM Langenbeck, of Göttingen.[6] Wrisberg's paper and Paletta's case report encouraged him to undertake this difficult task. His patient was a multiparous 50-year-old woman. On examination there was some uterine prolapse and the cervix was found to be hard, nodular and ulcerated. The cervical canal was vascular and ulcerated, and from it escaped a bloody and offensive discharge. The irritating vaginal discharge had caused erosions of the external genitalia and the ulceration of the cervical canal extended deeply into the cavity of the uterus. Digital exploration of the cervical canal and uterine cavity revealed an ulcerated surface with induration of the cervix and body of the uterus, and was followed by haemorrhage. As Langenbeck had no precedent to follow, he had to devise his own plan for removal of the uterus. The patient was placed with the pelvis on the edge of the bed with the thighs separated and the feet resting upon two stools. Langenbeck sat between the patient's thighs and dissected the vagina from the cervix, the dissection being continued until the peritoneal envelope of the uterus was reached. Special care was taken not to open the peritoneal cavity. To reach the fundus of the uterus, the broad and round ligaments and the fallopian tubes had to be divided. The last part of the operation consisted of the subperitoneal enucleation of the fundus of the uterus. He had no one to assist him except a surgeon suffering from severe gout, who, when called upon to render much needed aid, could not rise from his chair. Towards the end of the operation the haemorrhage became alarming, when the following conversation occurred: Langenbeck: 'Herr, so humpeln Sie doch jetzt herbei' ['Sir, could you just try and limp over here']. Assistant: 'Ich kann nicht' ['I cannot']. With severe haemorrhage and approaching collapse of the patient, Langenbeck grasped and compressed the bleeding part with his left hand, and with his right hand he passed a needle armed with a ligature through the tissues behind the bleeding point. Having only one hand at his disposal, the ligature was tied by grasping one end between his teeth and the other with his right hand. At this stage the woman appeared to be dying. Dashing cold water over her face revived her. The long wide vagina was now pushed in an upward direction by introducing the whole hand. Above the vagina was a deep pocket, the walls of which were composed of the peritoneal investment of the uterus. The vagina and peritoneal pouch were continuous with each other and no opening into the peritoneal cavity could be detected. Through the peritoneum the intestinal coils could be distinctly felt. To prevent the inversion of this peritoneal bag by pressure against it of the intestines, a sponge was inserted. In spite of the critical condition of the patient at the close of the operation she made an uneventful recovery. Thus the first complete vaginal hysterectomy was performed without an anaesthetic, without assistance, and without the use of haemostatic forceps!

However, few of Langenbecks' peers and colleagues believed his accomplishment. His patient was suffering from dementia and was therefore deemed to be an unreliable witness, and his assistant had died two weeks after the procedure. The woman died on 17 June 1839, 26 years after the operation. The postmortem showed that the upper part of the vagina and the empty peritoneal pouch formed by the enucleation of the uterus were found inverted and formed a swelling in the vagina, which reached as far as the labia majora. Inspection of the peritoneal surface showed the fallopian tubes, their cut ends terminating in the peritoneal pouch. The inverted pouch appeared between rectum and bladder as a globular depression, the surface of which did not show signs of scar tissue anywhere. The description of the operation as given by Langenbeck was corroborated by the results of the postmortem, and the case will always remain in history as the first intentional complete vaginal removal of the uterus.

Between 1822 and 1830, a further 11 vaginal hysterectomies were undertaken by various surgeons, including Langenbeck.[1] Of these, nine died, a mortality of over 80% (75% for the first 12 patients). The experiences of these surgeons led to the development of the operation as we know it today. After the second total vaginal hysterectomy carried out by Sauter[1,7] on 28 January 1822, in a woman without prolapse, complications from haemorrhage and the development of a vesicovaginal fistula led him to make the following suggestions:

- horizontal positioning of the patient

- complete evacuation of the rectum and bladder

- pressure by the hand of an assistant over the abdomen above the pubes in the direction of the pelvis

- incision of the vaginal vault between the uterus and the bladder with a scalpel with a short convex blade

- enlargement of this opening around the whole cervix with the same knife

- section of the broad ligaments close to the uterus with curved scissors, guided by the fingers

- separation of the uterus from the rectum with curved scissors

- finally, bringing down the uterus with the whole hand and separation of remaining attachments.

Langenbeck, after the sixth total vaginal hysterectomy on 5 August 1825, which also resulted in the woman's death, placed great stress on opening the peritoneal cavity through the pouch of Douglas so that the bladder is exposed to less risk of being injured. He also insisted that the large pelvic vessels should be avoided by making the incisions close to the uterus. As an additional safeguard to protect the bladder and urethra, a catheter was held in position in the bladder by an assistant.[8]

The early pioneers of the operation thus established the basic premise of the procedure, which, with some modification, is what is undertaken in modern practice.

The late 19th century and the 20th century

Surgery in the late 19th century was associated with high morbidity and mortality, and was not performed unless absolutely necessary. In 1885 A Reeves Jackson[9] stated: 'Vaginal hysterectomy does not avert or lessen suffering; it destroys, and does not save, life. It is, therefore, not a useful but an injurious operation; and being such, it is unjustifiable, and ought to be abandoned.' In 1863, James Young Simpson[10] wrote in relation to vaginal hysterectomy for cancer of the cervix: 'Cases have been put on record where the operation was performed, but with such disastrous results as to hold no encouragement whatever to its repetition, but rather to serve as loud warnings against it.' It therefore took a number of decades for the techniques of vaginal surgery to be developed. The introduction of anaesthesia, improved surgical technique, and the introduction of aseptic surgery encouraged Freund in 1878[11] and Czerny in 1879[12] to revive, improve and report their methods and results of vaginal hysterectomy, although some credit for the modern operation should be given to Koeberle.[13] With improvements in antisepsis and the development of antibiotics in the next century, vaginal surgery advanced to the point that exponents considered the vaginal approach the best method to perform a hysterectomy. Friedrich Schauta,[14] treating carcinoma of the cervix, gave a boost to vaginal surgery in 1890. Before the turn of the century, brilliant French surgeons were most successful with the use of clamps and developed remarkable morcellation and bisection techniques.[15] The famous French surgeon Doyen[16] insisted in 1939 that "no one could call themselves a gynaecologist until he had performed a vaginal hysterectomy 'in private'". In the UK, ardent promoters of the technique were Green-Armytage,[16] Palmer,[17] Howkins,[18] Stallworthy[19,20] and

Watson.[21] Van Bastiaanse[22] from Amsterdam and Navratil[23] from Austria were eminent vaginal surgeons, while Mitra[24,25] and Purandare[26] were advocates from India. The superiority of hysterectomy by the vaginal route was not denied. The safety and efficacy of vaginal hysterectomy over abdominal hysterectomy was re-emphasised in the 1930s by both Babcock[27] and Heaney.[28] Dicker et al.[29] documented in 1982 that women who undergo vaginal hysterectomy experience significantly fewer complications than those who undergo abdominal hysterectomy. Why, therefore, did the use of the vaginal approach gain acceptance only in limited measure during this period?

Certainly, part of the problem may have related to training and attitudes in the UK. In the 1930s a visitor to leading Viennese clinics could see hysterectomy after hysterectomy performed with great skill by the vaginal route. At the same time a visitor to the famous Chelsea Hospital for Women, London, would have seen identical patients treated by abdominal hysterectomy with that effortless artistry for which Victor Bonney and his team were renowned. Certainly, during the 20th century in the UK, vaginal hysterectomy became an operation for prolapse, except in the hands of proponents of the procedure, and the abdominal approach to hysterectomy was actively encouraged in most centres except for prolapse. In addition, there was a vogue in the early part of the century for performing subtotal hysterectomy rather than the total procedure that became more accepted later. The encouragement of gynaecological trainees to train in surgery and achieve surgical fellowship may have been partially to blame. Even Professor Blair-Bell of Liverpool[30] actively encouraged the abdominal approach to enable the appendix to be removed at surgery, routinely through a midline incision. The issues are therefore likely to be related to training and experience. Stallworthy,[19] in 1957, made his views clear in relation to practitioners who adopted subtotal hysterectomy in preference to either abdominal or the vaginal total procedure: "Undoubtedly, many who adopted these views genuinely believed them, while others were possibly subconsciously endeavouring to rationalise the technique they practised because of their own inadequate training. An honest surgeon of limited experience may declare that in his hands … a subtotal hysterectomy is safer than either the total operation or vaginal extirpation of the uterus." His declaration is an indication of his personal integrity and operative ability, and not as fair comment on the respective merits of these operations.' He was thus supporting the view that many surgeons perform abdominal hysterectomy rather than vaginal hysterectomy because they are more comfortable with the abdominal procedure and it is therefore the safer operation in their practice.[31] The issue therefore seems to have been one of training. Certainly, by the end of the 20th century, the ratio of vaginal to abdominal procedures seems to have been at most 1:3 in the UK, and 1:5 in the USA.[32]

The modern era

Laparoscopically assisted vaginal hysterectomy

Over a decade ago, the first laparoscopic hysterectomy was described by Reich et al.[33] This was thought to herald a new chapter for the 'hysterectomy' as a way to avoid an abdominal procedure. There can be variation in the proportion of the procedure performed laparoscopically, although the endpoint is always the removal of the uterus through the vagina. The advent of this type of surgery essentially gave surgeons the confidence to attempt vaginal surgery, with less of the procedure being performed laparoscopically with increasing experience. The advantages of being able to perform the operation without recourse to a laparoscopically assisted procedure became apparent. There is no evidence that laparoscopically assisted vaginal hysterectomy (LAVH) has any advantage over vaginal hysterectomy in terms of morbidity measured by analgesia requirement, inpatient stay, discomfort and return to normal activity. There is a significant increase in operating time and operation costs because of the use of expensive disposable instruments with LAVH.[34,35] Thus, for the majority of vaginal surgeons, the role of the laparoscope is to allow assessment of a woman who is thought not to be suitable for vaginal hysterectomy. Therefore, if vaginal hysterectomy is achievable, it is a superior operation to both abdominal hysterectomy and LAVH. The consequence of this has been a fall in popularity of LAVH.

The return of subtotal hysterectomy

The end of the 20th century saw a resurgence in the use of subtotal hysterectomy. It was argued that total hysterectomy for benign conditions could be substituted by subtotal hysterectomy, particularly since cancers of the cervix were thought to be declining as a consequence of screening.[36,37] Subtotal hysterectomy is a safer and technically easier operation than total hysterectomy. It is said to be associated with a lower incidence of ureteric damage and vesico-urethral dysfunction. In addition, the uterosacral and cardinal ligaments remain intact, thus preserving the pelvic floor support. The cervix appears to play an important role in the arousal phase of intercourse and quality of orgasm in some women.[38–40] Additional benefits of the subtotal hysterectomy include less peri-operative blood loss and less postoperative infection and haematoma. Additionally, vault granulations do not complicate subtotal hysterectomy. The contemporary lifetime risk of cervical cancer in a monogamous woman with at least three normal Papanicolaou smears is 0.05%.[41]

The primary reason advanced for subtotal hysterectomy is to retain normal sexual function, but there are few convincing data to show that total hysterectomy is related to long-term sexual dysfunction. The preponderance of evidence suggests that detrimental effects on sexual function are rare with both total and subtotal hysterectomy, and that pre-operative sexual activity appears to be the most important factor in predicting postoperative sexual satisfaction. The data are both equally uncertain regarding postoperative bladder symptoms and inadequate to evaluate all other proposed advantages of subtotal hysterectomy.[41]

There are few published data on adverse effects of subtotal hysterectomy, but subsequent trachelectomy has been necessary in some patients because of continued bleeding, intraepithelial neoplasia, or prolapse of the cervical stump. Van der Stege and van Beek[39] reported that 10% of women who underwent laparoscopic supracervical hysterectomy suffered from discharge and 25% continued to menstruate (two were treated by vaginal cervical stumpectomy). In previous reports, 10% of women who underwent laparoscopic supracervical hysterectomy experienced menstrual bleeding[42] and, in my own series, 11% required further treatment, which consisted of either stump removal or loop excision of the transformation zone.[43] Routine cauterisation of the endocervical canal and/or excision of the endocervix by 'reverse conisation' should minimise the problems of vaginal bleeding. However, where residual endometrium exists there is the potential for continued menses and it is possible that endometrial carcinoma may develop, particularly if unopposed oestrogen is used for hormone replacement.

The alleged sexual and genitourinary benefits of subtotal hysterectomy over total hysterectomy are not proven, and well designed prospective trials are needed to address these issues. Women should understand that a second operation may he required to remove the cervix mainly because of continued menstruation and pelvic pain. The high rate of stump problems (11%) should be made clear to women before making the decision on whether to carry out total or subtotal abdominal hysterectomy. Total hysterectomy, preferably by the vaginal route, is better studied with longer follow-up, is less costly in the long term, and therefore remains the procedure of choice for most women. Vaginal subtotal hysterectomy by the Doderlein–Kronig technique,[44] originally described in 1907, may be used in women who want a vaginal procedure but who wish to retain the cervix.

INCREASING THE VAGINAL HYSTERECTOMY RATE IN MODERN PRACTICE

There are a number of conditions that have traditionally been regarded as relative or absolute contraindications to vaginal hysterectomy. Although such factors should still be regarded with caution, they do not necessarily exclude this operation.

Lack of uterine descent and nulliparity

The lack of uterine descent is not a contraindication to vaginal hysterectomy. Several large studies have been conducted showing that it is possible and safe in women with no uterine prolapse.[45–48] In practice, it is probable that vaginal access is more important. Limited access because of a narrow pubic arch, as found in an android shaped pelvis, is more likely to cause difficulty than a lack of uterine descent. Although this assessment is quite subjective, attempts have been made to quantify anatomical accessibility and define the necessary access as having a bituberous diameter of more than 9 cm, a pubic arch of more than 90 degrees and a vaginal capacity of more than two finger breadths.[49]

The main supports of the uterus are the cardinal and uterosacral ligaments. These are the most caudal of the pedicles and are relatively easy to divide to allow further descent.[50] This assessment of feasibility for vaginal hysterectomy can sometimes not be made fully until after examination under anaesthetic and division of these pedicles. It is therefore acceptable to commence a vaginal procedure and to complete it abdominally should the amount of uterine descent cause technical difficulties. The inability to perform vaginal hysterectomy because of uterine and adnexal immobility or inaccessibility occurred in only 1% of the series by Kovac,[47] although this figure will vary depending on the experience of the operator.

Nulliparity is related to lack of descent in that nulliparous women are less likely to have uterine descent. It is interesting that in one study[50] that retrospectively analysed the notes of women who had undergone hysterectomy (by any route) to assess their suitability for vaginal hysterectomy, a greater proportion of the women in the 'not suitable' group were nulliparous (34.7%) compared with the women deemed suitable for vaginal hysterectomy (16.5%). The only reasons for exclusion from suitability for vaginal hysterectomy used in that study were a uterine size equivalent to more than 20 weeks of gestation, known endometriosis, adnexal masses, cancer and those undergoing abdominal procedures such as colposuspension. The greater proportion of nulliparous women in the 'not suitable' group may therefore be because of the association of fibroids, endometriosis and endometrial carcinoma with nulliparity

The enlarged uterus

The enlarged uterus due to fibroids and menstrual disturbances secondary to this are common indications for hysterectomy.[51,52] However, an enlarged uterus due to adenomyosis can, in my experience, present a greater operative challenge. In one large series in the UK only 3.9% of hysterectomies for fibroids were carried out vaginally.[52] Several methods have been described for dealing with benign uterine enlargement to achieve vaginal hysterectomy.[53–56] These include bisection, morcellation and coring. These have been shown to be safe, with no added morbidity in terms of blood loss and visceral injury when compared with vaginal hysterectomy for uteri of normal size and abdominal hysterectomy.[57–59]

Furthermore, uterine volume can be reduced by pre-operative administration of gonadotrophin-releasing hormone analogues. Studies have shown that, in women with fibroid uteri of 12–18 weeks of gestation size, this increases the proportion of hysterectomies performed vaginally and, for those women who are initially anaemic (haemoglobin less than 11 g/dl), it reduces their risk of pre-operative transfusion; it also decreases estimated intraoperative blood loss.[60–62] It has been estimated that, if vaginal hysterectomy were performed on uteri of 14 weeks of gestation size in all cases, then the vaginal hysterectomy rate could be increased to 67% from the observed rate of 24%.[50]

Oophorectomy

If oophorectomy is indicated because of patient request, family history of ovarian cancer, endometriosis or premenstrual syndrome, most gynaecologists elect for abdominal hysterectomy, fearing technical difficulties with the vaginal route.[63] However, evidence suggests that bilateral (salpingo)oophorectomy at the time of vaginal hysterectomy is generally safely achievable.[64–67] A variety of techniques have been described to perform oophorectomy at vaginal hysterectomy and instruments have been specifically designed for this purpose.[66–69] These depend upon access and mobility of the adnexa. Using various techniques, a 97.5% success rate in oophorectomy for vaginal hysterectomy can be achieved.[64]

In the majority of women, the ovaries are easily accessible at the time of vaginal hysterectomy. The ovary can often be grasped with sponge forceps, and clamped and ligated with ease. Where there is difficulty, an endoloop or other endoscopic instruments may be used. Occasionally the laparoscope itself may be inserted vaginally to visualise the pedicle.

Previous pelvic surgery

There have been no prospective randomised controlled trials that have assessed the safety of vaginal hysterectomy compared with abdominal hysterectomy when there is a history of previous abdominal or pelvic surgery. However, previous pelvic surgery is the reason why an abdominal procedure is selected over a vaginal hysterectomy in 28% of patients.[50] Even Heaney,[55] one of the original proponents of the procedure, was reluctant to perform vaginal hysterectomy on women with a history of previous pelvic surgery. Such women are half as likely to undergo vaginal hysterectomy as abdominal hysterectomy.[31] There have since been a number of studies[70–73] attempting to demonstrate the safety of vaginal hysterectomy after previous abdominal and pelvic surgery. These have all been retrospective studies but the authors did surmise that vaginal hysterectomy remained a safe procedure in the majority of situations after previous surgery. One of the most common abdominal procedures that is considered by some to be a contraindication to vaginal hysterectomy is caesarean section. This has been assessed in isolation from other abdominal and pelvic surgery and no significant difference was found in complication rates in women with a history of caesarean delivery undergoing vaginal hysterectomy compared with those who had not had a caesarean delivery.[74] Morbidity was not affected by the number of previous caesarean deliveries; however, earlier studies did suggest that vaginal hysterectomy should he avoided in women who had more than two.[75] The main concern with a history of previous caesarean section is of bladder injury. However, vaginal hysterectomy allows the operator to start the dissection of the bladder in an area that is not scarred, and it is more likely that the correct tissue plane will be reached. When operating by the abdominal route, the uterovesical fold of peritoneum has been operated upon previously and initial dissection will therefore be more difficult. However, the abdominal route does give the option of performing a subtotal operation if scarring is severe.

Pelvic pain and tenderness

A history of pelvic pain and pelvic tenderness or uterine immobility at examination are also stated by some surgeons to be a contraindication to vaginal hysterectomy.[76,77] The unreliability of history and examination to predict the presence and extent of pelvic disease is well documented.[78,79] In one prospective study[47] of 617 women who were listed for hysterectomy, only 63 had risk factors from history or examination that might contraindicate vaginal hysterectomy. These women underwent laparoscopy before hysterectomy (LAVH). Laparoscopic surgery was necessary to permit a transvaginal operation in only 12 of 63 patients. Two women had abdominal hysterectomy after laparoscopic assessment because LAVH was not felt to be feasible. Thus, from this study it would appear that, when there is concern regarding endometriosis, pelvic inflammatory disease or other benign adnexal pathology, history and examination alone have a poor positive predictive value for women for whom vaginal hysterectomy is unsuitable. Therefore, an assessment with the laparoscope will exclude significant pathology before proceeding with a vaginal hysterectomy.

Personal data

Since 1998 I have endeavoured to reduce the number of women undergoing hysterectomy by the abdominal route. This practice was commenced because of the body of evidence that exists to suggest that recovery and patient satisfaction are improved if the procedure is undertaken vaginally. Previously, a large proportion of women had an abdominal procedure, many undergoing a subtotal operation, again because of its perceived advantages. However, our own data showed that more than 10% of these women had continued bleeding, discharge or pain from the residual cervix;[43] therefore, unless the woman specifically asks for a subtotal procedure, I would endeavour to perform a vaginal hysterectomy, with bilateral salpingo-oophorectomy if necessary. It was, however, the vaginal excision of the residual cervix (vaginal trachelectomy) subsequent to the subtotal operation and the performance of a vaginal hysterectomy on a nullipara with no prolapse that resulted in the realisation that vaginal hysterectomy is possible in circumstances that I would not have considered previously. This may be illustrated by the proportion of my patients undergoing various types of hysterectomy in 1997 and 2001. In 1997, of the hysterectomies performed under my care, 49% were subtotal procedures, 24% were total abdominal procedures and 27% were vaginal. However, when we look at the number performed for dysfunctional bleeding alone (excluding malignancy, prolapse and fibroids), we find that 65% were subtotal operations, 29% were total abdominal procedures and 6% were vaginal. In 2001, 14% were subtotal procedures, 17% were total abdominal procedures, and 69% were vaginal (48% vaginal hysterectomy, 21% vaginal hysterectomy and bilateral salpingo-oophorectomy). When we again exclude malignancy, prolapse and fibroids, we find 12% subtotal abdominal procedures, 12% total abdominal, and 76% vaginal (41% vaginal hysterectomy, 35% vaginal hysterectomy and bilateral salpingo-oophorectomy). During this period there were no major complications from surgery. Trends in type of hysterectomy over a five-year period can be seen in Figure 1.

This change in practice was not achieved by the purchase of expensive equipment or by additional training of theatre staff. The procedures were undertaken with one assistant and general theatre staff, with no additional expense or training being required. The skills that are necessary to perform vaginal surgery are those that all trained gynaecologists possess, although from my experience the ways to increase the proportion of hysterectomies performed vaginally are:

• Attend a course – listen to experienced exponents of the operation giving practical tips and advice.

- Initially choose multiparous women with a normal sized mobile uterus and slowly increase the technical difficulty as confidence increases.

- Warn the woman that an abdominal procedure may be required if the procedure is technically too difficult or there is unexpected bleeding. If successful the woman has had a vaginal procedure with its attendant benefits; if it fails, she has lost nothing.

- Assess the pelvis laparoscopically if there is a suggestion of adhesions, endometriosis or other pelvic pathology. If there is uterine enlargement, a sonographic assessment of size will help. Consider gonadotrophin-releasing hormone analogues if the uterus is more than 12 weeks of gestation size.

- Always follow the rules: there is no room for short cuts in vaginal surgery.

- Do not feel under pressure: ensure that there is enough time – although vaginal hysterectomy is often quicker than the abdominal route.

Vaginal hysterectomy should be considered the operation of choice for the majority of women with dysfunctional uterine bleeding[80,81] and may be contemplated for women with endometrial[82] or cervical[83] malignancy. Many of the traditional contraindications to vaginal hysterectomy are no longer valid[84] and the incidence of operative injury is low.[85] The vagina should be considered the route of choice for the majority of hysterectomies and an effort should be made to encourage the next generation of gynaecologists to acquire the appropriate skills.

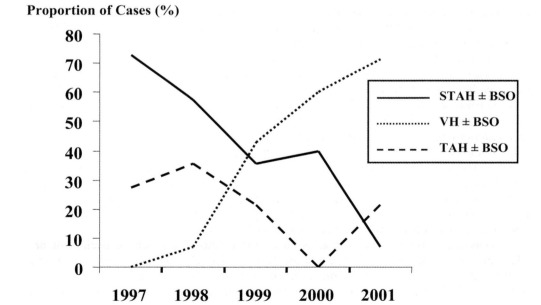

Figure 1 *Trends in hysterectomy type 1997–2001: BSO = bilateral salpingo-oophorectomy; STAH = subtotal abdominal hysterectomy; TAH = total abdominal hysterectomy; VH = vaginal hysterectomy*

References

1. Senn N. The early history of vaginal hysterectomy. *JAMA* 1895;25:476–82.

2. Windsor H. [Article title unknown] *Med Chir Trans* 1819;X:[page nos unknown].

3. Bernhard E. *Eine Extirpation der Gebärmutter aus Umoissenheit von einer Hebamme verrichtet; nebst Bermerkungen über die Extirpation der Gebärmutter, als neuerdings empfohlnes Heilmittel des Gebärmutter Krebses.* Leipzig: Lucina; 1802.

4. Wrisberg A. *Commentatio de uteri mox post-partum naturalem resectione non lethali, observatione illustrata cum brevissima principorum lethalitalis sciagraphia.* 1787.

5. Palletta P. Storia d'una matrice amputata. *Ann Univ Med Milano* 1822.

6. Langenbeck CJM. Geschichte einer von mir glucklich verrichteten extirpation der ganzen gebarmutter. *N Biblioth Chir Ophthalm* 1819–1820;1:551.

7. Sauter JN. *Die gänzliche Extirpation der Gebärmutter ohne selbst, entstandenen oder Rünstlich bewirkter Vorfall vorgenommen und glücklich vollführt mit näherer Anleitung, wie diese Operation gemacht werden kann.* Constanz; 1822.

8. Langenbeck CJM. *Nosologie u. Therapie der Chirurgischen Krankheiten*, B. 6. Göttingen; 1845.

9. Jackson AR. Vaginal hysterectomy for cancer. *JAMA* 1885;5:169–71

10. Simpson JY. Clinical lectures on diseases of women. 1863. p. 65. Cited in: Stallworthy J. The present status of hysterectomy. *Practitioner* 1957;178:291–7.

11. Freund WA. Volkmann's 'Sammlung Klin Vorträge'. 1878;(133).

12. Czerny V. Zur laparo-hysterotomie. *Wien Med Presse* 1879;20:1265–8.

13. Studd JWW. Hysterectomy and menorrhagia. *Baillieres Clin Obstet Gynaecol* 1989;3:415–24.

14. Schauta F. Die hauptindication der vaginalen total-exstirpation ist und bleibt des carcimoma uteri. *Wien Med Bl* 1890;13:551–3.

15. Sheth SS. Vaginal hysterectomy. *Prog Obstet Gynaecol* 1993;10:317.

16. Green-Armytage VB. Vaginal hysterectomy: new technique – follow-up of 500 consecutive operations for haemorrhage. *J Obstet Gynaecol Br Empire* 1939;46:848–56.

17. Palmer AC. Discussion on the role of vaginal hysterectomy in treatment of prolapse. *Proc R Soc Med* 1948;41:676.

18. Howkins J. Discussion on the role of vaginal hysterectomy in treatment of prolapse. *Proc R Soc Med* 1948;41:676–7.

19. Stallworthy J. The present status of hysterectomy. *Practitioner* 1957;178:291–7.

20. Stallworthy J. Donald Fothergill meeting. *J Obstet Gynaecol Br Cwlth* 1961;68:1061–5.

21. Watson PS. Late results in vaginal hysterectomy. *J Obstet Gynaecol Br Cwlth* 1963;70:29.

22. Van Bastiaanse BM. *Atti del Symposium Internazionale su i Virilismi in Ginecologis e su la Terapia del Cancero del Corpo dell'Utero.* Florence: Scienrifiche Salpietra; 1962.

23. Navratil E. The place of vaginal hysterectomy. *J Obstet Gynaecol Br Cwlth* 1965;72:841–6.

24. Mitra S. Radical vaginal hysterectomy and extraperitoneal pelvic lymphadenectomy for cancer of the cervix. *J Obstet Gynaecol Br Empire* 1955;62:672–5.

25. Mitra S. Extraperitoneal lymphadenectomy and radical vaginal hysterectomy for cancer of the cervix (Mitra technique). *Am J Obstet Gynecol* 1959;78:191–6.

26. Purandare BN. Vaginal hysterectomy with review of author's 203 cases. *J Obstet Gynecol* 1946;7:77–80.

27. Babcock WW. A technique for vaginal hysterectomy. *Surg Gynecol Obstet* 1932;54:193–9.

28. Heaney NS. A report of 565 vaginal hysterectomies performed for benign pelvic disease. *Am J Obstet Gynecol* 1934;28:751–5.

29.   Dicker RC, Greenspan JR, Strauss LT, Cowart MR, Scally MJ, Peterson HB, *et al.* Complications of abdominal and vaginal hysterectomy among women of reproductive age in the United States. The Collaborative Review of Sterilization. *Am J Obstet Gynecol* 1982;144:841–8.

30.   Peel J. *William Blair-Bell – Father and Founder.* London: Royal College of Obstetricians and Gynaecologists; 1986. p. 38.

31.   Dorsey JH, Steinberg EP, Holtz PM. Clinical indications for hysterectomy route: patient characteristics or physician preference? *Am J Obstet Gynecol* 1995;173:1452–60.

32.   Magos AL. The hysterectomy lottery. *J Obstet Gynaecol* 2001;21:166–70.

33.   Reich H, DeCaprio J, McGlynn F. Laparoscopic hysterectomy. *J Gynecol Surg* 1989;5:213–16.

34.   Richardson RE, Bournas N, Magos AL. Is laparoscopic hysterectomy a waste of time? *Lancet* 1995;345:36–41.

35.   Meikle SF, Nugent EW, Orleans M. Complications and recovery from laparoscopy-assisted vaginal hysterectomy compared with abdominal and vaginal hysterectomy. *Obstet Gynecol* 1997;89:304–11.

36.   Drife J. Conserving the cervix at hysterectomy. *Br J Obstet Gynaecol* 1994;101:563–4.

37.   Storm HH, Clemmensen IH, Manders T, Brinton LA. Supravaginal uterine amputation in Denmark 1978–1988 and risk of cancer. *Gynecol Oncol* 1992;45:198–201.

38.   Sutton C. Subtotal hysterectomy revisited. *Endosc Surg Allied Technol* 1995;3:105–8.

39.   van der Stege JG, van Beek JJ. Problems related to the cervical stump at follow-up in laparoscopic supracervical hysterectomy. *J Soc Laparosc Surg* 1999;3:5–7.

40.   Johns A. Supracervical versus total hysterectomy. *Clin Obstet Gynecol* 1997;40:903–13.

41.   Scott AR, Sharp HT, Dodson MK, Norton PA, Warner HR. Subtotal hysterectomy in modern gynecology: a decision analysis. *Am J Obstet Gynecol* 1997;176:1186–92.

42.   Nezhat CH, Nezhat F, Roemisch M, Seidman DS, Nezhat C. Laparoscopic trachelectomy for persistent pelvic pain and endometriosis after supracervical hysterectomy. *Fertil Steril* 1996;66:925–8.

43.   Ewies AA, Oláh KS. Subtotal abdominal hysterectomy: a surgical advance or a backward step? *BJOG* 2000;107:1376–9.

44.   Doderlein A, Kronig S. *Die Technik der Vaginalen Bauchholen-Operationen.* Leipzig: Verlag von S Hirzel; 1906.

45.   Magos A, Bournas N, Sinha R, Richardson RE, O'Connor H. Vaginal hysterectomy for the large uterus. *Br J Obstet Gynaceol* 1996;103:246–51.

46.   Davies A, O'Connor H, Magos AL. A prospective study to evaluate oophorectomy at the time of vaginal hysterectomy. *Br J Obstet Gynaecol* 1996;103:915–20.

47.   Kovac SR. Guidelines to determine the route of hysterectomy. *Obstet Gynecol* 1995;85:18–23.

48.   Sheth SS, Malpani A. Vaginal hysterectomy for the management of menstruation in mentally retarded women. *Int J Gynaecol Obstet* 1991;35:319–21.

49.   Kovac SR. Which route for hysterectomy? Evidence-based outcomes guide selection. *Postgrad Med* 1997;102:153–8.

50.   Davies A, Vizza E, Bournas N, O'Connor H, Magos A. How to increase the proportion of hysterectomies performed vaginally. *Am J Obstet Gynecol* 1998;179:1008–12.

51.   Amirikia H, Evans TN. Ten year review of hysterectomies: trends, indications and risks. *Am J Obstet Gynecol* 1979;134:431–7.

52.   Vessey MP, Villard-Mackintosh L, McPherson K, Coulter A, Yeates D. The epidemiology of hysterectomy: findings in a large cohort study. *Br J Obstet Gynaecol* 1992;99:402–7.

53.   Kovac SR. Intramyometrial coring as an adjunct to vaginal hysterectomy. *Obstet Gynecol*

1986;67:131–6.

54. Hoffman MS, Spellacy WN. *The Difficult Vaginal Hysterectomy – a Surgical Atlas*. London: Springer-Verlag; 1995.

55. Heaney NS. Vaginal hysterectomy – its indications and technique. *Am J Surg* 1940;48:284–8.

56. Grody MH. Vaginal hysterectomy: the large uterus. *J Gynecol Surg* 1989;5:30l–12.

57. Unger JB. Vaginal hysterectomy for the woman with a moderately enlarged uterus weighing 200 to 700 grams. *Am J Obstet Gynecol* 1999;180:1337–44.

58. Mazdisnian F, Kurzcl RB, Coe S, Bosuk M, Montz F. Vaginal hysterectomy by uterine morcellation: an efficient non-morbid procedure. *Obstet Gynecol* 1995;86:60–4.

59. Hoffman MS, DeCesare S, Kalter C. Abdominal hysterectomy versus transvaginal morcellation for the removal of enlarged uteri. *Am J Obstet Gynecol* 1994;171:309–13.

60. Stovall TG, Ling FW, Henry LC, Woodruff MR. A randomized trial evaluating leuprolide acetate before hysterectomy as treatment for leiomyomas. *Am J Obstet Gynecol* 1991;164:1420–3.

61. Stovall TG, Summit RL, Washburn SA, Ling FW. Gonadotrophin-releasing hormone agonist use before hysterectomy. *Am J Obstet Gynecol* 1994;170:1744–8.

62. Vercellini P, Crosignani PG, Mangioni C, Imparato E, Ferrari A, De Giorgi O. Treatment with a gonadotrophin releasing hormone agonist before hysterectomy for leiomyomas: results of a multicentre randomised controlled trial. *Br J Obstet Gynaecol* 1998;105:1148–54.

63. Kovac SR, Christie SJ, Bindbeutel GA. Abdominal versus vaginal hysterectomy: a statistical model for determining physician decision making and patient outcome. *Med Decis Making* 1991;11:19–28.

64. Davies A, O'Connor H, Magos AL. A prospective study to evaluate oophorectomy at the time of vaginal hysterectomy. *Br J Obstet Gynaecol* 1996;103:915–20.

65. Kovac SR, Cruikshank SH. Guidelines to determine the route of oophorectomy with hysterectomy. *Am J Obstet Gynecol* 1996;175:1483–8.

66. Sheth SS. The place of oophorectomy at vaginal hysterectomy. *Br J Obstet Gynaecol* 1991;98:662–6.

67. Smale LE, Smale ML, Wilkening RL, Mundy CE, Ewing TL. Salpingo-oophorectomy at the time of vaginal hysterectomy. *Am J Obstet Gynecol* 1978;131:122–8.

68. Wright RC. Vaginal oophorectomy. *Am J Obstet Gynecol* 1974;120:759–63.

69. Magos AL, Bournas N, Sinha R, Lo L, Richardson RE. Transvaginal endoscopic oophorectomy. *Am J Obstet Gynecol* 1995;172:123–4.

70. Ingram JM, Withers RW, Wright HL. Vaginal hysterectomy after previous pelvic surgery. *Am J Obstet Gynecol* 1957;74:1181–6.

71. Jacobs WM, Adels MJ, Rogers SE. Vaginal hysterectomy after previous pelvic surgery. *Obstet Gynecol* 1958;12:572–4.

72. Carpenter RJ, Silva P. Vaginal hysterectomy following pelvic operation. *Obstet Gynecol* 1967;30:394–8.

73. Coulam CB, Pratt JH. Vaginal hysterectomy: is previous pelvic operation a contraindication? *Am J Obstet Gynecol* 1973;116:252–60.

74. Unger JB, Meeks GR. Vaginal hysterectomy in women with history of previous cesarean delivery. *Am J Obstet Gynecol* 1998;179:1473–8.

75. Sheth SS, Malpani AN. Vaginal hysterectomy following previous caesarean section. *Int J Gynaecol Obstet* 1995;50:165–9.

76. Gupta JK, Frank TG, Nwosu CR. The Gupta–Frank clamp for salpingo-oophorectomy at vaginal hysterectomy. *Obstet Gynecol* 1998;92:144–7.

77. Kovac SR. Vaginal hysterectomy. *Baillieres Clin Obstet Gynaecol* 1997;11:95–110.

78. Lee NC, Dicker RC, Rubin CL, Ory HW. Confirmation of the preoperative diagnosis for hysterectomy. *Am J Obstet Gynecol* 1984;150:283–7.

79. Lundberg WI, Wall JE, Mathers JE. Laparoscopy in evaluation of pelvic pain. *Obstet Gynecol* 1973;42:872–6.

80. Varma R, Tahseen S, Lokugamage AU, Kunde D. Vaginal route as the norm when planning hysterectomy for benign conditions: a change in practice. *Obstet Gynecol* 2001;97:613–16.

81. Mehra S, Bhat V, Mehra G. Laparoscopic vs. abdominal vs. vaginal hysterectomy. *Gynecol Endocrinol* 1999;8:29–34.

82. Carriero C, Nappi L, Melilli GA, Di Gesu G, Cormio G, Di Vagno G, *et al.* Prognostic factors and selective use of vaginal hysterectomy in early stage endometrial carcinoma. *Eur J Gynaecol Oncol* 1999;20:408–11.

83. Angioli R, Martin J, Heffernan T, Massi G. Radical vaginal hysterectomy: classic and modified. *Surg Clin North Am* 2001;81:829–40.

84. Doucette RC, Sharp HT, Alder SC. Challenging generally accepted contraindications to vaginal hysterectomy. *Am J Obstet Gynecol* 2001;184:1386–91.

85. Mathevet P, Valencia P, Cousin C, Mellier G, Dargent D. Operative injuries during vaginal hysterectomy. *Eur J Obstet Gynecol Reprod Biol* 2001;97:71–5.

29

The role of intrauterine progestogens in menorrhagia

Nicholas Panay and Vineeta Verma

INTRODUCTION

Menorrhagia (heavy menstrual bleeding) is a common reason for women of reproductive age to seek medical advice. Especially in developed countries, women today experience a greater number of menstrual cycles. As increased use of effective contraception continues, the contributory factors include early menarche, lower number of lifetime pregnancies, and periods spent in lactation amenorrhoea. Furthermore, with changes in social position and attitudes, women now are less ready to accept the inconvenience of prolonged heavy bleeding and expect the health service to provide a range of effective treatments.

The traditional option of hysterectomy and even the techniques of endometrial destruction by minimally invasive techniques described in the early 1980s have their own risks and failure rates and are not suitable for the women who wish to retain their ability to conceive in the future. The addition of the levonorgestrel intrauterine system (LNG IUS), Mirena® (Schering Health Care Ltd, Burgess Hill, West Sussex, UK), to the medical armamentarium has been a significant development in the management of menorrhagia in this large subgroup of young women. They are also more likely to gain from the additional benefits of contraception, relief of dysmenorrhoea, and prevention of pelvic inflammatory disease and ectopic pregnancy.

There is however no such thing as a universal panacea and the current intrauterine system is not without its own problems, which will be discussed in the course of this chapter, as will the new developments in the field to overcome them.

STRUCTURE AND MECHANISM OF ACTION OF INTRAUTERINE SYSTEMS

Structure

Mirena and Progestasert® (Alza Corporation, Mount View, CA, USA) are the two intrauterine systems currently in use. A third novel 'frameless' intrauterine drug delivery system, the Fibro Plant™ LNG IUS (Contrel, Ghent, Belgium), is currently being evaluated in continuing pilot studies in Belgium.

The Mirena LNG IUS consists of a plastic T-shaped frame with a steroid reservoir around a vertical stem of polydimethylsiloxane. The stem contains 52 mg of levonorgestrel, the laevo–isomer of norgestrel, derived from the 19–nortestosterone progestogens, released at a rate of 20 µg per day. The Progestasert intrauterine progesterone system (PIPS) consists of a polymeric T-shaped platform with a reservoir containing 38 mg of progesterone released at a rate of 65 µg per day. The total quantity of progesterone contained in one Progestasert system is less than the amount

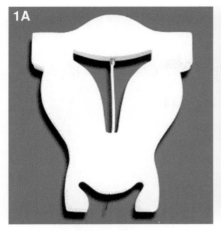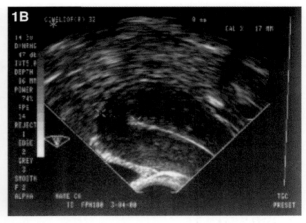

Figure 1 *The Fibro Plant LNG IUS in situ: (A) in a uterine model; (B) ultrasound picture (reproduced from: Wildemeersch D, Schacht E. The effect on menstrual blood loss in women with uterine fibroids of a novel 'frameless' intrauterine levonorgestrel-releasing drug delivery system: a pilot study. Eur J Obstet Gynecol Reprod Biol 2002;102:74–79.[2] © 2002, with permission from Elsevier Science)*

produced in one day by the corpus luteum during the latter part of the menstrual cycle. The drug is distributed in silicone (polydimethylsiloxane) fluid in both systems with a rate-limiting membrane allowing slow diffusion of the drug into the endometrium.[1] Both frames are rendered radio-opaque by impregnated barium sulphate. The LNG IUS is currently licensed in the UK for both contraception and more recently (in the 1990s) for use in menorrhagia for five years, but there are data for seven-year bioavailability; the PIPS is licensed in the USA for one-year usage with up to two-year bioavailability.

The Fibro Plant LNG IUS consists of a fibrous delivery system of 3 cm length and 1.2 mm diameter that releases 14 μg of levonorgestrel daily (Figure 1a). This is fixed to an anchoring filament by means of a metal clip positioned 1 cm from the anchoring knot, which is implanted into the myometrium of the uterine fundus using an insertion instrument. The stainless steel metal clip allows radiographic and ultrasound detection of the system. Measurement of the distance between the surface of the uterus and the metal clip (S–S distance) indicates whether the system has been correctly anchored (Figure 1b).

The Fibro Plant LNG IUS has no frame, so it is completely flexible and can adapt to uterine cavities of every size and shape. The duration of release is at least three years.[2]

Endometrial effects

Steroid hormones are major endocrine regulators of endometrial function, exerting effects through cellular receptors, which, when activated, induce gene expression of local regulatory factors. However, this interplay between oestrogen, progesterone, their receptors and local factors in endometrial function remains unclear.[3]

The 19-nortestosterone derivative, levonorgestrel, has a strong progestin effect on the endometrium. The LNG IUS has been shown to decrease endometrial proliferation and increase apoptosis of endometrial glands. An increase in Fas antigen expression, a mediator of apoptosis

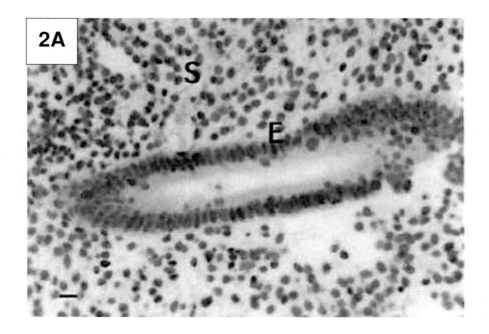

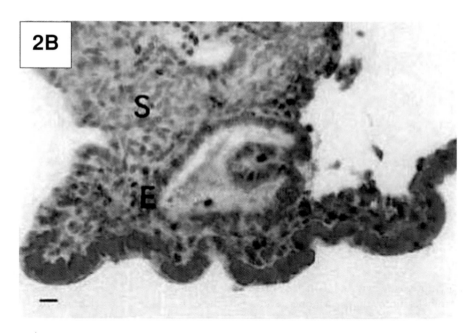

Figure 2 *Immunohistochemical localisation of Fas antigen in the endometrium (A) before and (B) 3 months after LNG IUS insertion; Fas antigen was present in the endometrial glands, but not in the stromal cells before LNG IUS insertion; Fas antigen expression became more abundant in both the endometrial glands and stroma 3 months after LNG IUS insertion; E = endometrial gland epithelium; S = endometrial stroma; scale bar = 10 μm; original magnification, ×400 (reproduced from: Maruo T, Laoag-Fernandez JB, Pakaninen P, Murakoshi H, Spitz IM, Johansson E. Effects of the levonorgestrel-releasing intrauterine system on proliferation and apoptosis in the endometrium. Hum Reprod 2001;16(10):2103–8.[4] © European Society of Human Reproduction and Embryology; reprinted by permission of Oxford University Press/Human Reproduction)*

(Figure 2) and a reduction in Bcl 2 protein expression, which promotes cell survival and blocks apoptosis in the endometrium (Figure 3), may be the underlying molecular mechanism for endometrial atrophy.[4]

After a few weeks, the endometrial glands atrophy, the stroma becomes swollen and decidual, the mucosa thins and the epithelium becomes inactive. The Doppler blood flow in the cervical branch of the uterine artery shows no change; however, subendometrial blood flow in the spiral artery is reduced and endometrial width decreases.[5] There is also capillary thrombosis and a local inflammatory response.[6] As a result of the high local levels of progestogen on the endometrium, despite no major change in uterine blood flow, the endometrium thinning occurs with reduced menstrual shedding. Continuous induction of plasminogen activator inhibitor by the LNG IUS may also contribute to the reduction in menstrual blood loss.[7] It has been shown that, in spite of the presence of oestrogen receptors and endogenous oestrogen production, not only the expression of progestogen receptors but also other oestrogen receptor mediated cellular functions appear to be suppressed in the levonorgestrel exposed endometrium.[8]

However, the decrease in epithelial and stromal progesterone receptors as well as epithelial proliferation marker Ki-67 expression has not been seen to vary in women experiencing breakthrough bleeding compared with controls, six months post-insertion of an LNG IUS.[3] No effect on endothelial factor VIII activity has been detected; this is reduced by ordinary intrauterine contraceptive devices, leading to a bleeding tendency.[9]

Endometrial biopsy studies indicate that continuous application of progestogens to the uterus results in changes indicative of an inactive endometrium. These changes are uniform within three cycles after insertion of the system,[10] with no further histological development over the long term.[11] After removal of the system, the morphological changes in the endometrium return to normal and menstruation returns within 30 days.[12] No cellular abnormalities have been attributed to use of the system.[13]

Endometrial suppression with decidual transformation is also the main mechanism of action with the PIPS, when there is an equally rapid return to normal of the morphological changes after discontinuation.[14]

Ovulation

During the first year of using the LNG IUS, some women may experience changes in ovarian function. After this, they usually have completely normal ovulatory cycles.[15] Menstrual bleeding does not reflect ovarian function, average oestradiol and progesterone levels being the same in amenorrhoeic and menstruating users.[16,17]

Studies of plasma hormone levels, menstrual patterns and blood chemistry in various patient groups using the PIPS demonstrated no systemic effects of the system, even on the progesterone sensitive hypothalamic–pituitary–ovarian axis.[18,19]

The LNG IUS has been shown to be associated with a higher incidence of ovarian cysts, mostly asymptomatic, with high rates of spontaneous resolution. The occurrence is not related to age or follicle-stimulating hormone levels, but there is a weak correlation with irregular bleeding.[20]

Pharmacokinetics

The plasma concentrations achieved by the LNG IUS are lower than those seen with a levonorgestrel implant, the combined oral contraceptive and the mini-pill.[21-24] Although there is marked interindividual variation in serum levonorgestrel levels (1–200 pg/ml) the serum and

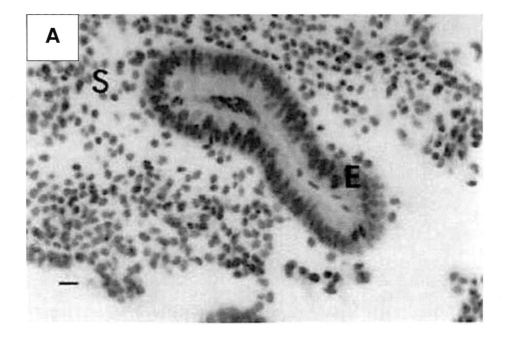

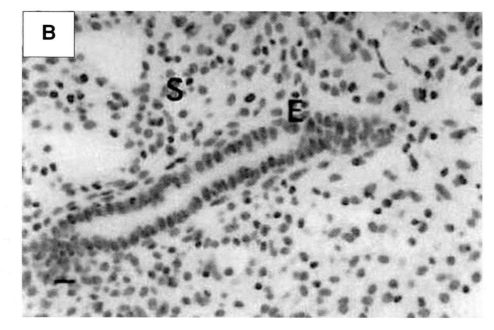

Figure 3 *Bcl-2 protein expression in the endometrium (A) before and (B) 3 months after LNG IUS insertion; Bcl-2 protein expression was noted in the cytoplasm of endometrial glands before LNG IUS insertion, but was scanty 3 months after LNG IUS use; E = endometrial gland epithelium; S = endometrial stroma; scale bar = 10 μm. Original magnification, ×400 (reproduced from: Maruo T, Laoag-Fernandez JB, Pakaninen P, Murakoshi H, Spitz IM, Johansson E. Effects of the levonorgestrel-releasing intrauterine system on proliferation and apoptosis in the endometrium. Hum Reprod 2001;16(10):2103–8.[4] © European Society of Human Reproduction and Embryology; reprinted by permission of Oxford University Press/Human Reproduction)*

endometrial levels remain stable for six to seven years. Unlike the oral contraceptives, the levels with the LNG IUS do not display peaks and troughs. Endometrial concentrations after six years are still in excess of the capacity of the local progesterone receptors.

Results of studies with baboons show that intrauterine systems delivering 65 μg/day of labelled progesterone do not produce detectable changes in concentrations of circulating progesterone. Progesterone released by the system is quickly metabolised to steroid intermediates. Unlike the metabolites of synthetic analogues, progesterone catabolites have little or no endocrine function and do not accumulate in the tissues.

ROLE OF INTRAUTERINE SYSTEMS IN THE MANAGEMENT OF MENORRHAGIA

Menorrhagia is experienced by up to 30% of women of reproductive age;[25] it accounts for 60% of general practice consultations for menstrual dysfunction[26] and 12% of gynaecology referrals,[27] and is the most common cause of the iron deficiency anaemia affecting 20–25% of healthy fertile women in the UK.[25,26]

The main focus of the treatment of menorrhagia is on reducing the blood loss to improve quality of life and prevent anaemia. Although defined as a blood loss of more than 80 ml per cycle (figure derived from population studies that have shown the average menstrual blood loss to be between 30 and 40 ml), in hospital practice only 40% of women with the symptom will actually have such a loss on objective measurement,[28,29] despite a convincing history.

Actual menstrual blood loss measurements are rarely carried out in daily clinical practice outside research trials. Pictorial charts have in some studies been demonstrated to measure menstrual blood loss objectively and are easy to use,[30] but others have failed to reproduce their validity.[31]

TRADITIONAL MANAGEMENT AND PITFALLS

Hysterectomy and resection/ablation of endometrium

Each year, 1 in 20 women aged 30–49 years consult their general practitioner with menorrhagia.[32] Sixty percent of women referred to secondary care are likely to have a hysterectomy within 5 years of the referral, as shown by Coulter et al.,[33] and in most of these women there is no demonstrable pelvic pathology.[26]

In the period 1993–1994, 73 517 hysterectomies were carried out in England; there was a decline in 1997–1998, when there were 63 345 operations.[34] Endometrial ablations rose markedly from 9945 to 36 440 in the same period.[35]

These data are not entirely surprising; endometrial destructive procedures are associated with lower complication rates and mortality, and high patient satisfaction.[36] However, these procedures may not always be successful; re-operation rates range from 11% to 40%[37] and approximately a third of these women will eventually require a hysterectomy.[38]

Despite high patient satisfaction with hysterectomy,[39,40] considerable morbidity and occasional mortality may occur. Complication rates up to 44% have been shown to be associated with abdominal hysterectomy, the most common route used in the UK, compared with 27% for vaginal hysterectomy.[41] Substantial costs are incurred and convalescence is longer.[34,40]

Medical therapies

Women warrant a trial of effective medical therapies before proceeding to definitive surgical treatment.[42] Many drug therapies, however, are ineffective and suffer from poor patient compliance.

A meta-analysis and survey of general practice prescription patterns showed that norethisterone was most widely used by 40.9% of general practitioners. Low-dose late luteal phase regimens given for six to ten days are often ineffective and may even increase the blood flow in some cases.[43]

The reductions of menstrual blood loss by different forms of medical treatment reported in various studies[44–47] are: 25% (mefenamic acid), 50% (tranexamic acid), 40% (oral contraceptive pill), 80% (danazol) and 75% (gonadotrophin-releasing hormone analogues).

EFFECTIVENESS OF MIRENA IN THE MANAGEMENT OF MENORRHAGIA

Observational studies

Andersson and Rybo[48] used the LNG IUS in 20 women with confirmed menorrhagia and observed a significant reduction in menstrual loss of 85% at three months' LNG IUS use and a further reduction up to 97% at 12 months. There was also a significant increase in mean serum ferritin level of 47% in the first year of use. Spotting was commonly reported in the first three months; however, 35% of these women were amenorrhoeic at one year.

In another observational study, in ten Chinese women who were anaemic and had an objectively measured blood loss of more than 80 ml, the LNG IUS resulted in significant reductions of menstrual blood loss of 54%, 87% and 95% in the first, third and sixth months of treatment, and an increase in mean haemoglobin by 19.2% at six months compared with pretreatment cycles.[49]

The progesterone releasing system has also been shown to reduce menstrual blood loss but not to the same extent as the LNG IUS (65% reduction 12 months after insertion).[50]

In a study by Wildemeersch and Schacht the Fibro Plant LNG IUS was inserted in 32 women with a normal uterus. A decreased menstrual blood loss of at least 80% occurred in the 1–23-month follow-up, with reduction seen as early as one month.[51]

Meta-analysis of Mirena in menorrhagia

Stewart et al.[52] conducted a systematic review to address the effectiveness of levonorgestrel-releasing systems in menorrhagia. Thirty-four studies were identified using the LNG IUS releasing 20 μg levonorgestrel and reporting menstrual loss. Only ten studies fulfilled the inclusion criteria because they had objective evidence of menorrhagia. Five studies were randomised controlled trials[53–57] and reported the use of the LNG IUS in 110 women with menorrhagia, and five case series[48,49,58–60] reported on use in a further 101 women. The main outcome measures were reduction in menstrual blood loss, serum ferritin/haemoglobin level, adverse effects, satisfaction with treatment at three months, and decision to cancel hysterectomy.

The results of the meta-analysis showed that the use of the LNG IUS could significantly reduce menstrual blood loss (range 74–97%) in women with confirmed menorrhagia (Table 1).

However, to establish the effectiveness and cost effectiveness relative to other treatments and effect on surgical waiting lists larger, more powerful randomised controlled trials with longer follow-up were noted to be required.

Table 1 *Summary of menstrual blood loss results*

Study	n	Baseline MBL	End of study MBL	MBL difference	MBL% reduction	Endpoint (months)
Controlled trials						
Crosignani et al., 1997[56]	30	LNG IUS:				12
		Mean score 184.8	Mean score 38.8	Score 146	79%[***]	
		SD 62.2	SD 37.1	(CI 123–169)		
	30	Endometrial resection:				
		Mean score 203.2	Mean score 23.5	Score 180	89%[***]	
		SD 77.4	SD 32.6	(CI 152–208)		
Irvine et al., 1998[53]	20	LNG IUS:				3
		Median 105 ml	Median 6 ml	99 ml	94%[***]	
		Range 82–780 ml	Range 0–284 ml	$z = 12.5$		
	16	Norethisterone:				
		Median 120 ml	Median 6 ml	100 ml	83%[***]	
		Range 82–336 ml	Range 4–137 ml	$z = 8.23$		
Kittelsen and Istre, 1998[57]	24	LNG IUS:				12
		Mean score 418	Mean score 42	Score 376	90%	
		SD 349	SD 99.7			
	29	Endometrial resection:				
		Mean score 378	Mean score 6.6	Score 371.4	98%[*]	
		SD 463	SD 15			
Milsom et al., 1991[54]	16	LNG IUS:				12
		Mean 203 ml	Mean 9 ml	194 ml	96%[***]	
		Range 81–381 ml	Range 0–33 ml			
		SEM ± 25.2	SEM ± 2.7			
	15	Flurbiprofen:				
		Mean 295 ml	Mean 223 ml	72 ml	21%[*]	
		Range 81–701 ml	Range 50–636 ml			
		SEM ± 52	SEM ± 44			
	15	Tranexamic acid:				
		Mean 295 ml	Mean 155 ml	140 ml	44%[**]	
		Range 81–701 ml	Range 36–511 ml			
		SEM ±52	SEM ± 33			
Case series						
Andersson and Rybo, 1990[48]	16	Median 176 ml	Median 5 ml	171 ml	83%[***]	12
		Range 80–381 ml	Range 0–33 ml			
Barrington and Bowen-Simkins, 1997[58]	42	Mean score 120	Mean score 31	Score 89	Mean 74%[***]	3
		Median score 85	Median Score 21		Median 75%	
		SD 98	SD 28			
Fedele et al., 1997[59]	23	Mean score 211	Mean score 44	Score 167	79%[***]	12
		SD 61	SD 18			
Scholten et al., 1989[60]	11	Mean 119 ml	Mean score 17	102 ml	86%[**]	7–12
		SD 72	SD 14			
Tang and Lo, 1995[49]	10	Mean 247 ml	Mean 26 ml	Mean 221 ml	Mean 89%	6
		Median 183 ml	Median 10 ml	Median 173 ml	Median 95%[**]	
		Range 82–563 ml	Range 0–143 ml			
		SD 158.1	SD 45.6			
		SE 52.7	SE 15.2			

[*]$P < 0.05$; [**]$P < 0.01$; [***]$P < 0.001$; MBL = menstrual blood loss; SD = standard deviation; CI = confidence interval; SEM = standard error of the mean; SE = standard error (reproduced from: Stewart A, Cummins C, Gold L, Jordan R, Phillipson W. The effectiveness of the levonorgestrel-releasing intrauterine system in menorrhagia: a systematic review. BJOG 2001;108:74–86.[52] © 2001, with permission from Elsevier Science)

Mirena versus other medical therapies

Only two of the randomised trials directly compared LNG IUS with other forms of medical treatment.[53,54] In the study by Irvine et al.[53] the efficacy and acceptability of the LNG IUS was compared with higher doses of norethisterone 5 mg three times daily, from days 5 to 26 of the cycle for three cycles. After three cycles, the reduction of menstrual blood loss by the LNG IUS was 94% and with oral norethisterone it was 87%. Seventy-six percent of the women in the LNG IUS group wished to continue with the treatment compared with 22% of the norethisterone group. It is interesting to note that, although 52% (10/19) in the LNG IUS group were still experiencing intermenstrual bleeding, a higher proportion of women than this objected to taking 64 tablets a month.[53]

In another randomised study, the mean menstrual blood loss reduction at 12 months was much higher with the LNG IUS, reducing blood loss by 96% compared with 21% with flurbiprofen and 44% with tranexamic acid.[54]

In the Cochrane Database review[61] no studies were found comparing intrauterine progesterone/progestogen with placebo or no treatment. In one small study Progestasert was compared with other medical treatments but no conclusions could be drawn on its effectiveness.

Use of Mirena to avoid surgery

A reduction in menstrual loss by the LNG IUS was demonstrated[58] in a group of 50 women who had failed medical therapy and were awaiting hysterectomy or trans-cervical resection of the endometrium. The treatment was so effective that it was possible to take 41 of these women off the waiting list (i.e. 82% were able to avoid major surgery). In another randomised controlled study of 56 women on the waiting list for hysterectomy for menorrhagia, 64% came off the list at six months because they were satisfied with their treatment, compared with only 14% of the control group (those continuing with current medical treatments).[55]

The results published in 2002 of Nagrani and Bowen-Simpkins'[62] 4–5-year long-term follow-up of the women recruited in their original study[58] demonstrated a continuation rate of 50% after a mean 54 months of follow-up. The more important observation from this study was that only 26.4% eventually underwent surgical treatment, despite 50% not continuing with the LNG IUS; overall, 67.4% avoided surgery.

Mirena versus endometrial resection

A randomised study on 75 premenopausal women published in 1997 compared the LNG IUS with endometrial resection.[56] A mean menstrual blood loss reduction of 79% with the LNG IUS at 12 months was significantly less than that achieved with endometrial resection (89%). Satisfaction was high in both: 85% and 94% in LNG IUS and resection groups respectively. Health related quality of life perception was not significantly different in the two treatment groups.

Another randomised study on 60 women reported a mean menstrual blood loss reduction of 90% with LNG IUS at one year compared with a 98% reduction for endometrial resection. The reduction was significant from baseline menstrual blood loss pretreatment but the difference was not statistically significant between the two groups.[57]

In a further randomised study,[63] treatment success was defined as a pictorial blood assessment chart score of ≤75 at 12 months. This was achieved in 67% (20/30) in the LNG IUS group and 90% (26/29) in the resection group. In a visual analogue scale assessment of the subjective

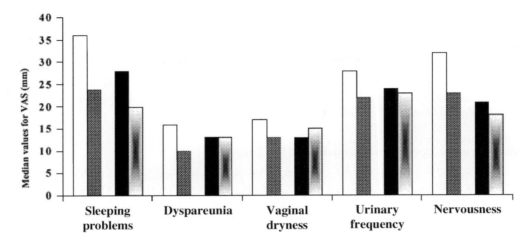

Figure 4 *Median values (mm) for visual analogue scale (VAS); open bars = baseline for LNG IUS; hatched bars = 12-month follow-up for LNG IUS; filled bars = baseline trans-cervical resection of the endometrium (TCRE); shaded bars =12-months follow-up for TCRE (reproduced from: Istre O, Trolle B. Treatment of menorrhagia with the levonorgestrel intrauterine system versus endometrial resection. Fertil Steril 2001;76:304–9.[63] © 2001, with permission from American Society for Reproductive Surgery)*

symptoms, sleeping problems were slightly improved in the trans–cervical resection of the endometrium group, a general feeling of genital health was increased, and menstrual pain decreased over time in both groups (Figures 4 and 5).

The SMART (Satisfaction with Mirena and Ablation) study aimed to determine women's

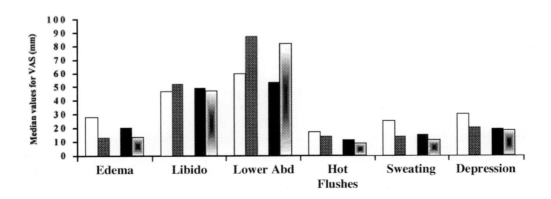

Figure 5 *Median values (mm) for visual analogue scale (VAS); open bars = baseline for LNG IUS; hatched bars = 12-month follow-up for LNG IUS; filled bars = baseline for trans-cervical resection of the endometrium (TCRE); shaded bars, 12-month follow-up for TCRE (reproduced from: Istre O, Trolle B. Treatment of menorrhagia with the levonorgestrel intrauterine system versus endometrial resection. Fertil Steril 2001;76:304–9.[63] © 2001, with permission from American Society for Reproductive Surgery)*

satisfaction and assessment of heaviness of bleeding by using pictorial charts at 12 months post-treatment. This study was terminated owing to a poor recruitment rate because of reluctance to be randomised to the Mirena arm.[64]

Johnson et al.[65] are more optimistic about a similar randomised trial, TALIS (Thermo-Ablation versus the Levonorgestrel Intrauterine System), in Auckland, where recruitment has been more successful. This is possibly owing to these women having a more favourable attitude towards research and the Mirena coil, to a better study design that allows more decision time and the use of one/two-stop menstrual disorder clinics in the research trial.

Mirena versus hysterectomy: quality of life issues

Hurskainen et al.[66] conducted a trial on quality of life and cost effectiveness of the LNG IUS versus hysterectomy for treatment of menorrhagia in 236 women. After 12 months, 68% of the women in the LNG IUS group continued to use the system, with 69% experiencing amenorrhoea or minimal bleeding. Twenty percent underwent hysterectomy in this group. Among those randomised for hysterectomy, 91% went on to have the operation. Health related quality of life and indices of psychosocial wellbeing improved significantly in both groups. There was no significant difference between the two groups except that women who underwent hysterectomy had less pain. Overall, costs were three times higher for the hysterectomy group than for the IUS group.[66]

PROBLEMS OF HORMONE-RELEASING INTRAUTERINE SYSTEMS

Fitting of systems

The initial drawback of both systems is their slightly wider diameter vertical stem, which is a consequence of the steroid reservoir. The insertion diameter is even greater in the case of the PIPS because the arms are initially folded down against the stem. These features can lead to difficulty in fitting of the systems, particularly in nulliparous women and may require some cervical dilatation prior to insertion. The requirement for dilatation can usually be determined at the time of uterine sounding, by judgement of the ease with which the sound passes. Should it be deemed necessary to dilate the cervix it is vital that adequate analgesia is administered first if the woman's confidence is to be retained and insertion is not to fail. This can usually be achieved either by the administration of a nonsteroidal analgesic (e.g. mefenamic acid 500 mg, one hour before insertion) or by use of a paracervical block via a dental syringe of either 1% lignocaine or 1% xylocaine without adrenaline five minutes before insertion. The same care should be taken when inserting the intrauterine systems as with other intrauterine devices; complications such as perforation, embedment, expulsion and fragmentation are all possible.

BLEEDING PROBLEMS

A problem with both the currently available intrauterine systems is that, even with a normal nonhyperplastic endometrium, it takes approximately three months for the endometrium to atrophy under the influence of the released hormone. During this time bleeding can be erratic and heavy at times but almost always settles after three to six months use.[67] Pre- and perimenopausal women experience more episodes of spotting and bleeding. Good counselling is vital if treatment discontinuation is to be avoided. It may be of benefit to use tranexamic acid for the first three months to reduce bleeding until atrophy of the endometrium has occurred under the influence of the intrauterine system hormone. If pathology has been excluded and bleeding continues for more than a year, it is unlikely that the system is not going to be effective and an alternative treatment should be sought.

Adverse progestogenic effects: physical and metabolic

In spite of the low constant serum levels of progestogen produced by the LNG IUS, some women still seem to experience adverse progestogenic effects. These can be both physical, such as oedema, headache, breast tenderness, acne and hirsuitism,[19] and metabolic, such as decreased low-density lipoprotein levels.[68] This is probably because of the 19-nortestosterone progestogen within the LNG IUS.

There appears to be no significant effect on carbohydrate metabolism, coagulation parameters or liver enzymes.[69] The physical effects have been shown to subside after the first few months of use. It is important that women are sympathetically counselled and reassured that most adverse effects are transient and reminded that the serum hormone levels are much lower than those produced by other hormonal contraceptives such as the progestogen-only pill. Adverse effects related to fluid retention such as oedema and bloating may respond to a mild diuretic such as 25 mg of either spironolactone or hydrochlorothiazide.[70] The addition of an androgen (e.g. a 100 mg testosterone implant every 6 months) may occasionally ameliorate breast tenderness.[71]

There do not appear to be adverse physical or psychological progestogenic effects with the PIPS and as such it is ideal for women who are exquisitely progestogen sensitive.

Functional ovarian cysts

Functional ovarian cysts have been shown to be more common in LNG IUS users than copper intrauterine contraceptive device users (1.2 versus 0.4 per 100 woman years).[72] This finding is not surprising considering the higher incidence of cysts in progestogen-only pill users. What must be remembered is that these cysts can almost always be managed conservatively.

Amenorrhoea

If inadequately counselled prior to insertion, a woman may regard the reduction in bleeding or the cessation of periods as being pathological. This has led to unnecessary system removal in some cases.[48,72] It is vital that patients and practitioners are aware that the amenorrhoea is purely due to a local effect of hormone on the endometrium producing atrophy. Women should be made aware of the health benefits of reduced bleeding. If a woman feels strongly about maintaining regular bleeds then the hormone releasing intrauterine systems are an inappropriate therapeutic option. As discussed earlier, ovulation is only rarely affected and oestrogen levels are identical in menstruating and nonmenstruating users.[16,17]

COST EFFECTIVENESS

The cost of the LNG IUS to the NHS is £99;[73] its licensed duration of use is five years, equating to just under £20 per year if used for the entire period. Other costs vary between primary care (insertion fees £54.70, follow-up visits £16.40) and secondary care (insertion fees £77, follow-up visits £52) removal and counselling.[74] LNG IUS costs in the primary care setting are lower than high-dose norethisterone or tranexamic acid, and in the secondary care setting they are higher than high-dose norethisterone but still cheaper than tranexamic acid.[73] The costs of hysterectomy are substantial, with average costs for 1997–1998 at £1702 and £547 for endometrial resection/ablation[35,52] in the same period. Hurskainen et al.[66] in an early report demonstrated the LNG IUS to be a cost-effective alternative to hysterectomy in the first year of use.

The direct costs incurred per woman from insertion or operation expenses, inpatient stay, readmissions, outpatient visits, travel, medications and productivity loss (absence from work) were significantly lower for the intrauterine system ($1530) compared with the hysterectomy group ($4222).[66]

The systematic review by Stewart et al.[52] was unable to establish cost effectiveness based on current available evidence from the five small randomised trials, where maximum study duration was one year for a product licensed for five years. However, the results of the continuing five-year follow-up of Hurskainen et al.'s study[75] need to be evaluated before firm conclusions can be drawn.

CONCLUSION AND FUTURE DEVELOPMENTS

The LNG IUS (Mirena) is a simple and effective alternative to the surgical management of menorrhagia and produces a concomitant reduction in surgical morbidity and mortality.[62] Fertility is preserved, reliable contraception provided and anaemia prevented. These are highly desirable benefits for women, particularly in developing countries, from a single procedure that requires only good insertion technique training and avoids the resources and training required for surgery.

The therapeutic effects are maintained for at least five years, and patient acceptability and continuation rates for use of the system are high. Minor adverse effects are common but are usually self-limiting and can be managed satisfactorily by counselling.

The use of natural progesterone as in Progestasert, and newer developments such as Fibro Plant, hold the potential to reduce the hormonal adverse effects experienced by some women on the currently available 20 μg/24 h releasing LNG IUS. Also, a lower dose LNG IUS (MLS®, Schering Health Care Ltd, Burgess Hill, West Sussex, UK); 10 μg/24 h) currently being developed for use in hormone replacement therapy may also be used in the treatment of menorrhagia. There is little compromise in efficacy of the contraceptive and menstrual blood reduction benefit with either Fibro Plant or MLS. Their flexible design allows them to adapt to cavities of every size, even if distorted, and the novel anchoring system reduces dislodgement and minimises complaints of pain, irregular bleeding and expulsion.[2,51] This can further improve compliance and satisfaction with treatment, thus reducing the need for hysterectomy for menorrhagia, which can be reserved for women with significant gynaecological disease.

Future work should focus on reinforcing efficacy and safety, and confirming the cost effectiveness of these systems through larger randomised controlled trials, thus building confidence among gynaecologists, general practitioners and patients concerning their first-line use for menorrhagia.

References

1.   Davie J. New hormone delivery systems. *Diplomate* 1996;3:184–90.
2.   Wildemeersch D, Schacht E. The effect on menstrual blood loss in women with uterine fibroids of a novel 'frameless' intrauterine levonorgestrel-releasing drug delivery system: a pilot study. *Eur J Obstet Gynecol Reprod Biol* 2002;102:74–9.
3.   Hurskainen R, Salmi A, Paavonen J, Teperi J, Rutanen E. Expression of sex steroid receptors and Ki-67 in the endometria of menorrhagic women: effects of intrauterine levonorgestrel. *Mol Hum Reprod* 2000;6:1013–18.

4. Maruo T, Laoag-Fernandez JB, Pakaninen P, Murakoshi H, Spitz IM, Johansson E. Effects of the levonorgestrel-releasing intrauterine system on proliferation and apoptosis in the endometrium. *Hum Reprod* 2001;16:2103–8.

5. Zalel Y, Shulman A, Lider A, Achiron R, Mashiach S, Gamzu R. The local progestational effect of the levonorgestrel-releasing intrauterine system: a sonographic and Doppler flow study. *Hum Reprod* 2002;17:2878–80.

6. Zhu P, Luo HZ, Xu RH, Cheng J, Wu SC, Chen JH, *et al.* The effect of intrauterine devices, the stainless steel ring, the copper T220, and releasing levonorgestrel, on the bleeding profile and the morphological structure of the human endometrium – a comparative study of three IUDs. A morphometric study of 96 cases. *Contraception* 1989;40:425–38.

7. Rutanen E, Hurskainen R, Finne P, Nokelainen K. Induction of endometrial plasminogen activator-inhibitor 1: a possible mechanism contributing to the effect of intrauterine levonorgestrel in the treatment of menorrhagia. *Fertil Steril* 2000;73:1020–4.

8. Rutanen EM, Salmi A, Nyman T. mRNA expression of insulin like growth factors (IGF-I) is suppressed and those of IGF-II and IGF-binding protein-1 are constantly expressed in the endometrium during the use of an intrauterine levonorgestrel system. *Mol Hum Reprod* 1997;3:749–54.

9. Zhu PD, Luo HZ, Shi WL, Wang JD, Cheng J, Xu GH, *et al.* Observation of the activity of factor VIII in the endometrium of women pre- and post-insertion of three types of IUDs. *Contraception* 1991;44:367–84.

10. Luukkainen T, Allonen H, Haukkamaa M, Lahteenmaki P, Nilsson CG, Toivonen J. Five years' experience with levonorgestrel releasing IUDs. *Contraception* 1986;33:139–48.

11. Silverberg SG, Haukkamaa M, Arko H, Nilsson CG, Luukkainen T. Endometrial morphology during long-term use of levonorgestrel-releasing intrauterine devices. *Int J Gynecol Pathol* 1986;5:235–41.

12. Nilsson CG, Lahteenmaki P. Recovery of ovarian function after the use of a d-norgestrel-releasing IUD. *Contraception* 1977;15:389–400.

13. Erickson RE, Mitchell C, Pharriss BB, Place VA. The intrauterine progesterone contraceptive system. In: *Advances in Planned Parenthood*. Princeton, NJ: Excerpta Medica; 1976. p. 167–74.

14. Hagenfeldt K, Landgren BM, Strom K, Johannisson E. Biochemical and morphological changes in the human endometrium induced by the Progestasert device. *Contraception* 1977;16:183–97.

15. Luukkainen T. Levonorgestrel-releasing intrauterine device. *Ann N Y Acad Sci* 1991;626:43–9.

16. Luukkainen T, Lahteenmaki P, Toivonen J. Levonorgestrel-releasing intrauterine device. *Ann Med* 1990;22:85–90.

17. Nilsson CG, Lahteenmaki PL, Luukkainen T. Ovarian function in amenorrheic and menstruating users of a levonorgestrel-releasing intrauterine device. *Fertil Steril* 1984;41:52–5.

18. Tillson SA, Marian M, Hudson R, Wong P, Pharriss B, Aznar R, *et al.* The effect of intrauterine progesterone on the hypothalamic–hypophyseal–ovarian axis in humans. *Contraception* 1975;11:179–92.

19. Wan LS, Hsu YC, Ganguly M, Bigelow B. Effects of the Progestasert on the menstrual pattern, ovarian steroids and endometrium. *Contraception* 1977;16:417–34.

20. Inki P, Hurskainen R, Palo P, Ejholm E, Grenman S, Kivela A, *et al.* Comparison of ovarian cyst formation in women using the levonorgestrel-releasing intrauterine system vs. hysterectomy. *Ultrasound Obstet Gynecol* 2002;20:381–5.

21. Diaz S, Pavez M, Miranda P, Johansson ED, Croxatto HB. Long term follow-up of women treated with Norplant implants. *Contraception* 1987;35:551–67.

22. Kuhnz W, al-Yacoub G, Fuhrmeister A. Pharmacokinetics of levonorgestrel and ethinylestradiol in 9 women who received a low-dose oral contraceptive over a treatment period of 3 months, and, after a wash-out phase, a single oral administration of the same contraceptive formulation. *Contraception* 1992;46:455–69.

23. Weiner E, Victor A, Johansson ED. Plasma levels of d-norgestrel after oral administration. *Contraception* 1976;14:563–70.

24. Nilsson CG, Lahteenmaki PL, Luukkainen T, Robertson DN. Sustained intrauterine release of levonorgestrel over five years. *Fertil Steril* 1986;45:805–7.

25. Reid B, Gangar K. The medical management of menorrhagia in general practice. *Diplomate* 1994;1:92–8.

26. McPherson A, Anderson AB, editors. *Women's Problems in General Practice*. Oxford: Oxford University Press; 1983. p. 21–41.

27. Bradlow J, Coulter A, Brooks P. *Patterns of Referral*. Oxford: Oxford Health Service Research Unit; 1992. p. 20–1.

28. Fraser IS, McCarron G, Markham R. A preliminary study of factors influencing perception of menstrual blood loss volume. *Am J Obstet Gynecol* 1984;149:788–93.

29. Chimbira TH, Anderson AB, Turnbull A. Relation between measured menstrual blood loss and patient's subjective assessment of loss, duration of bleeding, number of sanitary towels used, uterine weight and endometrial surface area. *Br J Obstet Gynaecol* 1980;87:603–9.

30. Higham JM, O'Brien PM, Shaw RW. Assessment of menstrual blood loss using a pictorial chart. *Br J Obstet Gynaecol* 1990;97:734–9.

31. Reid PC, Coker CA, Coltart R. Assessment of menstrual blood loss using a pictorial chart: a validation study. *BJOG* 2000;107:320–2.

32. Vessey MP, Villard-Mackintosh L, McPherson K, Coulter A, Yeates D. The epidemiology of hysterectomy: findings in a large cohort study. *Br J Obstet Gynaecol* 1992;99:402–7.

33. Coulter A, Bradlow J, Agass M, Martin-Bates C, Tulloch A. Outcomes of referrals to gynaecology outpatient clinics for menstrual problems: an audit of general practice records. *Br J Obstet Gynaecol* 1991;98:789–96.

34. Department of Health. *Hospital Episode Statistics: England Financial Year 1994–95,* Vol. 1. *Finished Consultant Episodes by Diagnosis Operation and Speciality.* London: HMSO; 1995.

35. National Health Service Executive. *National Schedule of Reference Costs: Collection of Retrospective Cost and Activity Data June 1999.* (HSC 1999/098.) London: Department of Health; 1999. Appendix 1A.

36. Dwyer N, Hutton J, Stirrat GM. Randomised controlled trial comparing endometrial resection with abdominal hysterectomy for the surgical treatment of menorrhagia. *Br J Obstet Gynaecol* 1993;100:237–43.

37. New Zealand Guideline Group. *Guidelines for Management of Heavy Menstrual Bleeding.* National Advisory Committee on Health and Disability. Wellington: National Health Committee; 1998.

38. Lilford RJ. Hysterectomy: will it pay the bills in 2007? *BMJ* 1997;314:160–1.

39. Coulter A, Peto V, Jenkinson C. Quality of life and patient satisfaction following treatment for menorrhagia. *Fam Pract* 1994;11:394–401.

40. Coulter A, Kelland J, Long A, O'Mears S. *The Management of Menorrhagia. Effective Health Care Bulletin,* Vol. 1, No. 9. London: RSM Press; 1995.

41. Varol N, Healey M, Tang P, Sheehan P, Maher P, Hill D. Ten-year review of hysterectomy morbidity and mortality: can we change direction? *Aust N Z J Obstet Gynaecol* 2001;41:295–302.

42. Duckitt K, Shaw RW. Is medical management of menorrhagia obsolete? *Br J Obstet Gynaecol* 1998;105:569–72.

43. Coulter A, Kelland J, Peto V, Rees MC. Treating menorrhagia in primary care. An overview of drug trials and a survey of prescribing practice. *Int J Technol Assess Health Care* 1995;11:456–71.

44. Bonnar J, Sheppard BL. Treatment of menorrhagia during menstruation: randomised controlled trial of ethamsylate, mefenamic acid, and tranexamic acid. *BMJ* 1996;313:579–82.

45. Fraser IS, McCarron G. Randomized trial of 2 hormonal and 2 prostaglandin-inhibiting agents in women with a complaint of menorrhagia. *Aust N Z J Obstet Gynaecol* 1991;31:66–70.

46. Chimbira TH, Cope E, Anderson AB, Bolton FG. The effect of danazol on menorrhagia, coagulation mechanisms, haematological indices and body weight. *Br J Obstet Gynaecol* 1979;86:46–50.

47. Thomas EJ, Okuda KJ, Thomas NM. The combination of a depot gonadotrophin releasing hormone agonist and cyclical hormone replacement therapy for dysfunctional uterine bleeding. *Br J Obstet Gynaecol* 1991;98:1155–9.

48. Andersson JK, Rybo G. Levonorgestrel-releasing intrauterine device in the treatment of menorrhagia. *Br J Obstet Gynaecol* 1990;97:690–4.

49. Tang GW, Lo SS. Levonorgestrel intrauterine device in the treatment of menorrhagia in Chinese women: efficacy versus acceptability. *Contraception* 1995;51:231–5.

50. Bergqvist A, Rybo G. Treatment of menorrhagia with intrauterine release of progesterone. *Br J Obstet Gynaecol* 1983;90:255–8.

51. Wildemeersch D, Schacht E. Treatment of menorrhagia with a novel 'frameless' intrauterine levonorgestrel-releasing drug delivery system: a pilot study. *Eur J Contracept Reprod Health Care* 2001;6:93–101.

52. Stewart A, Cummins C, Gold L, Jordan R, Phillipson W. The effectiveness of the levonorgestrel-releasing intrauterine system in menorrhagia: a systematic review. *BJOG* 2001;108:74–86.

53. Irvine GA, Campbell-Brown MB, Lumsden MA, Heikkila A, Walker JJ, Cameron IT. Randomised comparative trial of the levonorgestrel intrauterine system and norethisterone for treatment of idiopathic menorrhagia. *Br J Obstet Gynaecol* 1998;105:592–8.

54. Milsom I, Anderson K, Andersch B, Rybo G. A comparison of flurbiprofen, tranexamic acid, and a levonorgestrel-releasing intrauterine contraceptive device in the treatment of idiopathic menorrhagia. *Am J Obstet Gynecol* 1991;164:879–83.

55. Lahteenmaki P, Haukkamaa M, Puolakka J, Riikonen U, Sainio S, Suvisaari J, *et al.* Open randomised study of use of levonorgestrel releasing intrauterine system as alternative to hysterectomy. *BMJ* 1998;316:1122–6.

56. Crosignani PG, Vercellini P, Mosconi P, Oldani S, Cortesi I, De Giorgio O. Levonorgestrel-releasing intrauterine device versus hysteroscopic endometrial resection in the treatment of dysfunctional uterine bleeding. *Obstet Gynecol* 1997;90:257–63.

57. Kittelsen N, Istre O. A randomized study comparing levonorgestrel intrauterine system and the transcervical resection of the endometrium in the treatment of menorrhagia: preliminary results. *Gynecol Endosc* 1998;7:61–5.

58. Barrington JW, Bowen-Simpkins P. The levonorgestrel intrauterine system in the management of menorrhagia. *Br J Obstet Gynaecol* 1997;104:614–16.

59. Fedele L, Bianchi S, Raffaelli R, Portuese A, Dorta M. Treatment of adenomyosis-associated menorrhagia with a levonorgestrel-releasing intrauterine device. *Fertil Steril* 1997;68:426–9.

60. Scholten PC, Christiaens GC, Haspels AA. Treatment of menorrhagia by intrauterine administration of levonorgestrel. In: Scholten PC, editor. *The Levonorgestrel IUD: Clinical Performance and Impact on Menstruation*. Utrecht: Utrecht University Hospital; 1989. p. 47–55.

61. Lethaby AE, Cooke I, Rees M. Progesterone/progestogen releasing intrauterine systems versus either placebo or any other medication for heavy menstrual bleeding. *Cochrane Database Syst Rev* 2000;(2):CD002126.

62. Nagrani R, Bowen-Simpkins P, Barrington JW. Can the levonorgestrel intrauterine system replace surgical treatment for the management of menorrhagia? *BJOG* 2002;109:345–7.

63. Istre O, Trolle B. Treatment of menorrhagia with the levonorgestrel intrauterine system versus endometrial resection. *Fertil Steril* 2001;76:304–9.

64. Rogerson L, Duffy S, Crocombe W, Stead M, Dasu D. Management of menorrhagia – SMART study (Satisfaction with Mirena and Ablation: a Randomised Trial). *BJOG* 2000;107:1325–6.

65. Johnson N, Busfield N, Sadler L, Lethaby A, Farquhar C. The management of menorrhagia – SMART study (Satisfaction with Mirena and Ablation: a Randomised Trial). *BJOG* 2001;108:773–4.

66. Hurskainen R, Tepen J, Rissanen P, Aalto AM, Grenman S, Kivela A, *et al.* Quality of life and cost-effectiveness of levonorgestrel-releasing intrauterine system versus hysterectomy for treatment of menorrhagia: a randomised trial. *Lancet* 2001;357:273–7.

67. Nilsson CG, Lahteenmaki P, Luukkainen T. Levonorgestrel plasma concentrations and hormone profiles after insertion and after one year of treatment with a levonorgestrel-IUD. *Contraception* 1980;21:225–33.

68. Raudaskoski TH, Tomas EI, Paakkari IA, Kauppila AJ, Laatikainen TJ. Serum lipids and lipoproteins in postmenopausal women receiving transdermal oestrogen in combination with a levonorgestrel-releasing intrauterine device. *Maturitas* 1995;22:47–53.

69. Luukkainen T. Levonorgestrel-releasing IUCD. *Br J Fam Plann* 1991;19:221–4.

70. Gambrell RD. Progestogens in estrogen replacement therapy. In: Peterson CM, editor. *Clinical Obstetrics and Gynaecology.* Philadelphia, PA: Lippincott-Raven; 1995. p. 890–901.

71. Dimitrakakis C, Zhou J, Wang J, Belanger A, LaBrie F, Cheng C, *et al.* A Physiologic role for testosterone in limiting estrogenic stimulation of the breast. *Menopause* 2003;10;292–8.

72. Sivin I, Stern J. Health during prolonged use of levonorgestrel 20 micrograms/d and the copper TCu 380 Ag intrauterine contraceptive devices: a multicenter study. International Committee for Contraception Research (ICCR). *Fertil Steril* 1994;61:70–77.

73. British Medical Association, Royal Pharmaceutical Society of Great Britain. *British National Formulary* 2003;(46): ss 7.3.2.

74. Department of Health, Welsh Office. National Health Service General Medical Services. *Statement of Fees and Allowances Payable to General Medical Practitioners in England and Wales.* London: HMSO, 1999.

75. Hurskainen R, Paavonen J, Teperi J. The effectiveness of the levonorgestrel-releasing intrauterine system in menorrhagia: a systematic review. *BJOG* 2003;110 87–8.

30

The psychology of the infertile couple

Michael Pawson

PREAMBLE

A woman who was on clomifene for hypothalamic anovulation returns to the fertility clinic for review and breaks down in tears. Her husband has become impotent, but only when he knows she is ovulating. He is treated successfully but then she in turn loses all interest in sex at the time of ovulation. Why? Why had she stopped ovulating previously? Was there a deep subconscious barrier preventing her from conceiving for good reasons that were then overridden by clomifene and she had to find another way of avoiding conception?

A Roman Catholic woman had unexplained infertility in her two marriages of six and seven years respectively. Why? One day she has a violent emotional catharsis in the clinic and shares with me the secret that she has hidden from the world for 18 years. She had procured an illegal abortion at the age of 17. She had passed the gestation sac and foetus during the night while her parents were asleep in the next room. She broke the tissue up and flushed it all down the toilet. Two years later she came home from college to find her father dying on the floor of the same toilet and being administered the last rites. 'Now you know why I can't conceive', she cried. Her religious sense of guilt was profound and she insisted on going on the pill as a sort of self-inflicted punishment. However, she found a priest to whom she felt she could confess and seek absolution. She then came off the pill, conceived within a few cycles and again two years later. Why? How?

A Buddhist couple with ten years of infertility sadly admitted that their marriage was unconsummated. Why? The woman had been sexually abused by her grandfather's servant as a child. Both partners received psychosexual counselling and she conceived by artificial insemination by the husband. Her second conception was natural.

A political refugee from Columbia had secondary infertility. Her banker husband had agreed to give evidence in a drug trial. When she was at 20 weeks in her first pregnancy she received threats through the post that the dealers would 'get' her baby in revenge. She went into premature labour that week and lost her baby. Why could she not now conceive again? There was nothing physically wrong, but she did finally conceive by *in vitro* fertilisation.

In addressing the title of this chapter I am taking psychology to mean both the conscious and the unconscious nature and functioning of the mind. This inevitably includes emotions and feelings.

It would seem to be 'natural', in the sense of being related to nature, to want children. It is therefore probably normal to be distressed if one is not able to conceive. The concept of what is normal, however, changes and it is becoming more normal for couples and individuals to choose not to have children.

THE MOTIVATION TO CONCEIVE

What it is that motivates us to reproduce is more complicated than it appears superficially. The reasons that women in particular give on attending a fertility clinic are that they are ready for a child, that a child will be something that completes and cements their relationship with their partner. Other reasons less frequently voiced are that it is natural to have children, that it is normal and what most people do. Occasionally the couple are responding to their own parents' need for grandchildren. As Adam Phillips[1] has pointed out, contemporary culture has a longing for sameness and there is a need and a desire to be the same as other people, and most people want and have children. As an aside, cloning, if it ever becomes established, will solve the problem of being different. That a sheep was the first animal to be cloned seems appropriate.

There is, however, a more profound motive, which is an attempt to achieve a degree of immortality by perpetuating ourselves. Spinoza remarked that 'everything endeavours to persist in its own being' and Plato was even more specific: 'What is lost and what decays always leaves behind a fresh copy of itself. This is the mechanism by which mortal creatures can taste immortality so it is not surprising that everything naturally values its own offspring. They all feel this concern, and this love, because of their desire for immortality.'

Human beings are the only creatures with foreknowledge of their own death. This foreknowledge goes back in legend to the Garden of Eden when Eve plucked the apple from the tree of knowledge and Man then paid the price of understanding his mortality. As the angel said on expelling Adam and Eve from Eden: 'Thou shalt surely die.'

There are a number of givens in our existence, which include:

• the inevitability of death

• that we are alone in this world

• that there is no known purpose or meaning to our lives.

To some extent a child will alleviate these existential problems (but not cure them). A child will be the nearest most of us get to immortality, will dilute our aloneness and will provide some purpose in our lives.

We are safeguarded from the awareness of our mortality and from the other fears of our existence by two protective mechanisms. One is the belief that 'I am different, I am special', which is true genetically and experientially, but in no other way. This is the belief of the smoker that 'It won't happen to me', and of the career woman who delays pregnancy in the belief that she will be able to conceive easily at age 40. This very important defence mechanism is destroyed by failing to conceive. Not getting pregnant confronts you with the distressing realisation that you are not different, you are not special.

The second defence is that, even if you are in trouble or difficulty, you will be rescued. For those with a religious belief it is their God, and if they do not conceive they can blame their God. For others, their salvation or rescuer will be medicine, the doctor. When treatment fails this is also very traumatic because the person has not been rescued.

Then there is the problem of our aloneness, our existential isolation. Infertility may confront us with this in a very painful way.

Finally, for many women a very important purpose in their life is to have a child. If this does not happen they are left questioning why they are here at all. How often in a fertility clinic does a woman express the feeling that if she is not going to have a child then what is her life about?

For some, religious belief still provides a refuge from death by the reassurance of an afterlife. The rapid decline of Christian belief, spawned by Darwin's observations in an increasingly secular and scientific world, has removed that reassurance for many. We are now confronted by our mortality and a conviction that our life is finite. The immortality of a Mozart or Picasso is assured, but for most of us our only chance of immortality is to procreate. Failure to do so exposes us to the unavoidable recognition of our mortality and of our finitude.

AMBIVALENCE

Even for those who are prepared to go to extreme lengths, there is still a degree of ambivalence about having a child and the commitment involved. Sacrifices have to be made. A child costs money and may not turn out to conform to the idealised picture that the couple, particularly the woman, have had in their minds. A child is demanding and dependent. A woman or man may have to sacrifice career ambitions to accommodate a child. Such ambivalence is normal and it is important that it is recognised by the woman and that her doctor is reassuring to her about it.

There are other good reasons against having a child. A woman may want to prove her fertility by conceiving but then not feel able to face all that is subsequently involved. She may be fearful of labour, of having an unhealthy or stillborn child, either through her own experience or that of others, especially her own mother. Her own experience of being mothered may be painful and unhappy and many infertile women describe a poor relationship with their own mother. It may be that as many women who do conceive have a similar background but they have successfully come to terms with it. The infertile woman's relationship with her own mother is an important area to discuss with her in the initial history. Fears of repeating her own mother's failures and deficiencies may be very relevant to her not conceiving.

The woman who is able to recognise her own ambivalence and discuss it objectively will be easier to treat than the woman who pursues conception with a frenetic need and is unable to consider a patient 'wait and see' approach. There is also some evidence that women who recognise their ambivalence will cope better with parenting in the future.

DIFFERENCE BETWEEN VOLUNTARY AND INVOLUNTARY CHILDLESS COUPLES

Changes in social mores and the advances in and widespread acceptance of contraception have given women much more control over their fertility. They have separated the pleasure from the reproductive side of lovemaking. They have allowed women the choice of voluntary childlessness or delaying motherhood while they follow a career. Couples choosing to remain childless do not appear to be more materialistic or selfish than those who do have children. Some studies have suggested that voluntarily childless couples are happier in their marriages, more self-reliant and more aware of individual freedom. Voluntarily childless couples seem mature and contented.

Fertile women, those who want to have children and succeed, are still the 'normal'; they conform to the concept of the normal woman. They are confronted by all the difficulties and disadvantages of children but sustained by the fulfilment they experience.

It is those who want to conceive and do not succeed, involuntarily infertile women, who suffer emotionally. There is often an underlying guilt in their depression, their sadness and sometimes their remorse, where the cause of the infertility is apparent. Commonly, there is a pelvic infection from a previous relationship, or pregnancy has been deferred for career or material reasons, and now, suddenly, the biological clock has caught up with them. These are the women who are panicked inappropriately into assisted conception and pursue conception with a desperate consuming need. They need to talk their feelings through in the fertility clinic, preferably with a trained counsellor, to get a perspective on the problem that is free of guilt.

HOW DOES THE PSYCHE CONTRIBUTE TO FAILURE TO CONCEIVE?

The role of the psyche is difficult to explore scientifically. Is a problem in the psyche responsible for the infertility or is it the infertility that is causing the depression or psychopathology? The demand of science for proof in response to a hypothesis is very difficult to answer in this area. Indeed, the oldest and most fundamental problem of science is how one does arrive at the truth. Absolute truth is neither self-evident nor is it reached through belief or tradition. It was once regarded as absolute truth that the world was flat and that it was also the centre of the universe. At one time everybody believed it and everybody was wrong. In medicine, bloodletting was a cure. Such universal beliefs were wrong and the certain truths of today's medicine will as surely be disproved or adjusted in the future. Equally, what may be regarded as scientifically invalid or uncertain may become the truth of the future.

As we learn more about neuroendocrinology and brain function, some answers may start to appear to help to explain the role of the psyche in infertility. An example that I use with my patients is to ask them what they would think if a young female relative lost her husband and two children in a road accident and then had no periods for six months. I then go on to say that there are other less obvious conscious and subconscious areas in the much less obviously traumatised psyche that have a less dramatic effect than amenorrhoea but which still may affect neuroendocrine function.

In the few brief cases described at the beginning, I cannot prove that there was a psychological factor in their infertility, but neither can anyone prove that this is not the case. Although it is entirely appropriate that there should be a scientific and logical approach to the problem of infertility, it is also appropriate to apply experience and an instinctive feeling about psychological background to the management of the patient.

THE PSYCHOLOGICAL EFFECT IN THE MALE

The psyche affects male fertility through failure of sexual function, impotence, failure to sustain an erection and premature ejaculation. Although it is well recognised that lifestyle, alcohol, drugs, smoking, diet etc. affect the quality of the semen, it is not clear what effect the psyche may have. A history of sexual function is essential in the initial consultation. If there is a problem with the male partner, my practice has been to discuss it with the couple, then to refer the partner to a male fertility specialist, and after that for psychosexual counselling if appropriate. It is not uncommon for an impotent male to be able to masturbate and, provided that there is no contraindication, artificial insemination by the husband is an easy treatment for the infertility. Very occasionally the fact that his partner is visibly pregnant may cure the impotence. My experience of psychological impotence in the male is small; maybe these men seek advice elsewhere, do not marry or deliberately seek a platonic relationship. Impotence with a medical aetiology requires appropriate treatment for the underlying condition.

Failure to achieve pregnancy and the demands of the clinic, doctors and the female partner may often affect the male. Sex 'on demand' at ovulation may induce impotence at that time and certainly removes spontaneity and much of the pleasure of lovemaking. All those who have worked in *in vitro* fertilisation clinics will be familiar with the situation where the normal healthy male is unable to produce a specimen at the critical time. The feeling of failure in him and of being let down in his partner is intense and can be very destructive to the relationship.

The effect of stress, of the psyche, on the quality of semen and spermatogenesis is little researched. A bizarre report by Stieve[2] claimed that, at autopsy, the testicles of men executed for rape showed complete absence of spermatogenesis. De Watteville[3] reported reduced quality of semen in samples collected by masturbation as opposed to postcoital vaginal samples. It is also interesting that the semen analysis may improve a long time after all treatment has stopped. The psyche as a possible factor in the quality of semen remains a wide open area for research. The effect of the psyche on ovulation is so well recognised that it would be surprising if there was not a comparable effect in the male.

THE PSYCHOLOGICAL EFFECT IN THE FEMALE

The cortical–hypothalamic–pituitary–ovarian axis is vulnerable to psychological factors manifested by amenorrhoea and anovulation at its most obvious. Less obvious trauma and less obvious effects may still reduce fertility in ways that we do not understand. Women who are not ovulating should have a full psychosexual and family history taken before being treated with fertility drugs. Without a full psychological history, the doctor overrides nature at his or her peril.

The woman's own experience of parenting or mothering is often bad. A patient of the author who had been trying to conceive for seven years gave a history that her own twin had been stillborn, another sibling died of meningitis at three weeks, her parents separated when she was aged 16, and she had been raped at 18. I would not advocate that such a patient should not be offered conventional treatment for her infertility, but I would say that she should be referred to an experienced counsellor both before and during treatment. If she is reluctant I would try very hard to persuade her.

A woman's own experience of stillbirth, miscarriage or abortion may make her recognise that she does not want to conceive again. Such events, however, may inhibit her fertility without she herself recognising this. It is the responsibility of the doctor treating her to uncover such a history with probing but sensitive questions and explore it with her. If she rejects such a discussion, so be it, and for some women past trauma is best left buried, but for many it is a relief to share previous emotional pain and I believe that this can have a direct beneficial effect on their fertility.

Women and men have two levels of existence. On a superficial level we interact with the external, the physical and the secular. At a deeper level we interact with the nonmaterial, with ideals and with the spiritual. In all of medicine, and especially in the area of infertility, a patient has spiritual needs and, if these needs are unrecognised and not understood and discussed, the treatment and management will be incomplete.

MANAGEMENT OF THE PSYCHOLOGY OF INFERTILITY

I want now to focus on the management of infertility, on the approach that I think should be taken with all couples attending a fertility clinic and which should encourage the patient to open up about areas where there may be a psychological problem.

The doctor's approach to the patient has been based on the dualistic concept that started with Descartes (1596–1650). Before Descartes a patient was cared for by a healer, a doctor who saw the person as a whole, as a soul, a psyche and a body. The Cartesian philosophy divided science from religion, body from spirit, and the objective realm of facts and knowledge from the subjective realm of feelings, values and aesthetics. The healer who cared for the whole person therefore began to be replaced by the priest who cared for the soul, and medical progress has meant that doctors have concentrated increasingly on the body. Modern subspecialisation has led to management and treatment of infertile people that has become ever more reductionist.

The woman who seeks advice for her infertility will thus be perceived as a failing reproductive system and, within that system, a uterus, tubes, ovaries, hypothalamus and pituitary. The emphasis of investigation, treatment (and research) is increasingly reductionist. Now that subfertility is recognised as a specialty, couples will see fewer doctors than was once the case but the emphasis on the body remains. There is the advantage of this reductionist specialisation in that a doctor who is practising one skill all the time is likely to have better results than one who is mixing several skills.

I advocate that infertility would be better managed if we, the doctors, focused our attention on the whole person within the context of his or her family, culture and environment.

This is not a substitute for subspecialisation, but should complement it. Background culture is of increasing importance in our multicultural society. For some cultures secondary infertility means having no male child regardless of how many female children there may be. The perceived failure of a woman to produce a male child may be grounds to take another wife. Family, community and cultural pressures may be intense on a woman and must be understood and taken into account in the management. For example, the strict observance of the Jewish laws in relation to coitus and bleeding may be a major problem for the Jewish woman with intermenstrual or irregular bleeding.

I hope that I have made a case for a 'holistic' approach to the infertile couple. I want now to enlarge on that approach and make a plea for a serious consideration and application of the 'art' of medicine. I repeat that I do not criticise a scientific, reductionist approach, but I do believe that we must include in that approach what comes under the now, sadly, rather old fashioned term, 'the art of medicine'.

Hippocrates had some wise observations to make in respect of the medical art. He wrote that 'there are as many different diseases as patients'. If three women attend the clinic with a diagnosis of polycystic ovaries, they themselves are not all the same just because their hormone profiles, ultrasound scans and complaints are identical. They may come from different cultures; they will have different family backgrounds and different stresses within relationships and careers. There is a great temptation to see them under one polycystic ovaries heading and to treat them the same, but of course they are not the same. The Canadian novelist, Robertson Davies,[4] expressed this very well when one of his doctor characters reassured his patient that she was unique and that no one had ever suffered like her before because no one had ever been her before. We all recognise that every woman troubled by infertility is different physically, but the psyche is different also.

Hippocrates further said that the art of medicine involved the 'complete removal of the distress of the sick'. All too often we perceive sickness in general and infertility in particular as purely a somatic problem, but distress is also emotional and a problem of the psyche. There is a rider to the complete removal of the distress of sick people and Hippocrates urges his pupils to recognise that everything is not always possible to medicine. In treating the infertile couple there are sadly a lot of failures. The imperatives of our political masters that force us to aim for the maximal rather than the optimal, to see as many patients as possible, and to measure 'success' in league tables, mean that failures are rapidly forgotten and discarded. They are dropped in a medical wastepaper basket because no doctor likes to be confronted by failure. However, such patients merit our concern and care even more if we cannot help them, and one of the great gaps in our care of infertile couples is in helping those who do not and cannot conceive. Many women have a mental picture of the baby they believe they will have and losing that baby means that they go through a period of mourning; they grieve for the baby they are not going to have after all. We have come to recognise grief and mourning in relation to stillbirth and even miscarriage; we need to acknowledge and help a similar grief when all our efforts in the fertility clinic have finally failed.

In order to give care to the couple with infertility that incorporates both the psyche and the soma I want to offer a few guidelines that I hope will not appear too didactic or patronising.

Knowledge

No one can treat infertility without scientific knowledge of the subject but, as reductionism shows us, we cannot know everything. It is important to be aware of what you do not know and refer appropriately. This applies most especially in the area of the psychology of infertility and all specialist clinics now have a counsellor. Many doctors find it difficult to talk to patients about the emotions, if only sometimes because of the time it takes, but the counsellor is trained and equipped to deal with this aspect.

Observation

Looking at the woman when she enters the consulting room will often give clues about her feelings. If her partner has come too, their interactions will tell you a lot about their relationship. Thresholds are important in our lives, birth and death especially, and crossing the threshold of a hospital consulting room is a threatening and anxious experience for most people. If the computer on your desk has not completely taken you over, greeting the patient at the threshold and sitting her down goes a long way towards easing her anxiety and thereby obtaining a better history.

Listening

A full history may tell you more than numerous investigations; it certainly will do so about the patient's emotional state. Many years ago an editorial in the *British Medical Journal* stated that the most important diagnostic tool in medicine is the spoken word. The principle of this is still true and too often forgotten. A patient was referred to my clinic with a diagnosis of unexplained secondary infertility. What the referral letter failed to state was that the woman had her only child at the age of 16 after running away from a very unhappy and abusive home, the father of the child took it back to his own country at six months, and 17 years later she had still never seen her child again. I would not call such infertility unexplained, however normal the investigations had been. A proper listening history would have told the referring doctor a great deal more than all the investigations he had done.

CONCLUSION

One of the traditional symbols of medicine is the staff or caduceus of Hermes around which two snakes are entwined. The story goes that Hermes came across the two snakes fighting furiously on the ground and he thrust his staff between them. Harmony and peace were established as each serpent climbed the staff. One snake represents science, knowledge, what you learn and acquire, the other wisdom, what you take to your medicine. Both should be part of the doctor's makeup.

All sickness or 'dis-ease' is part soma and part psyche, although the ratio varies. In infertility the woman with extensive endometriosis or bilateral tubal damage has a predominantly somatic condition but the psyche will be much affected. The woman with unexplained infertility may have a significant psychological element manifesting itself as a somatic condition. The psyche is profoundly affected by infertility and may also be a major aetiological factor in not conceiving. We will serve our patients best if we remember this during the investigation and treatment of infertility and also after treatment if it is finally abandoned without success.

References

1.   Phillips A. *Darwin's Worms.* London: Penguin; 1999.
2.   Stieve H. *Der Einfluss des Nervensystems auf Bau und Tätigkeit der Geschlechtsorgane des Menschen.* Stuttgart: Thieme; 1952.
3.   de Watteville H. Psychologic factors in the treatment of sterility. *Fertil Steril* 1957;8:12–24.
4.   Davies R. *The Deptford Trilogy.* London: Penguin; 1983.

31

Reducing mother to child transmission of HIV-1 infection: the role of anti-retroviral therapy and caesarean delivery

Catherine Peckham, Pat Tookey and Marie-Louise Newell

INTRODUCTION

Most paediatric HIV infections are acquired through mother to child transmission (vertical transmission) and it has been estimated that, in 2002, worldwide there were 800 000 children aged less than 15 years newly infected with HIV, with 2000 infants acquiring infection each day.[1] More than 95% of these infections arise in sub-Saharan Africa where the prevalence of HIV in the pregnant population reaches 25% or higher in some settings. In these countries, paediatric infections continue to occur because few HIV infected women have access to prenatal testing and intervention programmes are not generally available.

The overall management of pregnancy is similar for HIV infected and uninfected women but specific HIV related issues need to be considered. In this chapter we focus our discussion on the role of anti-retroviral therapy and mode of delivery in the management of HIV infected women living in countries where antenatal testing is widespread and interventions to reduce mother to child transmission are routinely available. When making decisions about the management of delivery, knowledge of the woman's HIV clinical and immunological status and her anti-retroviral treatment history are essential, as well as results of laboratory investigations such as viral load. The proven benefit of interventions to reduce mother to child transmission has resulted in increased efforts to ensure that women are identified in pregnancy. In 2002, a panel of experts produced consensus recommendations for the management of HIV infection in pregnancy and in newborns that are appropriate to European healthcare systems.[2,3] British HIV/AIDS Association guidelines[4] and US recommendations[5] on the use of anti-retroviral drugs in pregnant women with HIV infection and interventions to reduce vertical transmission are also available.

NEWLY ACQUIRED PAEDIATRIC HIV INFECTION IN EUROPE

Heterosexual contact is now the most frequent transmission mode for adults in Western Europe, accounting for nearly half of all cases of newly diagnosed HIV reported in 2002.[5] The prevalence of HIV infection in pregnant women is generally less than 1% but this varies widely between and within European countries. There has been, for example, a rise in the overall HIV prevalence among pregnant women in the UK, with a ten-fold higher prevalence in London compared with elsewhere (Figure 1).[6]

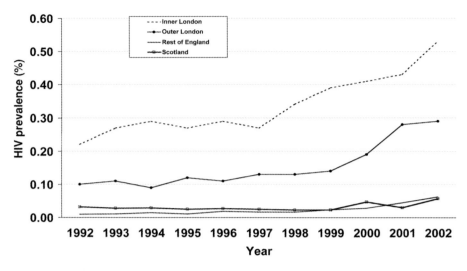

Figure 1 *Trends in prevalence of HIV infection in pregnant women in England and Scotland 1999–2002; data derived from the Unlinked Anonymous HIV Prevalence Monitoring Programme (adapted from: Health Protection Agency, SCIEH, ISD, National Public Health Service for Wales, CDSC Northern Ireland and the UASSG. Renewing the Focus. HIV and Other Sexually Transmitted Infections in the United Kingdom in 2002. London: Health Protection Agency; 2003,[6] used with permission from the Health Protection Agency)*

Risk of mother to child transmission

In the absence of interventions, the risk of mother to child transmission of HIV infection ranges from 15% to 40%.[7] It is likely that this range reflects not only differences in the stage of the epidemic but, more importantly, breastfeeding rates and duration. Indeed, of the 800 000 infants infected annually through mother to child transmission, it is estimated that more than a third acquire infection through breastfeeding. In Europe and North America, interventions to reduce mother to child transmission have had a major impact on the number of new cases of paediatric HIV infection and, with anti-retroviral therapy, elective caesarean section and refraining from breastfeeding, the rate of vertical transmission has been substantially reduced to less than 2%.

Factors associated with an increased risk of vertical transmission of HIV include: maternal progression of infection as measured by peripheral viral load or clinical and immunological markers; obstetric factors, including mode of delivery and rupture of the membranes; and breastfeeding.[8] Mothers with advanced clinical HIV disease or immune suppression are three times more likely to transmit infection than those who are clinically and immunologically normal. Both HIV RNA viral load and CD4 cell counts are independently associated with risk of transmission. For example, women with CD4 counts below 200 cells/ml are three times more likely to transmit HIV infection than those with higher cell counts, and women with a viral load above 100 000 copies per millilitre are four times more likely to transmit HIV than those with a lower viral load.[9–12] An elective caesarean delivery performed before the onset of labour and rupture of the membranes can substantially reduce the vertical transmission rate.[13] Premature delivery before 38 weeks of gestation is also associated with increased rates of vertical transmission.[14,15]

There are several possible mechanisms by which intrapartum transmission could occur. These include microtransfusions of maternal blood into the fetus during intrauterine contractions, infection of the amniotic fluid after rupture of the membranes, and ingestion of virus during labour through direct contact between the infant's skin and mucous membranes and maternal genital secretions. Although other obstetric factors such as the use of fetal scalp electrodes, intrapartum haemorrhage, episiotomy and vaginal tears have also been implicated, findings are not consistent across studies and their role remains unclear. Nevertheless, for women known to be HIV infected it is prudent to avoid invasive procedures whenever possible.[3,4]

The role of chorioamnionitis or the presence of other sexually transmitted diseases deserves consideration because these infections could act indirectly by precipitating early onset of labour, itself a risk factor, by causing an increase in viral load in the genital tract, or by increasing the friability of the placenta and facilitating virus replication. However, in terms of risk factors for vertical transmission in developed countries, these roles are less relevant.

The timing of vertical transmission

The infant may become infected *in utero*, during labour and delivery, or through breastfeeding. Knowledge of timing of mother to child transmission is important because it has a direct impact on the design and success of preventive strategies. A significant proportion of perinatal HIV transmission occurs during the intrapartum period. Based on the detection of the HIV-1 genome within 48 hours of delivery, by polymerase chain reaction or virus isolation, an estimated 35–40% of non-breastfed infants are infected *in utero*, most of these in late pregnancy.[16] In a review of the timing of mother to child transmission, Newell[17] concluded that about one-third of non-breastfed infants acquire HIV infection *in utero*, and the remaining two-thirds in the intrapartum period. In breastfeeding populations, less than a quarter acquire infection *in utero*, around half in the intrapartum period, and about one-third postpartum. These estimates are based on information gathered prior to the introduction of anti-retroviral prophylaxis and, with the introduction of interventions to reduce transmission, the proportion of infants acquiring infection at the different stages will be altered.

PREVENTION OF MOTHER TO CHILD TRANSMISSION

In the light of knowledge about the timing and risk factors for vertical transmission, approaches to prevention include: the reduction of maternal viral load through anti-retroviral therapy, elective caesarean section to avoid contamination with maternal vaginal secretions during passage through the birth canal, and the avoidance of infant exposure to HIV through breastfeeding.

Anti-retroviral therapy

In 1994, the results from a randomised placebo controlled trial (ACTG 076) demonstrated that zidovudine administered to HIV infected pregnant women starting at between 14 and 34 weeks of gestation, then intravenously during delivery and orally to the newborn for the first six weeks of life, reduced the risk of transmission of HIV from mothers to infants from 26% to 8% in a non-breastfeeding population.[18] This schedule was rapidly introduced into practice in Europe and North America, and was soon shown to be effective in the general HIV infected pregnant population. A subsequent placebo controlled trial of a short course regimen of zidovudine given during late pregnancy and labour in Thailand demonstrated a 51% reduction in vertical transmission in formula fed infants.[9] Two similar trials of short-course zidovudine in predominately breastfeeding populations in the Cote d'Ivoire and Burkina Faso also demonstrated effectiveness.[9,19] Subsequently, four different zidovudine schedules were compared in a non-breastfeeding population in Thailand.[20] Treatment started at either 28 weeks or at 35 weeks of pregnancy and was continued with a three-day or six-week postnatal regimen for the infant. The short pregnancy and infant regimens were significantly less effective than the longer regimens and were discontinued at the first interim analysis, whereas the other three arms of the trial (long-short, short-long, long-long) showed comparable transmission rates of between 6% and 8%. Observational studies suggest that, when women receive no antepartum or intrapartum zidovudine therapy, postexposure prophylaxis given to the neonate within 72 hours of birth reduces vertical transmission.[21,22]

Several trials have assessed the efficacy of anti-retroviral therapy given around the time of delivery. The HIVNET012 study[23] compared the efficacy of two short regimens: a single oral dose of nevirapine given to the mother at the start of labour, and to the infant within 72 hours of birth, compared with zidovudine given orally to the mother during labour and to the infant for one week. The transmission rate at 14–16 weeks in the nevirapine arm was significantly lower than in the zidovudine arm, with a relative efficacy of nearly 50%. In a South African trial,[24] two regimens starting from onset of labour were compared: a nevirapine regimen similar to that used in HIVNET012 (with an additional postpartum dose for the mother), and zidovudine plus lamivudine from onset of labour to one week postpartum for the mother and for one week for the infant. Transmission rates with the two regimens were similar at 12.3% and 9.3% at eight weeks respectively. The American/European (PACTG 316) trial[25] was an attempt to evaluate the additional effect of a single oral dose of nevirapine at delivery (plus a single oral dose to the neonate at 48–72 hours) in women who were already receiving other anti-retroviral therapy, many of whom were delivered by elective caesarean section. However, the trial was stopped early because the rate of vertical transmission was only 1.5% in both arms and the required sample size was not achievable.

The zidovudine regimen has now been superseded by the use of combination therapy, although no randomised controlled trial comparing the efficacy of monotherapy with combination therapy has been conducted. In France, the efficacy and safety of combined zidovudine and lamivudine was evaluated in a prospective cohort study.[26] In the absence of breastfeeding, the transmission rate was 2.5%. Three different regimens of zidovudine plus lamivudine (prepartum, intrapartum and postpartum to mother and child for one week) were compared with placebo in the PETRA trial in Africa.[27] The regimen starting from 36 weeks was more effective than that starting in labour (5.7% versus 8.9%), although not significantly so, while intrapartum treatment alone showed no reduction in transmission rate compared with the 15.3% in the placebo arm.

Since the mid-1990s, highly active anti-retroviral therapy (HAART) to delay progression of the disease in HIV infected adults has become the standard of care, although in some countries there is a move to defer treatment until CD4 cell counts fall below 200 cells/ml. Such regimens are now usually applied at an earlier stage in the disease so that an increasing number of HIV infected women are receiving complex anti-retroviral regimens at the time of conception. There is also anecdotal evidence to suggest that more HIV infected women now choose to become pregnant and that those who do so are less likely to have the pregnancy terminated because their own disease is well managed and interventions are available to reduce the risk of vertical transmission.

The choice and timing of therapy depends on the woman's clinical and immunological status and has to take into account both delaying her own disease progression and preventing vertical transmission. Management decisions need to be based on treatment history, clinical signs and symptoms, and available prognostic markers such as CD4 count, lymphocyte count, and plasma HIV and RNA levels. Regardless of the antenatal regimen, intravenous zidovudine is currently recommended for the intrapartum period, with oral zidovudine for the newborn for four to six weeks.[3,4]

Women who are known to be HIV infected and who present late in pregnancy or in labour should be offered zidovudine as soon as possible, with consideration given to the addition of nevirapine. Data published in 2003 suggest that infants who are born less than two hours after the administration of maternal nevirapine have lower cord blood concentrations and should therefore receive a dose of nevirapine immediately after birth in addition to the standard dose at 48–72 hours.[28] Rapid HIV testing should be considered for women of unknown infection status who present around the time of labour and are perceived to be at high risk. However, given the lack of time, special consideration should be given to issues relating to informed consent.

Possible adverse effects of therapy

In vitro and primate research suggests that exposure to anti-retroviral therapy *in utero* or early life could have an adverse effect on the infant.[29] No teratogenic effects resulting from anti-retroviral therapy have been observed in clinical practice, even in infants born after exposure to zidovudine in the first trimester of pregnancy,[30] although efavirenz is contraindicated in women who may become pregnant because significant teratogenic effects have been observed in primate studies.[5] Anaemia is well documented in infants who are exposed to zidovudine *in utero* but there are few data on toxicity in the medium and long term. Blanche *et al.*[31] described possible mitochondrial disorder in eight uninfected children exposed *in utero* to maternal zidovudine with or without lamivudine. Two children developed severe neurological disease and died, three had mild/moderate symptoms, and three showed transient biochemical abnormalities. Later research from Barret *et al.*[32] (from the same group) reported circumstantial evidence of mitochondrial dysfunction in 12 children, which included six from the original report who fulfilled the stricter definition used. All presented with neurological symptoms, often associated with abnormal magnetic resonance image and/or a significant episode of hyperlactataemia. The 18-month incidence was 0.26% compared with 0.01% for paediatric neuromitochondrial diseases in a Finnish population. Although follow-up still remains relatively short, no similar events have been reported from any of the other European or US prospective cohorts to date.[33–36] In a systematic review of deaths occurring in five large prospective US cohorts that included more than 16 000 uninfected children exposed to maternal HIV infection, with and without anti-retroviral therapy exposure, there were no deaths attributable to mitochondrial dysfunction.[37] However, none of these studies included specific laboratory testing for mitochondrial function.

It has been suggested that zidovudine incorporation into cord blood leucocyte DNA may produce damage and initiation of mutagenic effects that could lead to carcinogenesis, although there is no clinical evidence to support this.[38] Poirier *et al.*[39] reported mitochondrial DNA damage present at birth and persisting to two years in asymptomatic uninfected children exposed to HIV infected mothers receiving zidovudine. The presence of HIV infection in the mother and the exposure to zidovudine were independently associated with depleted mitochondrial DNA in infant leucocytes. These findings highlight the need for the follow-up of uninfected children exposed to anti-retroviral therapy *in utero*, but, as adverse affects are likely to be rare, large numbers of children will need to be followed up in the long term.

Data from observational studies are conflicting with regard to the effect of anti-retroviral therapy and premature delivery. In a joint analysis of nearly 4,000 mother–child pairs in the European Collaborative Study and the Swiss mother to child cohort study there was an increased rate of prematurity (<37weeks) among infants exposed to combination therapy, particularly when a protease inhibitor was included and when treatment was started before or in early pregnancy.[33,40,41]

However, studies from the USA have not identified prematurity as an adverse effect of anti-retroviral therapy.[42]

The safety of therapy is a key issue in the management of HIV infected pregnant women but there is still a lack of information on the impact of anti-retroviral prophylaxis during pregnancy on disease progression. Evidence from the PACT076 study suggests that limited exposure to zidovudine monotherapy has no impact on disease progression or response to later therapy. The rebound in HIV RNA during the postpartum period in women continuing or stopping therapy requires further study.[43] There have been initial reports of three cases of lactic acidosis resulting in maternal death and four nonfatal cases in pregnant women. All these women had received a combination of drugs including didanosine and stavudine,[5] and lactic acidosis is a known toxic effect of nucleoside analogues. Clinicians need to be alert to this because the symptoms and signs may be similar to those of pre-eclampsia. Widespread anti-retroviral therapy, particularly monotherapy, has been associated with increased drug resistance, which raises concerns about the longer term effectiveness of anti-retroviral prophylaxis and its impact on later treatment options for these women.[44]

THE MANAGEMENT OF AN HIV INFECTED WOMAN IN LABOUR

Before considering management of the delivery, consideration must be given to the woman's clinical status, her viral load, and her past and current treatment regimens.

Caesarean section

The benefit of caesarean delivery over vaginal delivery was demonstrated in a European randomised controlled trial in which 436 women were randomised, before the onset of labour and rupture of the membranes, to either a vaginal or a caesarean delivery.[13] Vaginal delivery was associated with a more than two-fold increased risk of vertical transmission of HIV infection, independent of the use of prophylactic zidovudine. The transmission rate was 1.8% in women randomised to caesarean section and 10.5% for those randomised to vaginal delivery, which represents 80% efficacy. The results from a large meta-analysis of individual data from 8653 mother–child pairs from 15 American and European studies showed similar benefits.[45] Caesarean section more than halved the risk of infection, independent of the use of zidovudine, with transmission rates of 8.2% in the caesarean section group and 16.7% in the group undergoing other modes of delivery. These seminal studies confirmed the previously reported findings from several observational European studies in the mid-1980s,[45,46] which had already influenced the management of delivery in Europe and resulted in an increase in caesarean sections for HIV infected women in the USA, thus highlighting the rapid impact of study results on obstetric practice.[47]

In the light of these findings, recommendations were made in Europe and the USA to offer all HIV infected women the option of an elective caesarean section performed at 38 weeks of gestation to avoid the initiation of labour and rupture of the membranes.[3] Figure 2 shows trends in caesarean section in the UK over time. In 2002, 86% of diagnosed HIV infected women were delivered by caesarean section compared with 21% of the general population.[48] However, with the increasing use of HAART during pregnancy, caesarean section for women with an undetectable or low viral load at the time of delivery has been questioned because the benefits of reducing infection may no longer be sufficient to outweigh the potential adverse effects of the procedure.[49] However, there is no HIV-1 RNA threshold below which transmission does not occur and there is evidence from observational studies that caesarean section has an independent effect in halving

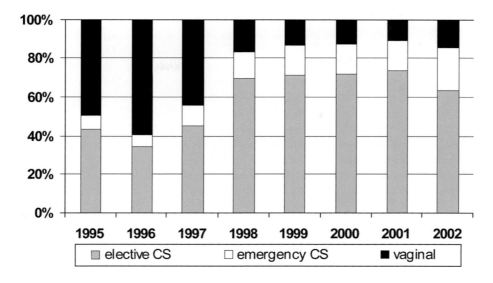

Figure 2 *Mode of delivery for women diagnosed with HIV infection reported to the National Study of HIV in Pregnancy and Childhood, UK 1995–2002; CS = caesarean section*

the rate of vertical transmission, even in women with a low viral load and in those treated with combination therapy.[41,46,50] Although plasma RNA concentration is the most important factor associated with genital HIV-1 shedding, some women receiving HAART, and who have a suppressed plasma viral load, still have high concentrations in their genital tract, suggesting a separate reservoir of HIV-1 replication.[51] Exposure to HIV infected genital secretions and the presence of HIV infected cells in the infant's oropharyngeal cavity have independently been associated with intrapartum and early postpartum infection.[52–54]

Caesarean section, particularly when carried out as an emergency procedure, carries well known risks of postoperative complications for the mother. Much of the morbidity is due to the underlying obstetric or medical condition leading to the indication for a caesarean section rather than the operation itself. Complications are increased in HIV infected women, particularly in those with more severe disease, irrespective of mode of delivery.[55–58] In the European mode of delivery trial[13] there was no significant increase in serious infection complications in HIV infected women delivered by caesarean section compared with those delivered vaginally. In a retrospective study of 401 HIV infected women who delivered at a single centre,[56] the incidence of postpartum morbidity, fever or serious complications after vaginal, emergency or elective caesarean delivery was 4%, 6.4% and 12% respectively, but this did not differ significantly between women who planned to deliver by caesarean section and those who planned to deliver vaginally. These findings are comparable with those reported in the European mode of delivery trial. However, the risk of complications after an emergency caesarean delivery was significantly higher. This risk is reduced with the use of optimal antibiotic prophylaxis and strict aseptic procedures to limit the incidence of infection from scheduled caesarean section, as well as intravenous zidovudine prophylaxis. Blood loss should be kept to a minimum, drainage should be used sparingly and connected to a closed suction system, and the bladder catheter should be removed as soon as possible.[2]

Rupture of the membranes

Prolonged rupture of the membranes has been associated with an increased risk of HIV transmission. In a meta-analysis of available evidence from ten American and five European cohort studies, a one-hour increase in the duration of ruptured membranes was estimated to be associated with a relative increase of 2% in the risk of vertical transmission. However, in women with AIDS, the risk increased from about 8% with one hour's duration of ruptured membranes to over 30% after 24 hours.[59] If premature labour with or without rupture of membranes occurs at or after 34 weeks of gestation, it is advisable to deliver by caesarean section immediately. If the pregnancy is of less than 30 weeks' duration, conservative handling to delay the delivery is recommended because the risk of complications of prematurity are greater than the risk of HIV transmission. When the premature labour occurs at between 30 and 34 weeks, the best course of action depends on the individual circumstances of the mother and the fetus.[2,3]

SURVEILLANCE OF OBSTETRIC AND PAEDIATRIC HIV IN THE UK AND IRELAND

Surveillance is required to monitor the impact of interventions and to detect any adverse events that may arise. In the UK and Ireland, women known to be HIV infected in pregnancy, paediatric cases of HIV infection and children born to infected women, are reported to the National Study of HIV in Pregnancy and Childhood (NSHPC) through parallel reporting schemes run under the auspices of the Royal College of Obstetricians and Gynaecologists and the Royal College of Paediatrics and Child Health.[58] Obstetric and paediatric reports are linked and contribute the paediatric data to the overall national surveillance of HIV and AIDS carried out by the Health Protection Agency and the Scottish Centre for Infection and Environmental Health. By the end of 2003, more than 4000 pregnancies in women with HIV infection had been reported, with the numbers increasing from about 100 a year during the period 1995–1997 to over 800 in 2002.

The majority of diagnosed HIV infected pregnant women reported to the NSHPC since 1999 received combination therapy; the number of women on combination therapy at the time of conception and in early pregnancy is rising steadily. The situation is constantly changing, with women receiving new combinations of drugs and many different drug combinations being prescribed in pregnancy. With the increasing number of fetuses and newborn infants exposed to multiple potentially toxic drugs, the possible risks to an uninfected child need to be addressed. Decisions about the use and choice of an anti-retroviral regimen should be individualised and based on discussions with the woman concerned. More than 95% of children exposed to potent anti-retroviral drugs in fetal and early neonatal life will not be infected with HIV and will need to be followed up for evidence of possible adverse effects, both in the short and long term.

ANTENATAL TESTING AND TARGETS

Although antenatal testing has been officially recommended for all women in high prevalence areas in the UK since 1992, throughout the 1990s most HIV infected pregnant women remained unidentified and the scope for prevention was limited. In 1998 intercollegiate guidelines were published recommending that the offer of antenatal HIV testing be normalised and integrated into the routine antenatal screening framework. The following year the Department of Health advised that a routine offer and recommendation of antenatal HIV testing should be made to all pregnant women in England. By the end of 2002 the aim was for 90% of maternal infections to be diagnosed before delivery, which was expected to reduce vertical transmission rates by 80%.[60] Detection rates improved first in London, where the universal offer was already being implemented in most units during the late 1990s. Since 1999, similar improvements in both uptake and detection have occurred throughout England and in the other countries of the UK, where similar policies are being implemented. At least 75% of HIV infected pregnant women giving birth in 2002 were aware of their HIV status and able to benefit from interventions to reduce the risk of infection in their infant, although it is not yet known whether the ambitious targets have been met.[6] Most diagnosed women opt for treatment and the transmission rate in this group is under 2%. Thus, despite the increase in the number of births to HIV infected women, the number of infected infants born each year has declined (Figure 3). As most reported infants have been born to diagnosed women, nearly all the children described as being of indeterminate status will in fact be uninfected.

CONCLUSION

The management of most aspects of pregnancy in HIV infected women is similar to that for noninfected women. However, treatment options need to be discussed with infected women, including the potential risks of anti-retroviral therapy to the child. The most important factors influencing treatment decisions are the mother's clinical and immunological status and the viral load. Prophylactic zidovudine, caesarean section and the avoidance of breastfeeding reduce the risk of vertical transmission to about 2%. Combination therapy is increasingly used for the prevention of vertical transmission to reduce further the viral load, thereby lowering the risk of transmission. Nevertheless, it is unlikely that transmission can be eliminated completely because viral load is not the only risk factor.

The management of delivery must be individualised and the risks and benefits of a caesarean section discussed with the woman so that she can make an informed decision. The European

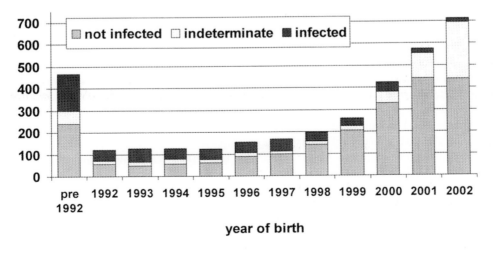

Figure 3 *Children born in the UK and Ireland to HIV infected women and reported to the National Study of HIV in Pregnancy and Childhood by the end of 2003*

consensus guidelines recommend that all HIV infected women are offered caesarean section.[3] However, the question that remains is whether the benefit of caesarean section in reducing the risk of vertical infection from about 1–2% to 0.5–1% in women who are on HAART and/or those with an undetectable viral load justifies the increased individual risk of postpartum complications. Given the low rate of vertical transmission in this situation, many caesarean sections will need to be performed to prevent one infection and the risks of the procedure need to be balanced against the benefits. However, this should be seen in the context of the current caesarean section rate of about one in five deliveries in the UK.[61] The benefits of treatment by both anti-retroviral therapy and caesarean section must be weighed up against the risk of adverse effects in the mother and the fetus, and subsequently the child.

References

1.   World Health Organization, UNAIDS. *AIDS Epidemic Update December 2002*. Geneva: WHO; 2003 [http://www.unaids.org/worldaidsday/2002/press/Epiupdate.html].

2.   Tovo P-A, Newell ML, Mandelbrot L, Semprini A, Giaquinto C. *Recommendations for the Management of HIV Infected Women and Their Infants – a European Consensus.* Brussels: European Commission; 1999. p. 1–37.

3.   Coll O, Fiore S, Florida M, Ciaquinto C, Grosch-Worner I, Guilano M, *et al.* Pregnancy and HIV infection. A European consensus on management. *AIDS* 2002;16 Suppl 2:S1–18.

4.   Lyall EG, Blott, M, de Ruiter A, Hawkins D, Mercy D, Mitchla Z, *et al.* Guidelines for the management of HIV infection in pregnant women and the prevention of mother-to-child transmission. *HIV Med* 2001;2:314–34.

5.   European Centre for the Epidemiological Monitoring of AIDS. *HIV/AIDS Surveillance in Europe. End-year Report 2002.* No. 68. Saint Maurice: Institut de Veille Sanitaire; 2003.

6.   Health Protection Agency, SCIEH, ISD, National Public Health Service for Wales, CDSC Northern Ireland and the UASSG. *Renewing the Focus. HIV and Other Sexually Transmitted Infections in the United Kingdom in 2002.* London: Health Protection Agency; 2003 [http://www.hpa.org.uk/infections/topics_az/hiv_and_sti/publications/annual2003/annual2003.htm].

7.   Dabis F, Msellati P, Dunn D, Lepage P, Newell ML, Peckham C, *et al.* Estimating the rate of mother-to-child transmission of HIV. Report of a workshop on methodological issues, Ghent (Belgium), 17–20 February 1992. The Working Group on Mother-to-Child Transmission of HIV. *AIDS* 1993;7:1139–48.

8.   Nduati R, John G, Mbori-Ngacha D, Richardson B, Overbaugh J, Mwatha A, *et al.* Effect of breastfeeding and formula feeding on transmission of HIV-1: a randomised clinical trial. *JAMA* 2000;283:1167–74.

9.   Shaffer N, Chuachoowong R, Mock PA, Bhadrakom C, Siriwasin W, Young NL, *et al.* Short-course zidovudine for perinatal HIV-1 transmission in Bangkok, Thailand: a randomised controlled trial. Bangkok Collaborative Perinatal HIV Transmission Study Group. *Lancet* 1999;353:773–80.

10.   Mofenson LM, Lambert JS, Stiehm ER, Bethel J, Meyer WA III, Whitehouse J, *et al.* Risk factors for perinatal transmission of human immunodeficiency virus type 1 in women treated with zidovudine. Pediatric AIDS Clinical Trials Group Study 185 Team. *N Engl J Med* 1999;341:385–93.

11.   Maternal viral load and vertical transmission of HIV-1: an important factor but not the only one. European Collaborative Study. *AIDS* 1999;13:1377–85.

12. Garcia PM, Kalish LA, Pitt J, Minkoff H, Quinn TC, Burchett SK, *et al*. Maternal levels of plasma human immunodeficiency virus type 1 RNA and the risk of perinatal transmission. Women and Infants Transmission Study Group. *N Engl J Med* 1999;341:394–402.

13. Elective caesarean-section versus vaginal delivery in preventing vertical HIV-1 transmission: a randomised clinical trial. The European Mode of Delivery Collaboration. *Lancet* 1999;353:1035–9.

14. Thomas C, Newell ML, Dunn D, Peckham C. Characteristics of pregnant HIV-1 infected women in Europe. European Collaborative Study. *AIDS Care* 1996;8:33–42.

15. Landesman SH, Kalish LA, Burns DN, Minkoff H, Fox HE, Zorrilla C, *et al*. Obstetrical factors and the transmission of human immunodeficiency virus type 1 from mother to child. *N Engl J Med* 1996;334:1617–23.

16. Dunn DT, Brandt CD, Krivine A, Cassol SA, Roques P, Borkowsky W, *et al*. The sensitivity of HIV-1 DNA polymerase chain reaction in the neonatal period and the relative contributions of intra-uterine and intra-partum transmission. *AIDS* 1995;9:F7–F11.

17. Newell ML. Mechanisms and timing of mother-to-child transmission of HIV-1. *AIDS* 1998;12:831–7.

18. Connor EM, Sperling RS, Gelber R, Kiselev P, Scott G, O'Sullivan MJ, *et al*. Reduction of maternal–infant transmission of human immunodeficiency virus type 1 with zidovudine treatment. Pediatric AIDS Clinical Trials Group Protocol 076 Study Group. *N Engl J Med* 1994;331:1173–80.

19. Wiktor SZ, Ekpini E, Karon JM, Nkengasong J, Maurice C, Severin ST, *et al*. Short-course oral zidovudine for prevention of mother-to-child transmission of HIV-1 in Abidjan, Cote d'Ivoire: a randomised trial. *Lancet* 1999;353:781–5.

20. Lallemant M, Jourdain G, Le Coeur S, Kim S, Koetsawang S, Comeau AM, *et al*. A trial of shortened zidovudine regimens to prevent mother-to-child transmission of HIV-1. Perinatal HIV Prevention Trial (Thailand) Investigators. *N Engl J Med* 2000;343:982–91.

21. Wade NA, Birkhead GS, Warren BL, Charbonneau TT, French PT, Wang L, *et al*. Abbreviated regimens of zidovudine prophylaxis and perinatal transmission of the human immunodeficiency virus. *N Engl J Med* 1998;339:1409–14.

22. Bulterys M, Orloff S, Abrams E, Nesheim S, Palumbo P, Vink P, *et al*. Impact of zidovudine post-perinatal exposure prophylaxis on vertical HIV-1 transmission: a prospective cohort study in 4 US cities. Second Conference on Global Strategies for the Prevention of HIV Transmission from Mothers to Infants, 1–6 September 1999, Montreal, Canada 1999. Abstract 015.

23. Guay LA, Musoke P, Fleming T, Bagenda D, Allen M, Nakabiito C, *et al*. Intrapartum and neonatal single-dose nevirapine compared with zidovudine for prevention of mother-to-child transmission of HIV-1 in Kampala, Uganda: HIVNET 012 randomised trial. *Lancet* 1999;354:795–802.

24. Moodley D, Moodley J, Coovadia H, Gray G, McIntyre J, Hofmyer J, *et al*. A multicenter randomized controlled trial of nevirapine versus a combination of zidovudine and lamivudine to reduce intrapartum and early postpartum mother-to-child transmission of human immunodeficiency virus type 1. *J Infect Dis* 2003;187:725–35.

25. Dorenbaum A, Cunningham CK, Gelber RD, Culnane M, Mofenson L, Britto P, *et al*. Two-dose intrapartum/newborn nevirapine and standard antiretroviral therapy to reduce perinatal HIV transmission: a randomized trial. *JAMA* 2002;288:189–98.

26. Mandelbrot L, Landreau-Mascaro A, Rekacewicz C, Berrebi A, Benifla JL, Burgard M, *et al*. Lamivudine-zidovudine combination for prevention of maternal-infant transmission of HIV-1. *JAMA* 2001;285:2083–93.

27. Petra Study Team. Efficacy of the three short-course regimens of zidovudine and lamivudine in preventing early and late transmission of HIV-1 from mother to child in Tanzania, South Africa and Uganda (Petra study): a randomised, double-blind, placebo-controlled trial. *Lancet* 2002;359:1178–86.

28. Mirochnick M, Dorenbaum A, Blanchard S, Cunningham CK, Gelber RD, Mofenson L, *et al*. Predose infant nevirapine concentration with the two-dose intrapartum neonatal nevirapine regimen: association with timing of maternal intrapartum nevirapine dose. *J Acquir Immune Defic Syndr* 2003;33:153–6.

29. Mofenson LM, Munderi P. Safety of antiretroviral prophylaxis of perinatal transmission for HIV-I infected pregnant women and their infants. *J Acquir Immune Defic Syndr* 2002;30:200–15.

30. White A, Eldridge R, Andrews E. Birth outcomes following zidovudine exposure in pregnant women: the Antiretroviral Pregnancy Registry. *Acta Paediatr Suppl* 1997;421:86–8.

31. Blanche S, Tardieu M, Rustin P, Stama A, Barret B, Firtion G, *et al*. Persistent mitochondrial dysfunction and perinatal exposure to antiretroviral nucleoside analogues. *Lancet* 1999;354:1084–9.

32. Barret B, Tardieu M, Rustin P, Lacroix C, Chabrol B, Desguerre I, *et al*. Persistent mitochondrial dysfunction in HIV-1-exposed but uninfected infants: clinical screening in a large prospective cohort. *AIDS* 2003;17:1769–85.

33. European Collaborative Study. Exposure to antiretroviral therapy *in utero* or early life: the health of uninfected children born to HIV-infected women. *J Acquir Immune Defic Syndr* 2003;32:380–7.

34. Sperling RS, Shapiro DE, McSherry GD, Britto P, Cunningham BE, Culnane M, *et al*. Safety of the maternal-infant zidovudine regimen utilized in the Pediatric AIDS Clinical Trial Group 076 study. *AIDS* 1998;12:1805–13.

35. Culnane M, Fowler M, Lee SS, McSherry G, Brady M, O'Donnell K, *et al*. Lack of long-term effects of *in utero* exposure to zidovudine among uninfected children born to HIV-infected women. Pediatric AIDS Clinical Trials Group Protocol 219/076 Teams. *JAMA* 1999;281:151–7.

36. Bulterys M, Nesheim S, Abrams EJ, Palumbo P, Farley J, Lampe M, *et al*. Lack of evidence of mitochondrial dysfunction in the offspring of HIV-infected women. Retrospective review of perinatal exposure to antiretroviral drugs in the Perinatal AIDS Collaborative Transmission Study. *Ann NY Acad Sci* 2000;918:212–21.

37. Nucleoside exposure in the children of HIV-infected women receiving antiretroviral drugs: absence of clear evidence for mitochondrial disease in children who died before 5 years of age in five United States cohorts. *J Acquir Immune Defic Syndr* 2000;25:261–8.

38. Hanson IC, Antonelli TA, Sperling RS, Oleske JM, Cooper E, Culnane M, *et al*. Lack of tumors in infants with perinatal HIV-1 exposure and fetal/neonatal exposure to zidovudine. *J Acquir Immune Defic Syndr Hum Retroviral* 1999;20:463–7.

39. Poirier MC, Divi RL, Al-Harthi L, Olivero OA, Nguyen V, Walker B, *et al*. Long-term mitochondrial toxicity in HIV-uninfected infants born to HIV-infected mothers. *J Acquir Immune Defic Syndr* 2003;33:175–83.

40. Thorne C, Fiore S, Rudin C. Antiretroviral therapy during pregnancy and the risk of an adverse outcome. *N Engl J Med* 2003;348:471–2.

41. European Collaborative Study; Swiss Mother and Child HIV Cohort Study. Combination antiretroviral therapy and duration of pregnancy. *AIDS* 2000;14:2913–20.

42. Tuomala RE, Shapiro DE, Mofenson LM, Bryson Y, Culnane M, Hughes MD, *et al*. Antiretroviral therapy during pregnancy and the risk of an adverse outcome. *N Engl J Med* 2002;346:1863–70.

43. Watts DH, Lambert J, Stiehm ER, Harris DR, Bethel J, Mofenson L, et al. Progression of HIV disease among women following delivery. *J Acquir Immune Defic Syndr* 2003;33:585–93.

44. Nolan M, Fowler MG, Mofenson LM. Antiretroviral prophylaxis of perinatal HIV-1 transmission and the potential impact of antiretroviral resistance. *J Acquir Immune Defic Syndr* 2002;30:216–29.

45. Caesarean section and risk of vertical transmission of HIV-1 infection. The European Collaborative Study. *Lancet* 1994;343:1464–7.

46. Kind C, Rudin C, Siegrist CA, Wyler CA, Biedermann K, Lauper U, et al. Prevention of vertical HIV transmission: additive protective effect of elective cesarean section and zidovudine prophylaxis. Swiss Neonatal HIV Study Group. *AIDS* 1998;12:205–10.

47. Dominguez KL, Lindegren ML, D'Almada PJ, Peters VB, Frederick T, Rakusan TA, et al. Increasing trend of cesarean deliveries in HIV-infected women in the United States from 1994 to 2000. *J Acquir Immune Defic Syndr* 2003;33:232–8.

48. Dobson R. Caesarean section rate in England and Wales hits 21%. *BMJ* 2001;323:951.

49. Rowland BL, Vermillion ST, Soper DE. Scheduled cesarean delivery and the prevention of human immunodeficiency virus transmission: a survey of practicing obstetricians. *Am J Obstet Gynecol* 2001;185:327–31.

50. Ioannidis JP, Abrams EJ, Ammann A, Bulterys M, Goedert J, Gray L, et al. Perinatal transmission of human immunodeficiency virus type 1 by pregnant women with RNA virus loads <1000 copies/mL. *J Infect Dis* 2001;183:539–45.

51. Kovacs A, Wasserman SS, Burns D, Wright DJ, Cohn J, Landay A, et al. Determinants of HIV-1 shedding in the genital tract of women. *Lancet* 2001;358:1593–601.

52. Mandelbrot L, Burgard M, Teglas JP, Benifla JL, Khan C, Blot P, et al. Frequent detection of HIV-1 in the gastric aspirates of neonates born to HIV-infected mothers. *AIDS* 1999;13:2143–9.

53. Ait-Khaled M, Lyall EG, Stainsby C, Taylor GP, Wright A, Weber JN, et al. Intrapartum mucosal exposure to human immunodeficiency virus type 1 (HIV-1) of infants born to HIV-1-infected mothers correlates with maternal plasma virus burden. *J Infect Dis* 1998;177:1097–100.

54. Gaillard P, Verhofstede C, Mwanyumba F, Claeys P, Chohan V, Mandaliya K, et al. Exposure to HIV-1 during delivery and mother-to-child transmission. *AIDS* 2000;14:2341–8.

55. Semprini AE, Castagna C, Ravizza M, Fiore S, Savasi V, Muggiasca ML, et al. The incidence of complications after caesarean section in 156 HIV positive women. *AIDS* 1995;9:913–17.

56. Marcollet A, Goffinet F, Firtion G, Pannier E, Le Bret T, Brival ML, et al. Differences in postpartum morbidity in women who are infected with the human immunodeficiency virus after elective cesarean delivery, emergency cesarean delivery, or vaginal delivery. *Am J Obstet Gynecol* 2002;186:784–9.

57. Rodriguez EJ, Spann C, Jamieson D, Lindsay M. Postoperative morbidity associated with cesarean delivery among human immunodeficiency virus-seropositive women. *Am J Obstet Gynecol* 2001;184:1108–11.

58. Watts DH, Lambert JS, Stiehm ER, Bethel J, Whitehouse J, Fowler MG, et al. Complications according to mode of delivery among human immunodeficiency virus-infected women with CD4 lymphocyte counts of < or = 500/microL. *Am J Obstet Gynecol* 2000;183:100–7.

59. International Perinatal HIV group. Duration of ruptured membranes and vertical transmission of HIV-1: a meta-analysis from 15 prospective cohort studies. *AIDS* 2001;15:357–68.

60. Nicoll A, Peckham C. Reducing vertical transmission of HIV in the UK. *BMJ* 1999;319:1211–12.

61. National Social Audit Report [http://www.RCOG.org.uk].

32

Abdominal pregnancy

Prakashbhan S Persad

Although extrauterine pregnancy has attracted a great deal of attention, and the serial literature of our profession is rich in the records of individual experience, the natural history of the accident is not generally understood...

John S Parry (1876)

INTRODUCTION AND HISTORICAL PERSPECTIVES

Abdominal pregnancies are rare but notorious variants of reproduction. The occurrence of these curious experiments of nature proves that the uterus itself is not a necessary prerequisite for pregnancy and that our understanding of the mechanisms of human reproduction is far from complete. The existence of abdominal pregnancies has been documented not only in humans but also in dogs, cats and golden hamsters.[1–3]

The Arab surgeon, Abucasis (1013–1106), is accorded with the first documentation of abdominal pregnancies in the book entitled *Al Tasif*.[4] There were further reports in the 16th century by Cornax (1545), Felix Platter (1584) and Jacob Noierus (1595). The first successful laparotomy for an abdominal pregnancy is generally attributed to Jacob Nufer in Switzerland in 1500.[5] The patient was his wife and, fortunately, both mother and baby lived.

Parry[6] presented the first series of 500 cases from various sources in his classic text *Extra-uterine Pregnancy* in 1876. In it, Parry advised that the important function of the doctor when called to such a case was 'smoothing the stormy passage to the grave'. He further advised: "The only remedy that can be proposed... is gastrotomy – to open the abdomen, tie the bleeding vessels, or to remove the sac entire". The legendary Robert Lawson Tait (1845–1899)[7] accepted this advice and presented his classic paper in the *BMJ* in 1884 of his first five cases with only one death and, from this time, early surgery became the hallmark for the management of all extrauterine pregnancies. The criteria for differentiating primary and secondary peritoneal pregnancies were developed by Studdiford in 1942.[8]

One of the greatest problems in deciding the correct management of abdominal pregnancy is that the literature is replete with reports of cases that were often managed on an emergency basis. In this era of randomised controlled trials, there is little likelihood that any group would manage sufficient numbers of abdominal pregnancies for a comparison of different interventions to be made.

INCIDENCE AND AETIOLOGY

The occurrence of ectopic pregnancy, and therefore its peritoneal subtype, varies widely in the literature, depending on the particular geographical location of the population, the historical timing of the report, and the degree of development of the particular country. Thus it is generally accepted that the incidence of abdominal pregnancy is increased in developing countries;[9,10] in the Bantu tribe a figure of 1:1100 to 1:2000 deliveries has been reported.[11]

In the USA, Atrash *e. al.*[12] estimated that the incidence of abdominal pregnancy was 10.9 per 100 000 live births and 9.2 per 1000 ectopic gestations. This figure was based on an estimated 5221 abdominal pregnancies occurring between 1970 and 1983. The same authors also reviewed the previously published data, and a ratio of 29.2 abdominal pregnancies per 100 000 live births was reported in the period before their analysis, confirming a falling incidence with time.

Two other rare forms of abdominal pregnancy need to be kept in mind. The first is that occurring after abdominal hysterectomy, a possibility that has to be entertained if functioning ovarian tissue is left behind.[13,14] The second is the heterotopic pregnancy; that is, the occurrence of one pregnancy *in utero* and a second *ex utero*. The incidence of this in naturally occurring conceptions is about 1:30 000 but, with the advent of assisted reproductive techniques, the incidence is reported to be 1 in 500 in this subpopulation.[15–18]

It is interesting to note that, although the incidence of ectopic pregnancy is rising, that of abdominal pregnancy seems to be falling. As most abdominal pregnancies are thought to result from tubal rupture and secondary implantation of the chorion into adjacent structures, it is reasonable to assume that routine early ultrasound scanning would detect tubal pregnancies and thus forestall rupture. Improved antenatal care and early routine ultrasound scanning, together with heightened awareness of the possibility of ectopic pregnancy and the more rapid recourse to laparoscopy could explain this.

It is therefore not surprising that many authors have looked to the 'traditional' aetiological factors for tubal ectopic implantation for the cause of abdominal pregnancy. A prior history of infertility or previous ectopic pregnancy are considered to be important markers of underlying tubal and pelvic pathology. The general use of antibiotics has resulted in partially treated pelvic infections and partially obstructed, and thus poorly functioning, tubes rather than absolute tubal occlusion.[19]

Access to health care may also make an important contribution because modern gynaecological practice allows early diagnosis of tubal implantation before rupture and secondary nidation on to peritoneal surfaces. It may be the lack of this access that may be the factor responsible for the reported increased incidence in the Bantu population.[11] Pregnancy in the presence of an intrauterine contraceptive device is also more likely to be not intrauterine.[20,21]

Thus there has been some association between pelvic pathology (salpingitis, tubal surgery and endometriosis) and the occurrence of peritoneal pregnancy. Many other factors (past obstetric and gynaecological history, patient's age, disadvantaged socio–economic conditions) considered in extrauterine gestations have been shown to have only inconsistent links.

Certainly in the developed world, the increasing use of assisted reproductive technologies with embryo transfer must be viewed as an iatrogenic aetiological factor resulting in an increased likelihood of all types of extrauterine pregnancy.[15–18] Overall, however, most patients with an abdominal pregnancy will not have any discernible aetiological factor.

CLASSIFICATION AND NOMENCLATURE

Although the incidences vary in different series, about 98% of all pregnancies are intrauterine; of the extrauterine pregnancies, 98% are tubal (Figure 1).

An abdominal pregnancy may be defined as an ectopic gestation that implants in the peritoneal cavity; tubal, ovarian and interligamentary pregnancies are excluded. Some authors use the term peritoneal pregnancy; this is to differentiate gestations that are implanted directly on to the parietal or visceral peritoneum from those that are implanted intra-abdominally on structures such as the

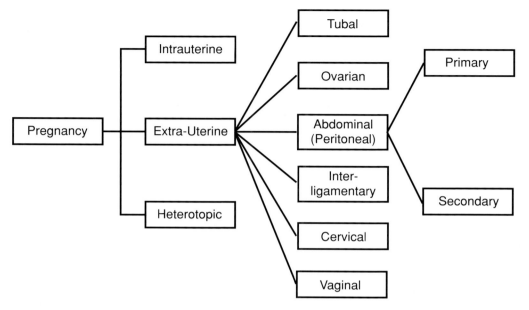

Figure 1 *Type of pregnancy identified by location*

ovaries. An advanced abdominal pregnancy is generally taken as one that has progressed to beyond 24 weeks of gestation.

Abdominal pregnancies are generally subdivided into primary and secondary types, although many authors doubt the occurrence of the former category. Studdiford[8] established the widely accepted criteria on which diagnosis of a primary abdominal pregnancy rests:

- that both tubes are normal with no evidence of recent or remote injury

- the absence of any uteroperitoneal fistula

- the presence of a pregnancy related exclusively to the peritoneal surface and young enough to eliminate the possibility of secondary implantation after primary nidation in the tube.

Placentation is complete only after 12 weeks, so a diagnosis of primary abdominal pregnancy should not be considered before this time. This would prevent the erroneous classification of tubal miscarriages as abdominal pregnancies.[22]

Secondary implantation of the conceptus on to the adjacent peritoneum after rupture of a 'primary' tubal pregnancy is therefore thought to account for the majority of abdominal pregnancies.

IMPLANTATION AND PLACENTATION

One of the most intriguing aspects of abdominal pregnancy relates to placentation on peritoneal surfaces. Although the site of implantation of the placenta is a source of great management dilemmas, the mechanism of implantation creates academic concerns that are worth exploring.

The fertilised ovum will implant on day 6 on any structure to which it is adjacent. Under normal circumstances this is the endometrium. Here, the blastocyst produces human chorionic gonadotrophin and this in turn stimulates decidua formation and a hypersecretory endometrium (Arias–Stella phenomenon). The blastocyst therefore becomes completely embedded in the endometrium, while at the same time the maternal blood vessels and myometrium are protected from trophoblastic invasion. Haemochorial placentation is established at about the 21st day and until that time the zygote receives nutrition from the decidua.

Pregnancies have been reported in every part of the peritoneal cavity, including the liver and spleen, yet the peritoneum cannot allow the blastocyst to become embedded as would occur in the endometrium and to a lesser extent in the endosalpinx. There is no decidua to nourish the pre-implantation embryo and there can be no decidual reaction and Arias–Stella phenomenon to prevent maternal haemorrhage, and thus disruption, of the implantation site. The inevitable fate of most extrauterine pregnancies must therefore be haemorrhage and miscarriage. Trophoblastic invasion and secondary implantation of viable chorionic villi can continue only after the 12th week, after a partial tubal miscarriage, tubal rupture or expulsion of the conceptus from the uterus via a rent in the myometrium. It would seem logical therefore that a primary abdominal pregnancy must be a rare event if it occurs at all.

Despite this logic, however, many advanced abdominal pregnancies are recorded where the implantation site is distant from the pelvis and in the absence of endometriosis. Furthermore, the occurrence of abdominal pregnancy after hysterectomy would lead us to conclude that fertilisation can and does occur in the peritoneal cavity and also that implantation can and does occur in the absence of endometrium.

In the case history described by Noren and Lindblom,[23] there was a 3 cm long, 2 cm wide stalk containing four or five arteries and veins between the uterine fundus and the amniotic sac as the only connection between the fetus and the mother. The amniotic sac was composed of thickened chorio-amniotic membranes with islands of placenta dispersed throughout. There was no evidence of any uteroperitoneal fistulas or tubal disruption. We can therefore safely conclude that the mechanism of placentation of primary peritoneal pregnancy awaits further elucidation. Our inability to produce an animal model of this phenomenon has greatly hindered exploration of implantation mechanisms in this scenario.

DIAGNOSIS

That abdominal pregnancy represents a diagnostic challenge to the clinician is an understatement. This is reflected in the fact that only one in nine to one in five patients who reach hospital alive have an accurate pre-operative diagnosis.[12] The vast majority of abdominal pregnancies are in fact diagnosed intraoperatively or at postmortem, which incidentally makes effective planning of management often a moot point. A high index of suspicion remains the most important facet in pre-operative diagnosis but even if abdominal pregnancy is suspected, confirmation presents many diagnostic dilemmas.

CLINICAL FEATURES

The clinical history is often inconclusive and nonspecific. Symptoms reported include nausea and vomiting, amenorrhoea, lower abdominal pain, painful fetal movements, vaginal bleeding, rectal bleeding, and bowel obstruction. Physical examination may reveal the classic picture of a ruptured ectopic pregnancy (a tender abdomen with rebound, a closed uneffaced cervix) if significant intraperitoneal bleeding has occurred. In an early abdominal pregnancy, a pelvic mass distinct from the uterus on bimanual examination can sometimes be palpated.

In advanced cases, the appreciation of a consistently abnormal fetal lie and easily palpable fetal parts may arouse suspicion. However, Costa et al.[24] reviewed 199 cases and found that more than 60% of the patients had no specific physical findings that could lead to the diagnosis of an intraperitoneal pregnancy. In the same series, the fetal lie was abnormal in only 15% of cases.

LABORATORY INVESTIGATIONS

Laboratory studies are generally not useful, although there have been reports of grossly elevated maternal serum alpha–fetoprotein in the absence of any discernible fetal or maternal cause.[25,26]

DIAGNOSTIC TESTS

Ultrasonography

Modern sonography, because of its general availability, remains the most likely technique that will detect an abdominal pregnancy. However, the literature is replete with cases of advanced abdominal pregnancy missed despite several scans.[24,27,28] The sonographer therefore also requires a high index of suspicion.

Criteria for the sonographic diagnosis of an abdominal pregnancy were put forward by Kobayashi[29] and Allibone et al.:[30]

- a pelvic mass, identified as the uterus, separate from the fetus

- no uterine wall visible between the fetus and the maternal bladder

- placental location outside the confines of the uterine cavity

- fetal parts close to the maternal abdominal wall

- persistent abnormality of fetal lie

- no amniotic fluid between the placenta and the fetal chest or head.

Using these criteria, Costa et al.[24] reviewed 78 cases and found that the diagnosis was missed in 50%! At the same time, false positive ultrasound diagnosis of abdominal pregnancy may occur in the presence of pedunculated fibroids, pregnancy in a bicornuate uterus, and an early pregnancy in a sharply retroflexed or anteflexed uterus.[31]

Radiography

Before the advent of ultrasonography, abdominal radiology was widely used. Mbura and Mgaya[10] found a diagnostic sensitivity of 90% for radiology compared with 83% for ultrasonography for abdominal pregnancy at the Muhumbili Medical Centre in Tanzania.

Radiological signs described in advanced abdominal pregnancy would include the absence of a uterine shadow around the fetus, intermingling of maternal bowel shadows with the fetal parts, and overlapping of fetal bones with the maternal spine on a lateral film. However, none of these are diagnostic.

Computed tomography and nuclear magnetic resonance imaging

There are only a few studies reporting the use of these modalities in the diagnosis of abdominal pregnancy. They seem to provide superior resolution in placental localisation antenatally[32] (Figure 2) and placental resorption postnatally, if the placenta is left *in situ*. Generally, they complement sonography when it is difficult to define the fetus, placenta or uterus because of intervening intestinal loops.

Tocography

Historically, it was Chessin and Zussman[33] who used parental administration of oxytocin in 1954 to prove the existence of an advanced abdominal pregnancy. Nowadays, the absence of uterine contractions after stimulation of the myometrium by intravenous oxytocin or intravaginal prostaglandin is often an event noted, albeit retrospectively, when advanced abdominal pregnancy is diagnosed. The technique has no place in modern practice and would not be useful in early abdominal gestation.

Invasive testing

Hysterosalpingography has been used in cases where fetal death has occurred, but, like thermography and pelvic angiography, is of historical interest only.

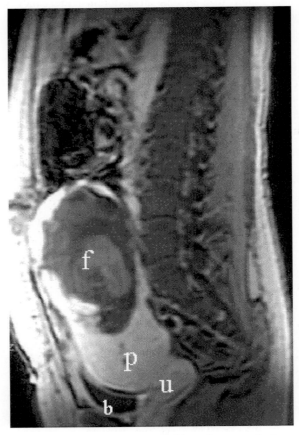

Figure 2 *Magnetic resonance imaging scan of maternal abdomen with abdominal pregnancy: f = fetus; p = placenta; u = uterus; b = bladder*

PROGNOSIS

As previously mentioned, the vast majority of abdominal pregnancies are diagnosed on the operating table. As such, discussion about prognosis is usually of academic interest. It is only occasionally that we have the luxury of planning the management of an abdominal pregnancy and it is in these cases that the following considerations become central to the discussion.

Maternal

Virtually every patient with an advanced abdominal pregnancy will suffer a major medical complication.[24] This includes massive haemorrhage with transfusion sequelae (disseminated intravascular coagulation, adult respiratory distress syndrome); when the placenta is left *in situ*, there is the strong possibility of pelvic and subphrenic abscesses. Perforation and fistula formation with abdominal viscera has been reported, as well as pulmonary embolism.

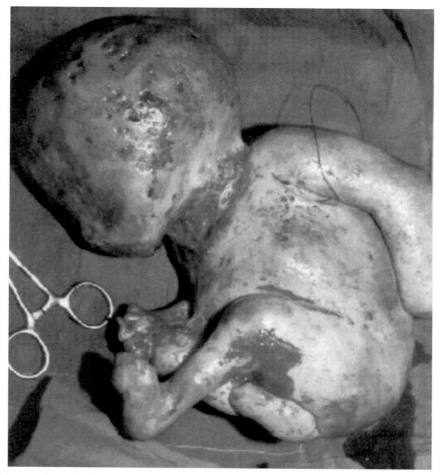

Figure 3 *Lithopaedion: 32-week intra-abdominal pregnancy with death and calcification of the fetus: the woman stated that she had been pregnant about three years previously, but 'the baby never came out' (reproduced courtesy of Andrew Folley and www.obgyn.net)*

Atrash *et al.*[12] estimated that the maternal mortality from abdominal pregnancy is 5.1 per 1000 cases, which is 7.7 times the risk of death from ectopic and 89.8 times that of intrauterine pregnancy.

Fetal

A live infant is born in only 25% of advanced abdominal pregnancies and, of these, 20–40% will have malformations as a result of compression due to oligohydramnios.[34] Thus, torticollis, facial asymmetry, flattening of the limbs and head, and pulmonary hypoplasia[35] are common problems.

If the fetus dies *in abdomino*, there is gradual resorption of amniotic fluid, mummification, calcification and lithopaedion formation (Figure 3).

MANAGEMENT

In many instances the diagnosis of an extrauterine pregnancy is made only on the operating table and there has been no opportunity to plan. In the emergency situation, the most important considerations relate to the management of the placental attachment, as described below. Given the maternal prognostic factors above, every woman with an abdominal pregnancy should be give a full course of broad-spectrum antibiotics (particularly if placental tissue is left *in situ*) and appropriate anticoagulation therapy, according to local guidelines.

There are three scenarios where, the diagnosis having been made pre-operatively, management options need to be debated in terms of timing of delivery. In all these scenarios, decisions regarding the placenta will need to be made at the time of delivery but planned beforehand. Furthermore, in all cases where the diagnosis is being considered, the woman is best transferred to a tertiary centre where more resources are available for the myriad of complications that can and do occur.

Early abdominal pregnancy

Most authors would agree that the diagnosis of any extrauterine pregnancy before 20–24 weeks of gestation should be followed by immediate surgical intervention. This is because of the poor prognosis for both the fetus and the mother.[36,37] The temptation to continue, in the face of an impending intra-abdominal catastrophe, should be resisted at all costs. There are no reports in the literature of the conservative management of extrauterine pregnancy after early diagnosis, although the many cases of viable advanced abdominal pregnancies illustrate that they can and do continue to term rather uneventfully, albeit occasionally.

Laparoscopic management of early abdominal pregnancy was first reported in 1994 in the French literature by Abossolo *et al.*,[38] who commented on the difficulty in maintaining haemostasis. Since then there have been several reports of the successful use of the laparoscope in primary abdominal pregnancy.[39–41] Probably more importantly, it should be pointed out that, when performing a laparoscopy for suspected tubal pregnancy and there is no visible pathology on either tube, careful evaluation of the whole abdominal cavity is necessary so as to not to overlook an abdominal pregnancy.

Advanced abdominal pregnancy: fetus dead

If an abdominal pregnancy has been diagnosed and the fetus is not alive, then immediate delivery would be warranted. However, some authors have suggested that a delay of seven days to eight weeks may be prudent.[42] This time would allow placental circulation to decrease, thus minimising the quantum of haemorrhage at the time of operation. However, this delay allows for a greater chance of a surgical emergency and increases the incidence of infectious morbidity.

Advanced abdominal pregnancy: fetus alive

Because of the unpredictability of the situation, many authors would recommend immediate laparotomy if a diagnosis of abdominal pregnancy is made. However, after 24 weeks of gestation, there may be merit in waiting for fetal maturity. In all cases the risks to the mother must be thoroughly discussed, particularly the possibility of sudden onset, life-threatening intra-abdominal haemorrhage. This approach will also mean that the woman has to be managed as an inpatient in a tertiary centre with rapid access to an operating theatre and cross-matched blood. Antenatal steroids should be administered from 26 weeks of gestation according to the local protocol.

The presence of oligohydramnios is associated with a high incidence of fetal abnormality (usually from pressure deformation) and with pulmonary hypoplasia.[35] There is therefore little advantage in procrastination in these situations because the fetal prognosis is grim anyway.

For a conservative approach in the management of an abdominal pregnancy the following criteria should be met:

- a live fetus

- an ultrasound scan documenting normal liquor volume and ruling out any fetal abnormality

- no signs of peritonism, which would be suggestive of intra-abdominal bleeding

- woman's willingness to stay in hospital and accept the risks associated with a conservative approach

- rapid access to an operating theatre, senior anaesthetic and surgical personnel, and cross-matched blood.

How long one waits depends on the level of neonatal services in the particular location, although after 34 weeks there will be little advantage in delaying delivery. The fetus should be serially monitored by daily cardiotocography and weekly ultrasound scans for liquor volume and biometry. While waiting, advantage should be taken to localise precisely the placental site using magnetic resonance imaging. Any signs of maternal distress or fetal compromise would warrant immediate delivery.

Laparotomy

When it is decided to proceed to laparotomy, a surgical team should be assembled to deal with all eventualities (bowel, vascular and genitourinary complications). In addition a paediatrician should be present in theatre.

Depending on the site of placental implantation, the woman may need to undergo bowel preparation, and serious consideration should be given to the placement of ureteric stents prior to laparotomy. Two large-bore intravenous access lines should be established, with at least four units of blood available. Some authors have advocated the use of a cell-saver and a military antishock trouser suit in these women, in anticipation of massive haemorrhage.[43]

A vertical midline skin incision is made and the fetal membranes incised in an avascular area, usually diametrically opposite to the placental attachment to avoid the fragile venous sinuses. The fetus is delivered carefully, minimising disruption of the placenta and membranes and thus reducing bleeding, and handed over to the attending paediatrician.

Placenta

As a rule the woman has fewer complications and recovers faster if the placenta is removed at the time of laparotomy, but this is not always possible, nor is it generally wise. Massive, and sometimes uncontrollable, haemorrhage is most likely to occur during its attempted or partial removal. Therefore, the decision to remove the placenta should be decisive: either remove it altogether or leave it alone.

The vascularity of the placenta depends on the site of implantation, its viability and its blood supply. In the series of Martin et al.,[44] six women with advanced abdominal pregnancy received a total of 28 units of blood. Thus in situations where blood is generally unavailable, or where the diagnosis is made at laparotomy, it may be best not to disturb the placenta or else wait on the operating table until at least four units of blood are available before attempting its removal.

If the blood supply to the placenta can be identified, isolated and ligated, it is generally agreed that removal would result in a smoother postoperative recovery. In their analysis of 101 cases, Hreshchyshyn et al.[45] were able to remove the placenta totally in 64.6% of cases. After removal, the placental bed may bleed diffusely and this can be controlled by direct pressure or the application of haemostatic sponges.

However, if any questions exist about the feasibility of placental removal, it is safer to ligate the cord close to the placental surface and leave the entire structure in situ.[44,46] This is particularly so if the implantation is on the dorsal peritoneal surface, or on a vascular structure such as the liver. It is important not to attempt too much manipulation unless it has been definitely decided to proceed with total removal.

Absorption without bleeding generally results, although the placenta can remain functional for up to 50 days.[47] Placental involution can be followed by serial ultrasonography and total resorption is usual by four months, although involution times of up to 5.5 years have been documented.[48,49] In some women, a second laparotomy is required to remove the avascular placental remnants, particularly if abdominal symptoms persist.

The use of methotrexate to hasten placental involution is controversial because it has been associated with the accumulation of necrotic debris, infection and abscess formation.[44] In any event the mature placenta has minimal hyperplastic growth and thus, in advanced abdominal pregnancies, methotrexate would have little effect. Complications of the retained abdominal placenta include secondary haemorrhage, hypofibrinogenaemia, ileus, intestinal obstruction, abscess formation, wound dehiscence, amniotic fluid cyst formation and pre-eclampsia.[50]

CONCLUSIONS

Abdominal pregnancy still presents diagnostic and management dilemmas more than a century after Parry's classic text. In spite of this, a high index of suspicion, the early diagnosis of tubal pregnancy on routine ultrasound scanning, and rapid recourse to laparoscopy has resulted in a declining incidence and mortality. No longer do we have simply to 'smooth the passage to the grave'. The management of the placenta in the advanced abdominal pregnancy remains the critical determinant in maternal outcome but in general it is best left alone unless it can be easily and completely removed.

References

1.   Buckley P, Caine A. A high incidence of abdominal pregnancy in the Djungarian hamster (Phodopus sungorus). J Reprod Fertil 1979;56:679–82.

2.   Carrig CB, Gourley IM, Philbrick AL. Primary abdominal pregnancy in a cat subsequent to ovariohysterectomy. *J Am Vet Med Assoc* 1972;160;308–10.

3.   Peters LJ. Abdominal pregnancy in a golden hamster (*Mesocricetus auratus*). *Lab Anim Sci* 1982;32:392–3.

4.   Ang LPS, Tan AJC, Yeo SH. Abdominal pregnancy: a case report and literature review. *Singapore Med J* 2000;41:454–7.

5.   King G. Advanced extrauterine pregnancy. *Am J Obstet Gynecol* 1954;67:712–19.

6.   Parry JS. *Extra-Uterine Pregnancy: Its Causes, Species, Pathological Anatomy, Clinical History, Diagnosis, Prognosis and Treatment*. Philadelpia, PA: Henry C Lea; 1876.

7.   Tait L. Five cases of extrauterine pregnancy operated upon at the time of rupture. *BMJ* 1884;i:1250–2.

8.   Studdiford WE. Primary peritoneal pregnancy. *Am J Obstet Gynecol* 1942;44:487–91.

9.   Leiken,E, Randall HW Jr. Hydrocephalic fetus in an abdominal pregnancy. *Obstet Gynecol* 1987;69:498–501.

10. Mbura JS, Mgaya, H. Advanced abdominal pregnancy in Muhumbili Medical Centre in Tanzania. *Int J Gynaecol Obstet* 1986;24:169–76.

11. Ombelet W, Vandermerwe JV, Van Assche FA. Advanced extrauterine pregnancy: description of 38 cases with literature survey. *Obstet Gynecol Surv* 1988;43;386–97.

12. Atrash HK, Friede A, Hogue CJR. Abdominal pregnancy in the United States: frequency and maternal mortality. *Obstet Gynecol* 1987;69:333–7.

13. Aurora VK. Abdominal pregnancy following total hysterectomy. *Int Surg* 1983;68:253–5.

14. Brown WD, Burrows L, Todd CS. Ectopic pregnancy after cesarean hysterectomy. *Obstet Gynecol* 2000;99 Suppl 1:933–4.

15. Bassil S, Pouly JL, Canis M, Janny L, Vye P, Chapron C, *et al*. Advanced heterotopic pregnancy after *in-vitro* fertilization and embryo transfer, with survival of both babies and the mother. *Hum Reprod* 1991;6:1008–10.

16. Fisch B, Peled Y, Kaplan B, Zehavi S, Neri A. Abdominal pregnancy following *in vitro* fertilization and embryo transfer in a patient with previous bilateral salpingectomy. *Obstet Gynecol* 1996;88:642–3.

17. Deshpande N, Mathers A, Acharya U. Broad ligament twin pregnancy following *in-vitro* fertilization. *Hum Reprod* 1999;14852–4.

18. Scheiber MD, Cedars MI. Successful management of a heterotopic abdominal pregnancy following embryo transfer with cryopreserved-thawed embryos. *Hum Reprod* 1999;14:1375–7.

19. Maas DA, Slabber CF. Diagnosis and treatment of advanced extra-uterine pregnancy. *S Afr Med J* 1975;49:2007–10.

20. Kasby C, Krins A. Primary peritoneal pregnancy in association with intrauterine contraceptive devices: two case reports. *Br J Obstet Gynaecol* 1978;85:794–5.

21. Muzsnai D, Hughes T, Price M, Bruksch L. Primary peritoneal pregnancy associated with the IUD (2 case reports). *Eur J Obstet Gynecol Reprod Biol* 1980;10:275–8.

22. Persad PS, Dwarakanath LS. Primary abdominal pregnancy: disregarding clinical features leads to misdiagnosis. *Am J Obstet Gynecol* 1996;174:296–7.

23. Noren H, Lindblom B. A unique case of abdominal pregnancy: what are the minimal requirements for placental contact with the maternal vascular bed? *Am J Obstet Gynecol* 1986;155:394–6.

24. Costa SD, Presley J, Bastert G. Advanced abdominal pregnancy. *Obstet Gynecol* 1991;48:515–25.

25. Hage ML, Wall LL, Killam A. Expectant management of abdominal pregnancy: a report of

two cases. *J Reprod Med* 1988;33:407–9.

26. Tromans PM, Coulson R, Lobb MO, Abdulla U. Abdominal pregnancy associated with an extremely elevated serum alpha-protein (case report). *Br J Obstet Gynaecol* 1984;91:296–8.

27. Moonen-Delarue MW, Haest JW. Ectopic pregnancy three times in line of which two advanced abdominal pregnancies. *Eur J Obstet Gynecol Reprod Biol* 1996;66:87–8.

28. White RG. Advanced abdominal pregnancy – a review of 23 cases. *Ir J Med Sci* 1989;158:77–8.

29. Kobayashi M. *Illustrated Manual of Ultrasonography in Obstetrics and Gynaecology.* 2nd ed. New York: Izaku-Shoin; 1980. p. 174.

30. Allibone GW, Fagan CJ, Porter SC. The sonographic features of intra-abdominal pregnancy. *J Clin Ultrasound* 1981;9:383–7.

31. Stanley JH, Horger EO, Fagan CJ, Andriole JG, Fleischer AC. Sonographic findings in abdominal pregnancy. *AJR Am J Roentgenol* 1986;147:1043–6.

32. Cohen JM, Weinreb JC, Lowe TW, Brown C. MR imaging of a viable full-term abdominal pregnancy. *AJR Am J Roentgenol* 1985;145:407–8.

33. Chessin H, Zussman L. The tokodynamometer: a diagnostic aid in late abdominal pregnancy. *Obstet Gynecol* 1954;4:440–2.

34. Strafford JC, Ragan WD. Abdominal pregnancy: review of current management. *Obstet Gynaecol* 1977;50:548–56.

35. Cartwright PS, Brown JE, Davis RJ, Thieme GA, Boehm FH. Advanced abdominal pregnancy associated with fetal pulmonary hypoplasia: report of a case. *Am J Obstet Gynecol* 1986;155:396–7.

36. Bouis PJ Jr, Messina AM, Inman W. Abdominal pregnancy: making the diagnosis by ultrasound. *Contemp Obstet Gynecol* 1981;18:160–4.

37. Hallat JG, Grove JA. Abdominal pregnancy: a study of 21 consecutive cases. *Am J Obstet Gynecol* 1985;54:444–9.

38. Abossolo T, Sommer JC, Dancoisne P, Ovain E, Tuaillon J, Isoard L. First trimester abdominal pregnancy and laparoscopic surgical treatment. 2 case reports of evolving abdominal pregnancy treated with laparoscopy at 10 and 12 weeks. *J Gynecol Obstet Biol Reprod (Paris)* 1994;23:676–8.

39. Ben-Rafael Z, Dekel A, Lerner A, Ovieto R, Halpern M, Powsner E, *et al.* Laparoscopic removal of abdominal pregnancy adherent to the appendix after ovulation induction with human menopausal gonadotrophin. *Hum Reprod* 1995;10:1804–5.

40. Morita Y, Tsutsumi O, Kuramochi K, Momoeda M, Yoshikawa H, Taketani Y. Successful laparoscopic management of primary abdominal pregnancy. *Hum Reprod* 1996;11:2546–7.

41. Chung MT, Lin YS, Wu MP, Huang KF. Laparoscopic surgery for omental pregnancy. *J Am Assoc Gynecol Laparosc* 2002;9:84–6.

42. Zuspan FP, Quilligan EJ, Rosenblum JM. Abdominal pregnancy. *Am J Obstet Gynecol* 1957;74:259–63.

43. Sandberg EC, Pelligra R. The medical antigravity suit for the management of uncontrolled bleeding associated with abdominal pregnancy. *Am J Obstet Gynecol* 1983;146:519–25.

44. Martin JN Jr, Sessums JK, Martin RW, Pryor JA, Morrison JC. Abdominal pregnancy: current concepts of management. *Obstet Gynecol* 1988;71:549–57.

45. Hreshchyshyn MM, Bogen B, Loughran CH. What is the actual present day management of the placenta in the late abdominal pregnancy? Analysis of 101 cases. *Am J Obstet Gynecol* 1961;81:303–10.

46. Delke I, Veridiano N, Tancer ML. Abdominal pregnancy: review of current management and addition of 10 cases. *Obstet Gynecol* 1982;60:200–4.

47. Ahmed AG, Jandial D, Klopper A. Postpartum decline in serum concentration of placental proteins in an abdominal pregnancy. *Arch Gynecol* 1985;237:27–30.

48. Belfar HL, Kurtz AB, Wapner RJ. Long-term follow-up after removal of an abdominal pregnancy: ultrasound evaluation of the involuting placenta. *J Ultrasound Med* 1986;5:521–3.

49. Spanta R, Roffman LE, Grissom TJ, Newland JR, McManus BM. Abdominal pregnancy: magnetic resonance identification with ultrasonographic follow-up of placental involution. *Am J Obstet Gynecol* 1987;157:887–9.

50. Attapattu JA, Menon S. Abdominal Pregnancy. *Int J Gynaecol Obstet* 1993;43:51–5.

33

The urinary system in pregnancy

Samantha J Pretlove and Philip M Toozs-Hobson

INTRODUCTION

Today's expectations of pregnancy and childbirth are high. Consequently, many women feel disillusioned and find it difficult to accept when complications occur. Even hospital-based parent education classes do not always discuss depression (affecting 21% of pregnant women),[1] problems with sexual intercourse (49%),[2] urinary incontinence (34%)[3] or faecal incontinence (4%).[4] There is no standard repository of knowledge for parent education classes and information is presented on an *ad hoc* basis with the subject matter being determined by the individual teacher. Parent education classes are based around consumer demand for topics, and subjects such as incontinence do not feature highly. This may be because women do not perceive it to be a major problem associated with childbirth or because those who do understand its significance are too embarrassed to raise this issue in a group situation. As a result, valuable opportunities to discuss and teach pelvic floor exercises are lost.

This leads to a situation where, despite healthcare structures being in place, we do women a disservice by not informing them of the potential complications of childbirth.[5] Is this because it seems a pointless discussion when the only alternative is a major abdominal operation, or does the medical profession believe that incontinence is an inevitable part of life for multiparous women as opposed to a preventable and treatable disease?

Despite the literature containing many studies demonstrating the significance of antenatal symptoms and the possible role of collagen in incontinence, the myth persists that only what happens on the day of delivery is significant, and the other 289 days of pregnancy are ignored.

A large longitudinal study spanning decades is needed to elucidate the factors involved in what seems to be a 'multifactorial physiological insult', assessing the antenatal factors. The cost of a project like this would be prohibitive because it would involve much time consuming tagging of notes and large amounts of data collection. Although the Government in their White Paper have identified continence as one of their priorities, it is still difficult to obtain funding for this type of work because continence research does not save lives, despite its potential vastly to improve quality of life for a great number of women.

PHYSIOLOGICAL CHANGES TO THE URINARY SYSTEM IN PREGNANCY

Women are aware that their entire body undergoes significant physiological change during pregnancy, which has an impact on every system, including increased cardiac and renal output, and increased oxygen consumption.

The changes to the pelvis and lower genitourinary tract are different from most systems because, postnatally, they may not return to the prepregnancy state. There are a variety of reasons for this, such as hormonal changes and pressure from the pregnant uterus. Connective tissue has been shown to be weaker in pregnancy[6] and changes have been demonstrated in the rectus sheath of pregnant women undergoing caesarean section. These changes are due to increases in glycosaminoglycans and a reduction in total collagen[7] as a consequence of tissue remodelling. These effects may be further exacerbated by stretching of the tissues during pregnancy and delivery. If these changes occur in the endopelvic fascia, the support mechanisms of the bladder and urethra could potentially be affected, resulting in bladder neck mobility and stress incontinence.[8] It is perhaps not surprising, given these changes, especially to the bladder, urethra and particularly the urethrovesical junction,[9] that pregnant and postnatal women commonly experience urinary symptoms.

ANATOMICAL CHANGES IN PREGNANCY

The gravid uterus becomes an abdominal mass during pregnancy, with pressure effects on both the pelvic floor muscles and the lower urinary tract. Distortion occurs in the position of the bladder, bladder neck, urethra and pelvic floor, which has been demonstrated both with cystography[10,11] and perineal ultrasound.[9,12] The bladder appears lower at rest, with increased bladder neck opening and mobility.[8] However, in practice, the development of incontinence and urinary symptoms during pregnancy is most probably multifactorial because no association between the engagement of the vertex and symptoms of stress incontinence has been demonstrated.[13]

HORMONAL EFFECTS

Although there does not appear to be a direct correlation between levels of progesterone and oestrogen in pregnancy and continence,[14] hormonal effects are thought to play a part. Progesterone increases bladder capacity and compliance and appears to inhibit alpha-adrenergic activity at the bladder base and urethra[15] and, although this may account for reduced maximal urethral closure pressure (MUCP) in pregnancy,[16] no correlation has been demonstrated between 17-OH-progesterone levels and changes in urethral pressure in pregnancy.[17] The findings remain controversial as they contradict other studies that suggest that the MUCP is increased in continent pregnant women.[18]

Relaxin, a peptide hormone from the family of insulin-like growth factors, is produced by the placenta and may also have a role in continence, although the mechanism of action is not clear.[14]

ANTENATAL PERIOD

Symptoms in pregnancy

Urine production in pregnancy

In the initial weeks of pregnancy, the osmotic threshold for antidiuretic hormone and thirst decreases. This means that thirst is increased and the woman drinks more and the body fluids become more dilute. When the osmolality falls below the new threshold, the steady state is resumed.[19] This increase in drinking may be responsible for the changes in voiding pattern that many women experience during pregnancy.[10]

Bladder storage during pregnancy

Animal studies on the effect of pregnancy on the bladder suggest that progesterone reduces vesical contraction and increases bladder capacity.[20] Human studies have used simple cystometry to assess bladder capacity and tone in pregnancy, with conflicting results. Some have found that by the third trimester there is bladder atony and reduced intravesical pressure for any given volume. Other studies have shown the reverse, with decreasing bladder capacity towards term and evidence of increased bladder tone.[10] However, at six weeks postpartum, bladder tone appears to return to normal,[21,22] although the studies that confirm this were performed some time ago.

Frequency and nocturia in pregnancy

Urinary frequency is one of earliest symptoms of pregnancy and is often noticed before the first missed period. Published reports on incidence of frequency and nocturia in pregnancy show different incidences, perhaps because of variation in definitions[10,23] (Table 1).

In Parboosingh and Doig's study[23] most of the women accepted nocturia as a normal part of pregnancy and less than 4% were distressed by it. Stanton et al.[13] defined frequency as seven or more daytime voids and nocturia as two or more night-time voids. More nulliparous women had frequency than multiparous women but this reached statistical significance at only 38 and 40 weeks. Cutner et al.[24] showed that 91% of women had an increased voiding pattern overall. This explains why frequency is an expected symptom of pregnancy; it appears to be almost universal. It causes little distress because it almost always resolves postnatally.[13]

It would be expected that pressure from an enlarged uterus would be relieved at night, allowing the bladder to fill properly, and frequency to be more marked during the day. However, nocturia remains a problem and there may be more to frequency in pregnancy than pressure and space effects of the uterus alone.[13]

Sodium excretion is increased at night, raising urine production and causing nocturia. This reduces in the third trimester but the reduced bladder capacity at this stage in pregnancy means that there is no improvement in symptoms.[23,25]

The definition of 'night time' needs to be precise because the amount of 'night-time' voiding that is reported in pregnancy depends on how long the woman spends in bed rather than the number of voids over a fixed time period.[23]

Although the studies may have different definitions, the broad sweep of the literature is that the majority of women have frequency during pregnancy, which gets worse as the pregnancy progresses. This is largely perceived as normal and generally resolves after delivery.

Table 1 *Summary of results from studies of nocturia and frequency in pregnancy*

Study	Definition	1st trimester	2nd trimester	3rd trimester	
Francis, 1960[10]	Frequency = 7 or more daytime voids + 1 night void	59.5%	61%	81%	
Parboosingh and Doig, 1973[23]	Nocturia = night-time voiding at least 3 times per week	60%	57%	66%	
Stanton et al, 1980[13]	Frequency = 7 or more daytime voids	<16/40 Nullip 11%	Nullip	38/40 54%	40/40 68%
	Nocturia = 2 or more night-time voids	Multip 13%	Multip	34%	42%

Urgency and urge incontinence

The symptoms of urgency and urge incontinence are frequently due to detrusor musculature overactivity. In pregnancy there is often a poor correlation between lower urinary tract symptoms and a urodynamic diagnosis. There appears to be increased detrusor overactivity in pregnancy, which resolves postpartum.[26,27] Urge incontinence has a peak incidence of 19% in multiparous women. It has been suggested that these changes are due to pressure effects from increasing uterine size.[13] In a study using New Zealand white rabbits as an animal model, there was increased bladder compliance when pregnant but, perhaps more importantly, a change in the threshold for the sensation of bladder fullness. It has been postulated that this change is responsible for the symptom of urgency during pregnancy and is due to the changes in the sex steroid levels.[28]

Possibly the most important thing about lower urinary tract symptoms during pregnancy is that antenatal symptoms are predictive of postnatal symptoms.

Management of the woman with proven detrusor overactivity during pregnancy

No formal clinical trials have been conducted to determine the safety of anticholinergics in human pregnancy and so only anecdotal information is available. Oxybutynin is an older drug, so there is more experience of it being used in pregnancy. A small risk of teratogenesis cannot be excluded but a high risk of congenital abnormality is unlikely. In animal studies, over 250 times the human dose had to be administered to pregnant rats before teratogenesis occurred.[29] Oxybutynin has become the drug of choice for women with severe detrusor overactivity who would have severe impairment of their quality of life during pregnancy without treatment for the bladder. However, as this is a low molecular weight molecule, it would be expected to cross the placenta.

Thirty-four reports have been received worldwide by Pharmacia regarding women who inadvertently took tolterodine immediately prior to or during a pregnancy. In 16 women the outcome is still awaited; seven had a miscarriage, two chose to terminate the pregnancy, and the remaining nine women delivered live healthy infants. Although no obvious malformations have occurred in this group and the number involved is small, the current recommendation is that tolterodine should not be prescribed in pregnancy (data from Pharmacia, Milton Keynes, Bucks).

Stress incontinence

Stress incontinence appears to result from increased parity, but whether pregnancy or vaginal delivery is the major determining factor remains unclear. Large population studies have been performed in this area,[30,31] which have confirmed that parity is related to the symptoms of stress incontinence. The argument that pregnancy rather than delivery is the major contributing factor is supported by studies that demonstrate significant numbers of parous women with stress incontinence who were delivered by elective caesarean section.[32] Furthermore, symptoms of stress incontinence are often present antenatally. In one study, 8.5% of women with stress incontinence reported that it commenced prepregnancy, 23% had permanent incontinence that started antenatally, and 50% had temporary incontinence that started in the second half of pregnancy and resolved spontaneously after delivery. Only 19% described stress incontinence that started postnatally and in 8% it was temporary.[33]

In women who developed symptoms of stress incontinence postnatally, some studies did not demonstrate a significant difference between them and a group of continent women with respect to length of labour, mode of delivery and infant weight, although Krue *et al.*[34] found an increased incidence of stress incontinence in obese women who delivered a baby weighing more than 4 kg vaginally. Studies have confirmed that 53% of nulliparous women and 84% of multiparous women admit to stress incontinence antenatally; therefore, stress incontinence rarely occurs for the first time postnatally.[13,35] Stress incontinence is also undoubtedly influenced by maternal weight, achieving statistical significance with a body mass index of more than 30 kg/m².[36]

Problematic stress incontinence prior to pregnancy is associated not only with a decrease in the amount of collagen in the tissues but also with the presence of fewer cross-links, resulting in reduced tensile strength.[35] Genetic factors may also be implicated in the aetiology of stress incontinence because its incidence in women whose mothers had suffered from it was five times that of the control group.[16,32] To complicate matters further, the onset of stress incontinence is often poorly recalled by women, with only 26% being able to remember accurately five years after delivery when it started.[37] This makes disentangling the cause even more difficult because the onset of stress incontinence may be wrongly attributed by the woman to specific events such as childbirth.

Urodynamics in pregnancy

Urethral pressure profiles

Urethral pressure profiles provide insight into the development of stress incontinence during pregnancy and after delivery. Continent women have a gradual increase in functional urethral length and MUCP during pregnancy, which returns to prepregnancy measurements after delivery. Women who develop stress incontinence during delivery do not increase their functional urethral length and have a low mean urethral closure pressure during pregnancy.[16] Vaginal delivery itself appears to be associated with a decrease in functional urethral length and MUCP. However, the duration of the second stage, episiotomy and baby weight do not appear to influence the measurements. Caesarean section has been reported to preserve MUCP and functional urethral length.[17]

Imaging of the bladder neck and urethra

It is now possible to measure urethral sphincter volume,[38] a reduction of which appears to be associated with stress incontinence.[39] Reduced MUCP correlates with a decrease in volume and maximal cross-section of the urethra in women who develop stress incontinence after delivery. Vaginal delivery is associated with a decrease in sphincter volume in comparison with caesarean section.[40,41] Perineal ultrasound has been used to investigate the position of the bladder neck and the proximal urethra. The advantages of perineal ultrasound include less distortion of the anatomy than when using a vaginal probe.[42] Using these techniques, some studies have demonstrated a significant increase in bladder neck movement on the Valsalva manoeuvre in women who are incontinent and who have had forceps deliveries.[43] It is already known that bladder neck hypermobility predisposes to stress incontinence[44] and it appears that women who have postnatal stress incontinence have a hypermobile bladder neck antenatally.[44]

Urinary tract infections in pregnancy

The presence of asymptomatic bacteriuria is probably the same in the pregnant population as in the nonpregnant population, at 5.3%.[45] The difference between the two populations is that 14–63% of pregnant women with asymptomatic bacteriuria will develop a symptomatic urinary tract infection (UTI).[46] As a result of this predisposition to UTI in pregnancy, all pregnant women are screened for bacteriuria.[47] The cheapest way to do this is with reagent strips to test for nitrites, leucocyte esterase, protein and blood. These have a positive predictive value of 10.5% for UTI and a negative predictive value of 99.3%. Protein and blood alone have a positive predictive value of 19.7% and a negative predictive value of 98.1%. After initial screening, only women with a positive result then have a mid-stream urine sent for culture and sensitivity. This is cost-effective because the reagent strips are much cheaper than microscopy, culture and sensitivity being performed on many negative specimens.[47] Bacteriuria is defined as 10^5 organisms from a clean mid-stream urine. Although acute pyelonephritis occurs in only 1–2% of pregnant women, screening for asymptomatic bacteriuria will prevent 75% of cases.[45] In addition to the usual symptoms of nausea, vomiting, pyrexia, loin pain and rigors that occur with acute pyelonephritis, there is also the possibility of uterine contractions and subsequent premature labour. Treatment is with intravenous antibiotics, rehydration and analgesia. Empirical treatment is usually commenced while results of cultures and sensitivities are awaited. Two percent of women who have a negative culture at booking will subsequently develop a significant bacteriuria and therefore it is important to retest those who have symptoms of a UTI even though symptoms such as frequency are common in normal pregnancy.

Urinary calculi

Although there is urinary stasis and increased urinary infection rates in pregnancy, this is offset by increased diuresis and ureteric dilatation, so the rate of urinary calculi in pregnancy is similar to that in the nonpregnant population.[48]

Voiding difficulties during pregnancy

Urinary retention in pregnancy is uncommon. It is most likely in women with a retroverted uterus that becomes caught under the sacral promontory as it expands. The problem generally resolves after 16 weeks of gestation, when the uterus becomes an abdominal organ. The obstruction is usually attributed to the enlarged uterus obstructing the opening to the internal urethral meatus. Management is with an indwelling catheter and correction of the position of the uterus using a ring or Hodge pessary. When the catheter is removed, the risk of retention occurring again must be explained to the woman because overdistension of the bladder can lead to long-term damage. Occasionally, if normal voiding does not restart it may be necessary to continue with the catheter for the duration of the pregnancy.

Symptoms of voiding disorders are common in pregnancy; up to 25% of pregnant women complain of a poor stream and 30% feel they have incomplete emptying. The symptoms persist throughout pregnancy.[24,49] These women may feel symptomatic but it is possible that they are passing small volumes more frequently, leading to dribbling and a feeling of incomplete emptying, although some studies have demonstrated reduced flow rates during pregnancy.[27]

INTRAPARTUM CARE

Perhaps the most startling finding in this area is the lack of evidence for current obstetric practice, particularly when bearing in mind the frequency with which both childbirth and urinary incontinence occur.

The area that ignites the most interest is the debate surrounding the contribution of vaginal delivery to incontinence. The development of initial postnatal urinary symptoms in primiparous women is linked to the length of the second stage of labour but, although caesarean section appeared to confer some protection against developing incontinence, by three months postnatally all the obstetric correlations had disappeared, mostly linked to the resolution of much of the incontinence.[50] Wilson *et al.*[3] have shown that, although having one caesarean section seems to confer some protection from urinary incontinence (5–11% for caesarean section versus 24% for vaginal delivery), after three caesareans the rate rises to 35%.

The impact of using regional analgesia on continence

Epidural and spinal analgesia for labour and delivery have an impact on bladder function. Normal voiding may be delayed because the afferent sensory impulses from the bladder, which normally give the sensation of fullness, are suppressed. This is supported statistically as 2.7% of women who have had an epidural have retention of urine compared with 0.1% of those who have not had a regional block.[51] This evidence needs to be interpreted with caution because many confounding factors exist and were not controlled for in the study concerned. Epidurals are more likely to be used for instrumental deliveries because these are more painful. They are also more likely to be requested by primigravidae and in cases of high infant birth weight because, again, this may make the labour more painful. Women who have had an epidural are more likely to sustain perineal injury for all these reasons. The evidence remains conflicting, with studies split between those showing an association between epidurals and asymptomatic retention of urine[52] and others demonstrating the opposite.[53] To add further to the debate, women who subsequently have continence surgery are more likely to have had an epidural for delivery.[54]

The case for epidurals being associated with stress incontinence is also controversial, with some studies showing a reduction in stress incontinence with an epidural,[55] but others demonstrating an increase in nulliparous women who have had an epidural when compared with nulliparous women delivering without.[56]

Practical management of labour to avoid bladder problems

The key to avoiding bladder problems in pregnancy is to give obstetric staff an awareness of the care of the bladder during labour and the common pitfalls. Voiding is not always a reliable indicator of bladder function because emptying may be incomplete and retention painless owing to anaesthesia. Using an indwelling Foley catheter for women who are administered regional anaesthesia during labour and delivery reduces overdistension and voiding difficulties[57] and reduces the risk of infection from repeated catheterisation.[58] Other methods of quantifying bladder volume such as using ultrasound scanning are also available. Unfortunately, automated bladder scanners are not useful immediately postpartum because they cannot differentiate between the postpartum uterus and the bladder. 'In and out' catheters can be counterproductive as there is a 1% risk of UTI with each catheterisation and during a long labour women may need to be catheterised several times. It is easy to see how damage can occur because, after epidural analgesia has been used, the bladder may take up to eight hours to regain sensation, during which time the woman can have produced a large amount of urine. When a policy was introduced in our unit that all women undergoing regional anaesthesia should have an indwelling Foley catheter for labour and delivery, it was initially met with resistance and used as an example of another attempt to medicalise childbirth. However, as staff have seen the prevention of urinary problems and a reduction in the number of women returning with postpartum voiding difficulties, the policy has been accepted as an important part of care during labour.

It is also important to ensure that postnatal voiding is confirmed, even in women without risk factors for voiding difficulties. A policy for voiding after delivery where a void of more than 200 ml within four hours of delivery is needed to avoid catheterisation motivates both staff and women to ensure that voiding occurs. The policy is also helpful for correcting dehydration because women often need to be encouraged to drink appropriately after labour and delivery in a hot hospital environment.

MODE OF DELIVERY

Instrumental delivery

Instrumental delivery is often cited as a factor in the development of urinary symptoms. Ten to 24% of women in England have an assisted delivery, with the rate varying regionally.[59] Given how frequently this is used, there are few data available to suggest how such deliveries may be implicated in the development of stress incontinence. A postal study showed that women who had delivered instrumentally had ten times the rate of stress incontinence of those having a spontaneous vaginal delivery.[60] Arya *et al.*[61] studied primiparous women delivering vaginally, excluding those who were incontinent antenatally, and found that there was no association at two weeks between urinary incontinence and maternal age, ethnicity, infant birth weight, length of first and second stages of labour, and any type of perineal trauma or episiotomy. However, at 3 and 12 months, differences appeared between the groups. There was an increased incidence of incontinence in the group delivered with forceps compared with the ventouse and normal delivery groups, and the incontinence was more severe and more likely to persist. Forceps delivery increasing the likelihood of developing stress urinary incontinence has also been demonstrated by other studies.[62]

Other research has shown that perhaps the mode of delivery is less important than originally thought. Pregnancy longer than 20 weeks of gestation, regardless of mode of delivery, leads to an increase in incontinence, prolapse and pelvic floor surgery.[63]

Perineal ultrasonography of bladder neck mobility after vaginal delivery or caesarean section demonstrated that women who had undergone vaginal delivery had increased mobility of the bladder neck when compared with those undergoing a caesarean section. This was associated with a nonsignificant rise in stress incontinence in the vaginal delivery group. Women who had had three caesarean sections had the same level of bladder neck mobility as their counterparts who had delivered vaginally.[64]

Problems during delivery

Delivery has been thought to be the main culprit for urinary incontinence because this is when direct injury to the musculature and surrounding connective tissue occurs. This may stem partially from the era when profound injuries and fistulas occurred as a result of obstructed labour, producing instant and catastrophic incontinence. Vesicovaginal fistulas still remain a problem in the developing world, with extensive morbidity for the women who suffer with continual urinary incontinence.

Vaginal delivery is associated with a reduction in the urethral sphincter volume.[40,41] Despite this, the increase in the functional length of the urethra and maintenance of the mean urethral closure pressure may preserve continence.[16] If these parameters are not maintained, incontinence may be precipitated.

Vaginal delivery itself has been shown in some studies to have an effect on the bladder. Weil *et al.*[65] performed urodynamic studies on 27 primiparous women two to five days postpartum. They were divided into three groups: vaginal delivery without an epidural, vaginal delivery with an epidural, and lower segment caesarean section. The caesarean section group had a lower bladder capacity compared with other two groups; the group who had a vaginal delivery plus epidural analgesia had the most hypotonic bladders. Although these results are interesting, they may be due to the catheterisation policy, which differed between the groups, rather than to the effect of the mode of delivery.

POSTPARTUM

Voiding difficulties postpartum

Acute retention of urine is common after childbirth and drainage with an indwelling Foley catheter avoids overdistension of the detrusor musculature. If urinary retention remains undiagnosed, UTI, upper urinary tract damage and permanent voiding difficulties can develop. Problems such as oedema, localised haematoma, pain or the fear of pain usually resolve quite quickly. Only 0.05% of women[66] are still unable to void three days after delivery and leaving a Foley catheter *in situ* for a further two weeks may be the best option because it allows the woman to go home with a leg bag. The vast majority of voiding difficulties resolve during this period. Long-term follow-up of these women has not revealed a significant increase in urinary symptoms when compared with women who did not experience voiding difficulties postpartum.[52,67]

Postnatal symptoms

Within this group of women who suffer with postnatal urinary incontinence, perhaps the most interesting are those who develop new symptoms postnatally but did not have them antenatally. These symptoms could be regarded as pathological because they have arisen from the delivery alone. However, overall, women who have the most marked symptoms postnatally are those who appear to have a predisposition to urinary incontinence and have had symptoms antenatally.

Stress incontinence is usually less severe postnatally than antenatally.[68] Although women's perceptions and reporting of symptoms and definitions vary, particularly in the early postpartum period, 6% have demonstrable postnatal stress incontinence.[69] Again, antenatal stress incontinence is the biggest predictor of symptoms of stress incontinence postnatally.[45,70] Women who have symptoms of stress incontinence that persist for three months postnatally are particularly likely to have long-lasting symptoms, with 92% remaining incontinent at five years.[70]

Pelvic floor exercises

Pelvic floor exercises should be encouraged in all women and should become part of teaching in schools and a standard part of exercise classes for women. They are noninvasive, do no harm and can be performed by almost all women.

Pelvic floor exercises have been shown to reduce stress urinary incontinence when used antenatally[3,71] or postnatally.[72–75] However, the advice and practical instructions that unselected women receive seem to vary widely[76] and targeting women who are particularly at risk may be more effective. Chiarelli and Cockburn[77] performed a randomised controlled trial of pelvic floor exercise teaching in postnatal women who had either had an instrumental delivery or had delivered a baby heavier than 4 kg. One group were given the usual advice from a booklet while the second group had supervised exercises and were also taught behavioural techniques to help them to remember to perform them. In the group receiving the additional support, 84% were doing pelvic floor exercises regularly compared with 58% in the control group. Thirty-one percent reported incontinence compared with 38% in the control group and the number of women classed as severely incontinent of urine was reduced from 17% to 10%).[77] Given this evidence it seems a shame that only 6% of midwives observe the perineal area when teaching a woman pelvic floor exercises and usually rely on verbal advice or giving a leaflet.[78] How the exercises are taught is crucial because the woman's perception of her ability to perform the exercises and the severity of the incontinence denote how consistently they are performed.[79] A team of skilled, enthusiastic physiotherapists or specially trained midwives may seem like an expensive resource but, in comparison with using caesarean section to maintain pelvic floor health and continence, over time they may prove to be money well invested. However, difficulties are encountered when attempting to teach pelvic floor exercises. Certain groups of women, particularly teenagers, do not attend parent education classes regularly. Early postnatal discharge from hospital means that women may not have the chance to see a physiotherapist and, even if they do, they may not continue the exercises at home when they become busy with the new baby. Finally, many women do not see continence as an issue that may affect them personally.

Perineal massage

Unfortunately, another simple intervention, perineal massage during pregnancy, although it may reduce perineal trauma at delivery, does not have an effect on continence when measured at three months.[80]

PREGNANCY IN WOMEN WHO HAVE UNDERGONE CONTINENCE SURGERY

Artificial urethral sphincters

Artificial urethral sphincters are usually inserted in patients with an underlying neurological deficit such as spina bifida or spinal cord injury, but they are also occasionally used in female adolescents with non-neurogenic intrinsic sphincter weakness. Artificial urethral sphincters are used because they have success rates exceeding 60% continence in series with long-term follow-up. Experience of these devices in pregnancy and labour is limited but small case series have been published.[81] Women with artificial urethral sphincters have delivered both vaginally and by caesarean section. The early devices could not be turned off and artificial sphincters were used without any complications during pregnancy or delivery. The current recommendation is to deactivate the sphincter for pregnancy and delivery to reduce the pressure on the cuff and bladder neck.[82]

Augmentation cystoplasty

Augmentation cystoplasty is used as a last resort for gross detrusor overactivity when medical treatment has failed. In pregnancy there is increased morbidity, including from UTI, deteriorating renal function, ureteric dilatation or obstruction, bowel obstruction and premature labour.[83] In women who have had augmentation cystoplasty, caesarean section should be avoided apart from for the usual obstetric indications because it is easy for the unwary to injure either the bladder or the pedicle of the augmenting bowel. A classic upper segment caesarean section is usually required because the lower segment cannot be accessed easily.[84]

Other continence procedures

So far there have been only anecdotal reports of pregnancy after the tension-free vaginal tape procedure. In a case report from Germany there were no complications during pregnancy, with the tape remaining in the correct position throughout. The woman was delivered by caesarean section and remained continent.[85]

A questionnaire study of 87 women who had a pregnancy and delivery after a variety of different continence procedures showed a higher rate of continence in those delivered by caesarean section (95%, $n = 47$) compared with those who delivered vaginally (75%, $n = 40$).[86] Although this is observational evidence, it suggests that there may be a role for caesarean section in protecting a continent repair.

ANAL INCONTINENCE

Although this chapter is largely concerned with the effect of pregnancy on the lower urinary tract and urinary incontinence, anal incontinence is an important area that has largely been ignored for many years. Women are more susceptible to anal incontinence than men and even nulliparous women have a higher prevalence than their male counterparts. It has been reported that, overall, 10.9% of women experience incontinence of flatus compared with 6.8% of men; 3.5% of women admit to incontinence of solid or liquid faeces in comparison to 2.3% of men.[63] Pregnancy and delivery compounds this further as the denervation and direct muscle injuries also affect the anal sphincter. Sultan *et al.*[87] demonstrated by using endoanal ultrasonography that, at six weeks postpartum, 35% of primiparous women have defects in the anal sphincter. These findings have caused much debate about whether the injuries are 'missed' at the time of delivery or are genuinely occult. Work is currently continuing in our unit to answer these vital questions. Many women still find anal incontinence a taboo subject and often the onus rests on the obstetrician or the gynaecologist to elucidate the history.

CONCLUSIONS

For many years it has been assumed that vaginal delivery was the sole cause of urinary incontinence. In reality the evidence for an assumption such as this does not exist. It is impossible and unethical to perform a randomised controlled trial of vaginal delivery and caesarean section to try to determine cause and effect. It remains possible that women who undergo an emergency caesarean section have a more rigid type of collagen than those who deliver vaginally. Women with more lax connective tissue would be more at risk of stress incontinence and more likely to deliver vaginally.

Given that a randomised controlled trial is not a realistic proposition, how do we improve current clinical practice? We should aim to be teaching healthy bladder habits. Pelvic floor exercises should be taught to all women, with reinforcement techniques. We should aim to be honest and open with women about the difficulties they may face, not only in the first few weeks and months after they deliver but also in later life. We should not jump into blanket policies such as avoiding forceps or rotational delivery nor encourage the performance of caesarean section for indications that lack evidence. We need to press on with the research in areas where it can be performed with due regard to ethical issues, so that we are able to give women the information to decide what is best for themselves and for their baby.

References

1.   Glazener CM, Abdalla MI, Stroud P, Naji SA, Templeton AA, Russell IT. Postnatal maternal morbidity: extent, causes and treatment. *Br J Obstet Gynaecol* 1995;102:282–7.

2.   Glazener CM. Sexual function after childbirth: women's experiences, persistent morbidity and lack of professional recognition. *Br J Obstet Gynaecol* 1997;104:330–5.

3.   Wilson PD, Herbison RM, Herbison GP. Obstetric practice and the prevalence of urinary incontinence three months after delivery. *Br J Obstet Gynaecol* 1996;103:154–61.

4.   MacArthur C, Bick DE, Keighley MR. Faecal incontinence after childbirth. *Br J Obstet Gynaecol* 1997;104:46–50.

5.   Bick DE, MacArthur C. Attendance, content and relevance of the six week postnatal examination. *Midwifery* 1995;11:69–73.

6.   Landon CR, Crofts CE, Smith AR, Trowbridge EW. Mechanical factors of fascia during pregnancy: a possible factor in the development of stress urinary incontinence. *Contemp Rev Obstet Gynaecol* 1990;2:40–6.

7.   Lavin JM, Smith AR, Anderson J, Grant M, Buckley H, Critchley H, et al. The effect of the first pregnancy on the connective tissue of the rectus sheath. *Neurourol Urodyn* 1997;16:381–2.

8.   Green TH Jr. Urinary stress incontinence: differential diagnosis, pathophysiology and management. *Am J Obstet Gynecol* 1975;122:897–900.

9.   Wijma J, Weiss Potters AE, de Wolf BT, Tinga DJ, Aarnoudse JG. Anatomical and functional changes in the lower urinary tract during pregnancy. *Br J Obstet Gynaecol* 2001;108:726–32.

10. Francis WJ. Disturbances of bladder function in relation to pregnancy. *J Obstet Gynaecol Br Cwlth* 1960;67:353–66.

11. Malpas P, Jeffcoate TN, Lister UM. The displacement of the bladder and urethra during labour. *J Obstet Gynaecol Br Empire* 1949;56:949–60.

12. Peschers UM, Schaer G, Anthuber C, De Lancey JO, Schuessler B. Changes in vesical neck mobility following vaginal delivery. *Obstet Gynecol* 1996;88:1001–6.

13. Stanton SL, Kerr-Wilson R, Harris. G V. The incidence of urological symptoms in normal pregnancy. *Br J Obstet Gynaecol* 1980;87:897–900.

14. Kristiansson P, Samuelsson E, Von Schoultz B, Svardsudd K. Reproductive hormones and stress urinary incontinence in pregnancy. *Acta Obstet Gynecol Scand* 2001;80:1125–30.

15. Swift SE, Ostergard DR. Effects of progesterone on the lower urinary tract. *Int Urogynecol J* 1993;4:232–36.

16. Iosif S, Ulmsten U. Comparative urodynamic studies of continent and stress incontinent women in pregnancy and in the puerperium. *Am J Obstet Gynecol* 1981;140:645–50.

17. van Geelan JM, Lemmens WAJG, Eskes TKAB, Martin CB. The urethral pressure profile in pregnancy and after delivery in healthy nulliparous women. *Am J Obstet Gynecol* 1982;144:636–49.

18. Iosif S, Ingermarsson I, Ulmsten U. Urodynamic studies in normal pregnancy and the puerperium. *Am J Obstet Gynecol* 1980;137:696–700.

19. Davison JM, Shiells EA, Phillips PR, Lindheimer M. Serial evaluation of vasopressin release and thirst in human pregnancy. Role of human chorionic gonadotrophin in osmoregulatory changes of gestation. *J Clin Invest* 1988;81:798–806.

20. Tong YC, Hung YC, Lin JS, Hsu CT, Cheng JT. Effects of pregnancy and progesterone on autonomic function in rat urinary bladder. *Pharmacology* 1995;50:192–200.

21. Muellner SR. Physiological bladder changes during pregnancy and the puerperium. *J Urol* 1939;41:691–5.

22. Youssef AF. Cystometric studies in gynaecology and obstetrics. *Obstet Gynecol* 1959;8:181–8.

23. Parboosingh J, Doig A. Studies of nocturia in normal pregnancy. *J Obstet Gynaecol Br Cwlth* 1973;80:888–95.

24. Cutner A, Carey A, Cardozo LD. Lower urinary tract symptoms in early pregnancy. *J Obstet Gynaecol* 1992;12:75–8.

25. Parboosingh J, Doig A. Renal nyctohemeral excretory patterns of water and solutes in normal human pregnancy. *Am J Obstet Gynecol* 1973;116:605–9.

26. Cutner A, Cardozo LD, Benness CJ, Carey A, Cooper D. Detrusor instability in early pregnancy. *Neurourol Urodyn* 1990;9:329.

27. Nel JT, Diedericks A, Joubert G, Arndt K. A prospective clinical and urodynamic study of bladder function during and after pregnancy. *Int Urogynecol J Pelvic Floor Dysfunct* 2001;12:21–6.

28. Lee JG, Wein AJ, Levin RM. Effects of pregnancy on urethral and bladder neck function. *Urology* 1993;42:747–52.

29. Edwards JA, Reid YJ, Cozens DD. Reproductive toxicity studies with oxybutinin hydrochloride. *Toxicology* 1986;40:31–44.

30. Thomas TM, Plymat KR, Blannin J, Meade TW. Prevalence of urinary incontinence. *Br Med J* 1980;281:1243–5.

31. Foldspang A, Mommsen S, Lam GW, Elving L. Parity as a correlate of adult female urinary incontinence prevalence. *J Epidemiol Community Health* 1992;46:595–600.

32. Iosif S, Ingermarsson I. Prevalence of stress incontinence among women delivered by caesarean section. *Int J Gynaecol Obstet* 1982;20:87–9.

33. Iosif S. Stress incontinence during pregnancy and in the puerperium. *Int J Gynaecol Obstet* 1981;19:13–20.

34. Krue S, Jensen H, Agger AO, Rasmussen KL. The influence of infant birth weight on post partum stress incontinence in obese women. *Arch Gynecol Obstet* 1997;259:143–5.

35. Keane DP, Sims TJ, Abrams P, Bailey AJ. Analysis of collagen status in premenopausal nulliparous women with genuine stress incontinence. *Br J Obstet Gynaecol* 1997;104:994–8.

36. Rasmussen KL, Krue S, Johansson LE, Knudsen HJ, Agger AO. Obesity as a predictor of postpartum urinary symptoms. *Acta Obstet Gynecol Scand* 1997;76:359–62.

37. Viktrup L, Lose G. Do fertile women remember the onset of stress incontinence? Recall bias 5 years after 1st delivery. *Acta Obstet Gynecol Scand* 2001;80:952–5.

38. Noble JG, Dixon PJ, Rickards D, Fowler CJ. Urethral sphincter volumes in women with obstructed voiding and abnormal sphincter electromyographic activity. *Br J Urol* 1995;76:741–6.

39. Athanasiou S, Khullar V, Boos K, Salvatore S, Cardozo L. Imaging the urethral sphincter with three-dimensional ultrasound. *Obstet Gynecol* 1999;94:295–301.

40. Toozs-Hobson P, Athanasiou S, Khullar V, Boos K, Anders K, Cardozo LD. Why do women develop incontinence after childbirth? *Neurourol Urodyn* 1997;16:384–5.

41. Toozs-Hobson P, Cardozo LD, Boos K, Khullar V. The urethral sphincter volume and pressure profile changes due to childbirth. *Br J Obstet Gynaecol* 1998;105 Suppl 17:29.

42. Wise BG, Burton G, Cutner A, Cardozo LD. Effect of ultrasound probe on lower urinary tract function. *Br J Urol* 1992;70:12–16.

43. Meyer S, De Grandi P, Schreyer A, Caccia G. The assessment of bladder neck position and mobility in continent nullipara, multipara, forceps-delivered and incontinent women using perineal ultrasound: a future office procedure? *Int Urogynecol J Pelvic Floor Dysfunct* 1996;7:138–46.

44. King JK, Freeman RM. Is antenatal bladder neck mobility a risk factor for postpartum stress incontinence? *Br J Obstet Gynaecol* 1998;105:1300–7.

45. Little P. The incidence of urinary tract infection in 5000 pregnant women. *Lancet* 1966;ii:925–8.

46. Whalley PJ. Bacteriuria of pregnancy. *Am J Obstet Gynecol* 1967;97:723–8.

47. Etherington I, James DK. Reagent strip testing of antenatal urine specimens for infection. *Br J Obstet Gynaecol* 1983;100:806–8.

48. Maikranz P, Lindheimer M, Coe F. Nephrolithiasis in pregnancy. *Baillieres Clin Obstet Gynaecol* 1994;8:375–86.

49. Cutner A, Cardozo LD, Benness CJ. Assessment of urinary symptoms in the 2nd half of pregnancy. *Int Urogynecol J* 1982;3:30–2.

50. Viktrup L, Lose G, Rolff M, Barfoed K. The symptom of stress incontinence caused by pregnancy or delivery in primiparas. *Obstet Gynecol* 1992;79:945–9.

51. Olofsson CI, Ekblom AO, Ekman-Ordeberg GE, Irestedt LE. Post-partum urinary retention: a comparison between two methods of epidural analgesia. *Eur J Obstet Gynecol Reprod Biol* 1997;71:31–4.

52. Andolf E, Iosif CS, Jorgensen C, Rydhstroem H. Insidious urinary retention after vaginal delivery: prevalence and symptoms at follow-up in a population-based study. *Gynecol Obstet Invest* 1994;38:51–3.

53. Weissman A, Grisaru D, Shenhav M, Peyser RM, Jaffa AJ. Postpartum surveillance of urinary retention by ultrasonography: the effect of epidural analgesia. *Ultrasound Obstet Gynecol* 1995;6:130–4.

54. Persson J, Wolner-Hanssen P, Rydhstroem H. Obstetric risk factors for stress urinary incontinence: a population-based study. *Obstet Gynecol* 2000; 96:442–5.

55. Dimpfl T, Hesse U, Schussler B. Incidence and causes of postpartum urinary stress incontinence. *Eur J Obstet Gynecol Reprod Biol* 1992;43:29–33.

56. Viktrup L, Lose G. Epidural anesthesia during labor and stress incontinence after delivery. *Obstet Gynecol* 1993;82:984–6.

57. Kerr-Wilson RHJ, Thompson SW, Orr JW Jr, Davis RO, Cloud GA. Effect of labor on the postpartum bladder. *Obstet Gynecol* 1984;64:115–18.

58. Brostrom S, Jennum P, Lose G. Morbidity of urodynamic investigation in healthy women. *Int Urogynecol J Pelvic Floor Dysfunct* 2002;13:182–4.

59. Drife JO. Choice and instrumental delivery. *Br J Obstet Gynaecol* 1996;103:608–11.

60. Chiarelli P, Campbell E. Incontinence during pregnancy. Prevalence and opportunities for continence promotion. *Aust N Z J Obstet Gynaecol* 1997;37:66–73.

61. Arya LA, Jackson ND, Myers DL, Verma A. Risk of new-onset urinary incontinence after forceps and vacuum delivery in primiparous women. *Am J Obstet Gynecol* 2001;185:1318–24.

62. Van Kessel K, Reed S, Newton K, Meier A, Lentz G. The second stage of labor and stress urinary incontinence. *Am J Obstet Gynecol* 2001;184:1571–5.

63. MacLennan AH, Taylor AW, Wilson DH, Wilson D. The prevalence of pelvic floor disorders and their relationship to gender, age, parity and mode of delivery. *BJOG* 2000;107:1460–70.

64. Demirci F, Ozden S, Alpay Z, Demirci ET, Ayas S. The effects of vaginal delivery and caesarean section on bladder neck mobility and stress urinary incontinence. *Int Urogynecol J Pelvic Floor Dysfunct* 2001;12:129–33.

65. Weil A, Reyes H, Rottenberg RD, Beguin F, Hermann WL. Effect of lumbar epidural on lower urinary tract function in the immediate postpartum period. *Br J Obstet Gynaecol* 1983;90:428–32.

66. Groutz A, Gordon D, Wolman I, Jaffa A, Kupferminc MJ, Lessing JB. Persistent postpartum urinary retention in contemporary obstetric practice. *J Reprod Med* 2001;46:44–8.

67. Yip S-K, Sahota D, Chang AM, Chung TK. Four-year follow-up of women who were diagnosed to have postpartum urinary retention. *Am J Obstet Gynecol* 2002;187:648–52.

68. Chaliha C, Kalia V, Stanton SL, Monga A, Sultan AH. Antenatal prediction of postpartum urinary and fecal incontinence. *Obstet Gynecol* 1999;94:689–94.

69. Sampselle CM, Delancey JO, Ashton-Miller JA. Urinary incontinence in pregnancy and postpartum. *Neurourol Urodyn* 1996;15:329–30.

70. Viktrup L, Lose G. The risk of stress incontinence 5 years after first delivery. *Am J Obstet Gynecol* 2001;185:82–7.

71. Sampselle CM, Miller JM, Mims BL, Delancey JO, Ashton-Miller JA, Antonakos CL. The effect of pelvic floor muscle exercise on transient incontinence during pregnancy and childbirth. *Obstet Gynecol* 1998;91:406–11.

72. Morkved S, Bo K. The effect of postpartum pelvic floor muscle exercise in the prevention and treatment of urinary incontinence. *Int Urogynecol J Pelvic Floor Dysfunct* 1997;8:217–22.

73. Morkved S, Bo K. Effect of postpartum pelvic floor muscle training in preventing and treatment of urinary incontinence: a one-year follow-up. *BJOG* 2000;107:1022–8.

74. Meyer S, Hohlfield P, Achtari C, De Grandi P. Pelvic floor education after vaginal delivery. *Obstet Gynecol* 2001;97:673–7.

75. Glazener CM, Herbison GP, Wilson PD, McArthur C, Lang GD, Gee H, *et al.* Conservative management of persistent postnatal urinary and faecal incontinence: randomised controlled trial. *BMJ* 2001;323:593–6.

76. Mason L, Glenn S, Walton I, Hughes C. The instruction in pelvic floor exercises provided to women during pregnancy or following delivery. *Midwifery* 2001;17:55–64.

77. Chiarelli P, Cockburn J. Promoting urinary incontinence in women after delivery: randomised controlled trial. *BMJ* 2002;324:1241.

78. Logan K. Audit of advice provided on pelvic floor exercises. *Prof Nurse* 2001;16:1369–72.

79. Alewijnse D, Mesters I, Metsemakers J, Adriaans J, Van der Borne B. Predictors of intention to adhere to physiotherapy among women with urinary incontinence. *Health Res* 2001;16:173–86.

80. Labreque M, Eason E, Marcoux S. Randomized trial of perineal massage during pregnancy: perineal symptoms three months after delivery. *Am J Obstet Gynecol* 2000;182:76–80.

81. Fishman IJ, Scott FB. Pregnancy in patients with the artificial urinary sphincter. *J Urol* 1993;150:340–1.

82. Toh K, Diokno AC. Management of intrinsic sphincter deficiency in adolescent females with bladder emptying function. *J Urol* 2002;168:1150–3.

83. Doyle BA, Smith SP, Stempel LE. Urinary undiversion and pregnancy. *Am J Obstet Gynecol* 1988;158:1131–2.

84. Greenwell TJ, Venn SN, Mundy AR. Augmentation cystoplasty. *BJU Int* 2001;88:511–25.

85. Gauruder-Burmester A, Tunn R. Pregnancy and labor after TVT-plasty. *Acta Obstet Gynecol Scand* 2001;80:283–4.

86. Dainer M, Hall CD, Choe J, Bhatia N. Pregnancy following incontinence surgery. *Int Urogynecol J Pelvic Floor Dysfunct* 1998;9:385–90.

87. Sultan AH, Kamm MA, Hudson CN, Thomas JM, Batram CI. Anal-sphincter disruption during vaginal delivery. *N Engl J Med* 1993;329:1905–11.

34

Magnetic resonance guided thermal ablation therapy for uterine fibroids

Lesley Regan and Jonathan T Hindley

BACKGROUND

Uterine fibroids are common, benign tumours of the female genital tract. Symptomatic fibroids are diagnosed in some 25% of women; however, they are present in as many as 50–60%.[1] Fibroids typically present in one of three ways:

- with heavy and/or prolonged menstruation

- with symptoms of a pelvic mass causing abdominal pain and urinary symptoms

- with reproductive dysfunction including infertility, miscarriage and complications of pregnancy such as red degeneration of fibroids, fetal malpresentation and postpartum bleeding.[2]

In summary, uterine fibroids cause significant personal, social and financial problems for many women of childbearing age.

We do not understand how uterine fibroids develop, nor why only a proportion of women with fibroids develop symptoms. However, there appears to be a genetic predisposition. Fibroids present more frequently in black women than in white women. Black women tend to present at a younger age, with larger fibroids, and are more likely to become anaemic. Furthermore, they experience more postoperative complications after surgical treatment, even when they are matched for fibroid volume/symptoms.[3]

For many years the mainstay of treatment for uterine fibroids has been surgical, either hysterectomy, or myomectomy for women who wish to preserve their fertility. Fibroids are the most frequently cited reason for hysterectomy, which itself is the most common elective operation undergone by women in the UK. A total of 47 000 hysterectomies were performed in England in the years 2000–2001. During the same time 1321 myomectomies were performed.[4]

Fibroids affect large numbers of young women, so it is not surprising that there has been an increasing demand for alternative approaches to treatment. Women now more often prefer minimally invasive treatments that give symptomatic relief without compromising their lifestyle or their fertility. A number of new treatment modalities have been introduced, most notably uterine artery embolisation, first described for the elective treatment of fibroids by Ravina *et al.* in 1995,[5] and now widely available in the USA and increasingly in the UK.

Thermal ablation of fibroids gained limited popularity via the laparoscopic approach in the early 1990s.[6] This technique achieved volume reductions in fibroids of up to 90% and symptomatic relief in 95% of affected women.[7] However, concerns have been raised regarding the high rate of dense pelvic adhesions caused by the laparoscopic laser ablation of fibroids. In one series, dense fibrous adhesions were reported between the uterus and the small bowel in 8 of 15 women (53%) at second–look laparoscopy.[8] It is easy to understand why adhesions are so common when the techniques used for laparoscopic myolysis are considered. Essentially, they involve the introduction of laser fibres into the fibroid at laparoscopy under general anaesthesia. The laser fibres are 'live' as they burn into the fibroid through the uterine serosa. A change in the appearance of the fibroid is used to assess when sufficient heat has been applied. In this way the serosal surface of the uterus is burned as the fibres are placed and the lack of thermal mapping will mean that further damage can occur if the lesion reaches the serosa before the heat is removed.

There are reports of uterine rupture during pregnancy in women who have undergone this treatment.[9,10] These complications occurred in the third trimester but prior to the onset of uterine contractions. Donnez et al.[7] suggest that laparoscopic myolysis is suitable only for those women who have completed their families.

MAGNETIC RESONANCE GUIDED LASER ABLATION OF UTERINE FIBROIDS

Magnetic resonance imaging (MRI) is an excellent imaging modality for the assessment of the uterus owing to its high resolution of soft tissue (Figure 1). Although this resolution means that MRI can be used to plan treatments for fibroids it is the unique ability of magnetic resonance thermal mapping that underlies the techniques described in this chapter. The changes that occur in tissues as the temperature rises cause variation in the MR image obtained. This allows a colourised map to be created to show the temperatures reached in real time throughout the heating process (Figure 2). The heating can therefore be controlled to treat as much of the fibroid as possible without damaging the myometrium, serosa or surrounding structures. In addition MRI does not involve any ionising radiation and therefore has no known harmful effects.

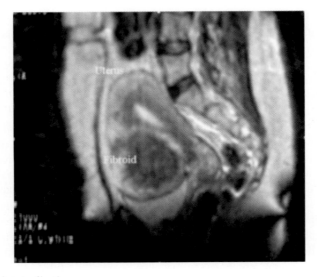

Figure 1 *MR image of uterine fibroids*

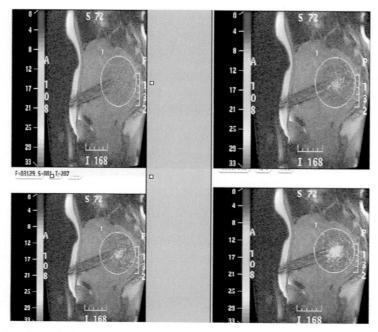

Figure 2 *MR thermal map showing rise in temperature to 55 degrees Celsius: colour changes from blue to green*

Traditional magnetic resonance systems are enclosed so that interventions have been hampered by the lack of access to the patient. At St Mary's Hospital, London, we have an 'open' magnetic resonance scanner (Signa SPIO 0.5T®, General Electrical Medical Systems, Milwaukee, WI). This system is different in that it is open in the vertical plane, thus allowing access to the patient while scanning (Figure 3). It enables us to place four needles into the fibroid through the anterior abdominal wall under real-time magnetic resonance guidance. The use of a 'Flash Point Tracker' (Signa SPIO 0.5T) allows the proposed path of the needle to be shown on the images, ensuring that the bladder or stray loops of bowel can be seen and avoided.

Once the needles are correctly positioned the laser fibres can be fed directly into the centre of the fibroids. This means that the heating begins distant from the serosal surface and thus limits the serosal damage to four needle punctures.

Irreversible tissue damage is achieved at 55 degrees Celsius and above[11] and this level can be rapidly appreciated using the thermal map.[12] Heat application is continued until a maximal area of green coloration is seen within the region of interest but stopped if the area of temperature rise threatens to reach outside the desired volume. This ensures that maximum thermal energy is applied to the target without any heating of the myometrium, the uterine surface or extrauterine structures.

An initial pilot study was performed in 12 women who were due to undergo hysterectomy subsequent to the magnetic resonance-guided laser ablation treatment.[13] Nine of the 12 (75%) stated that their symptoms had improved such that they did not wish to go ahead with surgery as planned. In those who had surgery there was good correlation between the histological findings and the lesions on the thermal maps. In contrast to laparoscopic laser ablation of fibroids, pelvic adhesions have not been seen subsequent to magnetic resonance-guided laser ablation (Figure 4) because serosal damage is avoided by using the guided technique.

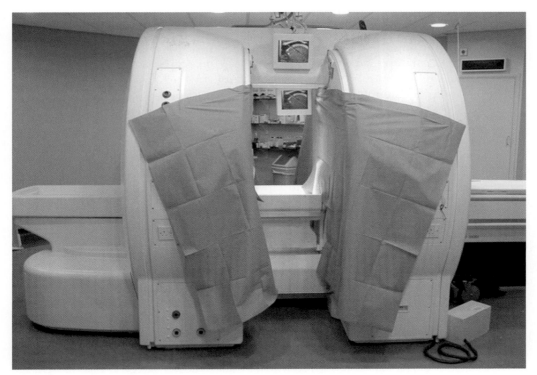

Figure 3 *Open magnetic resonance scanner at St Mary's Hospital, London*

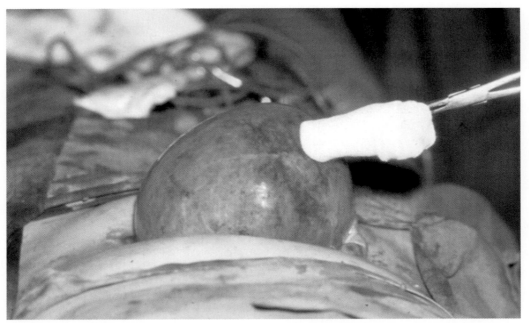

Figure 4 *Hysterectomy performed after magnetic resonance-guided laser ablation of uterine fibroids; there are no adhesions to the serosal surface*

Since carrying out this pilot study, over 100 magnetic resonance-guided laser ablation treatments of uterine fibroids have been performed in our unit and are being followed up. There have been no major adverse effects associated with this procedure, the only adverse events being urinary tract infections (six) and skin burns (three). Two of the skin burns were minor and had to be pointed out to the women by the physician. The third was a full thickness burn measuring 2 × 3 cm and caused the woman considerable distress.

Our early outcome data show that there is a significant and sustained reduction in fibroid volume of 30% at three months and 40% at one year (Figure 5).[14] More importantly, we used a validated outcomes questionnaire to measure satisfaction with this procedure. Sixty-nine percent of the women answered that their symptoms were much or a little better when compared with before magnetic resonance-guided laser ablation of the fibroids. Similarly, 69% felt better overall and 80% would recommend the treatment to a friend. In the same article we present a small series of menstrual blood loss measurements in women who complained of excessive menstrual bleeding and in whom there was a significant ($P = 0.012$) fall in measured menstrual blood loss after magnetic resonance-guided laser ablation of fibroids. This fall seems to be more marked in those with the highest initial monthly loss.

MAGNETIC RESONANCE-GUIDED FOCUSED ULTRASOUND SURGERY FOR UTERINE FIBROIDS

The earliest medical uses of ultrasound were therapeutic rather than diagnostic and the ability of ultrasound energy to cause a rise in tissue temperature was recognised as long ago as 1927.[15]

High-intensity ultrasound can be focused within a tissue to deliver energy to a specific spot and cause a temperature rise at that point to above 60 degrees Celsius. This is sufficient to kill cells in

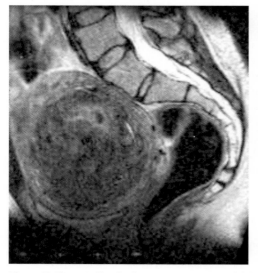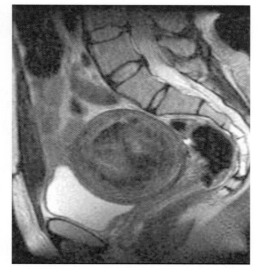

Figure 5 *Change in fibroids after magnetic resonance-guided laser ablation: (a) before; (b) after*

a cigar shape 1–2 cm long.[15] The tissue in the path of the ultrasound beam, but away from the focus, will be warmed but not to lethal temperatures. If sufficient time is left between sonications, then vascular perfusion will dissipate the heat, avoiding tissue damage except at the focus.[16]

We have been involved in the clinical development of a focused ultrasound surgery (FUS) system (ExAblate 2000™, InSightec-TXSonics, Haifa, Israel) that is fully integrated with our standard, closed MRI system. This consists of an ultrasound transducer that is built into the bed of the system. The FUS software enslaves the MRI and allows full magnetic resonance-guidance of the treatment. MRI monitoring once again offers several advantages:

- The excellent resolution of the magnetic resonance images allows the accurate selection of the fibroid to be treated. These images are passed automatically to the FUS system.

- The pathway that the high-energy ultrasound beam will take can be reviewed prior to treatment and, if necessary, adjusted to avoid structures that may be harmed, such as bowel, abdominal scars and air bubbles on the skin. Thus far we have avoided treating through the bladder but this is a potential pathway for the future.

- The essential advantage of integration of the FUS and magnetic resonance systems is, as in magnetic resonance-guided laser ablation, that of thermal monitoring. Real-time thermal monitoring fulfils three purposes:
  - It localises the thermal spot at a low power prior to treatment to ensure that the targeting and tissue compensation is correct and that the thermal dose is going to be delivered to the desired volume.
  - It minimises any damage to the normal tissue close to the targeted tissue. Real-time thermal monitoring allows control of the ultrasound energy delivery so that there is no damage to tissue outside the target fibroid.
  - The thermal map allows assessment of the therapeutic effect. Knowledge of the actual temperature reached in the target tissue enables the operator to ensure that a maximally effective lesion is created.

The treatment in magnetic resonance-guided FUS (MRgFUS) for symptomatic uterine fibroids proceeds through the creation of multiple cigar shaped burns within the fibroid. These continue until the central volume of the fibroid is completely destroyed. The thermal maps from each sonication are superimposed on to the latest image so that the volume of the fibroid that has been heated to a lethal dose can be easily appreciated (Figure 2).

St Mary's Hospital has been involved in an international multicentre trial of the application of this technology to the treatment of symptomatic uterine fibroids. We carried out a pilot study to assess the safety and practicality of this treatment.[17] This involved women who presented with symptomatic fibroids and were due to have a hysterectomy. They were treated with MRgFUS and then underwent the surgery. Of the 55 women reported in this study, 80% underwent the procedure. All were treated as outpatients and there were no major device related adverse events. There was good correlation between the target lesions created on the magnetic resonance images, the thermal maps recording the treated volume, and the histological lesions in those who underwent hysterectomy. The ethics committee at one site stipulated that the women treated there would be followed up for at least one month and then be offered hysterectomy or continuing follow-up. In this group, all but one declined surgery because their symptoms had improved sufficiently; their follow-up continues.

We have embarked on a further study to look at clinical and radiological outcomes after MRgFUS of fibroids using as patient centred outcome measures a general health and quality of life measure, the SF-36, and a fibroid specific outcomes measure, the Uterine Fibroid Symptom and Quality of Life questionnaire developed for the Cardiovascular and Interventional Radiology Research and Education Foundation.[18] We are using fibroid and uterine volumes measured from magnetic resonance images as secondary outcomes. Although we do not have any data to present from this study at this stage, anecdotal reports that we have received from participants appear encouraging.

The ExAblate2000 system is integrated into a standard magnet and thus, in comparison with MR guided laser ablation, which requires the much less readily available open magnetic resonance system, seems to offer advantages in terms of capital costs.

CONCLUSION

The two treatments described above are analogous in that they are both magnetic resonance-guided thermal ablative processes. A precise burn is created within the uterine fibroid and, as this resolves by coagulative necrosis, the fibroid shrinks; symptomatic improvements occur in two-thirds of women undergoing this process. There has been an early report of the use of magnetic resonance-guided cryotherapy for uterine fibroids.[19] This treatment seems to be associated with an unacceptably high complication rate, with three of nine women in the report suffering major adverse events. Further data are required before this modality can be considered.

Our treatment differs from previous ablative therapies because of the use of magnetic resonance-guidance to plan the procedure, target the ablative source, and map, in near real time, the progress of the ablation. This enables the operator to tailor the procedure to the individual woman and indeed to the individual fibroid. We have observed a marked heterogeneity among fibroids, not only in position, size and symptoms, but also in magnetic resonance signal characteristics and behaviour when exposed to a heating source, such that a didactic approach to ablation without online thermal mapping would, in our opinion, be unreliable and possibly unsafe.

We present these novel therapies as potential additions to the options available to women with fibroids and to the gynaecologist seeking to offer them a complete range of interventions. Unsolicited, we have been approached by women with symptomatic fibroids from as far afield as Uganda and Australia, suggesting that there is a cohort of women who are looking for a minimally or noninvasive approach to this problem. Our experience so far suggests that magnetic resonance-guided thermal ablation of fibroids may result in marked symptomatic relief for those with specific, fibroid related symptoms such as heavy prolonged periods or urinary frequency. However, it offers less satisfactory outcomes in those who have nonspecific symptoms or who are asymptomatic but wish to treat the mass that they have noted emerging from their pelvis. We have been aware that a volume reduction of 50% sounds more impressive than a reduction in diameter from 10 cm to 8 cm and have had to make clear to these women that this treatment will not rid them of their fibroids. In terms of recurrence we have reported that the fibroid volume reduction at three months appears to be maintained at one year without signs of regrowth. Magnetic resonance-guided thermal ablation treatments for fibroids are, however, localised therapies and will not prevent further growth in fibroids that are not treated. There are no known contraindications to multiple treatments of the same patient or of the same fibroid.

In the studies performed to date we have excluded women who plan to have further pregnancies and thus have no data on the safety of pregnancy after magnetic resonance-guided laser or FUS treatment of fibroids. We certainly do not have data to suggest that this treatment will play a role in fibroid related subfertility. It is however our belief that the problems with uterine rupture reported after laparoscopic myolysis[9,10] will not be repeated with these treatments because the magnetic resonance thermal mapping enables us to ensure that the lesion does not extend beyond the fibroid to affect the normal myometrium. In laparoscopic myolysis the heat is applied until a change in colour of the serosal surface of the fibroid, or the myometrium overlying the fibroid, signifies that the lesion has been made through the entire uterine wall.

We are aware of the advantages and high satisfaction rates associated with the surgical managements of fibroids, especially of hysterectomy.[20] We are also fully aware of the dearth of good quality data regarding the treatment of fibroids. The Agency for Healthcare Research and Quality report on the management of uterine fibroids for the US Department of Health and Human Services[21] concluded: 'Patients, clinicians and policy makers do not have the data that they need to make truly informed decisions about appropriate treatments.' With this ringing indictment we are determined to demonstrate the efficacy, cost efficiency and safety of MR guided laser and FUS ablation of symptomatic fibroids through well designed and regulated studies and through randomised controlled trials comparing these treatments with traditional and other novel treatments.

In conclusion, we believe that magnetic resonance-guided thermal ablation may represent an important additional therapeutic option for symptomatic uterine fibroids that thus far appears effective and, with no major adverse events in nearly 200 thermal treatments, safe. As an outpatient procedure giving a rapid return to normal activities it appears to be popular with our patients but further studies must be completed before this treatment can be considered a standard therapy.

Acknowledgement

Dr W Gedroyc, Consultant Radiologist, St Mary's Hospital, who developed the techniques of magnetic resonance-guided thermal ablation as applied to uterine fibroids.

References

1. Buttram VC Jr, Reiter RC. Uterine leiomyomata: etiology, symptomatology and management. *Fertil Steril* 1981;36:433–45.
2. Stewart EA. Uterine fibroids. *Lancet* 2001;357:293–8.
3. Kjerulff KH, Langenberg P, Seidman JD, Stolley PD, Guzinski GM. Uterine leiomyomas. Racial differences in severity, symptoms and age at diagnosis. *J Reprod Med* 1996;41:483–90.
4. Department of Health. Hospital Episode Statistics, England 2000–01 [www.doh.gov.uk/hes].
5. Ravina JH, Herbreteau D, Ciraru-Vigneron N, Bouret JM, Houdart E, Aymard A, *et al.* Arterial embolisation to treat uterine myomata. *Lancet* 1995;346:671–2.
6. Goldfarb HA. Nd:YAG laser laparoscopic coagulation of symptomatic myomas. *J Reprod Med* 1992;37:636–8.
7. Donnez J, Squifflet J, Polet R, Nisolle M. Laparoscopic myolysis. *Hum Reprod Update* 2000;6:609–13.
8. Nisolle M, Smets M, Malvaux V, Anaf V, Donnez J. Laparoscopic myolysis with the Nd:YAG laser. *J Gynaecol Surg* 1993;9:95–9.
9. Arcangeli S, Pasquarette M. Gravid uterine rupture after myolysis. *Obstet Gynecol* 1997;89:857.
10. Vilos G, Daly LJ, Tse B. Pregnancy outcome after laparoscopic electromyolysis. *J Am Assoc Gynecol Laparosc* 1998;5:289–92.
11. Jolesz F, Silverman SG. Interventional magnetic resonance therapy. *Semin Interv Radiol* 1995;12:20–7.

12. Gould SW, Vaughan NV, Gedroyc WM, Lamb G, Goldin R, Darzi A. Monitoring of interstitial laser thermotherapy with heat-sensitive colour subtraction magnetic resonance imaging: calibration with absolute tissue temperature and correlation with predicted lesion size. *Lasers Med Sci* 1999;14:1–7.

13. Law PA, Gedroyc WM, Regan L. Magnetic-resonance-guided percutaneous laser ablation of uterine fibroids. *Lancet* 1999;354:2049–50.

14. Hindley JT, Law PA, Hickey M, Smith SC, Lamping DL, Gedroyc WM, *et al.* Clinical outcomes following percutaneous magnetic resonance image guided laser ablation of symptomatic uterine fibroids. *Hum Reprod* 2002;17:2737–41.

15   ter Haar G. Therapeutic ultrasound. *Eur J Ultrasound* 1999;9:3–9.

16. Kuroda K, Chung AH, Hynynen K, Jolesz FA. Calibration of water proton chemical shift for noninvasive temperature imaging during focused ultrasound surgery. *J Magn Reson Imaging* 1998;8:175–81.

17. Stewart EA, Gedroyc WM, Tempany CM, Quade BJ, Inbar Y, Ehrenstein T, *et al.* Focused ultrasound treatment of uterine fibroid tumors: safety and feasibility of a noninvasive thermoablative technique. *Am J Obstet Gynecol* 2003;189:48–54.

18. Spies JB, Coyne K, Guaou Guaou N, Boyle D, Skyrnarz-Murphy K, Gonzalves SM. The UFS-QOL, a new disease-specific symptom and health-related quality of life questionnaire for leiomyomata. *Obstet Gynecol* 2002;99:290–300.

19. Cowan BD, Howard JC, Arriola RM, Robinette LG. Interventional magnetic resonance imaging cryotherapy of uterine fibroid tumors: preliminary observation. *Am J Obstet Gynecol* 2002;186:1183–7.

20. Carlson KJ, Miller BA, Fowler FJ Jr. The Maine Women's Health Study: I. Outcomes of hysterectomy. *Obstet Gynecol* 1994;83:556–65.

21. Agency for Healthcare Research and Quality. *Management of Uterine Fibroids.* (Evidence Report/Technology Assessment: No. 34; AHRQ Publication No. 01-E052.) Rockville, MD: AHRQ; 2001.

35

The Mirena intrauterine system

Lynne Rogerson and Sean Duffy

INTRODUCTION

The Mirena® intrauterine system (IUS) was developed by Leiras Pharmaceuticals (Leiras, Finland). It was launched in Finland in November 1990 and licensed in the UK in May 1995 with an extension in the time '*in situ*' from three to five years (Schering Health Care Ltd, Burgess Hill, West Sussex, UK). Initially the Mirena IUS was marketed as a contraceptive device but over the past few years it has become a versatile treatment option for a variety of clinical indications:

- contraception
- fibroids
- premenstrual syndrome
- hormone replacement therapy
- endometrial hyperplasia
- endometriosis
- adenomyosis
- tamoxifen
- endometrial preparation
- menorrhagia.

DESCRIPTION OF THE MIRENA IUS

The Mirena IUS comprises a T-shaped polyethylene frame carrying a white hormone cylinder 19 mm in length around the vertical arm, creating an outer diameter of 2.8 mm. The cylinder contains a mixture of polydimethylsiloxane (50%) and levonorgestrel (LNG) (50%) and is covered by a polydimethylsiloxane membrane, which regulates the release of the LNG. The total amount of LNG in the system is 52 mg. After insertion into the uterus, LNG is released from the reservoir at an initial rate of 20 µgl/24 h directly to the endometrium. The T-shaped frame is impregnated with barium sulphate to make the system X-ray detectable. Dark monofilament polyethylene threads are attached to the lower end of the vertical arm.

PRACTICAL ASPECTS WHEN FITTING A MIRENA IUS

Exclusion criteria that preclude insertion include: pregnancy, recent pelvic inflammatory disease, previous intrauterine device (IUD) expulsion, acute liver disease, and lower genital and uterine tract infection. The Mirena IUS may be inserted into a fibroid uterus when there is no significant distortion of the cavity but this may require hysteroscopy or a pelvic ultrasound scan to assess the cavity first.

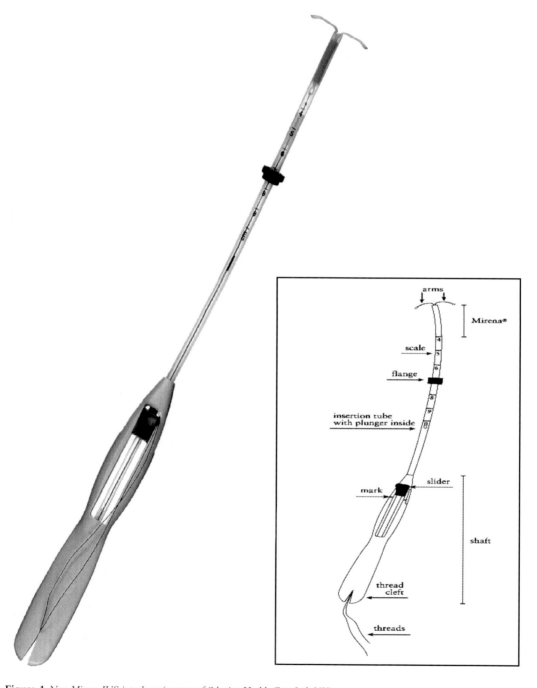

Figure 1 *New Mirena IUS introducer (courtesy of Schering Health Care Ltd, UK)*

Endometrial preparation is not necessary prior to treatment with Mirena IUS but the system should ideally be inserted within the first seven days of a woman's menstrual cycle or she should have abstained from sexual intercourse or used additional contraception for the previous five days to exclude an early pregnancy.

The IUS is usually inserted in an outpatient setting. The woman is placed in a modified lithotomy position and a pelvic examination performed to clarify the size and position of the uterus. After visualisation of the cervix using a speculum, the vagina and cervix are cleansed with warm antiseptic solution. The anterior lip of the cervix can then be grasped with a tenaculum to facilitate gentle traction to reduce the angle between the cervical canal and the uterine cavity. This allows the introduction of a uterine sound to assess the cavity's length and to ensure that it is unobstructed. Should the cervical canal be tight, cervical dilatation may be necessary and anaesthesia may therefore be required, such as 10 ml of local anaesthetic gel instilled into the cervical canal five minutes prior to insertion. In one study in which Mirena was inserted into 50 women (nine of whom were nulliparous) for menorrhagia, only three required anaesthesia, all of whom were parous.[1]

The Mirena IUS may then be inserted using an aseptic technique; with the new inserter (Figure 1) this technique is possible with one hand. The threads are then trimmed so that 2 cm remain visible outside the cervix to enable checking that the system is still *in situ* (especially after a heavy period), and also to allow removal when the time arises.

The whole procedure generally takes approximately 10–15 minutes and usually requires a doctor to insert the system and one assistant for psychological support for the woman. In a large contraceptive study in Finland,[2] pain scores at insertion of the system were recorded: 17% of women felt no pain, 49% minimum pain, 28% moderate pain, and 6% had severe pain.

The incidence of complications during insertion is small but they include syncope, usually due to dilatation of the cervical os. This normally settles with a head-down position but rarely atropine may have to be given. There is also a possibility of uterine perforation, which, again, usually occurs during cervical dilatation rather than on actual insertion of the Mirena IUS.

Other more long-term complications of the Mirena IUS include pelvic inflammatory disease because organisms can potentially be pushed up into the uterine cavity from the cervix and vagina. The Mirena IUS may also be spontaneously expelled, especially in women who have high menstrual blood loss.

The highest concentrations of LNG can be detected in the endometrium and the systemic levels are low (25% of peak level after taking a standard 30 μg LNG progestogen only pill), but systemic hormonal effects can occur. Adverse effects are most common during the first few months after the insertion and include irregular menstrual bleeding, intermenstrual spotting, and hormonal adverse effects such as mood changes, headache, nausea, breast tenderness and acne. Consequently, removal rates are higher for the Mirena than for other copper devices: 12.1/100 users at five years compared with 2/100.[3]

PRECLINICAL STUDIES

The pharmacological properties of LNG and its toxicity profile after oral administration are well known, and indicate that it is a safe drug. Less is known, however, about the effects of LNG in intrauterine use. The shape and size of the LNG IUS are unsuitable for the uteri of laboratory animals, so LNG releasing systems composed of similar components and materials have been tested. In spite of an apparently high endometrial LNG concentration, no local intolerance or systemic toxic reactions have been observed. Compared with the oral administration of LNG, administration directly into the uterine cavity allows a low systemic concentration in humans.

The inert polydimethylsiloxane carrier in the LNG IUS is a biocompatible material that has shown no *in vitro*, local or systemic toxicity. Similar material has been widely used in implantable valves and prostheses. There is also extensive experience of the polyethylene frame, gained from studies with a copper IUD, Nova T® (Schering Health Care Ltd, Burgess Hill, West Sussex, UK), which is used worldwide.

Few animal pharmacokinetic studies have been performed with the intrauterine LNG system but in a one-year study in rhesus monkeys systemic LNG blood concentrations were measured. Toxicological studies showed limited systemic pharmacological effects of LNG. The local effects on the endometrium were a typical strong progestogenic effect, including glandular atrophy, decidual changes and a foreign body reaction.[4-6] Safety evaluation of the silicone materials (membrane and core materials of the hormone reservoir) and polyethylene parts of the product (T body, removal threads and insertion tube) is based on assessments of genetic toxicology in standard *in vitro* and *in vivo* test systems. Biocompatibility has also been assessed in mice, guinea pigs, rabbits and *in vitro* test systems; all showed acceptable biocompatibility.

Embryonic/fetal toxicity and teratogenic potential of an intrauterine LNG system were studied in the rabbit. The treatment did not have any adverse effect on litter number, or embryonic or fetal development.[7]

Endometrial, myometrial and fallopian tube concentrations of LNG have been studied after four to six weeks' treatment with an LNG IUS.[8] The endometrial tissue concentration of LNG was more than 100 times higher than that achieved with orally administered LNG at a daily dose of 250 µg. After insertion of the Mirena IUS, LNG can be detected in plasma in 15 minutes and the highest concentrations are reached within a few hours.[9]

HOW DOES IT WORK?

The therapeutic effects of the Mirena IUS are based on local effects on the uterus. The progesterone release has a contraceptive action that complements the mechanical effect of the device but also has a direct effect on the function of the adjacent endometrium. Endometrial proliferation has been shown to be prevented by the local administration of LNG, which inhibits the function of oestradiol in the endometrium.[10] In addition, LNG thickens the cervical mucus thus also inhibiting sperm motility and function.[11] Suppression of ovulation may occur in some women using the Mirena IUS but, on average, 75% of cycles have been shown to be ovulatory.[11,12] The device may also have a weak foreign body effect.[10]

Endometrial histology during the use of the Mirena IUS has been studied for up to seven years after insertion in women of reproductive age. A few weeks after insertion, endometrial glands become atrophic with a thin, inactive epithelium and the stroma undergoes an intense decidual reaction. The histology of the endometrium does not change during prolonged use. In a long-term contraceptive study, endometrial histology was evaluated at the removal of the Mirena from 100 women;[13] 92% showed endometrial suppression, with focal proliferative changes in 24%. The endometrium recovered fully two to six months after removal.

CLINICAL INDICATIONS FOR THE MIRENA IUS

Contraception

The Mirena IUS has many features of the 'ideal' contraceptive method. It is not related to coitus and once *in situ* is effective for up to five years. The Mirena IUS is reversible, with a return of fertility as prompt as after removal of copper intrauterine contraceptive devices.[14,15] In one study,

79% of women wishing to conceive within one year did so; this was 87% within two years after removal of the Mirena.[14]

The Mirena IUS has been reported as being as effective as female sterilisation;[3,16] indeed, in many places, prescribing the Mirena IUS has become mandatory as an effective option in presterilisation counselling.

The occurrence of amenorrhoea may cause women concern and initially they may perform pregnancy tests for reassurance. However, this is usually short lived and, as long as the threads are checked regularly, women can be reassured that the system is in place and is functioning correctly.

The Mirena IUS is an ideal contraceptive choice for women who have either tried other methods that are not suitable or who have contraindications to other forms of contraception. It is also excellent where reliable long-term contraception is required but where sterilisation would not be appropriate such as in women with mental or physical handicaps. The Mirena can be inserted six weeks postnatally and is suitable for use in breastfeeding women.[17] The insertion of a Mirena should be considered at surgical termination of pregnancy, especially where an alternative contraceptive method has failed.

Ectopic pregnancy

In addition to its contraceptive action, the LNG system has a protective effect on the incidence of ectopic pregnancy. The system is so effective at preventing intrauterine pregnancy that, if conception does occur, the proportion of ectopic pregnancies is high at somewhere between 20–33%.[3] The actual ectopic rate with Mirena is 0.02 per 100 women years compared with 0.12–0.26 per 100 women years in those using no contraception.[18]

Pelvic inflammatory disease

There is variation in the incidence of pelvic inflammatory disease in Mirena users. Andersson *et al.*[3] reported a rate of removal for infection of 0.5 per 100 users by three years, but other groups[19–21] demonstrated rates comparable with copper devices. Certainly it appears that the Mirena is suitable to be used in a group of women previously excluded from the insertion of intrauterine contraceptive devices.

Premenstrual syndrome

Smith *et al.*[22] showed benefits in severe premenstrual syndrome when using oestradiol implants or continuous high-dose oestradiol skin patches to suppress the menstrual cycle. However, the symptoms may return during the days of artificial progestogen given to prevent the endometrial hyperstimulation associated with unopposed oestrogen. The Mirena IUS used as the progesterone is less likely to bring back the premenstrual symptoms or result in progestogenic adverse effects.[23]

Menorrhagia

Menorrhagia is one of the most common clinical problems encountered by both GPs and gynaecologists. Five percent of women between the ages of 30 and 49 years consult their GP each year with this problem, which represents 21% of all gynaecological referrals. Once referred to a gynaecologist, surgical intervention is likely, with 60% of women in one study undergoing a hysterectomy within five years of referral.[24]

Women presenting with menorrhagia whose symptoms are refractory to conventional medical therapy traditionally face the choice of undergoing either a hysterectomy or, since the late 1980s, some other alternative, less invasive surgical treatment. Endometrial resection is the alternative to hysterectomy that has been formally assessed in clinical trials.[25-28] The benefits to the woman include shorter hospital stay, less postoperative morbidity, quicker return to work, and quicker overall recovery. However, there are complications, such as the risks associated with general anaesthesia, fluid intravasation and dilutional hyponatraemia, and the risk of uterine perforation and subsequent intra-abdominal trauma.[28] Such complications have driven research into the development of alternative treatments for the management of menorrhagia.

By rendering the endometrium inactive, the Mirena IUS has a potential role in the treatment of women with heavy and irregular menstrual bleeding. There are supportive studies that have investigated this potential. One of the first reports of the effect on locally released progesterone (norgestrel) on reducing menstrual blood loss was by Nilsson in 1977.[29] Bergqvist and Rybo[30] recorded a 65% reduction in menstrual blood loss in women using the Progestasert® (Alza, Mountain View, CA, USA) device for contraception after 12 months of use. Andersson and Rybo[31] reported a 97% reduction in menstrual blood loss volume after 12 months of use in those women who continued to use the device. However, in this study, 20% of the initial women who had a device inserted were withdrawn, owing either to spontaneous expulsion of the device or unwanted adverse effects (irregular bleeding or progestogenic symptoms, such as breast tenderness and bloating). The latter study would therefore suggest a failure rate, after initial insertion, of 20%. In another study of women who were taken off a waiting list for hysterectomy and offered the Mirena system,[5] the failure rate (including primary expulsion of the device) was 24%. This study did not have a control group. A more recent attempt used controls,[32] but the study was flawed because the control group consisted of women already on a waiting list for definitive surgery; therefore, by definition, they were medical treatment failures and could not be classified as true controls.

There are two published randomised controlled trials of the Mirena system versus endometrial resection.[33,34] The first is that of Crosignani et al.,[33] which assessed the effect of the Mirena IUS in terms of a symptom chart score, patient satisfaction, effect on menstrual loss, and failure rate. The period of follow-up was for 12 months but the total study number of 70 (35 to each arm) was relatively small. The results are summarised in Table 1. The failure rate is defined by persistent menorrhagia and the unexpected loss of the Mirena by expulsion from the uterus. Blood loss was assessed using the pictorial blood loss assessment chart (PBAC).[35,36] Symptomatic improvement is defined as amenorrhoea or oligomenorrhoea at 12 months. Satisfaction was assessed by simple questionnaire, and responses of 'satisfied' or 'very satisfied' were recorded as successful outcomes. However, the study numbers would not be sufficient to demonstrate a clinically meaningful difference as statistically significant between the two groups.

The second study of endometrial resection versus the Mirena by Kittleson and Istre[34] was again relatively small, with only 60 women in total. There were substantial numbers of women who discontinued the Mirena prematurely (20%). In those who persisted with it, the mean blood loss score, as assessed by the PBAC, was reduced from 418 (standard deviation [SD] 349) at baseline to 42 (SD 99.7) at 12 months. In the resection group there were four failures (13%) and the mean PBAC score fell from 378 (SD 463) to 6.6 (SD 15.0). No data were provided on patient satisfaction.

There has not been a randomised controlled trial comparing the LNG IUS and hysterectomy, but one study[5] recruited 50 women with a history of failed medical treatment awaiting hysterectomy or transcervical resection of the endometrium. After insertion of the Mirena system, 41 (82%) were taken off the waiting list for surgery because of a reduction in mean blood loss score, a reduction in dysmenorrhoea (80%), and improvement in premenstrual syndrome (56%). The study of Lahteenmaki et al.[37] suggests that the Mirena IUS may be a valuable alternative for

Table 1 *Mirena vs. endometrial resection: data extracted from results of a randomised controlled trial by Crosignani et al.*[33]

	Mirena IUS (%) (n = 35)	Endometrial resection (%) (n = 35)
Failure rate	11	8
Change in mean PBAC score	79	89
Symptom improvement	65	71
Satisfaction	85	94

PBAC = pictorial blood loss assessment chart

hysterectomy in women with excessive bleeding because 60% of those who had a Mirena inserted cancelled their scheduled surgery, whereas only 15% in the control did so. Romer[38] stated that 75% of endometrial ablations could be replaced by treatment with a LNG IUD.

A larger randomised controlled trial comparing the LNG IUS with hysteroscopic surgery for menorrhagia and using quality of life assessments as its primary outcome measure is needed. One such multicentre study was commenced but had to be closed owing to poor patient recruitment as a result of patient preference for endometrial ablation.[39] A study is now ongoing to find out more about the reasons for patient preference.

Endometrial hyperplasia

The protective effect of progestogens on the endometrium and their use to treat endometrial hyperplasia is well known. Using Progestasert, a complete suppression of hyperplasia occurred in over 80% of study participants, with a 36% recurrence rate after removal.[40] Studies using Mirena have revealed that it achieves uniform endometrial suppression with, possibly, a reduced relapse rate.[41,42]

There may be a potential use of the Mirena IUS in combination with tamoxifen in the treatment of breast cancer. Tamoxifen is now used widely and is associated with typical hysteroscopic appearances, increased endometrial hyperplasia and endometrial cancer. It would seem sensible to give the progestogen locally at the site where it is needed.[43]

Hormone replacement therapy

An increasing amount of work is being done in this area, using the Mirena IUS as endometrial protection for women on continuous oestrogen. These studies have included the use of a smaller 10 mg system, which, in postmenopausal women has the added advantage of easier insertion. The Mirena effectively protects against endometrial hyperplasia, producing amenorrhoea in most women.[44,45]

CONCLUSIONS

The Mirena appears to be an easy and effective method of contraception and management for a host of clinical problems. It has many possibilities for an expanding role in gynaecology and is being used regularly by many clinicians, currently without the licence for certain indications. The potential advantage of the Mirena IUS is its ease of use and low complication rate, but its benefit will be of interest only if it is shown that it has a good success rate in terms of patient satisfaction and symptomatic improvement; it must also be of economic value. There is therefore a need to perform a large randomised controlled trial to assess the efficacy of and tolerance to the Mirena IUS against the established and effective methods before it can be used confidently supported by evidence based medicine.

References

1. Barrington JW, Bowen-Simpkins P. The levonorgestrel intrauterine system in the management of menorrhagia. *Br J Obstet Gynaecol* 1997;104:614–16.
2. Sommardahl C, Blom T. *Five-year Clinical Performance of the New Formulation of the Levonorgestrel Intrauterine System and Serum Levonorgestrel Concentration with the New Formulation Compared to that with the Original One*. Leiras study report 102-89532-07,1996. Turku, Finland: Leiras; 1996.
3. Andersson K, Odlind V, Rybo G. Levonorgestrel-releasing and copper-releasing (Nova T) IUCDs during five years of use: a randomized comparative trial. *Contraception* 1994;49:56–72.
4. Wadsworth PF, Heywood R, Allen DG, Sortwell RJ, Walton RM. Treatment of rhesus monkeys (*Macaca mulatta*) with intrauterine devices loaded with levonorgestrel. *Contraception* 1979;20:177–84.
5. Sethi N, Agarwal K, Singh RK, Bajpai VK. Effect of 24 mm levonorgestrel IUD on uterine endometrium of female rhesus monkeys, *Macaca mulatta*. *Contraception* 1988;37:99–108.
6. Schering UK. *One-year Local and Systemic Tolerance Study with a Levonorgestrel-releasing Intrauterine Device in the Rhesus Monkey and Determination of Plasma Concentration of Levonorgestrel Using a Radioimmunoassay Method*. Schering study report 9725, 1992. Burgess Hill, West Sussex: Schering UK; 1992.
7. Argus Research Laboratories. *Embryo/Fetal Toxicity and Teratogenic Potential Study of Levonorgestrel Administered via a Silastic Intrauterine Device to Pregnant New Zealand White Rabbits*. Turku, Finland: Leiras; 1984.
8. Nilsson CG, Haukkamaa M, Vierola H, Luukkainen T. Tissue concentrations of levonorgestrel in women using a levonorgestrel-releasing IUD. *Clin Endocrinol (Oxf)* 1982;17:529–36.
9. Luukkainen T. Levonorgestrel-releasing intrauterine device. *Ann N Y Acad Sci* 1991;626:43–9.
10. Silverberg SG, Haukkamaa M, Arko H, Nilsson CG, Luukkainen T. Endometrial morphology during long-term use of levonorgestrel-releasing intrauterine devices. *Int J Gynecol Pathol* 1986;5:235–41.
11. Barbosa I, Bakos O, Olsson SE, Odlind V, Johansson ED. Ovarian function during use of a levonorgestrel-releasing IUD. *Contraception* 1990;42:51–66.
12. Nilsson CG, Lahteenmaki PL, Luukkainen T. Ovarian function in amenorrheic and menstruating users of a levonorgestrel-releasing intrauterine device. *Fertil Steril* 1984;41:52–5.
13. Lahteenmaki P. *Evaluation of Endometrial Biopsies at the Time of and After the Removal of LNG IUS*. Leiras study report no. 1204. Turku, Finland: Leiras; 1991.
14. Andersson K, Batar I, Rybo G. Return to fertility after removal of a levonorgestrel releasing intrauterine device and NOVA T. *Contraception* 1992;46:575–84.

15. Sivin I, Stern J, Diaz J, Pavez M, Alvarez F, Brache V, et al. Rates and outcomes of planned pregnancy after use of Norplant capsules, Norplant II rods, or levonorgestrel-releasing or copper Tcu 380Ag intrauterine contraceptive devices. Am J Obstet Gynecol 1992;166:1208–13.

16. Toivonen J, Luukkainen T, Allonen H. Protective effect of intrauterine release of levonorgestrel on pelvic infection: three years' comparative experience of levonorgestrel- and copper-releasing intrauterine devices. Obstet Gynecol 1991;77:261–4.

17. Heikkila M, Luukkainen T. Duration of breast-feeding and development of children after insertion of a levonorgestrel-releasing intrauterine contraceptive device. Contraception 1982;25:279–92.

18. Franks A, Beral V, Cates W Jr, Hogue CJ. Contraception and ectopic pregnancy risk. Am J Obstet Gynecol 1990;163:1120–23.

19. Sivin I, Stern J. Health during prolonged use of levonorgestrel 20 micrograms/day and the copper TCu 380Ag intrauterine contraceptive devices: a multicenter study. International Committee for Contraception Research (ICCR). Fertil Steril 1994;61:70–7.

20. Sivin I, Stern J, Coutinho E, Mattos CE, el Mahgoub S, Diaz S, et al. Prolonged intrauterine contraception: a seven-year randomized study of the levonorgestrel 20 mcg/day (LNg 20) and the copper T380 Ag IUDs. Contraception 1991;44:473–80.

21. Luukkainen T, Allonen H, Haukkamaa M, Lahteenmaki P, Nilsson CG, Toivonen J. Five years' experience with levonorgestrel-releasing IUDs. Contraception 1986;33:139–48.

22. Smith RN, Studd JW, Zamblera D, Holland EF. A randomised comparison over 8 months of 100 micrograms and 200 micrograms twice weekly doses of transdermal oestradiol in the treatment of severe premenstrual syndrome. Br J Obstet Gynaecol 1995;102:475–84.

23. Sturridge F, Guillebaud J. Gynaecological aspects of the levonorgestrel-releasing intrauterine system. Br J Obstet Gynaecol 1997;104:285–9.

24. Coulter A, Bradlow J, Agass M, Martin-Bates C, Tulloch A. Outcomes of referrals to gynaecology outpatient clinics for menstrual problems: an audit of general practice records. Br J Obstet Gynaecol 1991;98:789–96.

25. Gannon MJ, Holt EM, Fairbank J, Fitzgerald M, Milne MA, Crystal AM, et al. A randomised controlled trial comparing endometrial resection and abdominal hysterectomy for the treatment of menorrhagia. BMJ 1991;303:1362–4.

26. Dwyer N, Hutton J, Stirrat GM. Randomised controlled trial comparing endometrial resection with abdominal hysterectomy for the surgical treatment of menorrhagia. Br J Obstet Gynaecol 1993;100:237–43.

27. Pinion SB, Parkin DE, Abramovich DR, Naji A, Alexander DA, Russell IT, et al. Randomised trial of hysterectomy, endometrial laser ablation, and transcervical endometrial resection for dysfunctional uterine bleeding. BMJ 1994;309:979–83.

28. O'Connor H, Broadbent JA, Magos AL, McPherson K. Medical Research Council randomised controlled trial of endometrial resection versus hysterectomy in management of menorrhagia. Lancet 1997;349:897–901.

29. Nilsson CG. Improvement of a d-norgestrel-releasing-IUD. Contraception 1977;15:295–306.

30. Bergqvist A, Rybo G. Treatment of menorrhagia with intrauterine release of progesterone. Br J Obstet Gynaecol 1983;90:255–8.

31. Andersson JK, Rybo G. Levonorgestrel releasing intrauterine device in the treatment of menorrhagia. Br J Obstet Gynaecol 1990;97:690–4.

32. Puolakka J, Nilsson C, Haukkamaa M, Riikonen U, Sainio S, Savonius H, et al. Conservative treatment of excessive uterine bleeding and dysmenorrhoea with levonorgestrel intrauterine system as an alternative to hysterectomy. Acta Obstet Gynecol Scand 1996;75:82.

33. Crosignani PG, Vercellini P, Mosconi P, Oldani S, Cortesi I, De Giorgi O. Levonorgestrel-releasing intrauterine device versus hysteroscopic endometrial resection in the treatment of dysfunctional uterine bleeding. *Obstet Gynecol* 1997;90:257–63.

34. Kittleson N, Istre O. A randomised study comparing levonorgestrel intrauterine system and transcervical resection of the endometrium in the treatment of menorrhagia: preliminary results. *Gynaecol Endosc* 1998;7:61–7.

35. Higham JM, O'Brien PM, Shaw RW. Assessment of menstrual blood loss using a pictorial chart. *Br J Obstet Gynaecol* 1990;97:734–9.

36. Janssen CA, Scholten PC, Heintz AP. A simple visual assessment technique to discriminate between menorrhagia and normal menstrual blood loss. *Obstet Gynecol* 1995;85:977–82.

37. Lahteenmaki P, Haukkamaa M, Puolakka J, Riikonen U, Sainio S, Suvisaari J, *et al.* Open randomised study of use of levonorgestrel releasing intrauterine system as alternative to hysterectomy. *BMJ* 1998;316:1122–6.

38. Romer T. Prospective comparison study of levonorgestrel IUD versus Roller-Ball endometrial ablation in the management of refractory recurrent hypermenorrhea. *Eur J Obstet Gynecol Reprod Biol* 2000;90:27–9.

39. Rogerson L, Duffy S, Crocombe W, Stead M, Dassu D. Management of menorrhagia – SMART study (Satisfaction with Mirena and Ablation: a Randomised Trial). *BJOG* 2000;107:1325–6.

40. Gasparri F, Scarselli G, Colafranceschi M, Taddei G, Tantini C, Savino L. Management of precancerous lesions of the endometrium. In: Ludwig H, Thomsen K, editors. *Gynaecology and Obstetrics.* Berlin: Springer-Verlag; 1986. p. 1232–36.

42. Scarselli G, Tantini C, Colafranceschi M, Taddei GL, Bargelli G, Venturini N, *et al.* Levonorgestrel-nova-T and precancerous lesions of the endometrium. *Eur J Gynaecol Oncol* 1988;9:284–6.

43. Perino A, Quartararo P, Catinella E, Genova G, Cittadini E. Treatment of endometrial hyperplasia with levonorgestrel-releasing intrauterine devices. *Acta Eur Fertil* 1987;18:137–40.

44. Neven P, De Muylder X, Van Belle Y, Campo R, Vanderick G. Tamoxifen and the uterus. *BMJ* 1994;309:1313–14.

45. Raudaskoski T, Tapanainen J, Tomas E, Luotola H, Pekonen F, Ronni-Sivula H, *et al.* Intrauterine 10 microg and 20 microg levonorgestrel systems in postmenopausal women receiving oral oestrogen replacement therapy: clinical, endometrial and metabolic response. *BJOG* 2002;109:136–44.

36

Workforce survey feedback

Robert Sawers

INTRODUCTION

'Planning the requirements for the medical workforce of the future has never been so difficult', wrote Richard Warren in his introduction to the 13th annual Royal College of Obstetricians and Gynaecologists (RCOG) Medical Workforce Report of April 2002.[1] Everyone involved in women's health services is only too familiar with the particular problems posed by changing patterns of care, women's expectations, medical training and working practices. These problems appear to be particularly acute in the UK because of the way in which health services have been provided for the last 50 years. In addition, the impact of changes in training and employment legislation was not adequately considered before they were imposed. The number of variables made the planning process difficult, but also the profession was given parameters for planning based on an expansion of consultant posts, which is only now beginning to take place. The profession must however shoulder some responsibility for failing to take a sufficiently radical view of staffing issues. What is the necessary professional and skill mix required to provide care in different circumstances? The RCOG has been active in promoting change but has frequently come under fire from other professional bodies, especially over the issue of different types of trained specialist.

The specialty of obstetrics and gynaecology is different from most others in two essential respects: it is extremely diverse, to the extent that it may well subdivide permanently; and the greater proportion of the work, maternity care, is a giant emergency service. The maternity services have a further problem. Society has the schizophrenic view that doctors should never interfere, but nothing should ever go wrong. The workforce therefore has to run on the one hand a gynaecology service, which is a combination of medicine and surgery, and on the other a maternity service providing constant surveillance and immediately available emergency care. There are now several RCOG publications on the standards of care that should be provided (e.g. *Towards Safer Childbirth*;[2] *Clinical Standards*[3]); these are helpful in the planning process.

The RCOG monitors medical staffing with the aid of its Medical Workforce Advisory Committee (now disbanded) and conducts an annual census[1] of units in the UK. It has also organised *ad hoc* working parties to examine manning issues in more detail, producing reports such as *Planning for the Future as Consultants in Obstetrics and Gynaecology*[4] and *A Blueprint for the Future*[5]. As an adjunct to the 2001 census, units in England and Wales were asked to complete an additional questionnaire on workforce changes. The principal findings were presented at the Present and Future Workforce meeting at the RCOG in April 2002.

THE QUESTIONNAIRE

The questions raised related to:

* consultant expansion

- changes in specialist registrar/senior house officer (SHO) posts

- compliance with the 'New Deal' on working hours for junior staff

- delivery suite and emergency gynaecology consultant sessions

- consultant cover and whether resident on call

- compliance with EU employment legislation

- hospital mergers

- perceived service deficits and stress.

Detailed questions were also asked about all the fixed sessions provided by all consultants, but information was incomplete and is not included in this report.

THE DATABASE

Included in the survey were 209 hospitals in 15 'deanery' regions in England and Wales. The units were classified by the annual number of deliveries, into less than 2500 (80 units), 2500–4000 (94 units) and more than 4000 (35 units). A total of 150 units responded (72%), with marked regional variation in response rate (46–94%), which was not obviously related to geography or number of units in a region.

The findings must be considered in the light of the response rate, but they give some indication of the pattern of change throughout the regions, and its impact as perceived on the ground. It is important to note that the figures from the feedback survey and the census sometimes differ considerably.

RESULTS

Size of unit by region

The size and distribution of units are fundamental to service provision, and also to manpower planning. Some regions have a preponderance of small units, delivering fewer than 2500 mothers per year, while some have none. This variation appears to be partly geographical in origin, affecting particularly the northern regions and Wales (Figure 1).

Consultant expansion

According to the census, the number of consultant posts increased by 95 from 1246 to 1341. Advisory Appointment Committee returns suggest 114 new posts. The survey recorded a net gain of 80 consultant posts in 2001, with a further 43 projected for 2002. About a quarter were said to be due to the Temple Plan (i.e. funded by a reduction in training posts), and the remainder were mainly to provide delivery suite cover (Table 1). The number of new posts did not, however, appear to correlate with either the number of hospitals in a region or the number of deliveries per whole-time equivalent consultant (Figure 2).

Specialist registrar and SHO changes

The survey reported a loss of 27 specialist registrar posts in 2001, with a further loss of 19.5

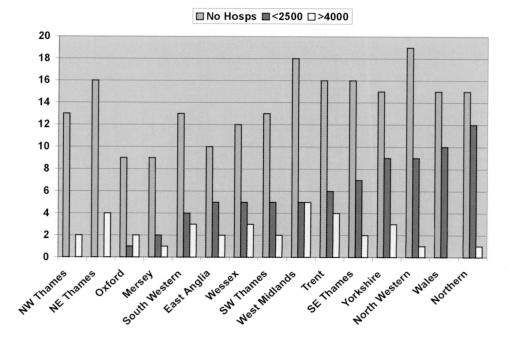

Figure 1 *Total number of maternity units in each deanery, and numbers of large and small units, delivering > 4000 and < 2500 respectively*

projected for 2002. In addition, 62 posts had been changed from type-1 trainees (national training numbers) to type-2 trainees (full-time training appointments). The census recorded a drop of 50 in the total number of specialist registrars from 910 to 860.

Forty-five SHO posts were lost, with a further projected reduction of 22 for 2002. The net gains and losses (as reported from the 150 responding units) are shown in Figure 3. There appears to be no obvious pattern to the changes, suggesting considerable local variation in implementation.

Table 1 *Consultant expansion achieved in 2001, planned for 2002, and principal reasons for posts already achieved, as reported from 150 units*

	Achieved 2001	Planned 2002
Gains	82.5	43
Losses	2.5	
Net gain:	80	
For labour and delivery suite	57	
Temple Plan	20.5	

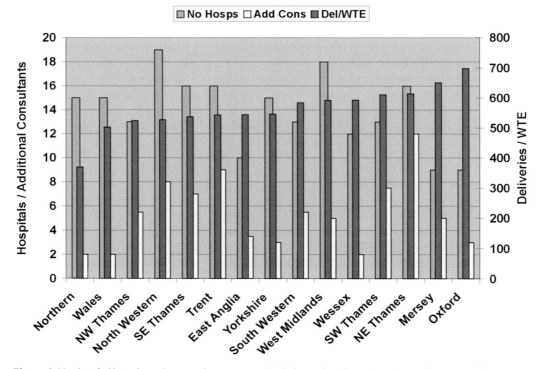

Figure 2 *Number of additional consultants per deanery compared with the number of maternity units and the number of deliveries per whole-time equivalent (WTE) consultant*

'New Deal' and 56-hour compliance

Sixty-seven units (45%) said they were noncompliant with the New Deal for specialist registrars; the figure for SHOs was 51 (34%). When asked about the impact of the 56-hour week, 15% said they had no plans to cope with it, 24% said they could cope with readjustment, and 51% planned an increase in staff. Fifty per cent predicted a service reduction (Table 2).

Table 2 *Number of units reporting non-compliance with the New Deal, and predicted impact of the 56-hour week, as reported from 150 units*

	Units (*n*)
Noncompliance	
Specialist registrars	67
SHOs	51
Impact of 56-hour week	
No plans	23
Cope with readjustment	36
Planned increase in staff	77
Predict service reduction	75

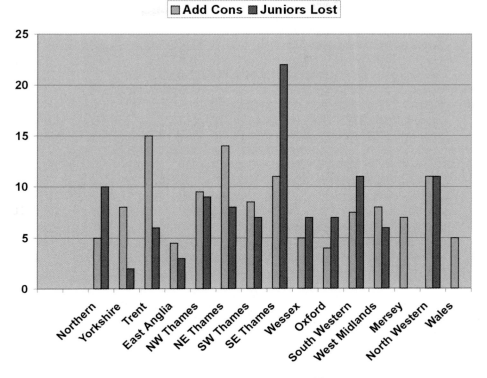

Figure 3 *Number of additional consultants and trainee losses, by deanery, as reported from 150 units*

Dedicated labour and delivery suite and gynaecology emergency sessions

Units were asked to report the number of 'fixed and dedicated' delivery suite or emergency gynaecology consultant sessions per week, and also their plans for the next year. Most units (95%) reported dedicated sessions, although a precise definition was not given in the questionnaire. The average number of sessions, for those units reporting them, was 7.4 per week (Figure 4).

Consultant on-call rotas

In most hospitals, consultant on-call rotas were combined for obstetrics and gynaecology and the predominant frequency was about 1:5 or 1:6, with a range of 1:3 to 1:10. Only 16 of the respondents had separate on call for obstetrics and gynaecology, and these were predictably large units delivering more than 4000 mothers per year. Only two units currently had consultants resident on call, and these were without mid-grade support. Six others were planning to have some consultants resident on call.

Increased disturbance and out of hours call-ins

Seventy-five percent of respondents reported increased call-ins and 78% increased disturbance (Figure 5).

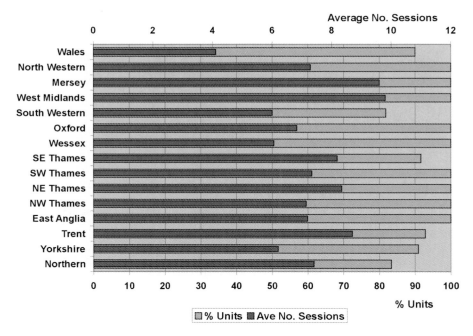

Figure 4 *Percentage of units by deanery with dedicated delivery suite or gynaecology emergency consultant sessions and average number of sessions per week*

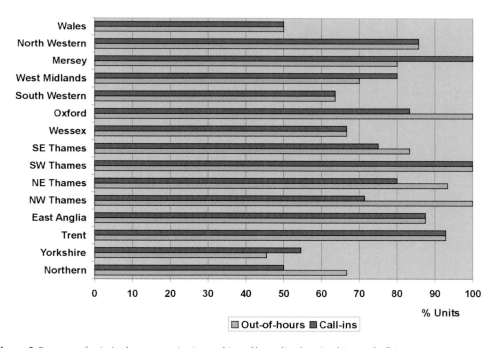

Figure 5 *Percentage of units by deanery reporting increased 'out of hours disturbance' and increased call-ins*

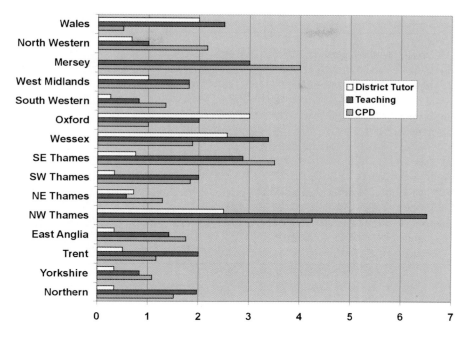

Figure 6 *Average number of dedicated consultant sessions per unit allocated to district tutor, teaching and continuing professional development (CPD), by deanery*

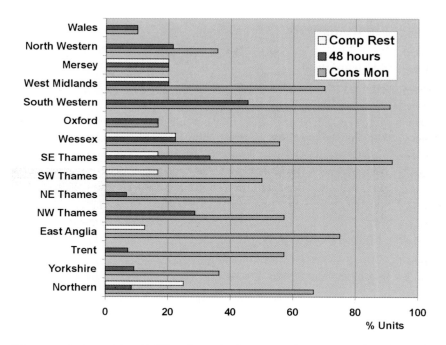

Figure 7 *Percentage of units complying with EU employment legislation on consultant monitoring, the 48-hour week, and compensatory rest periods, by deanery*

Table 3 *Perceived and actual consequences of EU legislation in terms of additional consultants required, hospital mergers already achieved, and those planned in the next 5 years by deanery, as reported from 150 units*

	Extra consultants	Mergers in previous 2 y	Mergers planned in next 5 y
Northern	6	4	1
Yorkshire	11	1	3
Trent	7	5	1
East Anglia	6	0	0
NW Thames	4	3	3
NE Thames	14	4	1
SW Thames	2	1	2
SE Thames	12	2	5
Wessex	2	0	0
Oxford	4	0	1
South Western	3	2	2
West Midlands	16	2	0
Mersey	17	2	2
North Western	8	0	7
Wales	7	1	3
Total	119	27	31

Dedicated sessions

The number of dedicated sessions for continuing professional development (CPD), clinical governance and audit, and teaching and district tutor duties, were recorded. Detailed information on every consultant was sought, but the information was incomplete and only the unit totals are analysed here. Around 50% of units had no dedicated sessions for CPD. The average number of sessions per unit per week dedicated to CPD, audit, clinical governance, teaching and tutoring was small in a majority of cases (Figure 6).

Consequences of EU legislation

The implementation of EU legislation on consultant monitoring, compensatory rest periods and the 48-hour working week was patchy (Figure 7). Some of the consequences predicted by respondents are shown in Table 3. A total of 119 new consultants were considered to be necessary; 27 mergers had occurred in the previous two years, and 31 were planned for the next five years.

Stress and service deficit

Most units reported increased stress levels and predicted a service deficit (Figure 8).

CONCLUSIONS AND DISCUSSION

The purpose of the survey questionnaire was to amplify the already extensive data of the annual census and to look beyond the numbers to some of the perceived effects of the manpower changes. The response rate of 72% was reasonable, but the results should be interpreted together with the full annual workforce report. The main conclusions that can be drawn are as follows:

- There are still many small units delivering fewer than 2500 mothers per year. Many of these may be dictated by geography, but not all. Rationalisation is probably urgently required if adequate staffing and support services, such as neonatology, are to be maintained.

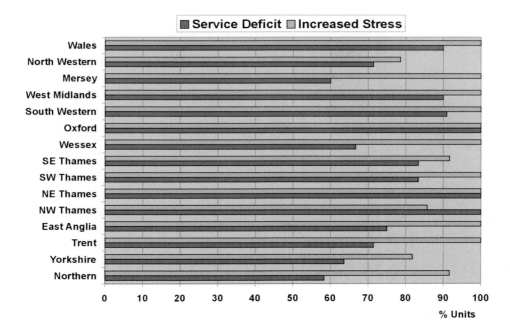

Figure 8 *Percentage of units claiming to be working under increased stress and already to have service deficits, by deanery*

- Consultant expansion has been uneven throughout the country, and does not appear to be related to need.

- Many units are still not compliant with the New Deal. This problem may be disguised where units are part of a large general hospital, but is clearly untenable.

- The numbers of consultants gained and trainees lost appear to be roughly equal, but this takes no account of the changes in working patterns of the remaining juniors, and the different contributions to care that consultants and trainees have traditionally made.

- Few units have, or are contemplating, consultants resident on call.

- Most units have some dedicated delivery suite or emergency gynaecology consultant sessions, but the number is small. The survey did not make clear what a 'dedicated' session entailed.

- The larger units have separate rotas for consultants on call for obstetrics and gynaecology.

- The average on call rota is 1:5 or 1:6.

- Most units report increased stress levels and believe that there are already service deficits in some areas.

A number of the questions, such as those on stress and service deficit, demanded highly subjective answers. More objective information regarding the impact on patient care is needed. Although the study recorded changes in medical staff numbers, it did not quantify actual changes in available working hours. It is these changes that have had most impact on working conditions and service. Although the consultant expansion is encouraging, it has been comparatively modest, and almost certainly does not compensate for the loss in available clinical time across all grades, or allow for the generally increased expectations of consultants in the delivery suite, outpatient departments and on call. It is also cause for concern that formal allowance for CPD, clinical governance and teaching is somewhat limited.

There are two overriding impressions from this survey. Most units perceive problems with manning and service provision, but change so far has been limited.

How may these issues be addressed? Surely it is time for radical solutions. There must be rationalisation of units to make best use of the manpower available. Where possible, low-risk may be separated from high-risk obstetrics, but in juxtaposition to allow safe transfer. The long discussed staffing changes must be accelerated. The basis for planning the workforce in obstetrics and gynaecology is clearly set out in the 'blueprint'[5] and the 'clinical standards'[3] documents. It is rightly expected that the medical component of care should be provided by trained specialists, but acute surgical specialties, and especially obstetrics, cannot be based entirely on traditional consultants. The answer has to be a specialist grade, attained after completion of basic specialist training. It has been suggested in the otherwise excellent 'blueprint'[5] report that consultants should progress smoothly through the different roles during the tenure of their post. The obvious weakness of this structure is that it does not allow for possible conflict between the career aspirations of consultants and the needs of hospital trusts, or take account of the age mix of the medical staff. It may seem cruel to the individual, but it must be in the interests of both the doctors and the service to maintain a degree of mobility during career development. If taken forward positively and enthusiastically, a specialist grade could strengthen our profession, and provide excellent opportunities for career development. If rejected, trusts are likely simply to expand the use of permanent nonconsultant career grades, which will be not a stepping stone but a cul-de-sac.

We now have much data and no shortage of recommendations. How can we push forward the changes?

References

1. Royal College of Obstetricians and Gynecologists. *Medical Workforce in Obstetrics and Gynecology: Thirteenth Annual Report.* London: RCOG Press; 2002.

2. Royal College of Obstetricians and Gynaecologists, Royal College of Midwives. *Towards Safer Childbirth: Minimum Standards for the Organisation of Labour Wards.* London: RCOG Press; 1999.

3. Royal College of Obstetricians and Gynaecologists. *Clinical Standards: Advice on Planning the Service in Obstetrics and Gynaecology.* London: RCOG Press; 2002.

4. Royal College of Obstetricians and Gynaecologists. *Planning for the Future as Consultants in Obstetrics and Gynaecology.* London: RCOG Press; 1999.

5. Royal College of Obstetricians and Gynaecologists. *A Blueprint for the Future: A Working Party Report on the Future Structure of the Medical Workforce and Service Delivery in Obstetrics and Gynaecology.* London: RCOG Press; 2000.

37

Intrapartum fetal ECG monitoring and the STAN S21 system

Neil K Shah and Chris Griffin

INTRODUCTION

Accurate fetal surveillance during labour constitutes one of the major challenges in perinatal medicine. The process of labour itself presents the greatest threat to intact survival for the vast majority of fetuses and current methods of fetal monitoring have been shown to be far from satisfactory.[1] It is interesting that the nonselective use of intrapartum electronic fetal monitoring (EFM) has led to an increase in medical intervention during labour, which is reflected by a higher rate of caesarean sections.[1,2]

Intrapartum EFM has not been shown significantly to reduce intrapartum or neonatal death rates compared with intermittent auscultation.[1,2] EFM has helped in reducing short–term serious neonatal morbidity (neonatal seizures), but there has been no effect on long–term neonatal outcome.[2,3] However, misinterpretation of fetal cardiotocograms (CTGs) is often a major factor in fetuses subjected to birth asphyxia.[4] Medico–legal litigation in obstetrics often focuses on 'inaccurate' interpretation of CTGs, despite the fact that experts may not be able to agree on the interpretation or significance of the same CTG pattern.

Fetal blood sampling should be used alongside EFM during labour to reduce unnecessary operative intervention.[1,5] However, blood sampling is not always possible owing to inadequate cervical dilation. In addition, it requires expertise, may need to be repeated, is expensive to maintain as a 'bedside test', and is generally not a procedure well liked by practising obstetricians or their patients. New methods to improve the sensitivity of fetal surveillance in labour have therefore been developed.

Changes of the ST waveform of the adult electrocardiogram (ECG) have been shown to reflect myocardial insufficiency during exercise.[6] In fetal lambs, ST segment and T wave changes have been associated with physiological responses to hypoxia.[7] In growth restricted guinea pigs, ST depression and T wave changes were observed during hypoxic episodes while their normally grown littermates showed ST elevation.[8] These observations prompted the development of a commercially available CTG plus ST waveform analyser (STAN). To understand how STAN may improve the sensitivity of fetal monitoring in labour we need to understand fetal physiology in response to hypoxia in conjunction with the fetal ECG.

FETAL PHYSIOLOGY

All fetuses face periods of relative oxygen deficiency during labour but few suffer long–term damage because of the multiple defence mechanisms employed to adapt to the varying levels of oxygen deprivation. Hypoxaemia is the initial phase of oxygen deficiency when oxygen saturation decreases and affects arterial blood but cellular and organ functions remain intact. The fetus acts against hypoxaemia by increasing cellular oxygen uptake and reducing body activity. This is demonstrated in the antepartum phase by an initial reduction or cessation of fetal breathing movements. When oxygen saturation falls further the fetus enters the hypoxic phase. This means that the degree of oxygen deficiency starts to affect peripheral tissues. In response to fetal hypoxia there is a surge of stress hormones from the fetal adrenal glands and a reduction in peripheral blood flow. This results in a redistribution of blood to the brain, heart and adrenals. Anaerobic metabolism is initiated in the peripheral tissues. Chronic anaerobic metabolism, when unchecked, results in lactic acidosis. It is appropriate for such metabolism to occur in the short term and it is a defence mechanism of the fetus. However, when this defence mechanism fails to maintain adequate oxygen levels, asphyxia will develop with the possibility of damage to the central nervous system.

During asphyxia the fetus reacts with maximum activation of the sympathetic nervous system and concomitant release of catecholamines. The central organs switch to anaerobic metabolism and glycogen reserves in the heart and liver are used for energy production. Central redistribution of blood becomes even more pronounced as the fetus tries to keep the cardiovascular system operating. In this final stage the system will collapse within minutes unless oxygen saturation levels improve.[9,10]

The ability of the fetus to deal with hypoxaemia and hypoxia varies depending on the condition of the fetus prior to labour and to events during labour that may affect its defence mechanisms.

FETAL ECG

Figure 1 illustrates the fetal ECG complex in relation to heart activity. The ST segment and T wave reflect repolarisation of myocardial cells in preparation for the next contraction.

The ability of the heart to pump blood is energy dependent. In circumstances where normal fetoplacental oxygen exchange occurs, fetal aerobic metabolism predominates and the ECG shows a normal ST waveform. During hypoxia, as oxygen availability decreases, the fetal ECG shows ST elevation and an increase in T wave height, quantified by the ratio between T and QRS amplitudes – the T/QRS ratio.[11,12]

The hypoxic fetal defence mechanisms maintain myocardial function as stated above, through initiation of glycogenolysis and redistribution of blood flow. This process produces potassium ions that affect myocardial cell membrane potentials and cause the rise in T wave height. This rise and the increase in T/QRS ratio therefore reflects the rate of utilisation of a key fetal defence against hypoxia.

ST depression with negative T waves, or biphasic ST events, reflect a myocardium that is not able or has not had time to mobilise its defence to hypoxia. They are caused by an imbalance of ionic status between the endocardial and epicardial layers of the heart. However, biphasic ST events occur not only in response to hypoxia but whenever the myocardium is exposed to factors that may decrease its ability to respond. These include fetal prematurity, intrauterine infections, maternal or fetal pyrexia, myocardial dystrophies, fetal cardiac malformations and chronic fetal stress.

Biphasic ST events signal a situation of potentially reduced myocardial performance and therefore the usual signs of fetal reaction may not occur.

ST waveform changes can occur in response to the surge of stress hormones produced during labour. These stimulate the heart to increase cardiac output but also induce glycogenolysis and high T waves. This general arousal in the healthy fetus will be indicated by a reactive CTG. If hypoxia becomes severe the ST waveform returns towards normal. This is seen together with a markedly reduced ability by the fetus to respond and an abnormal CTG. This last event is crucial in understanding the reason for early STAN monitoring in the presence of a normal CTG and not to apply STAN fetal monitoring when the CTG becomes abnormal.

ECG complex

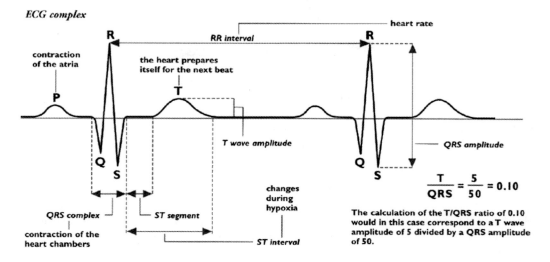

Figure 1 *The fetal ECG complex (courtesy Neoventa Medical AB, Moelndal, Sweden)*

STAN S21 SYSTEM

The STAN S21 fetal heart monitor, produced by Neoventa Medical AB (Moelndal, Sweden), combines standard CTG technology with ST waveform analysis of the fetal ECG. Both fetal ECG and heart rate are measured continuously via a scalp electrode placed on the presenting part. These measurements, together with uterine activity, measured via an external tocotransducer, are displayed on a large flat colour monitor as a horizontal rolling scroll. All information can be entered or accessed via two buttons, a trackball and a foldaway keyboard. The instrument is housed in an aluminium structure on wheels, slightly smaller than a conventional CTG machine. The ST waveform analysis is presented as a continuous T/QRS ratio. However, the system contains a log function to identify significant ST changes with the message 'ST event', which is printed on the screen. In order to find out about the type and degree of abnormality the event log has to be accessed, where this latter information is clearly identified. ST information should be used together with interpretation of the CTG in evaluating the fetal status. Simplified clinical guidelines to indicate when intervention is required (delivery or alleviation of the cause of fetal distress such as maternal hypotension) in response to ST and CTG changes have been produced. STAN has been used in term fetuses only and the event log requires 20 minutes of monitoring before automatic ST analysis can begin.

CLINICAL TRIALS

There have been two randomised controlled trials (RCTs) looking at term, cephalic deliveries and comparing ST + CTG waveform analysis with standard CTG monitoring. These two studies were reported from Plymouth in 1993[13] and from Sweden in 2001,[14] with the eight-year temporal advances in technological advancement and data presentation clearly evident in the Swedish study. Both contained the power to test their respective primary hypotheses.

The Plymouth RCT involved 2400 deliveries and tested the hypothesis that ST + CTG analysis would reduce operative interventions for fetal distress without placing the fetus at risk.[13] There was a 46% reduction in operative deliveries for fetal distress in the ST + CTG arm ($P < 0.001$) with no difference in operative deliveries for other reasons. Overall, 43% of operative interventions were judged unnecessary in the CTG arm compared with 5% in the ST + CTG arm of the trial. There were no significant differences in neonatal outcome but there was a significant reduction in the use of fetal blood sampling. However three babies in the ST + CTG arm showed evidence of asphyxia with ST events not being recognised. This highlighted the need to improve data presentation by providing continuous assessment of significant ST events, which is now done through the event log.

The Swedish multicentre RCT involved 4966 deliveries from three Swedish labour wards equipped with the STAN S21 system.[14] The primary hypothesis was that ST + CTG waveform analysis reduced the rate of metabolic acidosis at birth (cord artery pH < 7.05, base deficit >12 mmol/l) and operative deliveries for fetal distress compared with CTG alone. The CTG alone group had the ST analysis recorded in a blinded fashion to all participants at the time of fetal monitoring, while the combined CTG and ST group were not blinded. The baseline obstetric characteristics were similar in the two groups. There was a 61% reduction in metabolic acidosis ($P = 0.01$) and 28% fewer operative interventions for fetal distress ($P < 0.05$) in the STAN arm compared with the CTG arm. Initial interim analysis showed no significant differences in neonatal outcome measures (Apgar scores, admissions to neonatal intensive care unit, neonatal encephalopathy).

SECONDARY ANALYSIS OF CLINICAL TRIALS

A secondary analysis has now been performed examining findings related to cases with complicated/adverse neonatal outcomes in the Swedish RCT.[15] Of the 4966 term fetuses included in the trial, the cases of all 350 neonates admitted to the special care baby unit were examined by a paediatrician blinded to the trial group allocation. Twenty-nine babies had a complicated/adverse neonatal outcome; 22 of these 29 had ST + CTG patterns indicating a need for intervention according to the STAN clinical guidelines during labour. The ST waveform analysis data for the CTG arm was examined retrospectively. There was significantly less ($P = 0.02$) moderate (abnormal tone, profound lethargy) or severe (coma, seizures, abnormal tone) neonatal encephalopathy in the STAN group (0.04%, 1/2519) compared with the CTG group (0.33%, 8/2447).

Additional clinical data on STAN S21 are available through Neoventa. Two thousand cases were presented in April 2001. Only one baby had metabolic acidosis without ST events being noted (baby had no clinical evidence of hypoxia). A total of 715 cases using STAN S21 in Gothenburg, following on from the end of the Swedish RCT, have shown only three occurrences (0.4%) of cord metabolic acidosis.[11]

TRAINING

The Swedish RCT[14] provides convincing evidence of the need for expert training in the use of the STAN S21 system. This trial allowed for an interim analysis after 1600 cases, which showed that the clinical management guidelines in relation to ST events were, in many cases, being ignored and, consequently, a higher rate of neonatal acidosis and operative interventions was occurring. Retraining was performed and in the second half of the trial there was much better adherence to management protocols, with the overall significant decreases in neonatal acidosis and operative deliveries detailed above. Training issues in relation to obstetricians and midwives are therefore paramount when a new technology is introduced. With this in mind a multimedia based teaching programme has been developed. This is founded on the physiological and clinical basis of fetal monitoring, interactive analysis of recorded cases, written literature, and online access to STAN interpretation guidelines and important cases. Training of key personnel within a maternity unit who can then conduct small-group training on STAN with dissemination of information, access to the full training programme, regular update sessions, and personal STAN-user accreditation would seem the most efficient way of training labour suite staff. However, training costs should be factored into the overall costings of a unit that introduces STAN monitoring.

CURRENT WORKING STATUS OF STAN IN THE UK

Currently, six trusts in the UK have purchased the STAN system. We have taken the liberty, with their permission, of listing a main contact's email address. This, we hope, will promote active discussions about practical issues. To introduce STAN into a trust is no mean feat, from both funding and training perspectives. The issue of training is perhaps the most difficult owing to the large number of consultants, midwives and rotating doctors involved in providing intrapartum care. Our experience at Heartlands Hospital, Birmingham, has borne this out. Junior medical staff rotate on a yearly basis, work a shift pattern and, in the district general hospital setting, are mostly pre-MRCOG. Thus having a large enough core of medical staff trained in the use of STAN, as with the introduction of any new working practice, has been difficult. It is of interest that all the hospitals who have purchased the system to date have found the training issue of all staff to be the major hurdle to full implementation of STAN.

In our trust (6500 deliveries per year) a business case for the purchase of STAN was made on the financial savings from unnecessary caesarean sections performed for presumed fetal distress when fetal blood sampling was not possible owing to the degree of dilation of the cervix or was not performed for other reasons. In the discussions around the business case, it soon became evident that the grade A clinical evidence supporting STAN monitoring is far greater than that supporting the benefits of routine nontargeted anomaly scanning in pregnancy. Although our trust uses only two STAN machines at present, we are planning to move over entirely to the use of these machines as the preferred method of intrapartum fetal monitoring for the clinical reasons outlined above.

DISCUSSION

It does appear on the physiological and clinical evidence that ST + CTG waveform analysis can be used accurately to differentiate between the healthy, well oxygenated fetus, the healthy fetus being subjected to acute hypoxia, and the chronically hypoxic fetus, by analysing the most important defence mechanism the fetus has to withstand asphyxia: myocardial blood flow and glycogenolysis. Strong evidence from one well conducted study confirms that ST + CTG waveform analysis, in the form of the STAN system, does deliver a significant decrease in operative delivery rates and, more importantly, a significant decrease in severe neonatal morbidity in term pregnancies. With the methods of the clinical studies being of at least as good a standard as any other previous study on fetal monitoring in labour, then one would have to say that 'the writing is on the wall' for the traditional method of intrapartum CTG monitoring with fetal scalp pH testing.

However, no system will ever be ideal for all. The shortcomings recognised by current users in the UK are as follows:

- A unique user ID should be installed to log on to the system and to add annotation.

- Having to use a spiral fetal scalp electrode excludes the use of STAN when the potential for vertical transmission of infection exists.

- STAN can currently be used only in term pregnancies.

- STAN can currently be used only in labour, not antenatally.

- The cost of each STAN machine is approximately £20,000.

- Training of staff in the use of STAN is a long process but it can be accomplished. This change in practice needs to be championed by a team of highly committed practitioners from both the obstetric and midwifery fields within a trust.

- Discrepancies between ST analysis and the CTG may lead to inaccurate interpretation if the fetus is in a preterminal stage at the start of monitoring or if monitoring has been carried out for less than 20 minutes.

What, then, will make us change to a new system of fetal monitoring apart from what can now be considered robust clinical evidence? The following list is not exhaustive, but it is an example of why trusts are already using STAN:

- Legally, we are expected to store a CTG trace, preserved for all to see in the medical notes for two decades or more. Our current method of note storage does not in any way support this system. STAN, with its computerised data format, will fully meet this medico-legal requirement.

- Targeted fetal monitoring, as supported by NICE guidelines, will remove the shotgun approach to fetal monitoring and focus more clearly on the population of women who do require continuous fetal monitoring in labour.

- Clinical Negligence Scheme for Trusts is ensuring that users (lay women) are present and heard on labour suite forums. When the users learn the benefits of STAN intrapartum monitoring over CTG alone, a demand for more widespread use of STAN is likely to be made.

- Clinical Negligence Scheme for Trusts demands six-monthly CTG training schemes for staff. This can be accomplished more easily with the readily available clinical information that the STAN system provides for staff to access.

- The greater amount and degree of clinical information recorded using STAN in situations where estimation of fetal scalp pH is not possible will encourage obstetricians to use the system.

CONCLUSIONS

The next few years will, we feel, see a long overdue revolution in fetal monitoring in the UK. The strong clinical evidence now supporting the use of fetal ST waveform analysis, and the STAN system, should be viewed as a major clinical advancement in obstetrics. STAN has been shown significantly to decrease serious neonatal morbidity due to intrapartum hypoxia, neonatal acidosis, and operative delivery rates for presumed fetal distress in term cephalic deliveries. In the past, evidence based initiatives, such as the use of magnesium sulphate for the management of eclampsia or the use of corticosteroids for lung maturity in premature babies, were only adopted into widespread practice in the UK years after our European and American counterparts understood their benefits. Mothers should have confidence that, at the most vital time in any pregnancy (i.e. during labour), the best clinical care is being provided for both them and their baby.

    The authors have never received any financial aid or educational grants from Neoventa or any other groups associated with fetal monitoring.

Weblinks

For an online reference to all papers published to date about STAN: www.fetalstan.info
For information on STAN and training issues: www.neoventa.se

Current users of the STAN system in the UK

Mr D Tuffnell: derek.tuffnell@bradfordhospitals.nhs.uk
Ms C Sparey: colette.sparey@leedsth.nhs.uk
Professor S Arulkumaran: sarulkum@sghms.ac.uk
Ms S Hamilton: shona.hamilton@calderdale.nhs.uk
Mr C Griffin: christopher.griffin@heartsol.wmids.nhs.uk

References

1. Royal College of Obstetricians and Gynaecologists. *The use of Electronic Fetal Monitoring.* NICE Evidence Based Clinical Guideline No. 8. London: RCOG; 2001.
2. Thacker SB, Stroup DF. Continuous electronic heart rate monitoring for fetal assessment during labor. *Cochrane Database Syst Rev* 2000;(2):CD000063.
3. Nelson KB, Dambrosia JM, Ting TY, Grether J. Uncertain value of electronic fetal monitoring in predicting cerebral palsy. *N Engl J Med* 1996;334:613–18.
4. Westgate JA, Gunn AJ, Gunn TR. Antecedents of neonatal encephalopathy with fetal acidaemia at term. *Br J Obstet Gynaecol* 1999;106:774–82.
5. Westgate J, Greene K. How well is fetal blood sampling used in clinical practice? *Br J Obstet Gynaecol* 1994;101:250–1.
6. Miranda CP, Lehmann KG, Froelicher VF. Correlation between resting ST segment depression, exercise testing, coronary angiography and long-term prognosis. *Am Heart J* 1991;122:1617–28.
7. Greene KR, Dawes GS, Lilja H, Rosen KG. Changes in the ST waveform of the fetal lamb electrocardiogram with hypoxemia. *Am J Obstet Gynecol* 1982;144:950–8.
8. Widmark C, Jansson T, Lindecrantz K, Rosen KG. ECG waveform, short term heart rate variability and plasma catecholamine concentrations in response to hypoxia in intrauterine growth retarded guinea-pig fetuses. *J Dev Physiol* 1991;15:161–8.
9. Greene KR, Rosen KG. Intrapartum asphyxia. In: Levene MI, Bennett MJ, Punt J, editors. *Fetal and Neonatal Neurology and Neurosurgery.* Edinburgh: Churchill Livingstone; 1995. p. 265-72.
10. Neoventa Medical AB. Fetal surveillance with STAN [educational material]. Moelndal, Sweden: Neoventa Medical; 2000.
11. Rosen KG. Intrapartum fetal monitoring and the fetal ECG – time for a change. *Arch Perinat Med* 2001;7(2):7–12.
12. Greene K. Intrapartum fetal monitoring: CTG, ECG and fetal blood sampling. In: Rodeck CH, Whittle MJ, editors. *Fetal Medicine: Basic Science and Clinical Practice.* Edinburgh: Churchill Livingstone; 1999. p. 985–1003.
13. Westgate J, Harris M, Curnow JS, Greene KR. Plymouth randomized trial of cardiotocogram only versus ST waveform plus cardiotocogram for intrapartum monitoring: 2400 cases. *Am J Obstet Gynecol* 1993;169:1151–60.
14. Amer-Wahlin I, Hellsten C, Noren H, Hagberg H, Herbst A, Kjellmer I, *et al.*

Cardiotocography only versus cardiotocography plus ST analysis of fetal electrocardiogram for intrapartum fetal monitoring: a Swedish randomised controlled trial. *Lancet* 2001;358:534–8.

15. Noren H, Amer Wahlin I, Hagberg H, Herbst A, Kjellmer I, Marsal K, *et al*. Fetal electrocardiography in labor and neonatal outcome: data from the Swedish randomized controlled trial on intrapartum fetal monitoring. *Am J Obstet Gynecol* 2003;188:183–92.

38

Vaginal myomectomy

Malini Sharma, Alexander Taylor and Adam Magos

INTRODUCTION

Uterine leiomyomas (fibroids) are the most common benign tumours of the female genital tract. They occur in 20–25% of women over 30 years of age and are responsible for approximately one-third of all hospital admissions to gynaecology services.[1,2] Most women with fibroids are symptom free, but 20–50% have been estimated to suffer symptoms;[3] their symptomatology is related to the location, size and number of fibroids present. Approximately 30% of women with fibroids are reported to have some menstrual abnormalities, most frequently menorrhagia.[3] Other symptoms include dysmenorrhoea, acute pain (with degeneration, torsion or necrosis) and pressure symptoms on the bladder or bowel by larger fibroids. Fibroids can also be associated with subfertility and miscarriage. Consequently, they have a major financial and social cost to the community, especially in terms of hospital outpatient visits and surgery.

Traditionally, the mainstay of treatment for fibroids has been surgical. Medical treatment has a limited place. Gonadotrophin-releasing hormone analogues can be used pre-operatively to reduce the size and vascularity of fibroids, thereby reducing blood loss during surgery, or they can be used to help to correct anaemia. Surgical management options are dependent on the fertility needs of the woman as well as the number, site and size of the fibroids. Hysterectomy, both abdominal and, if suitable, vaginal, is appropriate management in women who no longer wish to conceive or are menopausal, or in those who have uncontrolled or debilitating symptoms from uterine fibroids. With women choosing to delay childbearing and seeking alternative treatment to hysterectomy, myomectomy is becoming an increasingly important option. Traditionally it has been performed at laparotomy, but it is now more often performed via laparoscopic and hysteroscopic routes. With laparotomy there is a high risk of haemorrhage and sepsis, with the added risks of blood transfusion and postoperative adhesion formation. Laparoscopic and hysteroscopic myomectomy also have potential limitations and complications (Table 1), and are traditionally reserved for women with only few relatively small fibroids that are either subserosal or submucous in origin.

Vaginal myomectomy is an alternative approach for the removal of uterine fibroids, and encompasses a variety of techniques that may be appropriate for women with larger and more numerous fibroids:[4]

- removal of a pedunculated submucous myoma via the cervix

- removal of a submucous myoma via Duhrssen's incision or vaginal hysterotomy

- removal of myoma via anterior or posterior colpotomy.

Several authors have reported series of myomectomies and it is evident that the proportion performed vaginally is relatively small.[5,6] However, in a series of 254 myomectomies by Ben Baruch *et al.*,[7] 18% were vaginal.

Table 1 *Problems with myomectomy*

Myomectomy	Problem
Abdominal	Requires laparotomy
	Haemorrhage
	Sepsis
	Postoperative adhesions
Laparoscopic	Technically difficult with intramural fibroids
	Limited to relatively small and few fibroids
	Long operative time
	Haemorrhage
	Weak uterine scar
Hysteroscopic	Suitable only for submucosal fibroids
	Limited to relatively small and few fibroids
	Uterine perforation
	Fluid overload

It would appear therefore that vaginal myomectomy is an underused technique that could potentially be applied to a greater proportion of women. It can be suitable not only for the obvious conditions such as a prolapsed submucous fibroid but also adapted for nonprolapsed submucous and subserous fibroids. In the following review, we wish to highlight the various applications of vaginal myomectomy.

HISTORICAL BACKGROUND AND LITERATURE REVIEW

Myomectomy was first described by Amussat in 1840 in Paris and, in 1845, WL Atlee[2] was the first surgeon to describe vaginal myomectomy in a woman with a prolapsed fibroid. Bonney[8] described his earliest experiences with myomectomy in 1931, consisting mainly of removing pedunculated myomas at laparotomy. In 1942 Rubin[5] described the removal of prolapsed small submucous fibroids that were protruding through the external os, either by avulsion as if it was a small polyp or, if the fibroid was on a thick pedicle, by ligating the pedicle before removal of the fibroid. He also described packing the uterine cavity with iodoform gauze if bleeding was present. Rubin suggested that if, in addition to the presence of an infected and degenerating prolapsed submucous fibroid, there were also intramural or subserous myomas, the prolapsed fibroid should be removed first; the other fibroids could be removed at a later date when the infection had subsided, to reduce the risk of postoperative sepsis. Rubin also described 11 cases of vaginal myomectomy for submucous fibroids; two were in nulliparous women with small submucous fibroids in whom he performed anterior vaginal hysterotomy, using a tenaculum to bring down the fibroid to a point where it could be incised and shelled out. Overall, 11 of 481 cases (2%) were managed vaginally, the remainder by laparotomy. Davids[6] also published a series in 1952 in which he reported on 1107 myomectomies, 43 of which (3.8%) were carried out via a vaginal route.

In 1979, Brooks and Stage[9] described a series of 17 women who underwent vaginal myomectomy using a Mayo renal pedicle clamp. The clamp was left in place for 24 hours then removed. The fibroids ranged from 2 to 10 cm in diameter.

In 1982, Riley reported on a series of 41 women with submucous myomas, of whom 28 were treated by vaginal myomectomy and the remaining 13 by abdominal hysterectomy.[10] These women presented with either a prolapsed or a nonprolapsed submucous fibroid and reported various symptoms (Table 2). In those undergoing vaginal myomectomy, the pedunculated fibroid was either twisted off or the pedicle was ligated and excised. Although this was a retrospective study, the number of women who had postoperative pyrexia or required blood transfusion was significantly lower in those who underwent vaginal myomectomy compared with those who had an abdominal hysterectomy. Hospital stay was also significantly shorter in the vaginal myomectomy group. The women in both groups were comparable in age, race, parity and presenting symptoms; however, the women in the vaginal fibroid group had a significantly lower haemoglobin (8.6 g/dl ± 2.7) compared with the unprolapsed fibroid group (11.4 g/dl ± 1.9). As a consequence the women in the vaginal fibroid group had a higher number of units of blood transfused (mean 2.3 units compared with 1.5 units in the nonprolapsed group).

TECHNIQUES OF VAGINAL MYOMECTOMY

Determining the operative approach to myomectomy has to take account not only of the position, size and number of fibroids, but also the inherent morbidity of the procedure. The ideal procedure should have the lowest risk of complications such as haemorrhage, febrile morbidity, postoperative adhesion formation, and, not least, hysterectomy.[11,12] The most obvious indication for vaginal myomectomy is a prolapsing submucous myoma, but the purpose of this review is to raise awareness that, in appropriately selected women, vaginal myomectomy can be performed for nonprolapsed submucous and subserous myomas.

Prolapsed fibroid in the vagina

Several authors have reported on their experiences with managing prolapsed pedunculated fibroids.[5-7,9,10,13] These fibroids can prolapse into the vagina, and have the potential to become necrotic and infected. The fibroid can be twisted off its pedicle or, if the pedicle is large, it can be ligated. Over a ten-year period, Brooks and Stage[9] found pedunculated fibroids in 17 of 1255 women who were due to undergo hysterectomy, giving an incidence of 1.3%. The fibroids ranged in diameter from 2 to 10 cm. The cervix was dilated in all cases. Bimanual examination revealed uterine size ranging from normal to that equivalent of 26 weeks of gestation. Four women had significant febrile morbidity. After correcting anaemia and treating infection, vaginal myomectomy was undertaken in 14 of these 17 women. As noted earlier, their technique involved clamping the pedicle, excising the fibroid, and removing the clamp 24 hours later.

Riley's retrospective study in 1982[10] described vaginal myomectomy in 28 of 41 women with prolapsed submucous fibroids. The remaining 13 underwent abdominal hysterectomy. In those managed by vaginal myomectomy the pedunculated fibroid was either twisted off or ligated and excised.

Table 2 *Submucous fibroids: presenting symptoms (after Riley, 1982[10])*

Symptom	n (%)
Vaginal fibroid group	
Abnormal vaginal bleeding	36 (88)
Lower abdominal pain	18 (44)
Abnormal vaginal discharge	18 (44)
Sensation of 'something coming down'	6 (15)
Headache, dizziness and other symptoms (probably relating to anaemia)	5 (12)
Unprolapsed fibroid group	
Lower abdominal discomfort	8
Abnormal vaginal bleeding	7
Sensation of abdominal mass	7

Dicker *et al.*[13] reported on a retrospective study of 142 women of whom 46 underwent vaginal myomectomy in a similar manner to the cases previously described. The others underwent abdominal myomectomy ($n = 12$) or hysterectomy ($n = 84$). They found no significant difference in postoperative morbidity or length of hospital stay between the study and control groups.

One study looked at the long-term outcome in 46 women who had previously undergone vaginal myomectomy for pedunculated prolapsed submucous fibroids.[7] Forty-three underwent successful vaginal myomectomy; in the other three the vaginal myomectomy failed and they required abdominal myomectomy. The study group was compared with a control group of 41 women who underwent abdominal myomectomy. Both groups were similar in age and menopausal status. Gravidity and parity were higher in the study group. Uterine size in the study group ranged from normal to moderately enlarged, and only five women had a uterine size of greater that 12 weeks (10.8%), in contrast to 21 (51%) in the control group. The mean haemoglobin was significantly lower in the study group (9.1 ± 1.1 g/dl versus 11.0 ± 1.0 g/dl). Vaginal myomectomy was carried out by grasping the fibroid and twisting it off its pedicle. The mean hospital stay was 2.4 days (range 1–13) in the vaginal myomectomy group, compared with 7.8 days in the control group (range 5–16). Thirty-four women in the study group were followed up for a mean of 5.5 years, with 27 having no subsequent symptoms related to fibroids. Three required repeat vaginal myomectomy for recurrent fibroids and only two required hysterectomy.

Vaginal myomectomy does seem to be the procedure of choice for pedunculated prolapsed submucous fibroids unless there are other indications requiring hysterectomy. However, when large prolapsed fibroids are occupying the pelvis, there may be limited space in the vagina for approaching and resecting the pedicle. Even in this situation, a vaginal approach may still be applicable. In 2001, Kanaoka *et al.*[14] published a case report involving morcellation of the centre of the fibroid to create a spherical intranodal space, which was further widened using an electrosurgical loop. When sufficient space between the vaginal wall and the surface of the fibroid was obtained, the myoma could be resected completely.

Nonprolapsed fibroids using *Laminaria*

Goldrath[15,16] performed a series of vaginal myomectomies using laminaria tents. *Laminaria japonica* had been used in obstetrics for many years to dilate the cervix to induce labour. In the 1970s laminaria tents were used to dilate the cervix before abortion.[17] Goldrath used the hydroscopic properties of *Laminaria* to dilate the cervix in preparation for myomectomy. This approach was used for submucous nonprolapsed pedunculated fibroids diagnosed at hysteroscopy. He used a paracervical block and placed two or three laminaria tents in the cervix. These were replaced by further tents after six hours, which were left *in situ* overnight. The *Laminaria* had the effect of dilating the cervix. After anaesthetising the woman with a paracervical block and sedation, the laminaria tents were removed and the fibroid was grasped and avulsed. Sometimes the fibroid was removed intact, but morcellation was occasionally required for larger myomas. If haemorrhage occurred a Foley catheter was inserted to achieve haemostasis. In his series of 151 women, this procedure was successful in 139 cases (92%). Goldrath's results are summarised in Table 3.

Nonprolapsed fibroids using Duhrssen's incision

The removal of a nonprolapsed submucous myoma can be achieved with a Duhrssen's incision.[2] Using the lithotomy position, the cervix is infiltrated with local anaesthetic. A longitudinal incision is made through the cervix to the point where the fibroid is exposed. The incision is either anterior or posterior depending on the location of the fibroid. The fibroid can then be avulsed or ligated

Table 3 *Results of vaginal myomectomy using* Laminaria *(after Goldrath, 1987[15])*

No. cases	151
Mean no. fibroids removed	2 (range 1–18)
Size of fibroids (cm)	2–5
Weight of fibroids (g)	10–180
Successful procedure	139 (92%)
Complications	
Uterine perforation	2 (1.4%)
Haemorrhage	7 (5.0%)
Cervical laceration	7 (5.0%)

and the incision repaired. This technique is suitable for fibroids that are considered to be too large for hysteroscopic resection because the incision can be extended to the lowest border of the fibroid. Once the fibroid has been removed the incision can be repaired with a continuous locked polyglactin suture. There are few data regarding the integrity of the cervix after a Duhrssen's incision, but clearly cervical incompetence or possibly stenosis could occur in any subsequent pregnancy.

Nonprolapsed fibroids using vaginal hysterotomy

When a submucous fibroid is located higher up in the uterine cavity it may be necessary to gain access via a hysterotomy. This is achieved by making a longitudinal incision through the cervix and extending into the myometrium. With an anterior approach there will be the need for bladder dissection. With posterior fibroids the hysterotomy can be made via a posterior approach. Once the fibroid is excised, the hysterotomy incision is closed in a similar fashion to the Duhrssen's incision. Again there are few data available on the outcome of subsequent pregnancies, and the same concerns apply as to the Duhrssen's incision, with the potential added risk of uterine rupture.

Intramural and subserous fibroids by colpotomy

The above techniques are not suitable for intramural or subserous fibroids. In this situation, vaginal myomectomy may still be possible using an anterior or posterior colpotomy to access the fibroids. This technique was first described by Magos *et al.* in 1994,[18] the concept of the procedure being based on the Doderlein–Kronig technique for vaginal hysterectomy from 1912.[19] The choice of anterior or posterior colpotomy is determined by the site of the dominant fibroid, a posterior approach being preferred whenever possible. Doderlein and Kronig used a nerve hook to deliver the uterine body through an anterior colpotomy; we use a No. 1 polypropylene suture, taking deep bites in to the myometrium to 'walk up' the uterine wall towards the fundus. Once in the colpotomy, the uterus is incised over the myoma, which is then excised in one piece or after morcellation, depending on its size. Once all the fibroids have been removed, the uterus can be pulled through the colpotomy incision toward the vaginal introitus, where it is repaired before being pushed back into the pelvis. This type of vaginal myomectomy is suitable when there is good uterine mobility, adequate vaginal access, and no evidence of adnexal pathology.

Table 4 *Results of 35 women undergoing vaginal myomectomy (after Davies et al., 1999[4])*

Outcome	Mean (%)	Range
Operating time (min)	77.9	65.9–89.9
No. fibroids removed per woman	2.5	1.7–3.4
Weight of fibroids removed (g)	113.8	84.2–143.4
Estimated blood loss (ml)	313.6	206.1–421.1
No. women requiring transfusion	4 (11.4%)	
No. women requiring laparotomy	3 (8.6%)	
Postoperative hospital stay (days)	3.9	3.1–4.7
No. readmissions to hospital	2 (5.7%)	

Davies et al.[4] updated the data on this type of vaginal myomectomy in 1999. Uterine size ranged from 6 to 16 weeks. The largest fibroid was 11 cm diameter, the mean measurement being 5.2 cm. In his series he employed the following steps for myomectomy:

- use lithotomy position

- catheterise bladder

- infiltrate cervix with lignocaine/adrenaline mixture

- anterior or posterior colpotomy

- deliver uterus into colpotomy incision

- perform myomectomy

- repair myometrium in layers

- replace uterus

- close colpotomy.

Surgical approach was by posterior colpotomy in 22 women (62%) and anterior colpotomy in nine (26%), with four having bilateral colpotomies. Of the 35 women in this study, 32 underwent successful vaginal myomectomy (91.4%), the remaining three procedures being converted to laparotomy. No woman had a hysterectomy. Postoperative complications included pelvic haematoma (four cases) and urinary tract infection (four cases). These women were followed up for a range of two to six months. Three went on to have successful pregnancies. Table 4 summarises the results of this study.

LAPAROSCOPIC ASSISTED VAGINAL MYOMECTOMY

A combined approach of laparoscopic/vaginal surgery has also been proposed for managing uterine fibroids, based on the colpotomy technique described above. A Chinese study reported that 31 women with symptomatic fundal and posterior wall fibroids were treated by laparoscopically assisted vaginal myomectomy (LAVM).[20] Laparoscopy was carried out to visualise the fibroids and to divide adhesions as necessary. A guide suture was placed in the largest fibroid for identification. A sponge holder with a swab was used to tent the posterior vagina, and laparoscopic unipolar scissors were used to make a transverse vaginal incision. A grasper was used to guide the suture into the vagina through the colpotomy, which was then widened laterally by digital pressure to allow delivery of the uterus

Table 5 *Results of laparoscopic assisted vaginal myomectomy (after Wang et al., 2000[20])*

Outcome	Mean	Range
Operating time (min)	79	50–103
No. fibroids removed per woman	1.74	1–9
Size of fibroids removed (cm)	7	4–12
Weight of fibroids removed (g)	102	40–400
Estimated blood loss (ml)	150	50–500
Haemoglobin decrease (g/dl)	1.16	0–2.7
Postoperative hospital stay (days)	3.1	1–6

into the vagina by grasping the stay suture. The serosa was incised and fibroids enucleated. The uterus was repaired transvaginally using conventional needle holders and sutures as at laparotomy. The uterus was replaced through the colpotomy incision, which was then closed. Finally, the pneumoperitoneum was recommenced and the suture lines examined laparoscopically for haemostasis.

The results of this study are summarised in Table 5. None of the women had previously undergone pelvic surgery. Five underwent concomitant ovarian cystectomy; none was converted to laparotomy. There were no major complications. One woman required a blood transfusion and two had postoperative pyrexia.

Compared with a purely vaginal approach to myomectomy, the addition of laparoscopy does provide a better view of the pelvis and allows for additional procedures such as adhesiolysis or the treatment of other pathology. Conventional instruments are used to repair the myometrium and the integrity of the uterine sutures can be more easily assessed compared with a purely laparoscopic technique.

Goldfarb and Fanarjian[21] also reported using LAVM in a woman who underwent a routine laparoscopic myomectomy followed by vaginal removal of the fibroid via colpotomy. The fibroid was grasped with a myoma screw, which was directed towards the cul-de-sac. A colpotomy was performed and the myoma grasped with a tenaculum and removed vaginally. He subsequently noticed that the dominant fibroid was projecting into the uterine cavity and went on to deliver the uterus through the colpotomy into the vagina. Myomectomy was then carried out using electrocautery and sharp dissection. The uterus was repaired in three layers, placed back into the pelvis and the colpotomy incision closed. Goldfarb went on to perform 11 additional LAVMs in a similar manner and his results are summarised in Table 6. Pelosi and Pelosi's group[22] also described their technique of LAVM using a posterior colpotomy.

Table 6 *Results of laparoscopically assisted vaginal myomectomy (after Goldfarb and Fanarjian, 2001[21])*

Outcome	Mean	Range
Operative time (min)	93	60–120
Size of dominant myoma (cm)	6	4–8
No. myomas removed	2	2–8
Estimated blood loss (ml)	125	75–300
Hospital stay (days)	1.3	1–3
Return to normal activity	10/11 women within 7 days	

VAGINAL MYOMECTOMY IN COMPARISON WITH OPEN AND LAPAROSCOPIC TECHNIQUES

There are relatively few comparative data of vaginal myomectomy compared with other routes of surgery. In contrast, there have been many reviews comparing open myomectomy with another 'minimal access' technique, laparoscopic myomectomy. This was first described by Kurt Semm in the late 1970s.[23] Since that seminal publication, several authors have reported their series of laparoscopic myomectomies.[24–32]

Stringer et al.[29] compared the results of 49 open and 49 laparoscopic myomectomies. In this study, uterine size was comparable in both groups, and the indications for both procedures were similar. The mean operating time for open myomectomy was 133 minutes; it was 264 minutes for the laparoscopic procedure. The mean blood loss was 340 ml for open myomectomy and 110 ml for laparoscopic myomectomy. Hospital stay was significantly shorter in the laparoscopy group. Postoperative pelvic adhesions were also evaluated and found to be lower in the laparoscopic group. Bulletti et al.[31] also looked at adhesions after open and laparoscopic myomectomy in a case–control study. They found significantly fewer adhesions after laparoscopic surgery.[31] Tulandi et al.[11] performed second-look laparoscopy six weeks after abdominal myomectomy and recorded adhesion scores using the American Fertility Society classification. They found that posterior uterine wall myomectomy was associated with significantly more adhesions than when fibroids were removed via an anterior uterine incision.

A particular concern after laparoscopic myomectomy is uterine integrity, in particular the risk of uterine dehiscence after laparoscopic suturing; sporadic cases have been reported.[22,33] Pelosi and Pelosi[22] suggested that electrosurgical dissection could contribute to suboptimal healing of the myomectomy site because it disrupts blood flow to the wound site, leading to uterine wall weakness and dehiscence.

Fertility after myomectomy has also been investigated. Fauconnier et al.[34] reported that the cumulative probability of conception was reduced after removal of a posterior or intramural fibroid, and after a sutured hysterotomy. In contrast, the cumulative probability of conception was greater after myomectomy for fibroids responsible for menorrhagia. This latter result is consistent with an observation published in 2001 that even small intramural fibroids can compromise fertility.[35]

Although none of these studies directly addressed vaginal myomectomy, the results of open and laparoscopic myomectomy could be extrapolated to some degree to vaginal myomectomy. Analgesia requirements, complications and recovery are likely to be less with vaginal surgery than laparotomy. Postoperative adhesion formation should not be a problem when prolapsed submucous fibroids are avulsed. Pelvic adhesions may be a risk when myomectomy is done through a colpotomy, particularly if the approach is via the posterior fornix. However, only anecdotal data are available. In the authors' experience, laparoscopy has been performed in two women after vaginal myomectomy; in neither case were there any pelvic adhesions.

Fertility after vaginal myomectomy has never been looked at in a setting of a randomised controlled study. As noted earlier, the use of Duhrssen's incision or vaginal hysterotomy may compromise the integrity of the cervix and risk cervical incompetence or stenosis, as seen occasionally after loop cone biopsy.

CONCLUSIONS

It is evident from this review that vaginal myomectomy encompasses a range of procedures to remove myomas from several sites. Traditionally, vaginal myomectomy has been used to avulse prolapsed submucous fibroids, but the indications may be extended by using the hysterotomy and colpotomy approach. Currently only a small proportion of myomectomies are carried out using these techniques, but vaginal myomectomy should be considered in cases of prolapsed submucous fibroids, large nonprolapsed submucous fibroids, and small to medium sized intramural and subserous fibroids, providing that there is adequate vaginal access and good uterine mobility. Posterior wall fibroids may be easier to remove vaginally, partly because there is more room for manipulation in the sacral hollow, and partly because a posterior hysterotomy or colpotomy is technically easier to perform and does not require bladder dissection. Laparoscopy can be used to assist with the procedure, particularly if adnexal pathology is suspected. An important advantage of vaginal myomectomy is that conventional instruments are used, and the uterine repair is likely to be considerably stronger than with laparoscopic suturing. Further studies are, however, needed to address postoperative outcomes such as adhesion formation and subsequent fertility. Only then can we accurately compare outcomes such as operating times, blood loss, complications, long-term symptom relief and recurrence of fibroids.

References

1. Whitfield CR. Benign tumours of the uterus. In: Whitfield CR, editor. *Dewhurst's Textbook of Obstetrics and Gynaecology for Postgraduates.* 5th ed. Oxford: Blackwell Science; 1995. p. 738–46.

2. Mattingly RF, Thompson JD. *Te Linde's Operative Gynecology.* 6th ed. Philadelphia, PA: Lippincott; 1985. p. 203–55.

3. Buttram VC Jr, Reiter RC. Uterine leiomyomata: etiology, symptomatology and management. *Fertil Steril* 1981;36:433–45.

4. Davies A, Hart R, Magos AL. The excision of uterine fibroids by vaginal myomectomy: a prospective study. *Fertil Steril* 1999;71:961–4.

5. Rubin IC. Progress in myomectomy. *Am J Obstet Gynecol* 1942;44:196–212.

6. Davids AM. Myomectomy. Surgical technique and results in a series of 1150 cases. *Am J Obstet Gynecol* 1952;63:592–604.

7. Ben Baruch G, Schiff E, Menashe Y, Menczer J. Immediate and late outcome of vaginal myomectomy for prolapsed pedunculated submucous myoma. *Obstet Gynecol* 1988;72:858–61.

8. Bonney V. The technique and results of myomectomy. *Lancet* 1931;i:171–7.

9. Brooks G, Stage AH. The surgical management of prolapsed pedunculated submucous leiomyomas. *Surg Gynecol Obstet* 1975;141:397–8.

10. Riley P. Treatment of prolapsed submucous fibroids. *S Afr Med J* 1982;63:22–4.

11. Tulandi T, Murray C, Guralnick M. Adhesion formation and reproductive outcome after myomectomy and second-look laparoscopy. *Obstet Gynecol* 1993;82:213–15.

12. Lamorte AI, Lalwani S, Diamond MP. Morbidity associated with abdominal myomectomy. *Obstet Gynecol* 1993;82:897–900.

13. Dicker D, Feldberg D, Dekel A, Yeshaya A, Samuel N, Goldman JA. The management of prolapsed submucous fibroids. *Aust N Z J Obstet Gynaecol* 1986;26:308–11.

14. Kanaoka Y, Hirai K, Ishiko O, Ogita S. An intranodal morcellation technique employing electrosurgical excision procedure for large prolapsed pedunculated myomas. *Oncol Rep* 2001;8:1149–51.

15. Goldrath MH. Vaginal removal of the pedunculated submucous myoma: the use of laminaria. *Obstet Gynecol* 1987;70:670–2.

16. Goldrath MH. Vaginal removal of the pedunculated submucous myoma. Historical observations and development of a new procedure. *J Reprod Med* 1990;35:921–4.

17. Manabe Y. Laminaria tent for gradual and safe cervical dilatation. *Am J Obstet Gynecol* 1971;110:743–50.

18. Magos AL, Bournas N, Sinha R, Richardson RE, O'Connor H. Vaginal myomectomy. *Br J Obstet Gynaecol* 1994;101:1092–4.

19. Doderlein A, Kronig G. *Operative Gynakologie*. Leipzig: Georg Thieme; 1912.

20. Wang C, Yen C, Lee C, Soong Y. Laparoscopic-assisted vaginal myomectomy. *J Am Assoc Gynecol Laparosc* 2000;7:510–14.

21. Goldfarb HA, Fanarjian NJ. Laparoscopic-assisted vaginal myomectomy: a case report and literature review. *JSLC* 2001;5:81–5.

22. Pelosi MA Sr, Pelosi MA. Spontaneous uterine rupture at thirty-three weeks subsequent to previous superficial laparoscopic myomectomy. *Am J Obstet Gynecol* 1997:177:1547–9.

23. Semm K. *Atlas of Gynaecologic Laparoscopy and Hysteroscopy*. Philadelphia, PA: Saunders; 1977.

24. Mais V, Ajossa S, Guerriero S, Mascia M, Solla E, Melis GB. Laparoscopic versus abdominal myomectomy: a prospective randomized trial to evaluate benefits in early outcome. *Am J Obstet Gynecol* 1996;174:654–8.

25. Rosetti A, Sizzi O, Soranna L, Cucinelli F, Mancuso S, Lanzone A. Long-term results of laparoscopic myomectomy: recurrence rate in comparison with abdominal myomectomy. *Hum Reprod* 2001;16:770–4.

26. Seracchioli R, Rossi S, Govoni F, Rossi C, Venturoli S, Bulletti C, *et al*. Fertility and obstetric outcome after laparoscopic myomectomy of large myomata: a randomized comparison with abdominal myomectomy. *Hum Reprod* 2000;15:2663–8.

27. Silva BA, Falcone T, Bradley L, Goldberg JM, Mascha E, Lindsey R, *et al*. Case–control study of laparoscopic versus abdominal myomectomy. *J Laparoendosc Adv Surg Tech A* 2000;10:191–7.

28. Miller CE. Myomectomy. Comparison of open and laparoscopic techniques. *Obstet Gynecol Clin North Am* 2000;27:407–20.

29. Stringer NH, Walker JC, Meyer PM. Comparison of 49 laparoscopic myomectomies with 49 open myomectomies. *J Am Assoc Gynecol Laparosc* 1997;4:457–64.

30. Parker WH. Myomectomy: laparoscopy or laparotomy? *Clin Obstet Gynecol* 1995;38:392–400.

31. Bulletti C, Polli V, Negrini V, Giacomucci E, Flamigni C. Adhesion formation after laparoscopic myomectomy. *J Am Assoc Gynecol Laparosc* 1996;3:533–6.

32. Dubuisson JB, Chapron C, Fauconnier A, Babaki-Fard K. Laparoscopic myomectomy fertility results. *Ann NY Acad Sci* 2001;943:269–75.

33. Dubuisson J, Chavet X, Chapron C, Gregorakis SS, Morice P. Uterine rupture during pregnancy after laparoscopic myomectomy. *Hum Reprod* 1995;10:1475–7.

34. Fauconnier A, Dubuisson JB, Ancel PY, Chapron C. Prognostic factors of reproductive outcome after myomectomy in infertile patients. *Hum Reprod* 2000;15:1751–7.

35. Hart R, Khalaf Y, Yeong CT, Seed P, Taylor A, Braude P. A prospective controlled study of the effect of intramural uterine fibroids on the outcome of assisted conception. *Hum Reprod* 2001;16:2411–17.

39

Ultrasound assessment of women with postmenopausal bleeding

Lil Valentin and Elisabet Epstein

ULTRASOUND MEASUREMENT OF ENDOMETRIAL THICKNESS IN WOMEN WITH POSTMENOPAUSAL BLEEDING CAN DISCRIMINATE BETWEEN THOSE WITH HIGH AND LOW RISK OF ENDOMETRIAL CANCER

There is strong scientific evidence that the risk of finding endometrial cancer in a woman with postmenopausal bleeding is small if the endometrium measures ≤4 mm at transvaginal ultrasound examination. In a meta-analysis comprising almost 6000 women with postmenopausal bleeding, this risk was estimated to be approximately 1:100 for women not on hormone replacement therapy (HRT) and 1:1000 for those on HRT.[1] This applies to an 'ordinary' population of women with postmenopausal bleeding, approximately 10% of whom have endometrial cancer.[1] The meta-analysis showed that, after the endometrium had been found to be ≤4 mm at ultrasound examination, the odds of endometrial cancer were only one-tenth of the odds before the measurement, irrespective of hormone use (negative likelihood ratio 0.10). This corresponded to an overall sensitivity with regard to endometrial cancer of 96% (95% confidence interval [CI] 94–98) and a false positive rate (defined as 1 minus specificity) of 39% (95% CI 27–41). Using the same cut off, the sensitivity and false positive rate with regard to any endometrial pathology were 92% (95% CI 90–93) and 19% (95% CI 17–21). This means that the use of a cut off of ≤4 mm to indicate a normal test result and ≥5 mm to indicate an abnormal test result resulted in 96% of all endometrial cancers and 92% of all endometrial pathology being detected at ultrasound examination, but that as many as 39% of women without endometrial cancer and as many as 19% of women without any endometrial pathology had a false positive test result.

In a Scandinavian multicentre study,[2] 1168 women with postmenopausal bleeding underwent ultrasound measurement of endometrial thickness on the day before or on the day of undergoing dilatation and curettage (D&C). None of 518 women with endometrium ≤4 mm had endometrial cancer versus 18% (114/620) of those with endometrium ≥5 mm. In an unpublished study, 257 women in the Scandinavian multicentre study with a benign D&C specimen were followed up for 10–13 years.[3] The results showed that women with postmenopausal bleeding and endometrium ≤4 mm did not run a higher risk of developing endometrial cancer than the general population, whereas women with postmenopausal bleeding and endometrium ≥5 mm had a higher risk, not only of having endometrial cancer diagnosed when they first presented with their bleeding, but also of having endometrial cancer diagnosed later in life. The increased risk of having endometrial cancer diagnosed later in life may be explained by thick endometrium reflecting a constitution associated with an increased risk of developing endometrial cancer, or by failure to diagnose an already existing cancer when the woman first presents with bleeding (the latter risk probably being higher if D&C instead of hysteroscopic resection is used as a diagnostic method; see below).

THE 5MM CUT OFF IS APPLICABLE TO BOTH USERS AND NON-USERS OF HRT

According to the meta-analysis of Smith Bindman et al.,[1] transvaginal ultrasound examination was equally good at detecting endometrial disease regardless of HRT use. Thus, using the 5 mm cut off, the sensitivity with regard to any endometrial disease was 95% (95% CI 93–97) in women not using HRT and 91% (95% CI 89–93) in HRT users (nonsignificant difference).[1] However, the false positive rate was much higher in women on HRT: 23% (95% CI 21–25) versus 8% (95% CI 6–10). According to the meta-analysis, the use of a 7 mm cut off in HRT users would have lowered the false positive rate to a level similar to that of the 5 mm cut off in nonusers, but then the detection rate of endometrial abnormalities among women on HRT would have decreased from 91% to 83% (95% CI 79–87). This shows that, if we decide to use a higher cut off for women on HRT than for women not on HRT, we must be willing to accept a lower detection rate of endometrial abnormalities in women on HRT. Smith Bindman et al.[1] did not analyse the detection rate of endometrial cancer in HRT users versus nonusers. However, the Scandinavian multicentre study did;[2] a cut off of 5 mm (≥5 mm indicating an abnormal test result) had a 100% detection rate of endometrial cancer irrespective of hormone use, but the false positive rate with regard to endometrial cancer was higher among HRT users: 63% versus 43%. If a cut off of 9 mm (≥9 mm indicating an abnormal test result) instead of 5 mm had been used among the HRT users, then the false positive rate would have decreased from 63% to 33%, but the detection rate of endometrial cancer would have decreased from 100% to 84% (these calculations were made by ourselves from data published in Karlsson et al.[2]). The results of the studies cited above[1,2] show that the use of a higher endometrial thickness cut off for women on HRT would result in a greater proportion of endometrial pathology, including endometrial cancer, being missed in these women. Thus, the 5 mm cut off is applicable to both users and nonusers of HRT, but we must accept a higher false positive rate among the HRT users. Because the endometrium in women on sequential HRT is at its thinnest on cycle days 1–7,[4] it may be possible to reduce the high false positive rate of ultrasound examination in HRT users without decreasing the detection rate by examining these women early in the cycle. Omodei et al.[5] measured endometrial thickness using ultrasound in 35 women with unscheduled bleeding during HRT treatment, taking the measurements 5–10 days after the last progestin tablet in women on sequential HRT. If the endometrium was ≥5 mm, the women underwent hysteroscopy and endometrial biopsy. Using this strategy, Omodei and colleagues detected all endometrial pathology (3/3; 95% CI 29–100) at a false positive rate of 25% (8/32; 95% CI 11–43). These figures are similar to those in the meta-analysis of Smith Bindman et al.,[1] where endometrial thickness was probably measured on any cycle day in women on sequential HRT. However, the number of women in the study of Omodei et al.[5] is too small for any firm conclusion to be drawn with regard to the sensitivity and false positive rate of their strategy (huge CIs; see above). Moreover, there was no endometrial cancer in their study, and they did not specify the number of women on sequential HRT therapy.

HOW SHOULD WE MANAGE WOMEN WITH POSTMENOPAUSAL BLEEDING AND ENDOMETRIUM ≤4 MM?

Because the risk of finding endometrial pathology in a woman with postmenopausal bleeding and endometrium ≤4 mm is small, it may be justified to refrain from invasive endometrial sampling in these women. Only 2–6% of endometrial cancers will be missed if we do not sample the endometrium in these circumstances (see above; detection rate 96%, 95% CI 94–98, thus false negative rate 4%, 95% CI 2–6[1]). The risk of missing an endometrial cancer by D&C or by a simple endometrial sampling device (e.g. Pipelle®, Prodimed, Neuilly en Thelle, France; or Endorette®, Medscand AB, Malmö, Sweden; or similar devices) in a woman with postmenopausal bleeding and endometrium ≤ 4 mm is unknown. If we choose to refrain from endometrial sampling in women with postmenopausal bleeding and endometrium ≤ 4 mm, do these women need to be followed up? If yes, how should they be followed up, how often, and for how long? Should they be followed by ultrasound measurements of endometrial thickness and be subjected to biopsy if the endometrium increases in thickness? Should they be submitted to endometrial sampling in case of re-bleeding, even if the endometrium remains thin at transvaginal ultrasound examination? There is little scientific evidence to answer these clinically relevant questions. The evidence that we have is the results of one randomised trial and one prospective study.[6,7] The results of both studies suggest that, if women with postmenopausal bleeding and endometrium ≤ 4 mm are managed by ultrasound follow-up, endometrial sampling should be performed if the endometrium increases in thickness to ≥ 5 mm during follow-up, but not necessarily if there is re-bleeding without a simultaneous increase in endometrial thickness to ≥ 5 mm. However, no endometrial cancer developed during the follow-up period (12 months) in either of the two studies.[6,7] What the two studies did show was that increasing endometrial thickness was a better predictor of *benign* pathology than isolated re-bleeding. We lack evidence that endometrial growth is a better predictor of malignancy than isolated re-bleeding.

POSTMENOPAUSAL BLEEDING MAY BE A SYMPTOM OF CERVICAL CANCER

Approximately 1% of all women with postmenopausal bleeding have cervical cancer.[2] However, the risk of cervical cancer may be higher in women with postmenopausal bleeding and thin endometrium, because in these women the cause of bleeding is less likely to be found in the endometrium. Small cervical cancers cannot be diagnosed by transvaginal sonography. Therefore, if one decides to refrain from fractionated D&C in women with postmenopausal bleeding and thin endometrium, one must not forget to take a cytological smear from the cervix.

WOMEN WITH POSTMENOPAUSAL BLEEDING WHO HAVE FOCAL LESIONS IN THE UTERINE CAVITY AND ENDOMETRIAL THICKNESS ≥ 5 MM SHOULD UNDERGO HYSTEROSCOPIC RESECTION OF THE FOCAL LESIONS

In a study comprising 105 consecutive women with postmenopausal bleeding and endometrium ≥ 5 mm at transvaginal ultrasound examination, we found that 80% had endometrial pathology, and that 25% had a uterine malignancy.[8] Moreover, 98% of the pathological lesions manifested a focal growth pattern at hysteroscopy under general anaesthesia.[8] Most (87%) of these focally growing lesions could not be removed or could be only partially removed at D&C.[8] This is in agreement with the results of other studies comprising both pre- and postmenopausal women, where 38–100% of focal lesions were partly or totally left in the uterine cavity after D&C.[9–12] We found that, in women who had focally growing lesions in the uterine cavity, the agreement between the diagnosis made on the basis of a D&C specimen and the final diagnosis made on the basis of hysteroscopically resected material and/or hysterectomy specimens was only 59%.[8] However, in those who did not have any focally growing lesions in the uterine cavity, the agreement was 94%.[8] On the basis of the results presented above we draw the conclusion that women with

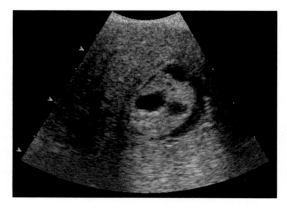

Figure 1 *Zoomed ultrasound image of the uterine cavity after infusion of sterile saline (hydrosonography); one focal lesion is seen*

postmenopausal bleeding who have focal lesions in the uterine cavity and endometrial thickness ≥ 5 mm should undergo hysteroscopic resection of the focal lesions under visual control. In women without focal lesions, D&C is probably an adequate sampling method.

FOCAL LESIONS IN THE UTERINE CAVITY CAN BE DETECTED BY HYDROSONOGRAPHY

Using hydrosonography, (i.e. infusion of sterile saline into the uterine cavity during vaginal ultrasound scanning), we can confidently detect focally growing lesions in the uterine cavity[13] (Figure 1). We have found excellent agreement between outpatient hydrosonography and hysteroscopy under general anaesthesia with regard to the presence or absence of focally growing lesions. The two methods disagreed in only 4 of 75 consecutive women with postmenopausal bleeding (κ-value 0.87).[13] Hydrosonography is quick and easy to perform, and it is better tolerated by women than outpatient hysteroscopy.[14]

MANAGEMENT OF WOMEN WITH POSTMENOPAUSAL BLEEDING

On the basis of the evidence presented above, we suggest that women with postmenopausal bleeding be managed in the following way (Figure 2):

- After undergoing a clinical examination including a cytological smear from the vagina and cervix to exclude cervical cancer, all women with postmenopausal bleeding should undergo transvaginal ultrasound examination with measurement of endometrial thickness.

- Women with postmenopausal bleeding and endometrial thickness ≤ 4 mm are at low risk of endometrial pathology, irrespective of hormone use, and it is safe to refrain from endometrial sampling in these women.

- Since only a small proportion (≤ 1%) of women with endometrium ≤ 4 mm have endometrial cancer, and because the risk that they will develop endometrial cancer in the future is likely to be low, it seems reasonable to refrain from follow-up examinations in these women, but to

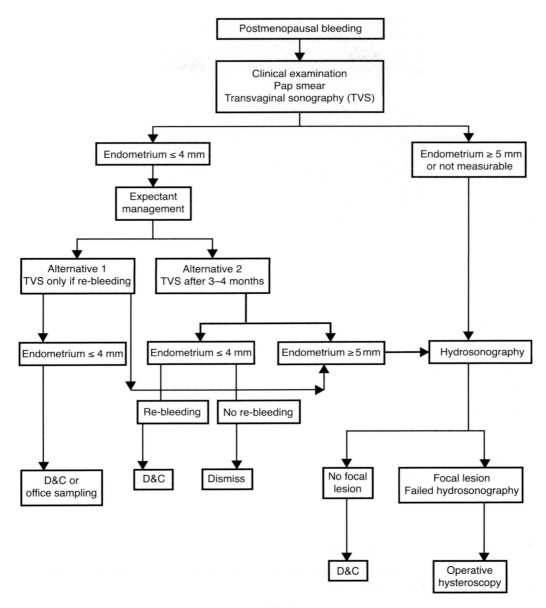

Figure 2 *Proposed management of women with postmenopausal bleeding*

advise them to come back if they bleed again. Whether one should sample the endometrium in re-bleeding irrespective of its thickness is a question to which there is no evidence based answer, but our personal opinion is that it is probably safest to take an endometrial sample in these women. A small proportion of women with endometrium ≤ 4 mm do have endometrial cancer, so some may believe that they should be offered follow-up. Ultrasound examination at

4–6 months, with sampling of the endometrium if it has increased in thickness to ≥5 mm (or if the woman reports re-bleeding) may be appropriate.

- If the endometrium is ≥5 mm, hydrosonography or office hysteroscopy should be carried out to detect focal lesions in the uterine cavity. If no focal lesions are found, then the woman should undergo D&C, or possibly endometrial sampling using an office based sampling device. If focally growing lesions are detected, then the woman should undergo hysteroscopic resection of the focal lesions under direct visual control.

MEASUREMENT TECHNIQUE AND REPRODUCIBILITY OF ENDOMETRIAL THICKNESS MEASUREMENTS

We suggest that women with postmenopausal bleeding be managed on the basis of results of endometrial thickness measurements. It is therefore important that the measurement technique is standardised, and that endometrial thickness measurements are reproducible. Endometrial thickness should be measured from a longitudinal sonogram through the thickest area of the endometrium, and from the outermost border of the endometrium on one side to that on the other. Thus, measurements of endometrial thickness should include both endometrial layers (Figure 3). In some studies, fluid in the uterine cavity was included in the measurements; in others it was not. Our personal opinion is that clear fluid in the uterine cavity and a thin, smooth endometrium throughout the whole uterine cavity is a normal finding, irrespective of the thickness of the whole uterine cavity.

We found excellent agreement between two experienced ultrasound examiners with regard to classifying postmenopausal women as having an endometrium ≤4 mm or ≥5 mm.[15] The classification of the two examiners disagreed in only 4 of 49 women, corresponding to a κ-value of 0.81. Thus, endometrial measurements in postmenopausal women are clinically acceptable if performed by experienced examiners. Our results suggest that it is enough to take one measurement.[15]

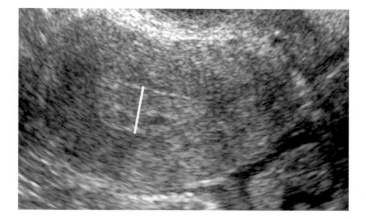

Figure 3 *Measurement of endometrial thickness (white line); the measurement should include both endometrial layers and any expansive process in the uterine cavity; it should be taken perpendicular to the endometrium*

CALCULATION OF INDIVIDUAL RISK OF MALIGNANCY USING MULTIVARIATE LOGISTIC REGRESSION MODELS

In the studies cited above, endometrial thickness alone was used to discriminate between women at low and high risk of endometrial cancer. Another approach is to use multivariate logistic regression models to calculate an individual risk of endometrial cancer in each woman. Such models could include clinical variables (e.g. information about age, body mass index, use of HRT, parity, diabetes, and blood pressure) as well as ultrasound variables (e.g. endometrial thickness and endometrial morphology) as independent variables. Ferrazzi et al.[16] calculated the background risk of endometrial cancer on the basis of the woman's age and body mass index. Then they used a likelihood ratio calculated on the basis of endometrial thickness to estimate the risk of endometrial cancer in each individual. They suggested that only women with a high risk of endometrial cancer be submitted to invasive endometrial sampling. Others, too, have suggested individual risk calculation using multivariate models.[17,18] It would be justified to test all these multivariate models prospectively, or to create even better models to estimate the individual risk of endometrial malignancy. Whether the use of multivariate models with individual risk calculation has clinical advantages over endometrial thickness measurements alone to discriminate between women with low and high risk of endometrial cancer remains to be determined.

NEITHER ULTRASOUND EXAMINATION NOR DIAGNOSTIC HYSTEROSCOPY CAN CONFIDENTLY DISCRIMINATE BETWEEN BENIGN AND MALIGNANT ENDOMETRIAL LESIONS OR PROVIDE A CORRECT SPECIFIC HISTOLOGICAL DIAGNOSIS

Even though ultrasound measurement of endometrial thickness can be used to estimate the risk of endometrial malignancy in women with postmenopausal bleeding, ultrasound examination of the endometrium cannot confidently discriminate between different histological diagnoses. In a prospective study comprising 105 consecutive women with postmenopausal bleeding and endometrial thickness ≥5 mm we found that at both outpatient hydrosonography and at hysteroscopy under general anaesthesia, benign endometrial polyps were sometimes confused with cancer and vice versa.[13] In the same study, distension problems with hydrosonography were associated with increased risk of endometrial malignancy, such problems being encountered in only 5% of women with a benign endometrium versus 29% of those with endometrial malignancy ($P = 0.004$) and in 71% of those with endometrial cancer invading >50% of the myometrium.[13] Thus, distension problems occurring during hydrosonography should raise the suspicion of endometrial malignancy.

THE ROLE OF POWER DOPPLER ULTRASOUND EXAMINATION IN THE DIAGNOSIS OF ENDOMETRIAL MALIGNANCY

Power Doppler ultrasound examination can contribute to the correct diagnosis of endometrial malignancy, especially if the endometrium measures 5–15 mm in thickness. Malignant endometrium has a higher colour content at power Doppler ultrasound examination than benign endometrium (Figure 4).[17] However, this modality needs further evaluation and refinement before its clinical value in the management of women with postmenopausal bleeding can be determined with certainty.

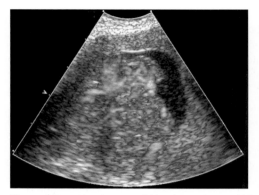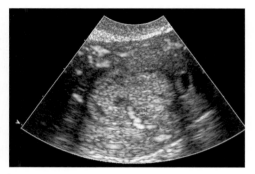

Figure 4 *Power Doppler image of (a) endometrial cancer, (b) benign polyp; note the higher colour content of the cancer*

CONCLUSIONS

- Ultrasound measurement of endometrial thickness in women with postmenopausal bleeding can discriminate between those with a low and a high risk of endometrial pathology.

- Women with endometrial thickness ≤4 mm have a low risk of endometrial pathology, including endometrial cancer; those with endometrial thickness ≥5 mm have a high risk.

- It is reasonable to refrain from endometrial sampling in women with postmenopausal bleeding and endometrium ≤4 mm.

- It is not clear if women with postmenopausal bleeding and endometrium ≤4 mm need to be followed up if endometrial sampling is not performed.

- In women with postmenopausal bleeding and endometrial thickness ≥5 mm, 98% of all endometrial abnormalities manifest a focal growth pattern.

- The presence of focally growing lesions in the uterine cavity can be confidently determined by using hydrosonography, which is better tolerated by women than office hysteroscopy.

- Because most focally growing lesions in the uterine cavity cannot be completely removed at D&C, they should be removed by hysteroscopic resection under direct visual control.

- At present, conventional transvaginal ultrasound examination, hydrosonography or diagnostic hysteroscopy cannot confidently predict the histological diagnosis of endometrial lesions.

Acknowledgements

Our studies were supported by grants from the Malmö General Hospital Cancer Foundation, Funds administered by the Malmö Health Care Administration, a government grant for clinical research ('ALF-medel' and 'Landstings finansierad regional forskning'), and the Swedish Medical Research Council (grant nos. B6-17X-11605-01A, K98-17X-11605-03A, and K2001-72X-11605-06A).

References

1. Smith-Bindman R, Kerlikowske K, Feldstein VA, Subak L, Scheidler J, Segal M, et al. Endovaginal ultrasound to exclude endometrial cancer and other endometrial abnormalities. *JAMA* 1998;280:1510–17.

2. Karlsson B, Granberg S, Wikland M, Ylostalo P, Torvid K, Marsal K, et al. Transvaginal ultrasonography of the endometrium in women with postmenopausal bleeding – a Nordic multicenter study. *Am J Obstet Gynecol* 1995;172:1488–94.

3. Gull B, Karlsson B, Milsom I, Granberg S. Can ultrasound replace dilatation and curettage? A longitudinal evaluation of postmenopausal bleeding and transvaginal sonographic measurement of the endometrium as predictors of endometrial cancer. *Am J Obstet Gynecol* 2003;188:401–8.

4. Gull B, Karlsson B, Milsom I, Wikland M, Granberg S. Transvaginal sonography of the endometrium in a representative sample of postmenopausal women. *Ultrasound Obstet Gynecol* 1996;7:322–7.

5. Omodei U, Ferrazzia E, Ruggeri C, Palai N, Fallo L, Dordoni D, et al. Endometrial thickness and histological abnormalities in women on hormonal replacement therapy: a transvaginal ultrasound/hysteroscopic study. *Ultrasound Obstet Gynecol* 2000;15:317–20.

6. Epstein E, Valentin L. Rebleeding and endometrial growth in women with postmenopausal bleeding and endometrial thickness <5 mm managed by dilatation and curettage or ultrasound follow-up: a randomized controlled study. *Ultrasound Obstet Gynecol* 2001;18:499–504.

7. Gull B, Carlsson S, Karlsson B, Ylostalo P, Milsom I, Granberg S. Transvaginal ultrasonography of the endometrium in women with postmenopausal bleeding: is it always necessary to perform an endometrial biopsy? *Am J Obstet Gynecol* 2000;182:509–15.

8. Epstein E, Ramirez A, Skoog L, Valentin L. Dilatation and curettage fails to detect most focal lesions in the uterine cavity in women with postmenopausal bleeding. *Acta Obstet Gynecol Scand* 2001;80:1131–6.

9. Englund S, Ingelman-Sundberg I, Westin B. Hysteroscopy in diagnosis and treatment of uterine bleeding. *Gynaecologia* 1957;143:217–22.

10. Goldfarb HA. D&C results improved by hysteroscopy. *N J Med* 1989;86:277–9.

11. Bettocchi S, Ceci O, Vicino M, Marello F, Impedovo L, Selvaggi L. Diagnostic inadequacy of dilatation and curettage. *Fertil Steril* 2001;7:803–5.

12. Gebauer G, Hafner A, Siebzehnrubl E, Lang N. Role of hysteroscopy in detection and extraction of endometrial polyps: results of a prospective study. *Am J Obstet Gynecol* 2001;184:59–63.

13. Epstein E, Ramirez A, Skoog L, Valentin L. Transvaginal sonography, saline contrast sonohysterography and hysteroscopy for the investigation of women with postmenopausal bleeding and endometrium ≥5 mm. *Ultrasound Obstet Gynecol* 2001;18:157–62.

14. Timmerman D, Deprest J, Bourne T, Van den Berghe I, Collins WP, Vergote I. A randomized trial on the use of ultrasonography or office hysteroscopy for endometrial assessment in postmenopausal patients with breast cancer who were treated with tamoxifen. *Am J Obstet Gynecol* 1998;179:62–70.

15. Epstein E, Valentin L. Intraobserver and interobserver reproducibility of ultrasound measurements of endometrial thickness in postmenopausal women. *Ultrasound Obstet Gynecol* 2002;20:486–91.

16. Ferrazzi E, Torri V, Trio D, Zannoni E, Filiberto S, Dordoni D. Sonographic endometrial thickness: a useful test to predict atrophy in patients with postmenopausal bleeding. An Italian multicenter study. *Ultrasound Obstet Gynecol* 1996;7:315–21.

17. Epstein E, Skoog L, Isberg PE, De Smet F, De Moor B, Olofsson PÅ, *et al.* An algorithm including results of gray-scale and power Doppler ultrasound examination to predict endometrial malignancy in women with postmenopausal bleeding. *Ultrasound Obstet Gynecol* 2002;20:370–6.

18. Randelzhofer B, Prompeler HJ, Sauerbrei W, Madjar H, Emons G. Value of sonomorphological criteria of the endometrium in women with postmenopausal bleeding: a multivariate analysis. *Ultrasound Obstet Gynecol* 2002;19:62–8.

40

Three-dimensional ultrasound in the diagnosis of fetal abnormality

Alec Welsh

INTRODUCTION

There has been much argument about the role of three-dimensional ultrasound (3DUS) in fetal medicine. Many potential benefits of 3DUS have been proposed, and many enthusiastic research teams have published data on 3DUS in the animal, adult and fetus. However, there are at present no clear clinical indications for fetal 3DUS and there have been no high-quality comparative studies on the usefulness of 2DUS versus 3DUS,[1] so this imaging modality remains in transition from research to clinical application.[2] Many feel that the expense of 3DUS machinery cannot be justified because experienced ultrasound practitioners already create a mental 3D image during conventional scanning. This review will discuss the background physics, potential advantages and problems, published research and clinical usefulness of 3DUS and then speculate about its future role in fetal medicine.

PHYSICS OF 3DUS

3DUS has been attempted in many forms since the early 1970s.[3-5] In order to understand its benefits and pitfalls, it is important to understand how 3D images are generated and some of the terminology used. Many modern ultrasound machines are now digital, meaning that the returning analogue acoustic echo is immediately converted into numerical information, which may be computer processed after acquisition ('post-processing'). 3DUS is one of many techniques for computer processing of ultrasound echoes.

All 3DUS relies upon the same underlying technique to generate or 'render' the 3D 'volume data set' from multiple 2D scan images. Computer software mathematically fills in the gaps or 'interpolates' between relative 2D points ('pixels') in the individual images, creating 3D volume points ('voxels'). It is for this reason that 3DUS relies heavily upon the underlying quality of the acquired 2D images, so much of the operator and subject dependence of high-quality fetal ultrasound is retained. Some groups have suggested overlapping or 'compounding' of ultrasound data to produce higher quality data sets.[6] Although this may be applicable to adult imaging of organs such as the gallbladder,[7] this cannot reliably be applied to the fetus, because of the likely fetal movement between acquisition of data sets.

Current methods of converting 2D images into 3DUS include

Purpose designed annular array ultrasound transducers

These use the 'swept-volume' technique and either fan or rotate the ultrasound probe from a fixed position to acquire images at predefined angular intervals. Abdominal transducers produce a pyramid-shaped volume and vaginal transducers a cone-shaped volume. Angular and spatial coordinates for each image and pixel are then used to create accurate 3D volumes. These transducers are easy to use and produce standardised volumes of densely sampled data without irregular gaps. They have been measured to have a mean absolute error of around 1% for distance and 6.4% for volume under experimental conditions using tissue-mimicking ultrasound phantoms in a water bath,[8] an accuracy confirmed in other studies.[9] These commercially available machines have been used for the vast majority of fetal research and clinical 3DUS imaging. Their main limitation is the maximum volume that can be measured owing to the position and size of the transducer.

Electromagnetic position sensing devices

These generate a 3D electromagnetic field, which is either DC or AC based, with a small receiver attached to the ultrasound transducer. This receiver interferes with the electromagnetic field, so its precise position in three physical dimensions ('x, y and z' planes) plus three angular dimensions ('yaw, pitch and roll') may be measured, allowing the individual 2D pixels to be plotted as 3D coordinates. This is described as a 'six degrees of freedom' method. This potentially allows for scanning of large areas and for overlapping images to be compounded for increased visual clarity. Position sensing devices allow the use of standard ultrasound transducers with minimal modification and are thus ideally suited to the varying shape of the maternal abdomen and size of the region of evaluation. Additionally they allow greater freedom of movement in image acquisition. An extremely high degree of accuracy has been reported, although this method is technically the most complex and requires accurate calibration.[10,11]

Mechanical transducer arms

These allow perfectly parallel images to be taken at predefined linear intervals,[12] but are not well suited to the curvature of the maternal abdomen.

Other 3DUS imaging

Other forms of 3DUS imaging rely on an assumption that images are equally spaced and parallel, and include commercially available systems as well as fully freehand image acquisition and offline computer processing techniques.[13]

Once acquired, the 3D volume of ultrasound information can be post-processed in a variety of ways, either on the machine or a personal computer to allow selective visualisation of parts of the data set.[14] These methods include: alterations in opacity and colour maps for all or part of the image; volume calculations by voxel counting; surface rendering to examine surface structures; lighting models to bring out various details with shadowing; varying intensity and transparency weightings in the rendering to enhance particular features such as fetal bone; movie generation to visualise the rotating volume in detail; multiple volume rendering to superimpose greyscale information on colour flow 3DUS; and image 'cropping' to remove overlying or adjacent structures.[14,15]

POTENTIAL ADVANTAGES OF 3DUS

- True volume measurements are obtained, rather than 2D approximations.

- High-quality volume data sets can be stored for later review and transfer for specialist opinion.

- More meaningful surface rendering is possible to improve physician and parental evaluation of fetal surface anomalies.

- There can be simultaneous display of all three orthogonal planes, including those planes perpendicular to the transducer that cannot otherwise be visualised. If fetal positioning precludes imaging in perfect anatomical planes, the volume data set may be rotated to allow their demonstration.

- Multiple display modalities may be used on the same volume data set after acquisition.

- Automated 3DUS acquisition systems may eventually reduce the operator dependency of 2DUS scanning.[16]

POTENTIAL PROBLEMS WITH 3DUS

Many physical properties of ultrasound limit 3DUS visualisation and volume measurement, and many artefacts have now been identified with 3DUS scanning:[7,17,18]

- The inherent 'speckle' in ultrasound images caused by interference between ultrasound pulses means that organ interfaces and vascular anatomy are not always demonstrated sufficiently clearly in 2D to allow 3D reconstruction. The sonographic appearance of the surface of an object in a fluid is defined by the point-spread function that depends on the resolution of the ultrasound beam, resulting in blurred boundaries.[19] The 'gold standard' against which 3DUS should be judged is three-dimensional magnetic resonance imaging (3DMRI), with its clear definition of organ boundaries. A small series using 3DMRI evaluated fetal volumes and longitudinal growth on 3–5 occasions until term, and demonstrated growth patterns for whole fetal as well as lung, liver and brain volumes.[20] Additional work has measured liver, brain and placental volumes with MRI.[21] However, equipment costs and availability, technical problems associated with fetal movement, and concerns about unproven safety have limited the fetal use of 3DMRI.

- Ultrasound attenuation means that imaging quality differs with depth within a 3D volume.

- Regions lacking signal may be filled in, appearing smaller, and those with strong echoes may appear broader.[22]

- Small structures may appear larger in 3DUS volumes than they actually are on the scan.

- Outlining of structures may result in overestimation of volumes proportional to the surface of the object being scanned.

- Changes in surface curvature may mean that boundaries have varying intensities.

- Shadowing from objects near the probe may affect 3D image quality.

- Resolution through a 3DUS volume may vary, depending on both the spacing between B-scans and the location within a B-scan.

- Rendered image quality is affected by organ orientation and beam pathway.

WHAT HAS BEEN SHOWN WITH FETAL 3DUS IMAGING?

A large body of research articles have now demonstrated the imaging potential of 3DUS in fetal medicine. These have predominantly used purpose designed transducers or electromagnetic position sensing devices for volume measurement, anatomical evaluation and vascular reconstruction. Many have documented the ease and speed of 3DUS imaging. In a study on real-time 3DUS in 57 normal fetuses and two with polyhydramnios, complete 3D fetal evaluation was possible in less than ten minutes.[23]

Volume measurement

Conventional 2D measurement and 3D swept-volume techniques have been compared to assess liver volumes, and the latter have been found to show significantly better intra- and interobserver reproducibility between 20 and 31 weeks.[24] A prospective cross-sectional study of normal fetal liver volume at 19–39 weeks of gestation allowed normal values and centile curves relative to gestational age to be plotted. However, technically acceptable liver volume measurement was possible at that time in only 25 of 34 participating women owing to fetal movement, position or maternal obesity.[25]

Lung volumes have been measured in 108 evaluations from 78 pregnancies to produce a gestational chart from 14 to 41 weeks using a purpose designed swept-volume system.[26] In the same year (1996), a position-sensing device based imaging system demonstrated an exponential increase in total lung volume in 20 pregnancies between 24 and 36 weeks of gestational age and a consistently greater volume of the right than the left lung.[27] A further longitudinal observational study on fetal lung volume on 58 women scanned at monthly intervals derived reference intervals for fetal lung growth,[28] although the lung volumes measured were not able to predict actual lung function.

A good correlation between renal volume and gestational age has been demonstrated, but no significant difference between right and left lung volumes.[29] A formula for fetal renal volume has been established.[30] Other fetal volume estimations include the heart,[31] thigh, abdomen[32] and arm to predict birthweight.[33] A combination of fetal upper arm, thigh and abdominal volumes has been shown to perform better than conventional fetal weight assessment in a cohort of 190 women.[34] Hafner et al.[35] evaluated placental volume in the second trimester using 3DUS in 382 women with singleton pregnancy at 16–23 weeks of gestation. Although variance between two observers for this slice tracing technique was shown to be only about 0.05%, there was no correlation between placental volume and small for gestational age fetuses, which had previously been suggested when using 2DUS.[36] A further publication from Hafner's team[37] showed little correlation between fetal and placental sizes in 356 singleton pregnancies between 15 and 17 weeks.

Surface and anatomical features

Preliminary results of 3DUS demonstration of fetal surface features were published in 1992, using two fetal specimens in a water bath with a linear movement system connected to a suspended transducer.[22] Although this early study demonstrated the feasibility of 3DUS, the water bath produced an artificially clear fetal surface and nonphysiological attenuation of the ultrasound beam, which reduced the clinical validity of the technique at this stage. Extensive research has subsequently been published on 3D fetal anatomical demonstration, although much of the published literature relates to case reports or small series. In 72 fetuses, 3DUS allowed complete fetal digital evaluation in 74.3% of cases versus 52.9% with 2D ($P < 0.05$), with particular accuracy between 20 and 28 weeks.[38] An isolated case of phocomelia was evaluated more clearly with 3DUS than with 2DUS, for both surface and skeletal features.[39] A further report from the same group evaluated four fetuses with facial abnormalities and found both surface rendering (for fetal skin) and transparent mode (for inner organs and skeleton) to be useful.[40]

Further publications have included normal[41] and abnormal[42,43] brain cavities, head and spine,[44,45] echocardiography with M-mode synchronisation,[46] first trimester diagnosis of ectopia cordis,[47] and nuchal translucency measurement.[48–50] The developmental stages of the early fetus have been studied in elegant detail using endovaginal 7.5 MHz 3DUS to examine 34 embryos with crown–rump lengths of 9.3–39 mm.[19]

In 2001, a team based at the University of California San Diego reported an evaluation of the feasibility of virtual patient examination using 2DUS and 3DUS data acquired at remote locations for a variety of indications.[51] They found that 3DUS could produce diagnostic-quality results comparable with 2DUS, although overall image quality was lower than 2DUS. Additionally, the role of a remote link for transmission of stored 3D volumes of the fetal heart to a tertiary centre has been evaluated in London in 30 normal singleton pregnancies.[52] This group accomplished a complete heart examination in 76.7% of cases, visualising the four-chamber view and cardiac situs in all cases, the right ventricular outflow tract in 96.7% and the left in 83.3%.

Fetoplacental vascular 3DUS

One of the problems with 2D evaluation of vascular structures is their branching and irregular nature, leading to difficulties with visual–spatial 3D recognition. Although it is possible to identify single vessels and follow their path, in a large vascular bed it may be impossible to generate a true mental 3D picture. The potential for 3D vascular reconstruction in obstetrics was initially proposed using a lamb kidney *in vitro*, with computer algorithms to separate greyscale and colour information.[53] With the introduction of commercial ultrasound machinery capable of 3D vascular reconstruction, the applications have widened. Adult and fetal research groups have examined the role of vascular 3DUS in evaluation of the breast,[54] carotid artery,[55] parenchymal organs,[56] tumour vascularity,[57] cardiological applications such as assessment of mitral regurgitation,[58] fetal vascular malformations such as vein of Galen aneurysm,[59] ovarian lesions[60] and for intraoperative assessment of vascular tumours.[61]

The placenta is an ideal site for evaluation of 3D vascular anatomy. Position-sensing device based imaging has been used to assess the number of vessels within the placenta, their branching pattern, the number of vessels on the placental surface, and the maternal component of the placental vascularity in 14 normal and one growth restricted fetus.[62] A progressive increase in the number of intraplacental vessels and vascular branches was seen with increasing gestation. Specific vessels could be identified and referenced relative to the placental substance, enhancing understanding of placental vascular anatomy. It has been proposed that power Doppler 3DUS could potentially be applied to the detection of placental vascular diseases, such as arterial and venous thromboses, maternal infarction, placental insufficiency, feto-fetal transfusion syndrome and placental abruption. Power Doppler may allow vessels to be demonstrated relatively equally, irrespective of the direction of blood flow and the angle of insonation.[62] Early research outlined the potential for 3D power Doppler angiography, using a position-sensing device based system.[56] Rendered images from 3DUS power Doppler of a transplanted kidney were superior to 2D imaging and initial images of placental vascularity were encouraging. Fully freehand 3DUS has also been applied to evaluation of gross fetoplacental vascularity,[13] as well as to the evaluation of anastomoses in monochorionic twin placentation.[63] In addition to normal placentation, a subsequent case report illustrated the use of 3DUS with power Doppler in the evaluation of placenta praevia percreta/increta.[64]

THE CLINICAL USEFULNESS OF 3DUS

Manufacturers of new machinery will always have a vested interest in the promotion of novel expensive techniques that may have little clinical use.[65] While new technologies are exciting for visualisation and picture generation, it is important that they are evaluated scientifically before being applied to clinical practice. For 3DUS to become accepted in routine clinical practice, it is important that performance of these machines should meet or exceed that of 2DUS systems.[66] They must additionally be quick and easy to use, reproducible and give clear added clinical benefit. Ideally the same machine used in clinical practice should be capable of 2D B-mode, M-mode and Doppler imaging (spectral and power), static 3D imaging (greyscale and Doppler) and real-time 3D (4DUS).

The imaging potential of 3DUS in fetal medicine has now been clearly proven, but it is in the area of clinical benefit that controversy persists about its role. One research and clinical 3DUS institution initially evaluated 3DUS, using swept-volume equipment, in 204 women at between 13 and 40 weeks of gestation with a fetal malformation. They found that 3DUS improved ultrasound diagnosis in 62% of cases, gave the same information in 36%, and confused the examination in 2% where movement artefacts interfered with the evaluation of cardiac malformations.[67] The same team later studied the fetal face in 618 pregnant women at between 9 and 37 weeks of gestation. They suggested that 3DUS was superior for demonstration of true mid-sagittal profiles in normal fetuses, which, in their study, had been visualised in only 69.6% of cases using 2DUS.[68] Only 20 of 25 facial anomalies were clearly demonstrated by 2D and 3D, and the diagnosis was revealed by 3DUS in the remaining five. In second and third trimester imaging, 3DUS has been proposed by another research team to be superior to 2DUS imaging. Of 247 fetuses referred with suspected anomalies, 170 anomalies were detected, with failed diagnosis in just three associated with oligohydramnios.[69]

However, despite the ability to demonstrate anatomy in detail, other clinical 3DUS groups have found that 2DUS remains superior for evaluation of fetal anatomy. In London it was found that a full anatomical survey was possible in the first trimester in 93.7% with 2DUS compared with 80.5% with 3DUS.[70] It has been proposed that 3DUS may have a role in the evaluation of fetal nuchal translucency measurements, with up to 100% seen in 3D and 85% in 2D.[48] Although this finding has been reproduced,[49,71,72] another group with a strong research and clinical programme in nuchal translucency screening found a 98.7% measurement success with 2DUS and only 91.8% with 3DUS.[73] The 3DUS resolution has been suggested to be too poor and to not allow clear discrimination between neck skin and amnion, seen best during fetal movement, thus precluding 3D study.[74]

The results of 3DUS evaluation of anomalies may be misleading and inaccurate because the vast majority of diagnoses made by 3D can be reliably made with 2D, and often the 2D diagnosis is made first before 3D evaluation.[75] For specific areas of examination such as the fetal skeleton, articles have been published showing no clear clinical benefit for either normal or abnormal anatomy, despite improved imaging.[76,77] Because of problems with artefacts, some areas such as the genitalia may be better evaluated in 2D.[78]

WHERE IS 3DUS NOW AND WHERE COULD IT BE IN THE FUTURE?

It is argued by many that current 3DUS systems have no role in routine clinical fetal care, and that 3DUS represents exciting technology in search of a clinical application. Real-time acquisition and viewing is now possible, albeit at a low frame rate, but it may not always be of high quality and is not 100% reliable. Both online and offline 3D imaging do, however, continue to improve rapidly, although a natural ceiling exists for 3D accuracy owing to the inherent limitations of ultrasound (noise). There remains a reluctance among fetal medicine practitioners in the UK to accept a role for 3DUS. In part this is because of their personal lack of need for enhanced 3D spatial awareness. It may also be related to the way in which 3DUS technology has been promoted to the public and the media as a means of generating quality pictures of normal fetal faces and digits. Ignoring these cosmetic uses of 3DUS and the unquantifiable benefits of enhanced bonding with the pregnancy,[1] one may propose logical applications for routine and research fetal medicine:

Parental understanding of fetal surface lesions or tumours

It is easy to overestimate parental perception of frozen 2D ultrasound images, which may hinder the counselling process. It has been shown that 3DUS increases parental understanding of certain lesions such as facial clefting[79,80] and, in routine scanning, parental perception of image quality is often much higher with 3DUS. Other surface lesions such as abdominal wall defects, sacrococcygeal teratomas or spina bifida may be more easily understood in 3DUS. Additionally, certain lesions such as cleft lip and palate, or talipes may at present require relatively broad counselling to cover a wide spectrum of severity. The use of 3DUS may allow some of these lesions to be more accurately categorised, directing counselling to a subset of the pathology.

Accurate volume measurements are highly likely to be superior to 2D distance approximation to volumes. Organ volumes may potentially be more accurately measured using 3DUS, particularly for irregularly shaped structures. Fetal surveillance commonly includes the measurement of 2D diameters and circumferences to approximate to volumes. Examples include measurement of head and abdominal circumferences as approximations to liver and brain volumes for growth monitoring, or lung measurement in fetuses with space-occupying lesions of the chest (diaphragmatic hernia, congenital cystic abnormality of the lung). It is logical that 3D measurement of actual volumes instead of 2D approximations would be more accurate and therefore clinically useful. Using MRI, fetal liver, but not brain or placental volumes, have been shown accurately to identify fetuses subsequently found to be small for gestational age.[21]

Assessment of regional perfusion

Vascular 3DUS has great potential for understanding the complexity of vessel branching and to assess volumetric perfusion.[81] As well as demonstrating the macroscopic vascularity of the placenta, with improvements in ultrasound image quality it may be possible to evaluate further the complexity of the placental villous tree. The degree and nature of its branching have been shown to be altered in fetuses with growth restriction,[82,83] although whether the resolution of current ultrasound would be sufficient to display vasculature at the necessary level is uncertain.

Quantification of regional blood flow may potentially be performed with 3DUS

At present, organ perfusion may be assessed only indirectly by measuring indices approximating to the resistance within individual blood vessels, or less accurately by multiplying mean velocities in large vessels by their cross-sectional area. 3D colour mapping, particularly using the relatively direction-independent power Doppler, allows the potential for quantification of regional blood flow although this may be technically complex. This has already been used in gynaecological applications such as vascular assessment of the ovary or endometrium[84–87] and, with appropriate standardisation for machine settings and attenuation, could be applied to fetal organ perfusion.[88,89] With the complex vascular branching pattern of the placenta, its relatively large surface area and relative immobility compared with fetal structures, it may be an ideal organ for quantification of flow. It could be predicted that 3D evaluation would be more accurate than 2D although variation in regional perfusion needs to be assessed.

Transfer of information to allied medical or paramedical staff

In the same way that we may overestimate parental perception, allied medical or paramedical staff, who are unused to examining ultrasound images, may find 2D ultrasound stills hard to interpret. The use of simple computer software may allow whole-volume data sets to be emailed to other medical staff who can view the lesion from any perspective with any rendering technique. This may include orthopaedic surgeons for talipes, neurosurgeons for spina bifida, and maxillofacial or plastic surgeons for cleft lip and palate.

Data storage for later review

The potential to store and repeatedly review high-quality data sets facilitates repeat review of ultrasound studies, which may, in turn, be stored for teaching purposes in local or distant institutions.

Training

These routine and research uses may be best suited to fetal medicine referral centres. Aside from the more cosmetic uses of 3DUS, the time required for training, as well as that spent on processing the ultrasound volumes, may preclude its use in centres performing routine scanning. Nothing has been published on the time taken to train staff in 3DUS techniques, but this is not inconsiderable. As well as having the appropriate 2DUS skills, care must be taken with the necessary image processing and interpretation, particularly in the light of recent literature highlighting potential problems with artefacts.[17,18]

SUMMARY

This review has assessed the physics, potential applications and pitfalls of this exciting new technology. Although the ability to visualise all or part of the fetal anatomy in 3D has been proven, its clinical benefit over 2D has not. However, ultrasound technology continues to advance at a significant pace, and new applications for 3DUS continue to be developed. A shift of focus from demonstration of normal fetal faces and hands to that of enhanced parental understanding of pathology and a more scientific application of 3DUS is likely to result in its greater acceptance. In the near future 3DUS will have an established role in fetal medicine, alongside 2DUS, as a valued adjunct for a percentage of cases to enhance diagnosis, counselling and education.

References

1.   Campbell S. 4D, or not 4D: that is the question. *Ultrasound Obstet Gynecol* 2002;19:1–4.
2.   Candiani F. The latest in ultrasound: three-dimensional imaging. Part 1. *Eur J Radiol* 1998;27 Suppl 2:S179–82.
3.   Rasmussen SN, Nielsen SS, Bartrum RJ Jr, Stigsby B, Holm HH. Three-dimensional imaging of abdominal organs with ultrasound. *Am J Roentgenol Radium Ther Nucl Med* 1974;121:883–8.
4.   McDicken WN, Lindsay M, Robertson DA. Three-dimensional images using a fibre optic ultrasonic scanner. *Br J Radiol* 1972;45:70–1.
5.   Szilard J. An improved three-dimensional display system. *Ultrasonics* 1974;12:273–6.

6. Pretorius DH, Nelson TR. Three-dimensional ultrasound. *Ultrasound Obstet Gynecol* 1995;5:219–21.
7. Rohling RN, Gee AH, Berman L. Automatic registration of 3-D ultrasound images. *Ultrasound Med Biol* 1998;24:841–54.
8. Riccabona M, Nelson TR, Pretorius DH. Three-dimensional ultrasound: accuracy of distance and volume measurements. *Ultrasound Obstet Gynecol* 1996;7:429–34.
9. Barry CD, Allott CP, John NW, Mellor PM, Arundel PA, Thomson DS, *et al*. Three-dimensional freehand ultrasound: image reconstruction and volume analysis. *Ultrasound Med Biol* 1997;23:1209–24.
10. Leotta DF, Detmer PR, Martin RW. Performance of a miniature magnetic position sensor for three-dimensional ultrasound imaging. *Ultrasound Med Biol* 1997;23:597–609.
11. Prager RW, Rohling RN, Gee AH, Berman L. Rapid calibration for 3-D freehand ultrasound. *Ultrasound Med Biol* 1998;24:855–69.
12. Griewing B, Schminke U, Morgenstern C, Walker ML, Kessler C. Three-dimensional ultrasound angiography (power mode) for the quantification of carotid artery atherosclerosis. *J Neuroimaging* 1997;7:40–5.
13. Welsh AW, Humphries K, Cosgrove DO, Taylor MJ, Fisk NM. Development of three-dimensional power Doppler ultrasound imaging of fetoplacental vasculature. *Ultrasound Med Biol* 2001;27:1161–70.
14. Riccabona M, Pretorius DH, Nelson TR, Johnson D, Budorick NE. Three-dimensional ultrasound: display modalities in obstetrics. *J Clin Ultrasound* 1997;25:157–67.
15. Riccabona M, Johnson D, Pretorius DH, Nelson TR. Three dimensional ultrasound: display modalities in the fetal spine and thorax. *Eur J Radiol* 1996;22:141–5.
16. Downey DB, Fenster A, Williams JC. Clinical utility of three-dimensional US. *Radiographics* 2000;20:559–71.
17. Hull AD, Pretorius DH, Lev-Toaff A, Budorick NE, Salerno CC, Johnson MM, *et al*. Artifacts and the visualization of fetal distal extremities using three-dimensional ultrasound. *Ultrasound Obstet Gynecol* 2000;16:341–4.
18. Nelson TR, Pretorius DH, Hull A, Riccabona M, Sklansky MS, James G. Sources and impact of artifacts on clinical three-dimensional ultrasound imaging. *Ultrasound Obstet Gynecol* 2000;16:374–83.
19. Blaas HG, Eik-Nes SH, Berg S, Torp H. *In-vivo* three-dimensional ultrasound reconstructions of embryos and early fetuses. *Lancet* 1998;352:1182–6.
20. Garden AS, Roberts N. Fetal and fetal organ volume estimations with magnetic resonance imaging. *Am J Obstet Gynecol* 1996;175:442–8.
21. Baker PN, Johnson IR, Gowland PA, Hykin J, Adams V, Mansfield P, *et al*. Measurement of fetal liver, brain and placental volumes with echoplanar magnetic resonance imaging. *Br J Obstet Gynaecol* 1995;102:35–9.
22. Nelson TR, Pretorius DH. Three-dimensional ultrasound of fetal surface features. *Ultrasound Obstet Gynecol* 1992;2:166–74.
23. Baba K, Okai T, Kozuma S, Taketani Y, Mochizuki T, Akahane M. Real-time processable three-dimensional US in obstetrics. *Radiology* 1997;203:571–4.
24. Chang FM, Hsu KF, Ko HC, Yao BL, Chang CH, Yu CH, *et al*. Three-dimensional ultrasound assessment of fetal liver volume in normal pregnancy: a comparison of reproducibility with two-dimensional ultrasound and a search for a volume constant. *Ultrasound Med Biol* 1997;23:381–9.
25. Laudy JA, Janssen MM, Struyk PC, Stijnen T, Wallenburg HC, Wladimiroff JW. Fetal liver volume measurement by three-dimensional ultrasonography: a preliminary study. *Ultrasound*

Obstet Gynecol 1998;12:93–6.

26.   Lee A, Kratochwil A, Stumpflen I, Deutinger J, Bernaschek G. Fetal lung volume determination by three-dimensional ultrasonography. *Am J Obstet Gynecol* 1996;175:588–92.

27.   D'Arcy TJ, Hughes SW, Chiu WS, Clark T, Milner AD, Saunders J, *et al*. Estimation of fetal lung volume using enhanced 3-dimensional ultrasound: a new method and first result. *Br J Obstet Gynaecol* 1996;103:1015–20.

28.   Bahmaie A, Hughes SW, Clark T, Milner A, Saunders J, Tilling K, *et al*. Serial fetal lung volume measurement using three-dimensional ultrasound. *Ultrasound Obstet Gynecol* 2000;16:154–8.

29.   Yu C, Chang C, Chang F, Ko H, Chen H. Fetal renal volume in normal gestation: a three-dimensional ultrasound study. *Ultrasound Med Biol* 2000;26:1253–6.

30.   Hsieh YY, Chang CC, Lee CC, Tsai HD. Fetal renal volume assessment by three-dimensional ultrasonography. *Am J Obstet Gynecol* 2000;182:377–9.

31.   Chang FM, Hsu KF, Ko HC, Yao BL, Chang CH, Yu CH, *et al*. Fetal heart volume assessment by three-dimensional ultrasound. *Ultrasound Obstet Gynecol* 1997;9:42–8.

32.   Chang FM, Liang RI, Ko HC, Yao BL, Chang CH, Yu CH. Three-dimensional ultrasound-assessed fetal thigh volumetry in predicting birth weight. *Obstet Gynecol* 1997;90:331–9.

33.   Liang RI, Chang FM, Yao BL, Chang CH, Yu CH, Ko HC. Predicting birth weight by fetal upper-arm volume with use of three-dimensional ultrasonography. *Am J Obstet Gynecol* 1997;177:632–8.

34.   Schild RL, Fimmers R, Hansmann M. Fetal weight estimation by three-dimensional ultrasound. *Ultrasound Obstet Gynecol* 2000;16:445–52.

35.   Hafner E, Philipp T, Schuchter K, Dillinger-Paller B, Philipp K, Bauer P. Second-trimester measurements of placental volume by three-dimensional ultrasound to predict small-for-gestational-age infants. *Ultrasound Obstet Gynecol* 1998;12:97–102.

36.   Wolf H, Oosting H, Treffers PE. Second-trimester placental volume measurement by ultrasound: prediction of fetal outcome. *Am J Obstet Gynecol* 1989;160:121–6.

37.   Hafner E, Schuchter K, van Leeuwen M, Metzenbauer M, Dillinger-Paller B, Philipp K. Three-dimensional sonographic volumetry of the placenta and the fetus between weeks 15 and 17 of gestation. *Ultrasound Obstet Gynecol* 2001;18:116–20.

38.   Ploeckinger-Ulm B, Ulm MR, Lee A, Kratochwil A, Bernaschek G. Antenatal depiction of fetal digits with three-dimensional ultrasonography. *Am J Obstet Gynecol* 1996;175:571–4.

39.   Lee A, Kratochwil A, Deutinger J, Bernaschek G. Three-dimensional ultrasound in diagnosing phocomelia. *Ultrasound Obstet Gynecol* 1995;5:238–40.

40.   Lee A, Deutinger J, Bernaschek G. Three dimensional ultrasound: abnormalities of the fetal face in surface and volume rendering mode. *Br J Obstet Gynaecol* 1995;102:302–6.

41.   Blaas HG, Eik-Nes SH, Kiserud T, Berg S, Angelsen B, Olstad B. Three-dimensional imaging of the brain cavities in human embryos. *Ultrasound Obstet Gynecol* 1995;5:228–32.

42.   Lai TH, Chang CH, Yu CH, Kuo PL, Chang FM. Prenatal diagnosis of alobar holoprosencephaly by two-dimensional and three-dimensional ultrasound. *Prenat Diagn* 2000;20:400–3.

43.   Wang PH, Ying TH, Wang PC, Shih IC, Lin LY, Chen GD. Obstetrical three-dimensional ultrasound in the visualization of the intracranial midline and corpus callosum of fetuses with cephalic position. *Prenat Diagn* 2000;20:518–20.

44.   Mueller GM, Weiner CP, Yankowitz J. Three-dimensional ultrasound in the evaluation of fetal head and spine anomalies. *Obstet Gynecol* 1996;88:372–8.

45.   Johnson DD, Pretorius DH, Riccabona M, Budorick NE, Nelson TR. Three-dimensional ultrasound of the fetal spine. *Obstet Gynecol* 1997;89:434–8.

46. Deng J, Gardener JE, Rodeck CH, Lees WR. Fetal echocardiography in three and four dimensions. *Ultrasound Med Biol* 1996;22:979–86.

47. Liang RI, Huang SE, Chang RM. Prenatal diagnosis of ectopia cordis at 10 weeks of gestation using two-dimensional and three-dimensional ultrasonography. *Ultrasound Obstet Gynecol* 1997;10:137–9.

48. Kurjak A, Kupesic S, Ivancic-Kosuta M. Three-dimensional transvaginal ultrasound improves measurement of nuchal translucency. *J Perinat Med* 1999;27:97–102.

49. Chung BL, Kim HJ, Lee KH. The application of three-dimensional ultrasound to nuchal translucency measurement in early pregnancy (10–14 weeks): a preliminary study. *Ultrasound Obstet Gynecol* 2000;15:122–5.

50. Eppel W, Worda C, Frigo P, Lee A. Three- versus two-dimensional ultrasound for nuchal translucency thickness measurements: comparison of feasibility and levels of agreement. *Prenat Diagn* 2001;21:596–601.

51. Nelson TR, Pretorius DH, Lev-Toaff A, Bega G, Budorick NE, Hollenback KA, et al. Feasibility of performing a virtual patient examination using three-dimensional ultrasonographic data acquired at remote locations. *J Ultrasound Med* 2001;20:941–52.

52. Michailidis GD, Simpson JM, Karidas C, Economides DL. Detailed three-dimensional fetal echocardiography facilitated by an internet link. *Ultrasound Obstet Gynecol* 2001;18:325–8.

53. Pretorius DH, Nelson TR, Jaffe JS. 3-dimensional sonographic analysis based on color flow Doppler and gray scale image data: a preliminary report. *J Ultrasound Med* 1992;11:225–32.

54. Carson PL, Adler DD, Fowlkes JB, Harnist K, Rubin J. Enhanced color flow imaging of breast cancer vasculature: continuous wave Doppler and three-dimensional display. *J Ultrasound Med* 1992;11:377–85.

55. Houi K, Mochio S, Isogai Y, Miyamoto Y, Suzuki N. Comparison of color flow and 3D image by computer graphics for the evaluation of carotid disease. *Angiology* 1990;41:305–12.

56. Ritchie CJ, Edwards WS, Mack LA, Cyr DR, Kim Y. Three-dimensional ultrasonic angiography using power-mode Doppler. *Ultrasound Med Biol* 1996;22:277–86.

57. Ohishi H, Hirai T, Yamada R, Hirohashi S, Uchida H, Hashimoto H, et al. Three-dimensional power Doppler sonography of tumor vascularity. *J Ultrasound Med* 1998;17:619–22.

58. De Simone R, Glombitza G, Vahl CF, Albers J, Meinzer HP, Hagl S. Three-dimensional color Doppler: a clinical study in patients with mitral regurgitation. *J Am Coll Cardiol* 1999;33:1646–54.

59. Heling KS, Chaoui R, Bollmann R. Prenatal diagnosis of an aneurysm of the vein of Galen with three-dimensional color power angiography. *Ultrasound Obstet Gynecol* 2000;15:333–6.

60. Kurjak A, Kupesic S, Sparac V, Kosuta D. Three-dimensional ultrasonographic and power Doppler characterization of ovarian lesions. *Ultrasound Obstet Gynecol* 2000;16:365–71.

61. Woydt M, Horowski A, Krauss J, Krone A, Soerensen N, Roosen K. Three-dimensional intraoperative ultrasound of vascular malformations and supratentorial tumors. *J Neuroimaging* 2002;12:28–34.

62. Pretorius DH, Nelson TR, Baergen RN, Pai E, Cantrell C. Imaging of placental vasculature using three-dimensional ultrasound and color power Doppler: a preliminary study. *Ultrasound Obstet Gynecol* 1998;12:45–9.

63. Welsh AW, Taylor MJ, Cosgrove D, Fisk NM. Freehand three-dimensional Doppler demonstration of monochorionic vascular anastomoses *in vivo*: a preliminary report. *Ultrasound Med Biol* 2001;18:317–24.

64. Chou MM, Tseng JJ, Ho ES, Hwang JI. Three-dimensional color power Doppler imaging in the assessment of uteroplacental neovascularization in placenta previa increta/percreta. *Am J Obstet Gynecol* 2001;185:1257–60.

65. Kossoff G. Three-dimensional ultrasound – technology push or market pull? *Ultrasound Obstet Gynecol* 1995;5:217–18.

66. Nelson TR. Three-dimensional imaging. *Ultrasound Med Biol* 2000;26 Suppl 1:S35–8.

67. Merz E, Bahlmann F, Weber G. Volume scanning in the evaluation of fetal malformations: a new dimension in prenatal diagnosis. *Ultrasound Obstet Gynecol* 1995;5:222–7.

68. Merz E, Weber G, Bahlmann F, Miric-Tesanic D. Application of transvaginal and abdominal three-dimensional ultrasound for the detection or exclusion of malformations of the fetal face. *Ultrasound Obstet Gynecol* 1997;9:237–43.

69. Kurjak A, Hafner T, Kos M, Kupesic S, Stanojevic M. Three-dimensional sonography in prenatal diagnosis: a luxury or a necessity? *J Perinat Med* 2000;28:194–209.

70. Michailidis GD, Papageorgiou P, Economides DL. Assessment of fetal anatomy in the first trimester using two- and three-dimensional ultrasound. *Br J Radiol* 2002;75:215–19.

71. Clementschitsch G, Hasenohrl G, Schaffer H, Steiner H. Comparison between two- and three-dimensional ultrasound measurements of nuchal translucency. *Ultrasound Obstet Gynecol* 2001;18:475–80.

72. Ohno M, Kanenishi K, Kuno A, Akiyama M, Yamashiro C, Tanaka H, *et al.* Three-dimensional sonographic features of nuchal edema. *Gynecol Obstet Invest* 2002;53:125–8.

73. Paul C, Krampl E, Skentou C, Jurkovic D, Nicolaides KH. Measurement of fetal nuchal translucency thickness by three-dimensional ultrasound. *Ultrasound Obstet Gynecol* 2001;18:481–4.

74. Michailidis GD, Economides DL, Schild RL. The role of three-dimensional ultrasound in obstetrics. *Curr Opin Obstet Gynecol* 2001;13:207–14.

75. Blaas HG, Eik-Nes SH, Berg S. Three-dimensional fetal ultrasound. *Baillieres Best Pract Res Clin Obstet Gynaecol* 2000;14:611–27.

76. Yanagihara T, Hata T. Three-dimensional sonographic visualisation of fetal skeleton in the second trimester of pregnancy. *Gynecol Obstet Invest* 2000;49:12–16.

77. Garjian KV, Pretorius DH, Budorick NE, Cantrell CJ, Johnson DD, Nelson TR. Fetal skeletal dysplasia: three-dimensional US – initial experience. *Radiology* 2000;214:717–23.

78. Hata T, Aoki S, Manabe A, Hata K, Miyazaki K. Visualization of fetal genitalia by three-dimensional ultrasonography in the second and third trimesters. *J Ultrasound Med* 1998;17:137–9.

79. Carlson DE. The ultrasound evaluation of cleft lip and palate – a clear winner for 3D. *Ultrasound Obstet Gynecol* 2000;16:299–301.

80. Lee W, Kirk JS, Shaheen KW, Romero R, Hodges AN, Comstock CH. Fetal cleft lip and palate detection by three-dimensional ultrasonography. *Ultrasound Obstet Gynecol* 2000;16:314–20.

81. Campani R, Bottinelli O, Calliada F, Coscia D. The latest in ultrasound: three-dimensional imaging. Part II. *Eur J Radiol* 1998;27 Suppl 2:S183–7.

82. Jackson MR, Walsh AJ, Morrow RJ, Mullen JB, Lye SJ, Ritchie JW. Reduced placental villous tree elaboration in small-for-gestational-age pregnancies: relationship with umbilical artery Doppler waveforms. *Am J Obstet Gynecol* 1995;172:518–25.

83. Krebs C, Macara LM, Leiser R, Bowman AW, Greer IA, Kingdom JC. Intrauterine growth restriction with absent end-diastolic flow velocity in the umbilical artery is associated with maldevelopment of the placental terminal villous tree. *Am J Obstet Gynecol* 1996;175:1534–42.

84. Sladkevicius P, Campbell S. Advanced ultrasound examination in the management of subfertility. *Curr Opin Obstet Gynecol* 2000;12:221–5.

85. Jarvela IY, Sladkevicius P, Kelly S, Ojha K, Nargund G, Campbell S. Three-dimensional sonographic and power Doppler characterization of ovaries in late follicular phase. *Ultrasound Obstet Gynecol* 2002;20:281–5.

86. Pan HA, Cheng YC, Li CH, Wu MH, Chang FM. Ovarian stroma flow intensity decreases by age: a three-dimensional power Doppler ultrasonographic study. *Ultrasound Med Biol* 2002;28:425–30.

87. Pan HA, Wu MH, Cheng YC, Li CH, Chang FM. Quantification of Doppler signal in polycystic ovarian syndrome using 3D power Doppler ultrasonography. *Hum Reprod* 2002;17:2484.

88. Rubin JM, Bude RO, Fowlkes JB, Spratt RS, Carson PL, Adler RS. Normalizing fractional moving blood volume estimates with power Doppler US: defining a stable intravascular point with the cumulative power distribution function. *Radiology* 1997;205:757–65.

89. Welsh AW, Fisk NM. Assessment of fetal renal perfusion by power Doppler digital analysis. *Ultrasound Obstet Gynecol* 2001;17:89–91.

41

Obstetric cholestasis

Catherine Williamson

INTRODUCTION

Cholestasis is described as a pathological state of reduced bile production or flow. Table 1 summarises the main causes of cholestasis in humans.

Obstetric cholestasis (OC), also called intrahepatic cholestasis of pregnancy, is the most common disorder of liver function unique to pregnancy and can have severe consequences for the mother and fetus. It is associated with maternal morbidity and with fetal morbidity and mortality.

EPIDEMIOLOGY

The prevalence of OC varies in different populations, with reported rates varying from 0.2% in France,[1] 1% in Poland[2] and 0.5–2% in Finland,[3–5] to 12% in Chile.[6] It affects 0.6% of pregnancies in UK white women[7,8] and double this proportion of Indian and Pakistani Asians.[7,8]

There is a seasonal variation in the prevalence of OC, with a greater number of cases reported in the winter months.[4,9] In addition, there has been a reduction in the number of reported cases in Chile and in Scandinavia since the 1990s.[9] The reasons for these epidemiological fluctuations are not clear, but they indicate that environmental factors must play a role in the aetiology of the condition. One Finnish study has demonstrated that OC occurs more commonly in women of relatively advanced age (>35 years).[5] In addition, the condition is more common in multiple pregnancy. This is thought to be due to the higher levels of oestrogen in such pregnancies.[10]

MATERNAL CLINICAL FEATURES

The classic maternal clinical feature of OC is generalised pruritus, which commonly develops in the third trimester, becoming more severe with advancing gestation and disappearing shortly after

Table 1 *Causes of cholestasis*

Obstructive cholestasis	Hepatocellular cholestasis
Biliary atresia	Drug induced (e.g. oestrogens, erythromycin, augmentin)
Congenital ductal abnormalities	Obstetric cholestasis
Cholelithiasis	Progressive familial intrahepatic cholestasis
Primary sclerosing cholangitis	Benign recurrent intrahepatic cholestasis
Infectious cholangitis	Infectious hepatitis
Infiltration (e.g. Langerhans cell histiocytosis)	Alpha-1-antitrypsin deficiency
Extrinsic compression	Inborn errors of bile acid synthesis
Ductal paucity	

delivery in the majority of affected women.[4] It is usually most marked on the trunk, soles and palms, and is not associated with any skin rash apart from dermatitis artefacta secondary to scratching. The severity of the pruritus is often sufficient to prevent women from sleeping. Eighty percent will develop pruritus after 30 weeks of gestation,[11] but symptoms can occur as early as the sixth week of pregnancy.[4] Rarer symptoms include anorexia, malaise, abdominal discomfort, pale stools and dark urine. If jaundice does develop, it tends to follow the pruritus by two to four weeks and to plateau relatively quickly.[12] An increased risk of postpartum haemorrhage has been reported.[13] This may be a consequence of malabsorption, with steatorrhoea[14] and resultant vitamin K deficiency.[13]

FETAL CLINICAL FEATURES

Although OC is associated with maternal morbidity, it causes perinatal morbidity and mortality. It causes fetal distress (defined as either meconium stained amniotic fluid or fetal heart rate abnormalities), spontaneous premature delivery and unexplained third trimester intrauterine death.[11,13,15,16] The major studies of the prevalence of fetal complications in OC are summarised in Table 2. The perinatal mortality rate has reduced from the 10–15% reported in older studies[11,13] to ≤ 3.5% in more recent series in which most women were delivered before 38 weeks of gestation.[11,15,16] Davies et al.[17] reported an uncontrolled series of 13 OC pregnancies that had been managed expectantly in the UK with resultant perinatal morbidity or mortality in 11. This included eight intrauterine deaths, two premature deliveries with fetal distress (one died in the perinatal period), and one emergency caesarean section for fetal distress. All but one of the pregnancies complicated by intrauterine death were delivered at ≤ 37 weeks of gestation.[17]

BIOCHEMICAL FEATURES

Abnormal liver function tests (LFTs) are necessary to make the diagnosis of OC. The serum total bile acid concentration is increased, which is largely due to primary bile acids.[18–20]

Serum bile acid levels do not change significantly during the course of a normal pregnancy,[18,21] although one study has reported reduced levels in the first trimester.[22] Several studies have demonstrated a slight rise in serum levels of specific bile acid levels in the third trimester,[18,21,22] but the overall levels did not differ significantly from the normal range. Cholic acid (CA) is the primary bile acid in pregnant women, while chenodeoxycholic acid (CDCA) and deoxycholic acid predominate in nonpregnant women.

Table 2 *Summary of the major studies of fetal outcome in OC*

Date of study	No. cases	% PMR or % IUD★	Meconium staining (%)	Preterm labour (%)	Delivery < 37–38/40 weeks	Reference
1964–69	87	9★	–	54	No	11
1965–79	56	11	27	36	No	13
Post-69	91	3★	–	–	Yes	11
1988	83	4	45	44	Yes	15
1994	320	2	25	12	Yes	16
1990–96	91	0	15	14.3	Yes	5
1999–2001	70	0	14	6	Yes	8

PMR = perinatal mortality rate; IUD = intrauterine death rate; – = data not given

In women with OC, CA is the most sensitive bile acid for early diagnosis and follow-up, and can rise as much as 100-fold.[23] It is the first bile acid to rise and this has been shown to precede the onset of symptoms in up to 50% of cases.[21,23] CDCA also increases, but this is less marked than the rise in CA, and occurs only in approximately 74% of these women.[23]

A study of 13 women that compared measurement of serum bile acid using either high-performance liquid chromatography, or an enzymic procedure that measured total bile acid, revealed that there was no difference in the total bile acid level measured by either procedure.[20] Therefore, although CA and CDCA are the main serum bile acids to rise in OC, many clinical laboratories use the simpler total bile acid assay, which is equally valid for diagnostic purposes.

The liver transaminases are also usually moderately raised (commonly two- to three-fold), although more marked elevation has been reported.[23,24] Both the alanine (ALT) and aspartate (AST) transaminases may be raised, and they are thought to be released as a result of hepatocyte damage. Some studies have shown an increase that occurs only after a rise in primary bile acids; this may reflect the severity of the disease with advancing hepatocyte damage.[25,26] ALT appears to rise first and is thought to be a more sensitive test.[23,25,27] When measuring the liver transaminases, it is important to use the reference ranges for pregnancy[28] (i.e. the upper end of the normal range should be reduced by about 20% compared with the quoted normal range for a laboratory). Normal ranges for LFTs in pregnancy are summarised in Table 3.[28,29]

Bilirubin was shown to correlate with raised primary bile acids in one study,[25] but has no value in early diagnosis or the follow-up of women with OC because it is usually normal.[22] gamma glutamyl transpeptidase is raised in 20–30% of cases.[30]

In one study of 21 women with OC, serum lipids (cholesterol, phospholipids, triglycerides and low-density lipoproteins) were increased, and high-density lipoproteins decreased, when compared with pregnant controls.[31] Another study found raised cholesterol levels in a cohort of pregnant women with raised glycocholic acid levels when compared with pregnant women with a normal glycocholic acid level.[22]

MANAGEMENT OF OBSTETRIC CHOLESTASIS

OC is a diagnosis of exclusion. Other causes of cholestasis, such as gallstones or extrahepatic obstruction, should be excluded by ultrasound examination. Investigations should also be performed to exclude infectious and autoimmune hepatitis. One large Italian study reported an increased prevalence of OC in women who were hepatitis C positive.[32]

The management of OC aims to avoid an adverse fetal outcome and improve the maternal morbidity. The mother should be counselled with regard to the fetal risks and the need for close surveillance. LFTs, including prothrombin time, should be checked regularly, and fetal wellbeing monitored at frequent intervals. There is accumulating evidence that the perinatal mortality is

Table 3 *Normal ranges for liver function tests in pregnancy (data from Girling et al., 1997[28] and Fagan, 2002[29])*

Liver enzyme	Nonpregnant	1st trimester	2nd trimester	3rd trimester
Aspartate transaminase (u/l)	7–40	10–28	11–29	11–30
Alanine transaminase (u/l)	0–40	6–32	6–32	6–32
Bilirubin (μmol/l)	0–17	4–16	3–13	3–14
Gamma glutamyl transpeptidase (u/l)	11–50	5–37	5–43	3–41
Alkaline phosphatase (u/l)	30–130	32–100	43–135	133–418

considerably reduced by induction of labour before 38 weeks of gestation.[11,15,16] There are currently no established forms of fetal surveillance that allow prediction of the at-risk fetus. Therefore, although women with OC are often seen several times a week for fetal assessment by cardiotocography, they are usually told this will give reassurance that there is no current problem but that it cannot exclude subsequent fetal complications. Two studies have shown that amniocentesis and/or amnioscopy can be of value to predict the at-risk fetus,[15,33] but this may be a more invasive approach than would be favoured by most obstetricians.

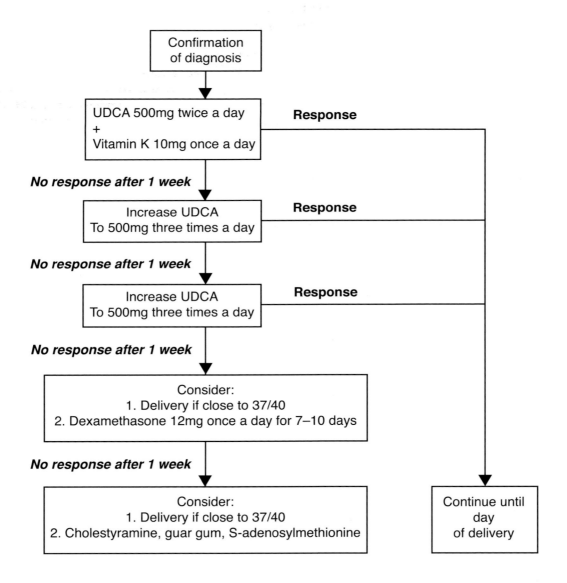

Figure 1 *Strategy for management of obstetric cholestasis: UDCA = ursodeoxycholic acid; o.d. = once daily; b.d. = twice daily; t.d.s. = three times daily; q.d.s. = four times daily*

Drug treatment

A variety of drug therapies have been used for the maternal pruritus; a recommended strategy for pharmacological treatment is given in Figure 1. The two most commonly used, ursodeoxycholic acid (UDCA) and dexamethasone, have been reported to improve both symptoms and LFTs. Other treatments that have been noted to be beneficial in some studies are S-adenosylmethionine (SAMe), colestyramine and guar gum. Vitamin K should be given to reduce the risk of postpartum haemorrhage.

UDCA is a hydrophilic bile acid. It acts by altering the bile acid pool and reducing the proportion of hydrophobic, and therefore hepatotoxic, bile acids. There have been several reports of the use of UDCA in OC in which women are given up to 2000 mg/day for periods of seven days to ten weeks, mainly during the third trimester. When the results of nine studies with a total of 85 affected women treated with UDCA are combined, 74 (87%) showed clinical or biochemical improvement, or both.[17,34-41] All babies born to mothers given UDCA were delivered safely and no problems attributable to treatment were reported. UDCA treatment has been shown to improve the serum bile acid levels measured in cord blood and amniotic fluid at the time of delivery.[38] In addition, there is little accumulation of UDCA in the amniotic fluid or in cord blood.[38] These findings are encouraging because several authors have postulated that raised maternal and fetal bile acids are the cause of the adverse fetal consequences of OC.[19,20,23,42] One study has demonstrated that, although bile acid levels were raised in the colostrum of women whose pregnancies were complicated by OC compared with controls, these were markedly reduced by UDCA treatment.[43]

Dexamethasone can also be an effective therapy. A Finnish study of ten women at between 28 and 37 weeks of gestation reported reduced pruritus and lowered bile acids and transaminases after treatment with dexamethasone 12 mg/day for seven days and a gradual reduction over three days.[44] The serum oestriol and oestradiol levels in these women reduced significantly after one day of treatment, and the authors postulated that this is the mechanism of action of dexamethasone in treating OC. Symptoms of cholestasis did not recur after cessation of therapy, even in one woman who delivered more than two months after treatment with dexamethasone. The results of this study are encouraging, but this is the only series of women treated with dexamethasone in the literature to date. There has been one case report of worsening of maternal pruritus and ALT levels after dexamethasone treatment,[45] but it is difficult to draw conclusions from a single case report.

SAMe reverses oestrogen induced cholestasis in rats. It has been reported to improve symptoms and LFTs in women with OC in some studies[39,46] but not in others.[36,47] In one Italian study, 30 women were randomised to receive either 800 mg of SAMe daily or placebo until delivery, for a mean period of 18 days. Treated women had significantly lower levels of serum bile acids, bilirubin and transaminases compared with both pretreatment levels and the placebo group.[46] In another study, 32 women with OC were subdivided into four groups treated with either UDCA, SAMe, both drugs or placebo for 20 days. Improvements in pruritus and serum bile acids were seen in all groups, but the serum glutamate-pyruvate transaminase (SGPT) did not improve in the placebo group.[39] The combination of UDCA and SAMe caused a greater reduction in pruritus, but not in serum bile acids or SGPT.[39] A Chilean double blind study in which 18 women with OC were randomised to receive either 900 mg SAMe daily or placebo did not demonstrate any difference in pruritus, nor in the levels of serum bile salts, ALT, total bilirubin or alkaline phosphatase between the groups.[47] An Italian study that compared the efficacy of SAMe and UDCA in the treatment of OC failed to show any significant changes in pruritus, serum bile acids, AST, ALT, or alkaline phosphatase tests after SAMe treatment, while UDCA resulted in a significant lowering of serum bile acids and improvement of pruritus.[36]

Colestyramine is an anion exchange resin that can bind bile acids in the intestine, thereby reducing their enterohepatic recirculation, and increasing their faecal elimination. It also binds cholesterol and is used as a cholesterol lowering therapy. There have been two studies of the use of colestyramine in OC. In one, five of seven women who were treated with 18 g daily had improved pruritus.[48] However, the only biochemical change of note was a reduction in the serum levels of one bile acid, CDCA, in four women, but not in the levels of CA, the main bile acid that is raised in OC.[48] There was no reduction in the serum transaminases, alkaline phosphatase or gamma-glutamyl transpeptidase, and there was an increase in conjugated bilirubin.[48] Another study in which ten women were treated with 8–12 g daily reported a reduction in both CA and CDCA in five, but there was no response in those who had the higher serum bile acid levels when treatment was commenced.[49] It is important to use colestyramine treatment with caution because it may bind vitamin K, and therefore reduce its absorption. This can result in exacerbation of the maternal vitamin K deficiency that can occur in OC, and may increase the risk of postpartum haemorrhage. In addition, there has been a case report in which fetal intracranial haemorrhage complicated colestyramine treatment in OC.[50] Colestyramine should not be given at the same time as UDCA therapy because it will prevent absorption of the UDCA.

Guar gum is a gel-forming dietary fibre that binds bile acids in the intestinal lumen and enhances their elimination. There have been two Finnish double blind placebo controlled studies in which up to 15 g guar gum per day was used to treat women with OC.[51,52] Both studies demonstrated an improvement in pruritus and the serum bile acids did not rise after treatment. However, in both studies the serum total bile acid level did not fall, remaining at approximately 20 μmol/l after treatment.[51,52]

Vitamin K is essential for normal coagulation. The active vitamin K dependent clotting factors (II, VII, IX and X) are formed from precursors in the liver, and people with liver disease are at risk of haemorrhage due to deficiency of these clotting factors. It is thought that the increased prevalence of postpartum haemorrhage in OC is caused by a vitamin K deficiency that develops as a result of impaired intestinal absorption secondary to steatorrhoea, but hepatic impairment may also contribute in some cases. There has been one report of a reduction in the prothrombin level to below 5% in a woman with OC[53] and, in a case report, fetal intracranial haemorrhage complicating colestyramine treatment was thought to be due to vitamin K deficiency.[50] Thus, vitamin K treatment is advised from approximately 32 weeks of gestation in OC.

POSTPARTUM COURSE

Biochemical and clinical features of OC resolve after delivery, but recurrence commonly occurs in subsequent pregnancies. Some women may report pruritus associated with the use of oestrogen-containing oral contraceptives and these should either be avoided or, if taken, the LFTs should be checked on a regular basis. In addition, gallstones are more common in women with OC and their relatives.

THE PATHOPHYSIOLOGY OF OBSTETRIC CHOLESTASIS

This condition has a complex aetiology, with hormonal, genetic and environmental factors all playing a role. The hormonal factors that contribute to the pathogenesis of OC include raised serum oestrogen and progestogen levels. It has also been demonstrated that the administration of oestrogens to women with a previous history of OC causes the symptoms and biochemical changes of OC.[54] In addition, a subgroup of women with pregnancy complicated by OC have been reported to develop symptoms after taking the combined oral contraceptive pill and in the second half of the menstrual cycle when not pregnant.[12] Oestrogens have also been shown to have a cholestatic effect in *in vitro* and animal models.[55,56] Progestogens may also play a role; 34 (68%) of 50 women in a French prospective series of OC were treated with oral micronised natural progesterone for risk of premature delivery.[57]

A genetic component to the aetiology of OC is supported by epidemiological studies, which suggest a founder mutation in certain populations (e.g. Chilean Araucanean Indian).[6] There are also a small number of reported pedigrees that show autosomal dominant sex-limited inheritance.[58–60] A preliminary study was conducted of the genetic epidemiology of OC in 81 women from Queen Charlotte's Hospital and the OC Patient Organisation. This demonstrated that 33% have a positive family history and a subgroup of women have a pedigree that demonstrates sex-limited dominant inheritance. In the other pedigrees the only affected woman is the index case. This could be because the other women in the pedigree who potentially have the OC phenotype are nonparous, or the condition has been inherited from male relatives. In this study, the relative risk for parous siblings (λ_S) was 24 and for parous daughters (λ_O) it was 30, assuming a population prevalence of 0.5% of pregnancies.

The only gene that has been shown to be mutated in OC to date is *MDR3*, and this is almost entirely in a rare subgroup of women identified as having a relative with the rare autosomal recessive childhood liver disease, progressive familial intrahepatic cholestasis type 3 (PFIC3).[61,62] In one pedigree in which a large consanguineous family had coexisting PFIC3 and OC, three of the six heterozygote female relatives had pregnancies complicated by unexplained intrauterine death.[61] There was also a report in 2001 of two additional *MDR3* mutations in three women with coexistent OC and a peculiar form of cholelithiasis (i.e. at least one episode of biliary colic, pancreatitis or cholangitis, chronic cholestasis, recurrence of symptoms after cholecystectomy and prevention of recurrence by UDCA therapy).[63] A trafficking mutation has also been identified in *MDR3* in a woman with OC and no family history of PFIC.[30]

Children with PFIC1 and PFIC2 have homozygous mutations in the *FIC1*[64] and *BSEP*[65] genes, respectively. *FIC1* mutations also cause benign recurrent intrahepatic cholestasis, a liver disease that is characterised by recurrent remitting episodes of cholestasis from childhood. The heterozygote mothers of children with PFIC1 and PFIC2 have not been reported to have symptoms of cholestasis in pregnancy.

No other candidate genes for OC have been investigated, although one study found no common HLA haplotypes in five female relatives.[60]

Environmental factors that may play a role in the aetiology of OC include selenium and erucic acid. Plasma selenium levels decrease with advancing gestation, but are maintained at usual levels if dietary intake is normal. Selenium levels were significantly reduced in pregnant women with OC compared with controls in a Finnish study,[66] and at approximately the same time a lower dietary intake of selenium was also demonstrated in Chile.[67] A Chilean study published in 2000 demonstrated that plasma selenium levels are lower in normal pregnant women near term, and that those with OC have significantly lower plasma selenium levels than women with a normal pregnancy.[68] This study also demonstrated that, in normal pregnancies, plasma selenium levels are higher in the summer. In the Finnish study, the activity of the selenoenzyme, glutathione peroxidase, had a significant positive correlation with selenium concentration, and it was also significantly lower in women with OC.[66] Oestrogens can cause oxidative damage but in normal pregnancy antioxidants prevent this. Glutathione peroxidase is an antioxidant that reduces the concentration of antioxidants (e.g. steroid hydroperoxides and other peroxides).[69] Thus it is possible that selenium deficiency in women with OC may contribute to oestrogen induced oxidant damage to hepatocytes. The Chilean study demonstrated that plasma selenium levels have increased in nonpregnant individuals since the 1980s, and the authors suggested that this may partly explain the reduction in the prevalence of OC in Chile since this time.[68]

It has also been reported that changes in the availability of dietary rapeseed oil, which has a high content of erucic acid, mirrored reductions in the prevalence of OC in Chile and Sweden from the 1960s.[70] It was therefore hypothesised that dietary erucic acid was involved in the pathogenesis of OC. A study in which rats and hamsters were fed diets containing a high proportion of erucic acid did not demonstrate an increased incidence of cholestasis, either during pregnancy or when not pregnant.[70] However, it is still possible that dietary erucic acid plays a role in the aetiology of the condition in genetically predisposed individuals.

THE AETIOLOGY OF INTRAUTERINE DEATH AND FETAL DISTRESS IN OBSTETRIC CHOLESTASIS

The pathophysiological mechanisms that cause intrauterine death in OC are currently not understood. The majority of stillborn infants are of appropriate weight with no evidence of uteroplacental insufficiency.[15,17] Thus, the evidence to date suggests that the intrauterine death is a sudden event. Two studies have demonstrated an abnormal fetal heart rate (≤ 100 or ≥ 180 beats/minute) in the children of women with OC.[19,71] A severe fetal bradycardia (<100 beats/minute) was noted in 16% of neonates in another study.[13]

Two studies have reported an association between raised maternal bile acid levels and fetal distress,[23,71] and several authors have postulated that raised bile acids are the cause of the adverse fetal consequences of OC,[19,20,23,42] although there has been no proven mechanism to date. Two studies have demonstrated increased bile acid levels in the fetus, which were uniformly lower than the maternal levels, suggesting that maternal bile acids cross the placenta and enter the fetal circulation and are then excreted from the fetus to the mother via the placenta in OC.[19,26] The fetal bile acid levels were raised and similar to maternal levels in 50% of these OC pregnancies,[19,26] suggesting that abnormal placental bile acid transport may predispose these fetuses to raised serum bile acids, and may result in associated fetal distress and intrauterine death.

Histological examination of placentas from OC pregnancies revealed nonspecific changes, including reduced syncytial sprout formation, maturation defects, villous oedema and trophoblastic swelling.[72,73] Measurement of intervillous blood flow has demonstrated both no change and a reduction in flow.[74] One study demonstrated a dose dependent vasoconstriction of the placental chorionic veins after the administration of bile acids.[75]

The cause of the increased incidence of spontaneous preterm labour is not fully understood. CA has been shown to cause a dose related increase in myometrial contractility in rat myometrium,[76] and it increases the incidence of preterm labour when given as an infusion to sheep.[77] The reason for the increased frequency of preterm labour is not clear, but it has been postulated that it may be a consequence of bile acid induced release of prostaglandins, which in turn may initiate labour.[77] There is also some evidence that in OC the myometrium is more responsive to oxytocin.[78]

In the study in which bile acids were given as an infusion to sheep, all the bile acid treated fetuses developed meconium stained amniotic fluid by the third day of infusion.[77] This may be because the bile acid infusion caused fetal distress and subsequent passage of meconium into the amniotic fluid. Alternatively, it may be due to bile acid induced increases in bowel motility because bile acids are implicated in diarrhoea in humans after extensive ileal resections,[79] and *in vitro* studies have demonstrated that deoxycholic acid activates luminal potassium and chloride secretion in rabbit distal colon.[80]

Studies using cultured neonatal cardiomyocytes as an *in vitro* model of the fetal heart at term have shown that the addition of the primary bile acid taurocholate to culture medium causes abnormal contraction and calcium dynamics.[81,82] It has been proposed that raised fetal bile acids may therefore cause a cardiac arrest and subsequent intrauterine death.

CONCLUSION

OC is an important complication of pregnancy because it can cause fetal morbidity and mortality. It affects 0.66% of pregnant women in the UK. Liver function tests, including serum bile acids, should be checked in women with pruritus in pregnancy, and these should subsequently be repeated if the initial test is normal and a woman continues to have symptoms. OC is a diagnosis of exclusion and other causes of cholestasis (e.g. hepatitis C infection or biliary obstruction) should be excluded. Once the diagnosis has been made, delivery before 38 weeks of gestation reduces the risk of intrauterine death. Management includes treatment with UDCA (recommended initial dose of approximately 500 mg twice daily) and regular fetal surveillance. The aetiology includes genetic and environmental factors, but is not yet fully understood.

References

1. Perreau P, Rouch R. Ictere cholestatique recidivant de la grosseusse. *Gynecol Obstet* 1961;60:161–79.
2. Wojcicka-Jagodzinska J, Kuczynska-Sicinska J, Czajkowksi K, Smolarczyk R. Carbohydrate metabolism in the course of intrahepatic cholestasis of pregnancy. *Am J Obstet Gynecol* 1989;161:959–69
3. Svanborg A, Ohlsson S. Recurrent jaundice of pregnancy: a clinical study of twenty-two cases. *Am J Med* 1959;27:40–9.
4. Berg B, Helm G, Petersohn I, Tryding N. Cholestasis of pregnancy. Clinical and laboratory studies. *Acta Obstet Gynecol Scand* 1986;65:107–13.
5. Heinonen S, Kirkinen P. Pregnancy outcome with intrahepatic cholestasis. *Obstet Gynecol* 1999;94:189–93.
6. Reyes H, Gonzalez MC, Ribalta J, Aburto H, Matus C, Schraum G, et al. Prevalence of intrahepatic cholestasis of pregnancy in Chile. *Ann Intern Med* 1978;88:487–93.
7. Abedin P, Weaver JB, Egginton E. Intrahepatic cholestasis of pregnancy: prevalence and ethnic distribution. *Ethn Health* 1999;4:35–7.
8. Kenyon AP, Piercy CN, Girling J, Williamson C, Tribe RM, Shennan AH. Obstetric cholestasis, outcome with active management: a series of 70 cases. *BJOG* 2002;109:282–8.
9. Reyes H. Review: intrahepatic cholestasis. A puzzling disorder of pregnancy. *J Gastroenterol Hepatol* 1997;12:211–16.
10. Gonzalez MC, Reyes H, Arrese M, Figueroa D, Lorca B, Andresen M, et al. Intrahepatic cholestasis of pregnancy in twin pregnancies. *J Hepatol* 1989;9:84–90.
11. Reyes H. The enigma of intrahepatic cholestasis of pregnancy: lessons from Chile. *Hepatology* 1982;2:87–96.
12. Lunzer MR. Jaundice in pregnancy. *Baillieres Clin Gastroenterol* 1989;3:467–83.
13. Reid R, Ivey KJ, Rencoret RH, Storey B. Fetal complications of obstetric cholestasis. *Br Med J* 1976;i:870–2.
14. Reyes H, Radrigan ME, Gonzalez MC, Latorre R, Ribalta J, Segovia N, et al. Steatorrhea in patients with intrahepatic cholestasis of pregnancy. *Gastroenterology* 1987;93:584–90.

15. Fisk NM, Storey GN. Fetal outcome in obstetric cholestasis. *Br J Obstet Gynaecol* 1988;95:1137–43.

16. Rioseco AJ, Ivankovic MB, Manzur A, Hamed F, Kato SR, Parer JT, et al. Intrahepatic cholestasis of pregnancy: a retrospective case–control study of perinatal outcome. *Am J Obstet Gynecol* 1994;170:890–5.

17. Davies MH, da Silva RC, Jones SR, Weaver JB, Elias E. Fetal mortality associated with cholestasis of pregnancy and the potential benefit of therapy with ursodeoxycholic acid. *Gut* 1995;37:580–4.

18. Sjovall K, Sjovall J. Serum bile acid levels in pregnancy with pruritus (bile acids and steroids 158). *Clin Chim Acta* 1966;13:207–11.

19. Laatikainen TJ. Fetal bile acid levels in pregnancies complicated by maternal intrahepatic cholestasis. *Am J Obstet Gynecol* 1975;122:852–6.

20. Bacq Y, Myara A, Brechot MC, Hamon C, Studer E, Trivin F, et al. Serum conjugated bile acid profile during intrahepatic cholestasis of pregnancy. *J Hepatol* 1995;22:66–70.

21. Heikkinen J, Maentausta O, Ylostalo P, Janne O. Changes in serum bile acid concentrations during normal pregnancy, in patients with intrahepatic cholestasis of pregnancy and in pregnant women with itching. *Br J Obstet Gynaecol* 1981;88:240–5.

22. Laatikainen T, Hesso A. Determination of serum bile acids by glass capillary gas-liquid chromatography. *Clin Chim Acta* 1975;64:63–8.

22. Lunzer M, Barnes P, Byth K, O'Halloran M. Serum bile acid concentrations during pregnancy and their relationship to obstetric cholestasis. *Gastroenterology* 1986;91:825–9.

23. Laatikainen T, Ikonen E. Serum bile acids in cholestasis of pregnancy. *Obstet Gynecol* 1977;50:313–18.

24. Misra PS, Evanov FA, Wessely Z, Rosenblum GA, Singh P. Idiopathic intrahepatic cholestasis of pregnancy. Report of an unusual case and review of the literature. *Am J Gastroenterol* 1980;73:54–9.

25. Heikkinen J. Serum bile acids in the early diagnosis of intrahepatic cholestasis of pregnancy. *Obstet Gynecol* 1983;61:581–7.

26. Shaw D, Frohlich J, Wittmann B, Willms M. A prospective study of 18 patients with cholestasis of pregnancy. *Am J Obstet Gynecol* 1982;142:621–5.

27. Fisk NM, Bye WB, Storey GN. Maternal features of obstetric cholestasis: 20 years' experience at King George V Hospital. *Aust N Z J Obstet Gynaecol* 1988;28:172–6.

28. Girling JC, Dow E, Smith JH. Liver function tests in pre-eclampsia: importance of comparison with a reference range derived for normal pregnancy. *Br J Obstet Gynaecol* 1997;104:246–50.

29. Fagan EA. Disorders of the liver, biliary system and pancreas. In: de Swiet M, editor. *Medical Disorders in Obstetric Practice.* 4th ed. Oxford: Blackwell Science; 2002. p. 282–345.

30. Dixon PH, Weerasekera N, Linton KJ, Donaldson O, Chambers J, Egginton E, et al. Heterozygous MDR3 missense mutation associated with intrahepatic cholestasis of pregnancy: evidence for a defect in protein trafficking. *Hum Mol Genet* 2000;9:1209–17.

31. Johnson P, Samsioe G, Gustafson A. Studies in cholestasis of pregnancy II. Serum lipids and lipoproteins. *Acta Obstet Gynecol Scand* 1975;54:105–11.

32. Locatelli A, Roncaglia N, Arreghini A, Bellini P, Vergani P, Ghidini A. Hepatitis C virus infection is associated with a higher incidence of cholestasis of pregnancy. *Br J Obstet Gynaecol* 1999;106:498–500.

33. Roncaglia N, Arreghini A, Locatelli A, Bellini P, Andreotti C, Ghidini A. Obstetric cholestasis: outcome with active management. *Eur J Obstet Gynecol Reprod Biol* 2002;100:167–70.

34. Berkane N, Cocheton JJ, Brehier D, Merviel P, Wolf C, Lefevre G, *et al.* Ursodeoxycholic acid in intrahepatic cholestasis of pregnancy. A retrospective study of 19 cases. *Acta Obstet Gynecol Scand* 2000;79:941–6.

35. Brites D, Rodrigues CM, Oliveira N, Cardoso M, Graca LM. Correction of maternal serum bile acid profile during ursodeoxycholic acid therapy in cholestasis of pregnancy. *J Hepatol* 1998;28:91–8.

36. Floreani A, Paternoster D, Melis A, Grella PV. S-adenosylmethionine versus ursodeoxycholic acid in the treatment of intrahepatic cholestasis of pregnancy: preliminary results of a controlled trial. *Eur J Obstet Gynecol Reprod Biol* 1996;67:109–13.

37. Mazzella G, Rizzo N, Salzetta A, Iampieri R, Bovicelli L, Roda E. Management of intrahepatic cholestasis in pregnancy. *Lancet* 1991;338:1594–5.

38. Mazzella G, Rizzo N, Azzaroli F, Sdimoni P, Bovicelli L, Miracolo A, *et al.* Ursodeoxycholic acid administration in patients with cholestasis of pregnancy: effects on primary bile acids in babies and mothers. *Hepatology* 2001;33:504–8.

39. Nicastri PL, Diaferia A, Tartagni M, Loizzi P, Fanelli M. A randomised placebo-controlled trial of ursodeoxycholic acid and S-adenosylmethionine in the treatment of intrahepatic cholestasis of pregnancy. *Br J Obstet Gynaecol* 1998;105:1205–7.

40. Palma J, Reyes H, Ribalta J, Iglesias J, Gonzalez MC, Hernandez I, *et al.* Effects of ursodeoxycholic acid in patients with intrahepatic cholestasis of pregnancy. *Hepatology* 1992;15:1043–7.

41. Palma J, Reyes H, Ribalta J, Hernandez I, Sandoval L, Almuna R, *et al.* Ursodeoxycholic acid in the treatment of cholestasis of pregnancy: a randomized, double-blind study controlled with placebo. *J Hepatol* 1997;27:1022–8.

42. Heikkinen J, Maentausta O, Tuimala R, Ylostalo P, Janne O. Amniotic fluid bile acids in normal and pathologic pregnancy. *Obstet Gynecol* 1980;56:60–4.

43. Brites D, Rodrigues CM. Elevated levels of bile acids in colostrum of patients with cholestasis of pregnancy are decreased following ursodeoxycholic acid therapy. *J Hepatol* 1998;29:743–51.

44. Hirvioja ML, Tuimala R, Vuori J. The treatment of intrahepatic cholestasis of pregnancy by dexamethasone. *Br J Obstet Gynaecol* 1992;99:109–11.

45. Kretowicz E, McIntyre HD. Intrahepatic cholestasis of pregnancy, worsening after dexamethasone. *Aust N Z J Obstet Gynaecol* 1994;34:211–13.

46. Frezza M, Centini G, Cammareri G, Le Grazie C, Di Padova C. S-adenosylmethionine for the treatment of intrahepatic cholestasis of pregnancy. Results of a controlled clinical trial. *Hepatogastroenterology* 1990;37 Suppl 2:122–5.

47. Ribalta J, Reyes H, Gonzalez MC, Iglesias J, Arrese M, Poniachik J, *et al.* S-adenosyl-L-methionine in the treatment of patients with intrahepatic cholestasis of pregnancy: a randomized, double-blind, placebo-controlled study with negative results. *Hepatology* 1991;13:1084–9.

48. Heikkinen J, Maentausta O, Ylostalo P, Janne O. Serum bile acid levels in intrahepatic cholestasis of pregnancy during treatment with phenobarbital or cholestyramine. *Eur J Obstet Gynecol Reprod Biol* 1982;14:153–62.

49. Laatikainen T. Effect of cholestyramine and phenobarbital on pruritus and serum bile acid levels in cholestasis of pregnancy. *Am J Obstet Gynecol* 1978;132:501–6.

50. Sadler LC, Lane M, North R. Severe fetal intracranial haemorrhage during treatment with cholestyramine for intrahepatic cholestasis of pregnancy. *Br J Obstet Gynaecol* 1995;102:169–70.

51. Gylling H, Riikonen S, Nikkila K, Savonius H, Miettinen TA. Oral guar gum treatment of

intrahepatic cholestasis and pruritus in pregnant women: effects on serum cholestanol and other non-cholesterol sterols. *Eur J Clin Invest* 1998;28:359–63.

52. Riikonen S, Savonius H, Gylling H, Nikkila K, Tuomi AM, Miettinen TA. Oral guar gum, a gel-forming dietary fiber relieves pruritus in intrahepatic cholestasis of pregnancy. *Acta Obstet Gynecol Scand* 2000;79:260–4.

53. Herre HD, Engelmann C, Wiken HP. Diagnosis and therapy of blood coagulation disorders in intrahepatic cholestasis. *Zentralbl Gynakol* 1976;98:217–19.

54. Kreek MJ, Weser E, Sleisenger MH, Jeffries GH. Idiopathic cholestasis of pregnancy. The response to challenge with the synthetic estrogen, ethinyl estradiol. *N Engl J Med* 1967;277:1391–5.

55. Schreiber AJ, Simon FR. Estrogen-induced cholestasis; clues to pathogenesis and treatment. *Hepatology* 1983;3:607–13.

56. Simon FR, Fortune J, Iwahashi M, Gartung C, Wolkoff A, Sutherland E. Ethinyl estradiol cholestasis involves alterations in expression of liver sinusoidal transporters. *Am J Physiol* 1996;34:G1043–52.

57. Bacq Y, Sapey T, Brechot MC, Pierre F, Fignon A, Dubois F. Intrahepatic cholestasis of pregnancy: a French prospective study. *Hepatology* 1997;26:358–64.

58. Holzbach R, Sivak DA, Braun WE. Familial recurrent intrahepatic cholestasis of pregnancy: a genetic study providing evidence for transmission of a sex-limited, dominant trait. *Gastroenterology* 1983;85:175–9.

59. Reyes H, Ribalta J, Gonzalez-Ceron M. Idiopathic cholestasis of pregnancy in a large kindred. *Gut* 1976;17:709–13.

60. Hirvioja ML, Kivinen S. Inheritance of intrahepatic cholestasis of pregnancy in one kindred. *Clin Genet* 1993;43:315–17.

61. Jacquemin E, Crestil D, Manouvier S, Boute O, Hadchouel M. Heterozygous non-sense mutation of the *MDR3* gene in familial intrahepatic cholestasis of pregnancy. *Lancet* 1999;353:210–11.

62. Jacquemin E, De Vree JM, Cresteil D, Sokal EM, Sturm E, Dumont M, *et al.* The wide spectrum of multidrug resistance 3 deficiency: from neonatal cholestasis to cirrhosis of adulthood. *Gastroenterology* 2001;120:1448–58.

63. Rosmorduc O, Hermelin B, Poupon R. MDR3 gene defect in adults with symptomatic intrahepatic and gallbladder cholesterol cholelithiasis. *Gastroenterology* 2001;120:1459–67.

64. Bull LN, van Eijk MJT, Pawlikowska L, DeYoung JA, Juijn JA, Liao M, *et al.* A gene encoding P-type ATPase mutated in two forms of hereditary cholestasis. *Nat Genet* 1998;18:219–24.

65. Strautnieks SS, Bull LN, Knisely AS, Kocoshis SA, Dah N, Arnell H, *et al.* A gene encoding a liver-specific ABC transporter is mutated in progressive familial intrahepatic cholestasis. *Nat Genet* 1998;20:233–8.

66. Kauppila A, Korpela H, Makila UM, Yrjanheikki E. Low serum selenium concentration and glutathione peroxidase activity in intrahepatic cholestasis of pregnancy. *Br Med J (Clin Res Ed)* 1987;294:150–2.

67. Agostini A, Gerli GC, Beretta L, Palazzini G, Buso GP, Hu XS, *et al.* Erythrocyte antioxidant enzymes and selenium serum levels in an Andean population. *Clin Chim Acta* 1983;133:153–7.

68. Reyes H, Baez ME, Gonzalez MC, Hernandez I, Palma J, Ribalta J, *et al.* Selenium, zinc and copper plasma levels in intrahepatic cholestasis of pregnancy, in normal pregnancies and in healthy individuals in Chile. *J Hepatol* 2000;32:542–9.

69. Ursini F, Maiorino M, Gregolin C. The selenoenzyme phospholipid hydroperoxide glutathione peroxidase. *Biochim Biophys Acta* 1985;839;62–70.

70. Reyes H, Ribalta J, Hernandez I, Arrese M, Pak N, Wells M, *et al.* Is dietary erucic acid hepatotoxic in pregnancy? An experimental study in rats and hamsters. *Hepatology* 1995;21:1373–9.

71. Laatikainen T, Tulenheimo A. Maternal serum bile acid levels and fetal distress in cholestasis of pregnancy. *Int J Gynaecol Obstet* 1984;22:91–4.

72. Laatikainen T, Ikonen E. Fetal prognosis in obstetric hepatosis. *Ann Chir Gynaecol Fenn* 1975;64:155–64.

73. Costoya AL, Leontic EA, Rosenberg HG, Delgado MA. Morphological study of placental terminal villi in intrahepatic cholestasis of pregnancy: histochemistry, light and electron microscopy. *Placenta* 1980;1:361–8.

74. Kaar K, Jouppila P, Kuikka J, Luotola H, Toivanen J, Rekonen A. Intervillous blood flow in normal and complicated late pregnancy measured by means of an intravenous 133Xe method. *Acta Obstet Gynecol Scand* 1980;59:7–10.

75. Sepulveda WH, Gonzalez C, Cruz MA, Rudolph MI. Vasoconstrictive effect of bile acids on isolated human placental chorionic veins. *Eur J Obstet Gynecol Reprod Biol* 1991;42:211–15.

76. Campos G, Guerra F, Israel E.]Effecto de los acidos biliares sobre la contractibilidad miometral en utero gestante aislado.] *Rev Chile Obstet Ginecol* 1988;53:229–33.

77. Campos GA, Guerra FA, Israel EJ. Effects of cholic acid infusions in fetal lambs. *Acta Obstet Gynecol Scand* 1986;65:23–6.

78. Israel EJ, Guzman ML, Campos GA. Maximal response to oxytocin of the isolated myometrium from pregnant patients with intrahepatic cholestasis. *Acta Obstet Gynecol Scand* 1986;65:581–2.

79. Hofmann AF. The syndrome of ileal disease and the broken enterohepatic circulation: cholerhetic enteropathy. *Gastroenterology* 1967;52:752–7.

80. Mauricio AC, Slawik M, Heitzmann D, von Hahn T, Warth R, Bleich M, *et al.* Deoxycholic acid (DOC) affects the transport properties of distal colon. *Pflugers Arch* 2000;439:532–40.

81. Williamson C, Gorelik J, Eaton BM, Lab M, de Swiet M, Korchev Y. The bile acid taurocholate impairs rat cardiomyocyte function: a proposed mechanism for intrauterine fetal death in obstetric cholestasis. *Clin Sci (Lond)* 2001;100:363–9.

82. Gorelik J, Harding SE, Shevchuk AI, Koralage D, Lab M, de Swiet M, *et al.* Taurocholate induces changes in cardiomyocyte contraction and calcium dynamics. *Clin Sci (Lond)* 2002;103:191–200.

42

Acupuncture

Ayman AA Ewies

INTRODUCTION

Traditional Chinese medicine includes acupuncture, acupressure, moxibustion, herbal therapy and specific exercises in an integrated system that has been practised in China for more than 2000 years.[1] Traditional Chinese medicine is now practised in one form or another by more than 300 000 practitioners in over 140 countries. The first hospital for traditional Chinese medicine in Europe was opened in Germany in 1990 and acupuncture is being more frequently adopted for use in Western medical clinics. British general practitioners are increasingly contracting out for acupuncture services, public health-insurance companies in Germany routinely refund part of the cost of acupuncture treatment provided by trained doctors, and in France acupuncture is a widely accepted part of healthcare provision. Degree programmes in traditional Chinese medicine are now offered at several British universities, and courses are established at many European medical schools. Tong Ren Tang, Beijing's oldest pharmacy, founded in the 17th century, opened a branch in central London in 1995.[2] The use of acupuncture in medicine is being promoted by organisations such as the British Medical Acupuncture Society and, as a result of patient demand,[3] about 2200 professional acupuncturists, who are members of the British Acupuncture Council, deliver approximately 2 million treatments per year in the UK.[4]

In spite of the increasing use, there is still a vast amount of prejudice with regard to acupuncture and techniques regarded as 'complementary' to traditional Western medicine. Because the mechanisms of action are not fully comprehended in physiological terms, the treatments are considered by many clinicians to be of no value. However, more research results support the use of acupuncture in medicine, including obstetrics and gynaecology.[3] The future of Chinese medicine in the West will depend on rigorous assessment of safety and efficacy. Addressing the equation of harm versus benefit involves subjective choices and is thus an intrinsically political problem. Ideally, these issues would be addressed by interdisciplinary research involving epidemiologists, anthropologists, sinologists and experts in the cultural studies of sciences, as well as clinicians.[2]

This chapter reviews the history and techniques of acupuncture and its various possible uses in obstetric and gynaecological practice. Safety issues are discussed critically, taking into account the best available evidence.

DEFINITION AND HISTORY

Acupuncture is defined from the Latin *acus* 'a needle', and *punctura* 'a puncture'.[5] It is an ancient system of healing in which the stimulation of certain points on the surface of the body affects the functioning of certain organs. These points are not scattered arbitrarily over the body, but follow a predictable and unchanging pattern, which can be used to diagnose organ involvement in a wide range of disorders. The line that can be drawn linking the points associated with any particular organ is known as a meridian.[6] Acupuncture typically involves penetration of the skin by fine, solid, metallic needles, which are manipulated manually or by electrical stimulation.[7]

Chinese medicine is an independent system of thought and practice that has been developed over centuries. Based on ancient texts, it is the result of a continuous process of critical thinking as well as of extensive clinical observation. Rooted in philosophy and logic, it has developed its own perception of the body, and of health and disease. The Chinese method is essentially holistic, based on the concept that no single part can be understood except in relation to the whole.[6] Fundamental to the concept of Chinese medicine is the idea of balance and harmony. Energy, or qi (pronounced chee), flows through the body from meridian to meridian. Pain and disease occur when there is a blockage in the flow of the qi. The body should be treated as an entity and attention should be paid to maintain the human body in harmonious balance within, and in relation to, its external environment.[5,6,8]

There are 12 meridians in total, relating to various organs such as the heart, bladder, kidney and lungs, and also to organs not recognised within Western medicine, such as the 'triple heater'. It is important to understand that the Chinese definition of organ differs from that in the West. To the Chinese, an organ comprises not only an organic structure but also its entire functional system (i.e. organs are identified in terms of function rather than the other way round). Acupuncture points (365 in number) lie along the meridians and it is at these points that needles are inserted, usually four to six in number and normally left in place for 15–20 minutes. The depth to which needles are inserted varies according to the position on the body. A thorough understanding of surface anatomy is essential to be able to locate acupuncture points precisely.[6]

Acupuncture is complementary rather than antithetical to Western medicine and the two can work well together and enhance each other. In China a close and mutually beneficial integration has long been established between the two systems.[6]

EVIDENCE OF BENEFIT

Many randomised controlled trials (RCTs) have been conducted in China to evaluate the effectiveness of traditional Chinese medicine, but much of the information is inaccessible to Western doctors. Tang et al.,[9] on reviewing the studies of traditional Chinese medicine, found that almost 10 000 RCTs were published in China before 1997. Although methodological quality has been improving over the years, many problems remain. The method of randomisation was often inappropriately described. Blinding was used in only 15% of trials. Few studies had sample sizes of 300 participants or more. Many trials used another Chinese medicine practice as a control whose effectiveness had not been evaluated. Most trials did not have data on compliance and completeness of follow-up, and effectiveness was rarely quantitatively expressed and reported. Intention to treat analysis was never mentioned. Over half did not report data on baseline characteristics or on adverse effects, with many trials being published only as short reports. Most trials claimed that the tested treatments were effective, indicating that publication bias may be common.

Depressingly, the conclusion of many systematic reviews published since 1999[1,3,9] has been similar to the first reviews carried out 15 years ago, in which findings were conflicting and the studies were too small and too few in number. Nevertheless, trial methods in acupuncture have improved substantially in the last decade, and there is some positive evidence emerging for its efficacy in treating many diseases.[10]

ACUPUNCTURE DURING PREGNANCY

Background

Acupuncture is, in theory, ideal for use in childbirth. Being 'drug free' and therefore having no harmful teratogenic effects, women may feel happier about receiving this type of treatment in their pregnancy. For many years caregivers have felt frustrated at not being able to offer women effective treatment for the minor ailments of pregnancy that can cause considerable distress.[6] Although the majority of the studies in this area are small, they seem to be promising enough to warrant further research to establish the role of acupuncture in the treatment of some pregnancy related problems.

Possible uses

Acupuncture has been used to treat morning sickness, carpal tunnel syndrome, headaches, migraine, backache, sciatica, breast soreness, discomfort due to sinus conditions, oedema, varicose veins, vulval varicosities, haemorrhoids, indigestion, heartburn, abdominal pain, constipation, diarrhoea, hyperemesis gravidarum, anaemia and hypertension. It has also been used in the correction of malpresentation, induction of labour and pain relief in labour.[6,11] It can be used postnatally to treat perineal pain, breast engorgement, mastitis, postnatal depression and insufficient lactation.[6]

Acupuncture for nausea and vomiting

A single blind, randomised, placebo controlled trial[12] included 593 women with nausea or vomiting in early pregnancy showed that acupuncture is an effective treatment for nausea and dry retching. A time-related placebo effect was found for some women receiving placebo acupuncture. There was no effect on vomiting, but it is possible that increasing the frequency of treatment would reduce the frequency and severity of vomiting. Daily treatments have previously been recommended in severe cases,[13] but this needs to be evaluated in future research. Another subject- and observer-masked, randomised, placebo controlled trial on 55 women in early pregnancy reported decreases in nausea in both acupuncture and placebo groups, and there was no significant difference between the groups.[14] A third placebo controlled, randomised, single blind, crossover study of 33 women suggested that active PC6 (pericardium 6) acupuncture, in combination with standard treatment, could hasten the improvement of hyperemesis gravidarum when compared with placebo acupuncture.[15] A review of the literature of acupressure for nausea of pregnancy[16] concluded that two studies found acupressure to be superior to no treatment, three found it superior to dummy acupressure, and one found it not superior to dummy acupressure.

Acupuncture for low back pain

A small prospective, randomised study showed that acupuncture relieved low back pain during pregnancy to a greater extent than physiotherapy. Acupuncture also diminished disability whereas physiotherapy did not. Overall satisfaction was good in both groups and there were no serious adverse events in any of the women.[17] However, the superiority of acupuncture may reflect the benefit of individual compared with group therapy.

Moxibustion and correction of breech presentation

A different technique is commonly used in fetal malpresentation. Although electro-acupuncture (EA)[18] and auricular plaster therapy[19] have also been used to induce cephalic version, a different technique is commonly employed to correct fetal malpresentation. This involves stimulating acupuncture points by heat rather than by needles. For example, moxibustion uses the heat generated by burning herbal preparations containing the plant *Artemisia vulgaris* (it is also called mugwort or moxa, the latter being derived from the Japanese *moe kusa,* which means 'burning herb') to stimulate the acupuncture points. The intensity of moxibustion is just below the individual tolerability threshold.[20,21] Women can be instructed in clinic to undertake this therapy themselves at home.[22,23] Moxibustion is simple, cheap, noninvasive and painless.[24,25]

Mechanism of action

The mechanism of action of moxibustion is not entirely clear and warrants further research. It was postulated that lighting moxa on the Zhiyin point causes adrenocortical stimulation, which results in increased placental oestrogens and changes in prostaglandin (PG) levels (an elevated PGF/PGE ratio due to reduction of PGE while PGF remains unchanged). Oestrogens increase myometrial sensitivity, which results in increased contractility in response to PGF. This stimulates fetal movements and makes version more likely. The increase in fetal movements, and subsequently fetal heart rate, is one of the most striking effects of moxibustion perceived by almost all women towards the second half of the stimulation period and persists even after the end of stimulation.[21,26] Stimulation performed in cases of intrauterine fetal death failed to produce version.[27] This clarifies that this type of version relies on active fetal participation and any explanation based purely on a dermatomeric reflex action of moxibustion acupuncture must be ruled out.[21,26]

Success rate

Encouraging results were reported in two published Chinese studies.[28,29] These were unrandomised and based on a mixed population of primigravidas and multiparas and treatment sessions were initiated between 28 and 36 weeks of gestation, when spontaneous version commonly occurs. No definitive conclusion could therefore be drawn. Nonetheless, the success rate in 880 women treated after 34 weeks was 84.6%.[29] In 1998, Cardini and Weixin[21] reported a randomised, controlled, open trial which included 260 primigravidas with breech presentation diagnosed by ultrasound scan in the 33rd week of pregnancy. Half of these women were randomised to the intervention group and received stimulation to the Zhiyin point with moxa, and the other 130 were randomised to the control group and received routine care but no intervention. In both groups, women with a persistent breech could undergo external cephalic version at any time between 35 weeks of gestation and delivery. The women were observed for one hour daily during the 35th week of gestation, and those in the intervention group experienced significantly more fetal movements than those in the control group. Of the 130 fetuses in the intervention group, 98 (75.4%) were cephalic compared with 62 (47.7%) in the control group ($P < 0.01$). After the 35th week all remaining breech presentations remained unchanged, except for 19 cases successfully treated with external cephalic version. This trial has been criticised because of lack of blinding or placebo. It has been argued that, in an open trial of any therapy versus no therapy, people receiving the treatment may adopt behaviours different to those not receiving it. This would effectively abolish the effect of randomisation since the groups would differ in more respects than just the intervention.[24]

Acupuncture for obstetric analgesia

A randomised controlled trial reported in 2002[30] involved 90 parturients and revealed that acupuncture treatment during labour significantly reduced the need for epidural analgesia and provided a significantly better degree of relaxation compared with the control group. No negative effects were found in relation to delivery outcome. However, further trials with larger numbers of women are required to clarify if the main effect of acupuncture during labour is analgesic or relaxing.[30]

EA has been used successfully to achieve pain relief during labour. Martoudis and Christofides[31] reported that 146 of 168 (85.7%) women treated by EA during the first or second stage of labour experienced some pain relief in a total of 192 acupuncture treatments. Treatment duration of 20 minutes was considered sufficient and the average application–maximum effect interval was 40 minutes, with a mean duration of analgesic effect of 6 hours. The method described was simple, practical, cheap and entirely safe to the mother and baby. It could be learned easily and practised satisfactorily by the obstetricians and midwives without specialised training in acupuncture.

A study of sacral acupuncture for pain relief in labour in Nigerian women[32] found that clinically adequate analgesia was produced in 19 (63.3%) of the 30 women included. The needles did not interfere with nursing or obstetric manoeuvres. However, the procedure was time consuming. It was also reported that acupuncture reduced the need for other methods of analgesia in childbirth and 94% of the women treated mentioned that they would consider acupuncture in future deliveries.[33]

Acupuncture for induction of labour

The limited observational studies to date suggest that acupuncture for induction of labour appears to be safe, has no known teratogenic effects and may be effective. Nonetheless, a 2001 Cochrane Database Systematic Review[34] found no well designed RCT to evaluate the role of acupuncture in induction of labour. Many investigators have studied labour induction using EA. In three studies, the majority of post-term pregnant women began labour during the treatment, although this often took more than 12 hours. However, none of these studies included control groups and thus progression to labour was not necessarily related to the treatment.[35–37] It was also shown that cervical maturation could possibly be improved if acupuncture sessions were carried out at the beginning of the ninth month of pregnancy.[38] A small randomised, placebo controlled study assessed the effect on uterine contractions (monitored by cardiotocography) of transcutaneous electrical nerve stimulation applied at acupuncture points over a four-hour period in post-term pregnant women. A significant increase in frequency and strength of uterine contractions was found in the electrically stimulated women compared with the placebo group. Electrical stimulation through acupuncture loci, if it is activating afferent nerve fibres, can initiate a number of physiological mechanisms, such as hormonal changes influenced through the ascending neuronal pathways to the hypothalamus or reflex activation of autonomic efferent nerves to the uterus.[39]

ELECTRO-ACUPUNCTURE IN ASSISTED REPRODUCTION

Effect on pulsatility index

Successful *in vitro* fertilisation and embryo transfer demand optimal endometrial receptivity at the time of implantation. Blood flow impedance in the uterine arteries, measured as the pulsatility index using transvaginal ultrasonography with pulsed Doppler curves, has been considered valuable in assessing endometrial receptivity. It was found that a pulsatility index greater than or equal to 3.0 at the time of embryo transfer could predict 35% of the failures to become pregnant.[40,41] No significant difference was observed between the pulsatility index measured on the day of oocyte retrieval compared with that on the day of embryo transfer. This lack of difference would allow prediction of nonreceptive endometria earlier in the cycle.[40] A prospective nonrandomised study found that EA reduced the high uterine artery blood flow impedance in ten infertile healthy women, an effect thought to be mediated by the central inhibition of sympathetic activity.[42] The vasodilatation resulting from acupuncture treatment may be caused by central sympathetic inhibition via the endorphin system,[43] by stimulation of sensory nerve fibres that inhibit the sympathetic outflow at the spinal level, or by antidromic nerve impulses that release substance P and calcitonin gene–related peptide from the peripheral nerve terminals.[43,44]

Use as an analgesic during oocyte retrieval

A multicentre RCT with 150 women compared the anaesthetic effect of lidocaine hydrochloride with either EA or intravenous alfentanil during ultrasound guided transvaginal oocyte aspiration. No differences in pain related to oocyte aspiration, adequacy of anaesthesia during oocyte aspiration, abdominal pain or degree of nausea were found between the two groups. Before oocyte aspiration, the level of stress was significantly higher in the EA group than in the alfentanil group, and the EA group experienced discomfort for a significantly longer period during oocyte aspiration. One possible explanation was that most of the women were unfamiliar with the EA procedure. No significant difference was found between the two groups in the mean number of oocytes retrieved, fertilisation rate or miscarriage rate. Compared with the alfentanil group, the EA group had a significantly higher implantation rate, pregnancy rate and 'take home baby' rate per embryo transfer, and the authors suggested that EA may be a good alternative to conventional anaesthesia during oocyte aspiration.[45] Although alfentanil was found in the follicular fluid shortly after an intravenous injection, it is not known whether opioids and sedatives negatively affect the follicles, the oocytes and/or endometrial receptivity,[46] whereas EA may exert some of its effects by activating endogenous opioid systems.[47]

ACUPUNCTURE FOR PRIMARY DYSMENORRHOEA

Acupuncture is thought to excite receptors or nerve fibres, which, through a complicated interaction with mediators such as serotonin and endorphins, block pain impulses.[7] A Cochrane Database systematic review[7] reported that there is insufficient evidence to determine the effectiveness of acupuncture in reducing primary dysmenorrhoea; however, a single small, but methodologically sound, trial of acupuncture suggested benefit for this modality. It was shown to be significantly more effective for pain relief than both placebo acupuncture and two control groups that received no treatment.

ACUPUNCTURE IN THE MENOPAUSE

There is no proven use for any of the traditional Chinese methods for common menopausal symptoms. An uncontrolled study[48] included 300 women with a variety of menopausal symptoms treated by acupuncture for various durations showed that 97% felt better and 51% were completely relieved of their symptoms. EA therapy may also reduce hot flushes in postmenopausal women.[49]

However, it has not been tested against placebo. It is interesting to note that the number of hot flushes was reduced by a mean of 70% in seven men who were being treated with androgen suppression for prostate cancer and had been given EA for seven weeks or more. In addition, at the third month after the last treatment, the mean reduction was approximately 50%.[50]

ACUPUNCTURE AS A TREATMENT FOR NAUSEA AND VOMITING

It is worth noting that some studies have shown favourable results with the use of point six (P6) acupressure techniques for relief of nausea and vomiting during chemotherapy, dialysis, recovery from anaesthesia and the postoperative period.[11] The first systematic review of the literature on acupuncture, acupressure and electrical stimulation for nausea included seven studies on acupressure for nausea of pregnancy, and concluded that all forms of stimulation of the relevant acupuncture points were effective for all forms of nausea.[51]

ACUPUNCTURE IN THE ONCOLOGY SERVICES

The results of a survey published in 2002[52] suggested that acupuncture may contribute to the control of symptoms of cancer, particularly pain, xerostomia, hot flushes and nausea/loss of appetite. Sixty percent of the 79 patients included demonstrated over 30% improvement in their symptoms, although about one-third had no change in severity of symptoms after a mean of five acupuncture visits. Standard allopathic care continued while these patients were receiving acupuncture. There were no adverse effects reported related to acupuncture and 86% of respondents considered it 'very important' that acupuncture services should continue.

Acustimulation of the PC6 point on the ventral surface of the wrist (acustimulation wristband) decreased the severity of delayed nausea when compared with placebo acustimulation and no acustimulation groups in a multicentre RCT using a three-level crossover design. Twenty-five women and two men with moderate to severe nausea after chemotherapy were included but the difference was not statistically significant, although less antiemetic medications were used by the treatment group. These findings provide ample justification for further study of acustimulation in clinical oncology.[53]

SAFETY ISSUES

Acupuncture

The apparent safety of acupuncture is its principal attraction for many people. Nevertheless, it is not free from risk. The early literature on safety aspects consisted entirely of case reports. Rampes and James[54] summarised all case reports published between 1966 and 1993 and found 395 instances of complications. Many were minor, such as bruising or fainting, but 216 were serious, including several cases of pneumothorax and injury to the spinal cord. Only one death was reported, in which a self-administered needle penetrated the pericardium.

In 1995, a survey in Norway found that 12% of doctors and 31% of acupuncturists had encountered adverse effects of acupuncture in their practice, including pneumothorax, nerve injury, infection, nausea, vomiting and fainting.[55] However, there was little indication of the period over which events were reported or the frequency with which complications occurred. Although such case reports and informal surveys are important in identifying potential problems, they are limited by the absence of a denominator. Assessing the degree of risk requires knowledge of both the frequency and the severity of the hazard.[10]

Safety is best established by prospective surveys. A systemic review[56] reported two cases of pneumothorax in nearly 250 000 treatments. Two reports,[4,57] the first systemically to examine both the rate and the nature of the adverse effects of acupuncture, were published in 2001; both suggested that the rate of complications was remarkably low and that most were transient, lasting two weeks at most.

In the York Acupuncture Safety Study,[4] a prospective survey of 34 407 treatments by 574 professional acupuncturists, there were no reports of serious adverse events. However, 43 minor adverse events were noted, a rate of 1.3 per 1000 treatments. The most common were severe nausea and fainting. Mild transient reactions occurred in 15% of treatments, the most common being 'feeling relaxed' and 'feeling energised'. Local reactions at the site of needling, such as mild bruising, pain or bleeding, were also reported. The second prospective survey[57] included 31 822 consultations with 48 doctors (members of the British Medical Acupuncture Society) and 30 physiotherapists (members of the Acupuncture Association of Chartered Physiotherapists), and showed no serious adverse events and 671 minor events per 10 000 acupuncture consultations. The most common were bleeding and needling pain.

Although these two studies give important evidence on the safety of acupuncture, the potential bias of self-reporting cannot be excluded. In addition, the surveys were restricted to immediate complications, so longer term deleterious effects on these patients' condition, or interactions with concurrent treatments, would probably not have been identified. Comparison of this adverse event rate for acupuncture with those of drugs routinely prescribed in primary care suggests that it is a relatively safe form of treatment.[58] It is worth noting that all the participants in these surveys had received training in acupuncture and were members of professional associations committed to high professional standards and patient safety. Rampes and James[54] pointed out that many of the problems in their case series could easily have been avoided by a competent practitioner.

Moxibustion

It has been reported that the smoke from burning the moxa herbal preparation can irritate the upper and lower respiratory tracts of patients, attendants or the therapist. Individuals with respiratory diseases such as allergic rhinitis and asthma could experience aggravation of their symptoms, although this is unusual.[21,25] Moxibustion can cause burn blisters, so there is also a possibility of permanent scarring from the procedure. Wong et al.[59] encountered individuals with residual lesions resulting from prolonged and repeated indirect moxibustion in addition to direct burning of moxa on the skin. It is not known if in utero exposure to moxa smoke would have any harmful effects.[25] No unintentional burning, placental abruption or intrauterine fetal demise among the participants in their RCT was observed. In addition, the number of cases of spontaneous rupture of membranes was similar in both treated and control groups.[21]

CONCLUSION

The World Health Organization sees the wealth of information favouring acupuncture as undeniable evidence that this modality should be considered as an important component of primary health care, fully integrated with conventional medicine.[5] Although many studies give encouraging results regarding the uses of acupuncture techniques in different fields, including obstetrics and gynaecology, a definitive conclusion cannot be reached. Most of the studies were small and not randomised. However, there is a great deal of public pressure to adopt these techniques and many claims that acupuncture is effective. Doctors therefore cannot dismiss acupuncture without good evidence.[3] Large and well designed RCTs on short- and long-term major outcomes should be performed. The best evidence should be systematically reviewed, summarised and disseminated, which in turn would lead to evidence based decision making in traditional Chinese medicine in general and acupuncture in particular.[9] The conclusion that acupuncture is a safe intervention in the hands of a competent practitioner seems justified on the evidence available.[10] We have moved a long way from the sterile and hostile debates between critics and advocates of complementary medicine and can look forward to a time when any proposed treatment is evaluated on the basis of its efficacy, risks, likely mechanisms, acceptability and cost effectiveness, regardless of its provenance.[10]

References

1. Ewies AA. A comprehensive approach to the menopause: so far, one size should fit all. *Obstet Gynecol Surv* 2001;56:642–9.

2. Scheid V. The globalization of Chinese medicine. *Lancet* 1999;354 Suppl:SIV10.

3. Ewies AA, Olah KS. The sharp end of medical practice: the use of acupuncture in obstetrics and gynaecology. *BJOG* 2002;109:1–4.

4. MacPherson H, Thomas K, Walters S, Fitter M. The York acupuncture safety study: prospective survey of 34000 treatments by traditional acupuncturists. *BMJ* 2001;323:486–7.

5. Yelland S. *Acupuncture in Midwifery*. Hale: Books for Midwives Press; 1996.

6. West Z. Acupuncture within the National Health Service: a personal perspective. *Complement Ther Nurs Midwifery* 1997;3:83–6.

7. Proctor ML, Smith CA, Farquhar CM, Stones RW. Transcutaneous electrical nerve stimulation and acupuncture for primary dysmenorrhoea. *Cochrane Database Syst Rev* 2002;(1):CD002123.

8. Ulett GA, Han S, Han JS. Electro-acupuncture: mechanisms and clinical application. *Biol Psychiatry* 1998;44:129–38.

9. Tang JL, Zhan SY, Ernst E. Review of randomised controlled trials of traditional Chinese medicine. *BMJ* 1999;319:160–1.

10. Vincent C. The safety of acupuncture. *BMJ* 2001;323:467–8.

11. Beal MW. Acupuncture and related treatment modalities. Part II: Applications to antepartal and intrapartal care. *J Nurse Midwifery* 1992;37:260–8.

12. Smith C, Crowther C, Beilby J. Acupuncture to treat nausea and vomiting in early pregnancy: a randomized controlled trial. *Birth* 2002;29:1–9.

13. Maciocia G. *Obstetrics and Gynecology in Chinese Medicine*. New York: Churchill Livingstone; 1998.

14. Knight B, Mudge C, Openshaw S, White A, Hart A. Effect of acupuncture on nausea of pregnancy: a randomized, controlled trial. *Obstet Gynecol* 2001;97:184–8.

15. Carlsson CP, Axemo P, Bodin A, Carstensen H, Ehrenroth B, Madegard-Lind I, *et al*. Manual acupuncture reduces hyperemesis gravidarum: a placebo-controlled, randomized, single-blind, crossover study. *J Pain Symptom Manage* 2000;20:273–9.

16. Atkins Murphy P. Alternative therapies for nausea and vomiting of pregnancy. *Obstet Gynecol* 1998;91:149–55.

17. Wedenberg K, Moen B, Norling A. A prospective randomized study comparing acupuncture with physiotherapy for low-back and pelvic pain in pregnancy. *Acta Obstet Gynecol Scand* 2000;79:331–5.

18. Li Q, Wang L. Clinical observation on correcting malposition of fetus by electro-acupuncture. *J Tradit Chin Med* 1996;16:260–2.

19. Qin GF, Tang H. 413 cases of abnormal fetal position corrected by auricular plastic therapy. *J Tradit Chin Med* 1989;9:235–7.

20. Cardini F, Marcolongo A. Moxibustion for correction of breech presentation: a clinical study with retrospective control. *Am J Chin Med* 1993;21:133–8.

21. Cardini F, Weixin H. Moxibustion for correction of breech presentation: a randomized controlled trial. *JAMA* 1998;280:1580–4.

22. West Z. *Acupuncture in Pregnancy and Childbirth*. Edinburgh: Churchill Livingstone; 2000.

23. Ewies A, Olah K. Moxibustion in breech version – a descriptive review. *Acupunct Med* 2002;20:26–9.

24. Ernst E. Moxibustion for breech presentation. *JAMA* 1999;282:1329.

25. Wong HC, Wong NY, Wong JK. Moxibustion for breech presentation. *JAMA* 1999;282:1329.

26. Cardini F, Basevi V, Valentini A, Martellato A. Moxibustion and breech presentation: preliminary results. *Am J Chin Med* 1991;19:105–14.

27. Wang W. Report number 78: Clinical analysis of moxibustion in correcting abnormal foetal position. In: *Advances in Acupuncture and Acupuncture Anaesthesia. Abstracts of the National Symposium of Acupuncture, Moxibustion and Acupuncture Anaesthesia; 1979 June; Beijing*. Beijing: The People's Medical Publishing House; 1980. p. 93–4.

28. Cooperative Research Group on Moxibustion Version of Jangxi Province. Studies of version by moxibustion on Zhiyin points. In: Xiangtong Z, editor. *Research on Acupuncture, Moxibustion and Acupuncture Anaesthesia*. Beijing: Science Press; 1980. p. 810–19.

29. Cooperative Research Group on Moxibustion Version of Jangxi Province. Further studies on the clinical effects and the mechanism of version by moxibustion. In: *Abstracts of the Second National Symposium on Acupuncture, Moxibustion and Acupuncture Anaesthesia; 1984 Aug 7–10; Beijing*. Beijing: The People's Medical Publishing House; 1985.

30. Ramnero A, Hanson U, Kihlgren M. Acupuncture treatment during labour – a randomized controlled trial. *BJOG* 2002;109:637–44.

31. Martoudis SG, Christofides K. Electro-acupuncture for pain relief in labour. *Acupunct Med* 1990;8:51–3.

32. Umeh BU. Sacral acupuncture for pain relief in labour: initial clinical experience in Nigerian women. *Acupunct Electrother Res* 1986;11:147–51.

33. Nilsson TKM. Acupuncture for pain relief during childbirth. *Acupunct Electrother Res* 1998;23:19–26.

34. Smith CA, Crowther CA. Acupuncture for induction of labour. *Cochrane Database Syst Rev* 2001;(1):CD002962.

35. Tsuei JJ, Lai YF. Induction of labor by acupuncture and electrical stimulation. *Obstet Gynecol* 1974;43:337–42.

36. Tsuei JJ, Lai YF, Sharma SD. The influence of acupuncture stimulation during pregnancy: the induction and inhibition of labor. *Obstet Gynecol* 1977;50:479–88.

37. Yip SK, Pang JC, Sung ML. Induction of labor by acupuncture electro-stimulation. *Am J Chin Med* 1976;4:257–65.

38. Tremeau ML, Fontanie-Ravier P, Teurnier F, Demouzon J. Protocol of cervical maturation by acupuncture. *J Gynecol Obstet Biol Reprod (Paris)* 1992;21:375–80.

39. Dunn PA, Rogers D, Halford K. Transcutaneous electrical nerve stimulation at acupuncture points in the induction of uterine contractions. *Obstet Gynecol* 1989;73:286–90.

40. Coulam CB, Stern JJ, Soenksen DM, Britten S, Bustillo M. Comparison of pulsatility indices on the day of oocyte retrieval and embryo transfer. *Hum Reprod* 1995;10:82–4.

41. Steer CV, Campbell S, Tan SL, Crayford T, Mills C Mason BA, *et al*. The use of transvaginal

color flow imaging after *in vitro* fertilization to identify optimum uterine conditions before embryo transfer. *Fertil Steril* 1992;57:372–6.

42. Stener-Victorin E, Waldenström U, Andersson SA, Wikland M. Reduction of blood flow impedance in the uterine arteries of infertile women with electro-acupuncture. *Hum Reprod* 1996;11:1314–17.

43. Reid JL, Rubin PC. Peptides and central neural regulation of the circulation. *Physiol Rev* 1987;67:725–49.

44. Anderson SA. The functional background in acupuncture effects. *Scand J Rehabil Med Suppl* 1993;29:31–60.

45. Stener-Victorin E, Waldenström U, Nilsson L, Wikland M, Janson O. A prospective randomized study of electro-acupuncture versus alfentanil as anaesthesia during oocyte aspiration in *in-vitro* fertilization. *Hum Reprod* 1999;14:2480–4.

46. Soussis I, Boyd O, Paraschos T, Duffy S, Bower S, Troughton P, *et al.* Follicular fluid levels of midazolam, fentanyl and alfentanil during transvaginal oocyte retrieval. *Fertil Steril* 1995;64:1003–7.

47. Andersson SA, Lundeberg T. Acupuncture – from empiricism to science: functional background to acupuncture effects in pain and disease. *Med Hypotheses* 1995;45:271–81.

48. Wu L, Zhou X. 300 cases of menopausal syndrome treated by acupuncture. *J Tradit Chin Med* 1998;18:259–62.

49. Moyad MA. Complementary/alternative therapies for reducing hot flashes in prostate cancer patients: reevaluating the existing indirect data from studies of breast cancer and postmenopausal women. *Urology* 2002;59(4 Suppl 1):20–33.

50. Hammar M, Frisk J, Grimas O, Hook M, Spetz AC, Wyon Y. Acupuncture treatment of vasomotor symptoms in men with prostatic carcinoma: a pilot study. *J Urol* 1999;161:853–6.

51. Vickers AJ. Can acupuncture have specific effects on health? A systematic review of acupuncture antiemesis trials. *J R Soc Med* 1996;89:303–11.

52. Johnstone PA, Polston GR, Niemtzow RC, Martin PJ. Integration of acupuncture into the oncology clinic. *Palliat Med* 2002;16:235–9.

53. Roscoe JA, Morrow GR, Bushunow P, Tian L, Matteson S. Acustimulation wristbands for the relief of chemotherapy-induced nausea. *Altern Ther Health Med* 2002;8:56–63.

54. Rampes H, James R. Complications of acupuncture. *Acupunct Med* 1995;13:26–31.

55. Norheim AJ, Fonnebo V. Adverse effects of acupuncture. *Lancet* 1995;345:1576.

56. Ernst E, White AR. Prospective studies of the safety of acupuncture: a systematic review. *Am J Med* 2001;110:481–5.

57. White A, Hayhoe S, Hart A, Ernst E. Adverse events following acupuncture: prospective survey of 32 000 consultations with doctors and physiotherapists. *BMJ* 2001;323:485–6.

58. Tranmer MR, Moore RA, Reynolds DJ, McQuay HJ. Quantitative estimation of rare adverse events which follow a biological progression: a new model applied to chronic NSAID use. *Pain* 2000;85:169–82.

59. Wong HC, Wong NY, Wong JK. Signs of physical abuse or evidence of moxibustion, cupping or coining? *CMAJ* 1999;160:785–6.

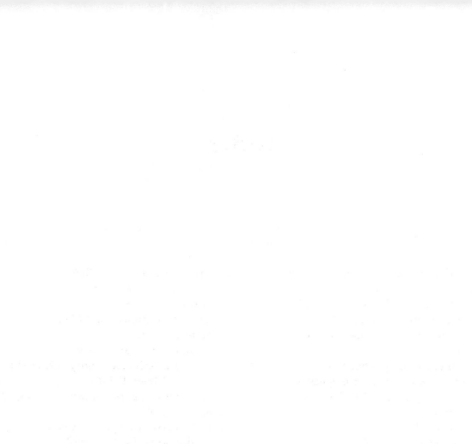

Index